A Clinician's Guide to Ophthalmology

A Clinician's Guide to Ophthalmology

Edited by Joanne Galbraith

hayle
medical

New York

Hayle Medical,
750 Third Avenue, 9th Floor,
New York, NY 10017, USA

Visit us on the World Wide Web at:
www.haylemedical.com

ISBN: 978-1-63241-706-0

Cataloging-in-Publication Data

A clinician's guide to ophthalmology / edited by Joanne Galbraith
    p. cm.
Includes bibliographical references and index.
ISBN 978-1-63241-706-0
1. Ophthalmology. 2. Eye--Diseases. 3. Ophthalmologists--Guidebooks. I. Galbraith, Joanne
RE48 .C55 2019
617.7--dc23

Table of Contents

Preface

The branch of medicine dealing with the structure, function and diseases of the eye is known as ophthalmology. The subspecialities which fall under ophthalmology deal with certain eye parts or specific diseases. Examples include glaucoma, anterior segment surgery, vitreo-retinal surgery, ocular oncology, neuro-ophthalmology, ophthalmic pathology, etc. Some of the common ways to assess the condition of the eye include ultrasonography, intraocular pressure, optical coherence tomography, slit lamp examination, fluorescein angiography, and retina examination. This book brings forth some of the most innovative concepts and elucidates the unexplored aspects of ophthalmology. The various sub-fields of ophthalmology along with technological progress that have future implications are glanced at in it. Those in search of information to further their knowledge will be greatly assisted by this book.

The researches compiled throughout the book are authentic and of high quality, combining several disciplines and from very diverse regions from around the world. Drawing on the contributions of many researchers from diverse countries, the book's objective is to provide the readers with the latest achievements in the area of research. This book will surely be a source of knowledge to all interested and researching the field.

In the end, I would like to express my deep sense of gratitude to all the authors for meeting the set deadlines in completing and submitting their research chapters. I would also like to thank the publisher for the support offered to us throughout the course of the book. Finally, I extend my sincere thanks to my family for being a constant source of inspiration and encouragement.

Editor

Conjunctival repair after glaucoma drainage device exposure using collagen-glycosaminoglycane matrices

André Rosentreter[1*] (iD), Alexandra Lappas[2], Randolf Alexander Widder[3], Maged Alnawaiseh[4] and Thomas Stefan Dietlein[2]

Abstract

Background: To report the results of the repair of conjunctival erosions resulting from glaucoma drainage device surgery using collagen-glycosaminoglycane matrices (CGM).

Methods: Case series of 8 patients who underwent revision surgery due to conjunctival defects with exposed tubes through necrosis of the overlying scleral flap and conjunctiva after Baerveldt drainage device surgery. The defects were repaired by lateral displacement of the tube towards the sclera, with a slice of a CGM as a patch, covered by adjacent conjunctiva.

Result: Successful, lasting closure (follow-up of 12 to 42 months) of the conjunctival defects was achieved without any side-effects or complications in all eight cases.

Conclusions: Erosion of the drainage tube, creating buttonholes in the conjunctiva after implantation of glaucoma drainage devices, is a potentially serious problem. It can be managed successfully using a biodegradable CGM as a patch.

Keywords: Episcleral drainage device, Baerveldt, Ahmed, Collagen-glycosaminoglycane matrix (CGM), Drainage tube, Conjunctival defect, Conjunctival repair, Conjunctival hole, Glaucoma drainage device, Biodegradable implant, Ologen implant

Background

Conjunctival defects after penetrating glaucoma surgery, e.g. trabeculectomy or insertion of episcleral glaucoma drainage devices, are rare but severe complications. The defects often lead to leakage and contact between the anterior chamber and surrounding surfaces with the risk of subsequent carry-over of bacteria, blebitis and endophthalmitis [1–5].

In the case of trabeculectomy, especially after use of antimetabolites such as mitomycin-C (MMC) and 5-fluoruracile (5-FU), conjunctival defects can even occur a long time after surgery. Antimetabolites, which are very useful for prevention of scarring, affect wound healing processes and lead to the formation of thin-walled blebs [6].

After implantation of an episcleral glaucoma drainage device (GDD, e.g. the non-valved Baerveldt (Advanced Medical Optics, USA) or the valved Ahmed (New World Medical, USA) etc.), complications such as erosion of the tube (GDD-specific) or even the plate of the implant through the conjunctiva occur in 2–7% cases [1–5]. As with late bleb leakage after trabeculectomy, erosion of the conjunctiva exposing the tube of the GDD makes revision surgery necessary [7]. Erosion of the conjunctiva on top of the tube or the implant is more frequent in eyes with a history of multiple intraocular surgeries.

To repair erosion of the conjunctiva, a patch is usually placed on top of the tube and the conjunctiva is closed above this patch. Due to the surrounding scar tissue and the fragile structure of the frequently inflamed tissue around the tube, specialist knowledge and skill are required to achieve long-lasting wound closure in conjunctiva surgery. As reported in a case report [8], we favour a combination of re-fixation of the tube to the sclera

* Correspondence: andre.rosentreter@googlemail.com
[1]Department of Ophthalmology, University of Würzburg, Josef-Schneider-Str. 11, 97080 Würzburg, Germany
Full list of author information is available at the end of the article

with prior lateral displacement of the tube, followed by patching of the implant with a slice of a biodegradable implant (ologen™ implant, Aeon Astron Corporation, The Netherlands) in combination with conjunctival advancement. The aim of the lateral displacement of the tube is to avoid mechanical problems between the tube and lid margin at the previous point of conjunctival erosion, which could trigger repeated conjunctival erosion.

Since only a small number of patients suffer from conjunctival erosion after glaucoma drainage device surgery (2–7%) [1–5], we present a case-series of just eight patients who underwent such surgery. We hereby focus not only on the surgical success in covering the defect, but also on intraocular pressure, antiglaucomatous medication, visual acuity and the need for further surgical interventions.

Methods

Patients and preoperative examination

Our study was based on a retrospective consecutive case series of eight patients who were treated for buttonholes [Fig. 1a] after glacuoma drainage device surgery between 2009 and 2016 in the Center of Ophthalmology, University of Cologne. Due to the retrospective study design and no further patient examinations, an ethics vote was considered unnecessary (§ 2 (1) and (2) of the Statutes of the Ethics Committee of the University of Lübeck). All surgeries were performed by an experienced glaucoma surgeon (TD). In all cases, an episcleral glaucoma drainage device was used after several preliminary operations (minimum 2) for intractable glaucoma. After a minimum of 1 month and a maximum of 6 years conjunctival erosion of the tube occurred.

Before surgical intervention, all patients underwent a baseline examination, which included measurement of best-corrected visual acuity (ETDRS charts, Lighthouse, Long Island, USA), visual field examination (30–2, Octopus perimeter 101, Haag-Streit, Switzerland), biomicroscopy, gonioscopy, and Goldmann applanation tonometry.

Surgical technique and follow-up

The surgical procedure was performed under either general or local anesthesia, according to the patient's preference. As described in our previous publication [8], the tubes were laterally displaced, fixed to the sclera with a horizontal mattress 10–0 nylon suture (knots recessed to the sclera), and covered with a slice of an ologen™ implant of 1–2 mm thickness. The conjunctiva was closed after mobilisation with a rotational flap of adjacent conjunctiva [Fig. 1b & c; 2]. Postoperatively, the patients received topical antibiotics three times a day for 2 weeks and low-dose steroids three times a day for 3 weeks.

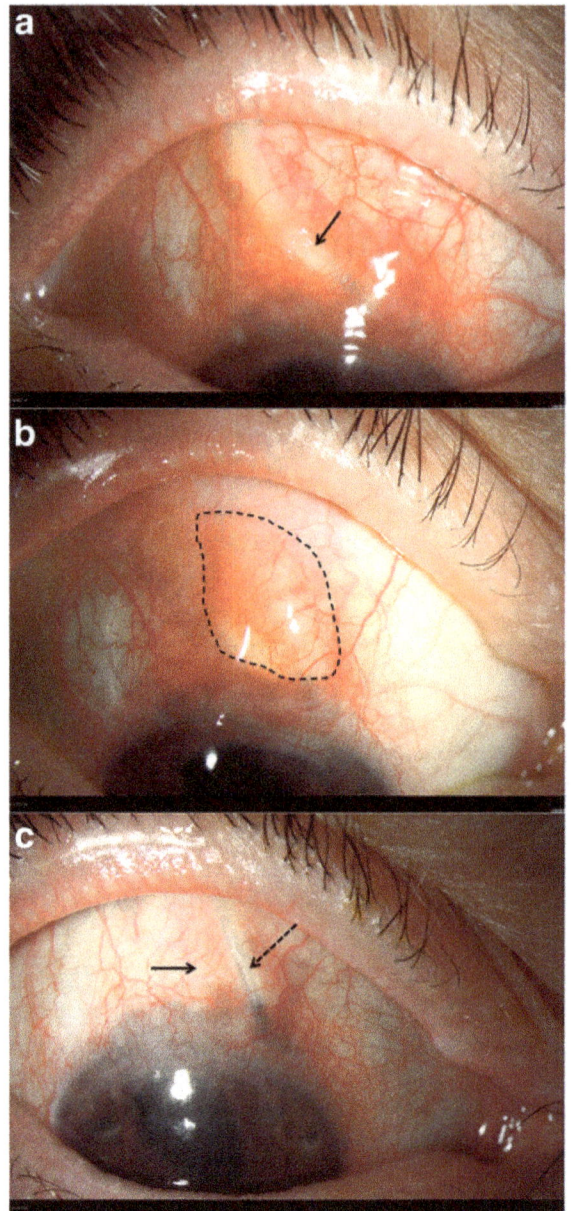

Fig. 1 Chronological order. **a** Conjunctival buttonhole of 1 × 0.5 mm with exposure of the tube; arrow indicates the area of exposure. **b** Conjunctival defect closed with conjunctival hyperemia and underlying ologen implant at 2 months after surgery; dashed line shows the size of the ologen slice. **c** Stable re-epithelialisation at 10 months following surgery; arrow indicates the former area of exposure, the dashed arrow shows the displaced tube. The ologen implant has already been resorbed at this time (Complete resorption is usually seen between the third and sixth postoperative months)

Postoperative examinations were performed on a daily basis during hospitalisation. After hospitalisation, follow-up visits were arranged at 1 and 4 weeks and 3, 6, 12 and 24 months after surgery. At each visit all the above-mentioned examinations, except for visual-field testing and gonioscopy, were repeated. Side-effects and complications were recorded during postoperative follow-ups.

Ologen™ implant

The ologen™ implant (Aeon Astron Europe B.V., the Netherlands) is a porous implant comprising > 90% lyophilized porcine atelocollagen and < 10% lyophilized glycosaminoglycan with a pore size of 20 to 200 μm [Fig. 2]. In our study we used a cylindrical (12 mm diameter) implant of 1 mm in height, either folded or unfolded, and in some cases cut down to a slice of 5 × 5 mm.

Atelocollagen is a highly purified pepsin-treated type I collagen. A collagen molecule has an amino acid sequence, known as a telopeptide, at both N- and C-terminals, which confers most of the collagen's antigenicity. Atelocollagen obtained by pepsin treatment is low in immunogenicity, because it is free of telopeptides [8, 9].

Statistics

Primary endpoint and surgical success were defined as complete wound closure without leakage of aqueous humour. Secondary endpoints were IOP control without the need for further revision surgery. Pre- and postoperative antiglaucomatous medication was classified according to a medication score [10].

The datasets used and/or analysed during the current study available are from the corresponding author on reasonable request. Statistical analysis was performed using Prism software (version 5, GraphPad software). Differences between preoperative and postoperative IOP and medication were compared by the non-parametric t-test, as the values were considered to be distributed non-parametrically (Mann-Whitney test, two-tailed). P-values of less than 0.05 were considered statistically significant.

Results

In most cases the buttonholes occurred directly adjacent to the lid margin. Patient characteristics are given in Table 1; showing that the patients had multiple preoperated eyes. Erosion of conjunctiva occurred after a minimum of one and a maximum of 70 months after glaucoma drainage

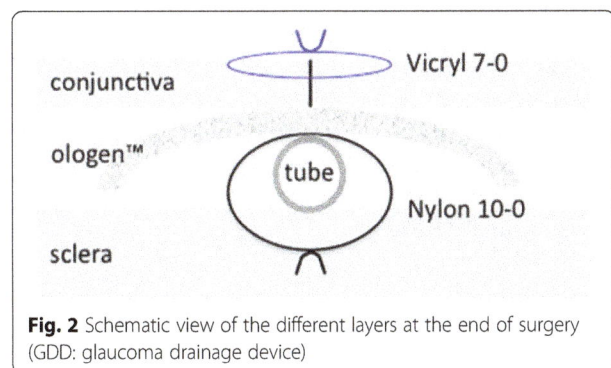

Fig. 2 Schematic view of the different layers at the end of surgery (GDD: glaucoma drainage device)

device surgery with a mean of 25.1 ± 30.8 months. We could not detect any ologen™ specific side-effects such as allergy or translocation of the implant on postoperative follow-up visits. No severe postoperative complications were detected and conjunctiva remained healthy and closed on follow-up.

The course of intraocular pressure changes and medication score is shown in Table 2. The mean follow-up time was 26.8 ± 9.0 months. Further glaucoma surgery was necessary in three cases: in one case (patient #2) an additional glaucoma drainage device was used, while in two cases (patient #4 & #6) additional cyclophotocoagulation was applied.

Discussion

Glaucoma drainage device surgery is a useful adjunct in the treatment of refractory glaucoma despite having a few serious complications [1, 11–13]. As a consequence of the results of the TVT study [14, 15], glaucoma drainage device surgery is now being used more frequently than in the past and at an earlier stage (typical situation: Pseudophakic eyes with one or two failed trabeculectomies). Since this surgical method is now carried out more frequently, an increasing number of typical side-effects should be taken into consideration. One such complication is thinning of the conjunctiva directly above the tube with complete erosion of the overlying tissue [5]. This may result in leakage and is always an indication for revision surgery, as this entrance gate is a potential source of endophthalmitis [7].

The exact mechanism of conjunctival erosion remains unclear since, as far as could be seen, the implants and the tubes were correctly positioned. The buttonholes are probably formed either due to mechanical stress at the lid margin or due to the gap between the tube and sclera posterior to the scleral flap arising through the architecture of the glaucoma drainage devices near the basal plate.

To prevent conjunctival erosion, the tube should be patched during primary surgery and the patch covered with conjunctiva. The tube can be patched either with a scleral flap or with bovine pericardium, human sclera or other materials. The use of patched tubes has decreased the exposure rate from 30% to less than 5% [5]. In our case series all tubes were patched with a scleral flap in primary surgery.

Should a penetrating defect in the conjunctiva nevertheless occur during follow-up, it can be difficult to achieve closure of conjunctiva. A few methods for closing these defects in the conjunctiva have been described previously: For direct suture of the defect and use of conjunctival autografts, the results in literature show different success rates: A simple conjunctival closure is inadequate [16]. Reports on conjunctival autografts and

Table 1 Patient characteristics for the presented case series of eight patients

#	Age [years]	Type of glaucoma	Preliminary surgeries	Erosion of conjunctiva after *xxx* months	BCVA [LogMAR]
P1	51	Angle closure	IE, Phaco, ppV, TE	70	0.20
P2	49	XFG	Phaco, TA, TE	2	0.20
P3	12	Uveitic	Phaco, TE	1	0.20
P4	57	Silicon oil	ppV, TE	4	0.80
P5	41	Silicon oil	ppV, TE	4	1.00
P6	81	Uveitic	Phaco, TE	60	Light perception
P7	18	Uveitic	Phaco, ppV	56	0.60
P8	44	Traumatic	2× TE	4	0.00
Mean ± SD	44.1 ± 21.8			25.1 ± 30.8	

BCVA best-corrected visual acuity, *IE* Iridectomy, *Phaco* Phacoemulsification, *ppV* pars plana vitrectomy, *SD* standard deviation, *TA* trabecular aspiration, *TE* trabeculectomy, *XFG* Pseudoexfoliation glaucoma

conjunctival closure with a patch graft provided better results (Success rates: acellular human dermis patch graft: 83%; autologous scleral lamellar graft: 100%) [5, 16]. Also good results have been reported with amniotic membranes and additional application of autologous serum in a few cases of conjunctival erosion (Three cases; 100% success; follow-up: 6–30 months) [17].

Table 2 Intraocular pressure and antiglaucomatous medication score preoperative and at different points of follow-up

Intraocular pressure [mmHg]

#	preOP	d1	12 m	Last follow-up (xx mo)
P1	15	13	15	16 (24 mo)
P2	19	23	15	13 (24 mo)
P3	25	10	12	14 (24 mo)
P4	17	–	15	9 (42 mo)
P5	25	24	17	16 (24 mo)
P6	19	11	19	19 (12 mo)
P7	16	21	6	9 (28 mo)
P8	14	–	12	19 (36 mo)
Mean ± SD	18.8 ± 4.2	17.0 ± 6,4	13.9 ± 3.9	14.4 ± 3.9

Medication score

#	preOP	d1	12 m	Last follow-up (xx mo)
P1	2	2	0	0 (24 mo)
P2	0	0	6	0 (24 mo)
P3	10	0	5	4 (24 mo)
P4	6	–	6	0 (42 mo)
P5	8	5	5	5 (24 mo)
P6	0	0	6	6 (12 mo)
P7	0	0	0	0 (28 mo)
P8	3	–	3	4 (36 mo)
Mean ± SD	3.6 ± 3.9	1.2 ± 2.0	3.9 ± 2.6	2.4 ± 2.6

12 m = 12 months after surgery; d1 = 1 day after surgery; IOP = intraocular pressure; MedScore = medication score; preOP = preoperative

Preliminary studies on bioengineered, biodegradable implants suggest that a porous collagen-glycosaminoglycane matrix (CGM; ologen™) will reduce conjunctival contraction and promote formation of an almost normal subconjunctival stroma [18–20]. Moreover, the use of the ologen™ implant was also described in primary glaucoma drainage device surgery as a patch with a good success rate [21]. This led us to try CGM in a single case of revision surgery after buttonhole formation on top of the drainage device tube [8]. After use of a total of eight CGM in revision surgery, we can confirm the persistent closure of conjunctival defects in all cases. No severe postoperative complications or CGM-specific side-effects were detected in our study series.

Except the patching of the tube with an ologen™ implant, the lateral displacement of the tube also appears to be decisive in our approach. This prevents the previously damaged conjunctiva from contact with the tube.

Conclusion

Our case series shows that the described method with lateral displacement of the tube and patching with CGM is a possible alternative in revision surgery for repair of eroded conjunctiva overlying the tube of the glaucoma drainage device. Possible positive effects of the CGM are the avoidance of direct contact between the conjunctiva and the tube and the fact that CGM acts as a wound healing scaffold for structurally more normal tissue rather than structurally deficient scar tissue. Moreover, CGM probably minimizes movement of the conjunctiva in relation to the tube thus facilitating wound healing.

Abbreviations

5-FU: 5-fluoruracile; CGM: Collagen-glycosaminoglycane matrices; GDD: Glaucoma drainage device; IOP: Intraocular pressure; MMC: Mitomycin-C; TVT study: Tube versus trabecuectomy study

Acknoledgements
No acknoledgement.

Authors disclosure
No external support.

Authors' contributions
Design and conception of the study: AR, AL, TD. Acquisition and analysis of data: AR, MA, RW, TD. Drafting and revising the manuscript: AR, AL, MA, RW, TD. Final approval: AR, TD. All authors read and approved the final manuscript.

Competing interests
The authors declare that they have no competing interests.

Author details
[1]Department of Ophthalmology, University of Würzburg, Josef-Schneider-Str. 11, 97080 Würzburg, Germany. [2]Center of Ophthalmology, University of Cologne, Cologne, Germany. [3]Department of Ophthalmology, St. Martinus-Krankenhaus Düsseldorf, Düsseldorf, Germany. [4]Department Of Ophthalmology, University of Muenster Medical Center, Muenster, Germany.

References
1. Ayyala RS, Zurakowski D, Smith JA, Monshizadeh R, Netland PA, Richards DW, et al. A clinical study of the Ahmed glaucoma valve implant in advanced glaucoma. Ophthalmology. 1998;105:1968–76.
2. Lim KS, Allan BDS, Lloyd AW, Muir A, Khaw PT. Glaucoma drainage devices; past, present, and future. Br J Ophthalmol. 1998;82:1083–9.
3. Aslanides IM, Spaeth GL, Schmidt CM, Lanzl IM, Gandham SB. Autologous patch graft in tube shunt surgery. J Glaucoma. 1999;8:306–9.
4. Siegner SW, Netland PA, Urban RC Jr, Williams AS, Richards DW, Latina MA, et al. Clinical experience with the Baerveldt glaucoma drainage implant. Ophthalmology. 1995;102:1298–307.
5. Heuer DK, Budenz D, Coleman A. Aqueous shunt tube erosion. J Glaucoma. 2001;10:493–6.
6. DeBry PW, Perkins TW, Heatley G, Kaufman P, Brumback LC. Incidence of late-onset bleb-related complications following trabeculectomy with mitomycin. Arch Ophthalmol. 2002;120:297–300.
7. Francis BA, DiLoreto DA Jr, Chong LP, Rao N. Late-onset bacteria endophthalmitis following glaucoma drainage implantation. Ophthalmic Surg Lasers Imaging. 2003;34:128–30.
8. Rosentreter A, Schild AM, Dinslage S, Dietlein TS. Biodegradable implant for tissue repair after glaucoma drainage device surgery. J Glaucoma. 2012;21:76–8.
9. Stenzel KH, Miyata T, Rubin AL. Collagen as a biomaterial. Annu Rev Biophys Bioeng. 1974;3:231–53.
10. Jacobi PC, Krieglstein GK. Trabecular aspiration. A new mode to treat pseudoexfoliation glaucoma. Invest Ophthalmol Vis Sci. 1995;36:2270–6.
11. Goulet RJ 3rd, Phan AD, Cantor LB, WuDunn D. Efficacy of the Ahmed S2 glaucoma valve compared with the Baerveldt 250 mm2 glaucoma implant. Ophthalmology. 2008;115:1141–7.
12. Syed HM, Law SK, Nam SH, Li G, Caprioli J, Coleman A. Baerveldt-350 implant versus Ahmed valve for refractory glaucoma. A case-controlled comparison. J Glaucoma. 2004;13:38–45.
13. WuDunn D, Phan AD, Cantor LB, Lind JT, Cortes A, Wu B. Clinical experience with the Baerveldt 250 mm2 glaucoma implant. Ophthalmology. 2006;113:766–72.
14. Gedde SJ, Schiffman JC, Feuer WJ, Herndon LW, Brandt JD, Budenz DL, Tube Versus Trabeculectomy Study Group. Treatment outcomes in the tube versus trabeculectomy (TVT) study after five years of follow-up. Am J Ophthalmol. 2012;153:789–803.
15. Gedde SJ, Herndon LW, Brandt JD, Budenz DL, Feuer WJ, Schiffman JC, Tube Versus Trabeculectomy Study Group. Postoperative complications in the tube versus trabeculectomy (TVT) study during five years of follow-up. Am J Ophthalmol. 2012;153:804–14.
16. Kalenak JW. Revision for exposed anterior segment tubes. J Glaucoma. 2010;19:5–10.
17. Ainsworth G, Rotchford A, Dua HS, King AJ. A novel use of amniotic membrane in the management of tube exposure following glaucoma tube shunt surgery. Br J Ophthalmol. 2006;90:417–9.
18. Chen HS, Ritch R, Krupin T, Hsu WC. Control of filtering bleb structure through tissue bioengineering: an animal model. Invest Ohthalmol Vis Sci. 2006;47:5310–4.
19. Hsu WC, Ritch R, Krupin T, Chen HS. Tissue bioengineering for surgical bleb defects: an animal study. Graefes Arch Clin Exp Ophthalmol. 2008;246:709–17.
20. Hsu WC, Spilker MH, Yannas IV, Rubin PA. Inhibition of conjunctival scarring and contraction by a porous collagen-glycosaminoglycan implant. Invest Ophthalmol Vis Sci. 2000;41:2404–11.
21. Stephens JD, Sarkisian SR Jr. The use of collagen matrix (Ologen) as a patch graft in glaucoma tube shunt surgery, a retrospective chart review. F1000Res. 2016;5:1898.

2

Comparison of hyperdry amniotic membrane transplantation and conjunctival autografting for primary pterygium

Xin Pan[1†], Daguang Zhang[2†], Zhifang Jia[2], Zhehui Chen[1] and Yuetian Su[1*]

Abstract

Background: The purpose of this study was to evaluate the safety and effectiveness of the hyperdry amniotic membrane transplantation compared with conjunctival autografting for the treatment of primary pterygium.

Methods: One hundred and forty-one eyes from 130 patients with primary pterygium were treated with excision followed by hyperdry amniotic membrane or conjunctival autografting after random selection. Seventy-nine eyes from 71 patients received hyperdry amniotic membrane transplantation (HD-AM group), and 62 eyes from 59 patients received conjunctival autografting (CG group). Patients were followed up at one week and one, three, six, and 12 months post-surgery. Recurrence rate, postoperative complications, and final follow-up patient visits were prospectively evaluated.

Results: The mean follow-up duration was 12.56 ± 4.35 months in the HD-AM group and 12.85 ± 3.90 months in the CG group. Recurrences were detected in four eyes (5.06%) in the HD-AM group and 13 eyes (20.97%) in the CG group. A statistically significant difference in frequency of recurrence between the two groups ($P = 0.003$) was observed. The cumulative non-recurrence rates at six and 12 months in all patients stratified by age and sex were not significantly different ($P = 0.642$ and $P = 0.451$, respectively, by log-rank test). Graft retraction and necrosis were not detected in the two groups during the follow-up period.

Conclusion: Hyperdry amniotic membrane transplantation was effective in preventing pterygium recurrence when compared with conjunctival autografting and can be considered a preferable and safe grafting procedure for primary pterygium.

Keywords: Primary pterygium, Hyperdry amniotic membrane transplantation, Conjunctival autografting, Recurrence rate

Background

Pterygium, a common benign ocular surface lesion, is a wing-shaped fibrovascular growth arising from subconjunctival tissue extending across the nasal limbus onto the cornea that can cause vision loss [1]. Epidemiologic studies indicate that the high rate of pterygium is strongly related to chronic exposure to ultraviolet radiation, dryness, heat, wind, dust, viruses, and oncogenes [2]. Surgical excision is considered the conventional

definitive treatment of pterygium [3]. The mainstay techniques presently in use include bare sclera excision followed by adjunctive mitomycin C and β-irradiation or covering the defect with graft tissue such as a conjunctival autograft and amniotic membrane (AM). The major problem associated with pterygium surgery is the incidence of recurrence, but none of the techniques have achieved complete success in completely preventing this recurrence. Currently, conjunctival autografting is the most commonly used technique with a lower recurrence rate and fewer complications despite the requirement for more technically demanding surgical skills and experience; it is more time-consuming to perform [4–6].

* Correspondence: yuetiansu2015@163.com
†Equal contributors
[1]The Second Hospital of Jilin University, No.218, Ziqiang Road, Changchun 130041, China
Full list of author information is available at the end of the article

Furthermore, it is not feasible to cover large defects created in large pterygia.

Hyperdry (HD)-AM was developed as a new matrix material that is suitable for tissue engineering applications in the form of a surgical patch [7]. It is a new type of AM that is expanded on a nitrocellulose filter paper with epithelial sheet facing upward, processed using consecutive far-infrared rays and microwaves (patented hyperdry method), and sterilized by cobalt-60 irradiation [8]. Thereafter, it was cut into all kinds of squares, vacuum packed, and stored safely at room temperature [9]. Recently, HD-AM has been exploited as a new ophthalmic tool for the management of many ocular surface diseases, including corneal perforations and bleb leaks [10].

This study was intended to evaluate the recurrence of primary pterygium after HD-AM transplantation compared with conjunctival autografting. To the best of our knowledge, this is the first report on the use of HD- AM for treatment of pterygium.

Methods
Study group
One hundred and forty-one eyes from 130 patients with primary pterygium were enrolled in this study between March 2015 and February 2016. In all cases, the size of the pterygium was at least 2 mm onto the cornea or causing extreme irritation. Most of the pterygium was translucent, and the episcleral vessels underneath the body of the pterygium could be identified, as previously reported by Tan [11]. Exclusion criteria included recurrent pterygium, dry eye, infection and inflammation of ocular area, glaucoma, and previous ocular surgery in the study eye. Patients were randomized into the hyperdry amniotic membrane transplantation or conjunctival autografting groups (HD-AM and CG groups, respectively) for pterygium excision. Informed consent for the surgery was signed by all patients. Patients with a < 6-month follow-up period were excluded.

Surgical methods
Pterygium excision: All surgical procedures were performed by the same surgeon using an operating microscope (Zeiss, Germany). After injection of 2% lidocaine hydrochloride containing 1:10000 adrenaline (epinephrine) into the body of the pterygium, the conjunctival sac was irrigated with gentamicin, and the lid speculum was inserted. The head was separated and removed from the cornea by blunt dissection. Residual tissue over the corneal defect area was shaved with toothed forceps. Subconjunctival fibrous tissue under the pterygium was removed as much as possible avoiding damage to the underlying muscle sheath. A rectangular area of bare sclera was created to which the graft could be directly attached.

Hyperdry amniotic membrane transplantation: The hospital ethics committee approved the use of HD-AM in pterygium surgery (2015 No. 063). After the preserved biological amniotic membrane (Jiangxi Ruiji BOI-Engineering Technology Co. Ltd.) was rinsed in physiological saline for 15 min (Fig. 1), it was cut into an appropriate size with scissors, peeled from the filter paper, and placed over the bare sclera area with epithelial basement membrane side facing up. The free edge of the HD-AM was sutured through the episcleral tissue to the edge of conjunctiva along the bare sclera border with 10–0 nylon sutures interrupted and was tightly pressed centrally to securely attach it to the bare sclera. The membrane was placed over the corneal lesion.

Conjunctival autograft transplantation: A conjunctival free graft of similar size was obtained from the superotemporal bulbar conjunctiva by splitting at the anatomic limbus. Careful excision was given to obtain a thin, tenon-free conjunctival graft. The limbal side of the autograft was sutured to the limbal side of the bare scleral bed by separate 10/0 nylon sutures. The donor site was later closed with a continuous suture of 10–0 nylon sutures.

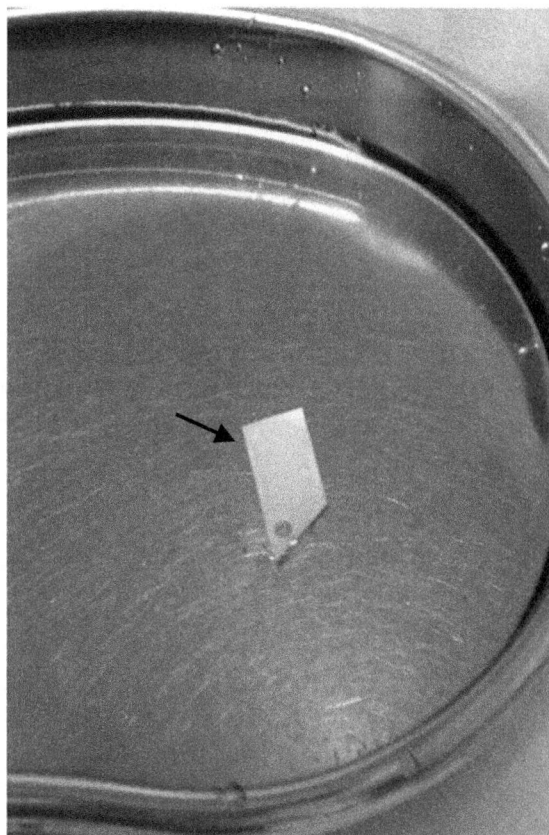

Fig. 1 The hyperdry amniotic membrane (HD-AM) (arrow) was expanded on a nitrocellulose filter paper and was rinsed in physiological saline

Post-operation and Follow-up: Postoperatively, all the patients received 0.1% fluorometholone (Santen, Osaka, Japan) and tobramycin (Alcon) drops four times daily. The drops were gradually tapered back within one month. Sutures were removed after one week. The patients were examined on the first postoperative day, followed by the first week and then one, three, six, and 12 months postoperatively. The minimum follow-up time was six months. The recurrence rate of pterygium after surgery was used as the primary outcome in this study. Recurrence was defined as the regrowth of the fibrovascular proliferation tissue invading the cornea again. Other complications such as pyogenic granuloma, inclusion cyst, or scleral thinning were recorded.

Statistical analyses

Statistical analysis was conducted using SPSS 18.0 software. The data were presented as means (±SD) or frequencies (%). χ^2 test was applied to compare the categorical data between the two groups and frequency of recurrence, whereas the unpaired t-test was used to analyze continuous variables such as age and graft size and follow-up times. The cumulative proportion of recurrence was analyzed by the Kaplan–Meier method and log-rank test. Significance was set at $P < 0.05$ using two-sided comparisons.

Results

The characteristics of patients in the two groups were compared in Table 1. There were no statistically significant differences regarding sex ($P = 0.963$), age ($P = 0.549$), and laterality ($P = 0.973$) between the two groups. The mean follow-up period was 12.56 ± 4.35 months for the HD-AM group and 12.85 ± 3.90 months for the CG group ($P = 0.674$). The size of the extension placed onto the cornea was 3.685 ± 0.848 mm in the HD-AM group and 3.469 ± 0.970 mm in the CG group ($P = 0.164$).

Four of 79 eyes (5.06%) in the HD-AM group developed pterygium recurrence compared with 13 of 62 eyes

Table 1 Comparison of patients' demographic data among amniotic membrane graft group and conjunctival autograft group

	HD-AM	CG	P
No. of patients (eyes)	71(79)	59(62)	–
Sex (M:F)	31:40	26:33	0.963
Mean age (SD)	62.32(7.030)	63.05(6.678)	0.549
Laterality (R:L)	38:41	30:32	0.973
Corneal extension (mm) (Range)	3.685 (0.848) (1.5–5.5)	3.469 (0.970) (1.0–5.6)	0.164
Mean follow up (SD)	12.56(4.35)	12.85 (3.90)	0.674
(Range)	(6–28)	(6–27)	
No. of recurrences (%)	4/79(5.06)	13/62 (20.97)	0.003

M male, *F* female, *R* right, *L* left, *FU* follow-up

(20.97%) in the CG group ($P = 0.003$). In the HD-AM group, four eyes had recurrence at three, seven, nine, and 12 months (mean, 7.75 months) postoperatively. In the CG group, all recurrence developed within six months (mean, 3.4 months) postoperatively. The cumulative recurrence-free proportions at 12 months were 0. 95 ± 0.03 in the HD-AM group and 0.78 ± 0.05 in the CG group, which were significantly different ($P = 0.003$) (Table 2 and Fig. 2). When stratified regardless of surgical groups, there were no significant differences in recurrence rates among patients < 55 years (four cases, 19.05%), between 55 and 65 years (seven cases, 10.95%), and > 65 years (six cases, 10.71%, $P = 0.642$). Also, when stratified by sex only, there were no significant differences in the recurrence rates between male (eight cases, 10.62%) and female patients (nine cases, 14.29%, $P = 0.45$; Table 3).

Three cases of Dellen ulcer and two cases of Tenon's cyst were observed in the CG group in the first postoperative week. Dellen cases were treated medically, and Tenon's cyst was punctured to drain the subconjunctival fluid or excised surgically. No complications were observed in the HD-AM group.

Discussion

Today, surgical excision is still main method for treating pterygium [5, 12]. The major and most important criteria for the success of the surgery is the rate of postoperative pterygium recurrence, which has been described as the development of fibro-vascular tissue on to the excision site [13]. In order to lower the recurrence rate, the use of antimetabolites has been suggested owing to their antifibrotic and antiangiogenic properties [14, 15].

Conjunctival autografting was first described in 1980 with recurrence rates reported to be between 2.9–39% in primary pterygium [16–20]. In this study, the recurrence rate was 20.97% after conjunctival autografting in the primary pterygium when compared with work done by other researchers. Variations in the recurrence rates of conjunctival autografting could be explained according to the surgical excision size, surgeon's experience, patient's age, and surgical technique. As for surgical technique, incomplete separation of Tenon's tissue from the graft can cause graft retraction and high recurrence rates [17].

While conjunctival autografting has gained worldwide acceptance for treatment of pterygium, it is not without its defects such as the long operation time, graft inversion, and iatrogenic injury to the rest of the conjunctiva [19]. Syam et al. found that 36.66% of patients developed conjunctival scarring at the site of the donor conjunctiva [21]. Therefore, it is not feasible to use this technique to cover wide ocular surface defects created in the cases of large or double-headed pterygia.

HD-AM is made with fresh human AM using the hyperdrying method and returns to a layered structure

Table 2 Comparison of cumulative non-recurrence rate among hyperdry amniotic membrane transplantation graft group and conjunctival autograft group

	Cumulative non-recurrence rate (%)		P Value
	6 months	12 months	
Hyperdry amniotic membrane transplantation graft	98.73	95.42	0.003
conjunctival autograft	83.83	77.81	

similar to that of fresh AM after absorbing water as shown in Fig. 1 [7, 8]. Okabe et al. found that the structures of collagen fibers in the connective tissues were not destroyed by the hyperdry device and were more stable than cryopreserved AM [7]. Allen et al. also showed that the biochemical composition of the dried AM, including the number of factors such as epidermal growth factor and TGF-β1, were similar to fresh AM [22]. Moreover, rabbit models have also shown that HD-AM can be at least as efficacious as cryopreserved AM when used as a substrate for ocular surface reconstruction [23].

The technique of HD-AM transplantation is increasingly being used for ocular surface reconstruction [8, 10]. It can be maintained at room temperature and cut easily to the desired size and shape just before application [7]. It is useful in the covering of wide ocular surface defects such as in the case of large or double-headed pterygium. Furthermore, many surgeons have stated that care for HD-AM is simple, and its use may lead to shorter operating times. When compared to available synthetic biomaterials and animal-derived alternatives, it has good mechanical properties that allow it to be directly surgically sutured [7].

In our study, the recurrence rate in the HD-AM group was significantly lower (5.06%) than recurrence rates in the CG group (20.97%; $P = 0.003$). The reported recurrence rates with amniotic membrane transplantation vary between 3.8 and 40.9% [24–26]. Inhibition of pathological neovascularization, prevention of excessive inflammation, and promotion of conjunctival epithelialization are the main reasons for the effectiveness of AM in pterygium surgery; therefore, use of HD-AM might help these processes and reduce recurrence of the condition [27–29].

It is interesting that the mean time to recurrence was 10.3 months in the HD-AM group as against 3.4 months in the CG group. This result correlated with a study by Kocamis, in which the average recurrence time was 4.5 months in conjunctival autografting [30]. This phenomenon suggests that conjunctival autografting provides a source of conjunctival epithelium and may eventually breach, whereas HD-AM seems to play a role in inhibiting the involvement of progenitor cells in pterygium recurrence [31].

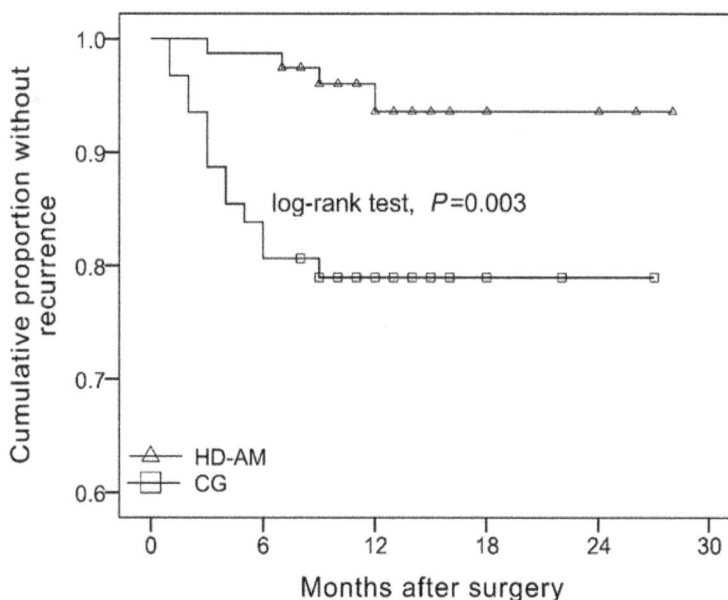

Fig. 2 Kaplan-Meier survival curve of recurrence after pterygium excision. The cumulative proportion recurrence-free at 12 months was 0.95 ± 0.03 in the HD-AMT group and 0.78 ± 0.05 in the CG group (P = 0.003)

Table 3 Comparison of cumulative non-recurrence rate for all patients stratified by age and sex only

	No. (%) of recurrences	Cumulative non-recurrence rate (%)		
		6 months	12 months	P Value
Age (years)				
< 55	4/21(19.05)	95.24	84.35	0.642
55–65	7/64 (10.94)	92.19	88.00	
> 65	6/56(10.71)	91.07	88.77	
Sex				
Male (eye)	8/78 (10.62)	90.48	84.01	0.415
Female (eye)	9/63 (14.29)	93.53	90.42	

To date, graft edema, necrosis of the graft, inclusion cysts, subconjunctival hematoma, Tenon's granuloma, corneal narrowing, and Dellen ulcers have been reported to be the most common postoperative complications of primary pterygium [32, 33]. Three cases of Dellen ulcer and two cases of Tenon's cyst were observed in the CG group in our study; whereas, none of these complications were observed in the HD-AM group during the follow-up period.

In addition to minimizing recurrence rates and surgical complications, it is expected that patients treated with HD-AM will have reduced postoperative pain and discomfort relative to conjunctival autograft surgery. These findings could be attributed to membrane covering of the corneal epithelial defect in addition to reducing inflammation [34].

Conclusions

In summary, HD-AM transplantation may be a superior treatment in primary pterygium owing to lower recurrence rate, shorter surgical times, and no major complications other than conjunctival autografting. HD-AM is a human-derived material that has potential safety issues in the context of viral and prion infection. Further studies are needed to reevaluate the safety and efficacy of HD-AM for excision of primary pterygium.

Abbreviations
AM: amniotic membrane; CG: conjunctival autografting; HD-AM: hyperdry amniotic membrane; TGF-β1: Transforming growth factor beta-1; UV: ultraviolet

Acknowledgements
The authors wish to acknowledge Drs. Chunyan Yu and Haitao Xu for their help with the operation.

Funding
This work was supported by the Plan of Jilin Education Department "Thirteen-Five" Science and Technology research[2016]No.473.

Authors' contributions
XP drafted this manuscript, collected the data, and reviewed the literature. XP and ZHC collected the data. XP, DGZ, ZFJ, and YTS were involved in the analysis. XP, DGZ, and YTS reviewed and revised the manuscript and produced the final version. All authors read and approved the final manuscript.

Competing interests
The authors declare that they have no competing interests.

Author details
[1]The Second Hospital of Jilin University, No.218, Ziqiang Road, Changchun 130041, China. [2]The First Hospital of Jilin University, No.71, Xinmin Road, Changchun 130021, China.

References
1. Jaros PA, Pinguecula DLVP. pterygia. Surv Ophthalmol. 1988;33:41–9.
2. Nemesure B, Wu SY, Hennis A, Leske MC. Nine year incidence and risk factors for pterygium in Barbados eye studies. Ophthalmology. 2008;115: 2153–8.
3. Mohammed I. Treatment of pterygium. Ann Afr Med. 2011;10:197–203.
4. Kim SH, Oh JH, Do JR, Chuck RS, Park CY. A comparison of anchored conjunctival rotation flap and conjunctival autograft techniques in pterygium surgery. Cornea. 2013;32:1578–81.
5. Ozer A, Yildirim N, Erol N, Yurdakul S. Long-term results of bare sclera, limbal-conjunctival autograft and amniotic membrane graft techniques in primary pterygium excisions. Ophthalmologica. 2009;223:269–73.
6. Tan Ang LP, Chua JL, Tan DT. Current concepts and techniques in pterygium treatment. Curr Opin Ophthalmol. 2007;18:308–13.
7. Okabe M, Kitagawa K, Yoshida T, Suzuki T, Waki H, Koike C, et al. Hyperdry human amniotic membrane is useful material for tissue engineering: physical, morphological properties, and safety as the new biological material. J Biomed Mater Res A. 2014;102:862–70.
8. Kitagawa K, Yanagisawa S, Watanabe K. A hyperdry amniotic membrane patch using a tissue adhesive for corneal perforations and bleb leaks. Am J Ophthalmol. 2009;148:383–9.
9. Toda A, Okabe M, Yoshida T, Nikaido T. The potential of amniotic membrane/amnion-derived cells for regeneration of various tissues. J Pharmacol Sci. 2007;105:215–28.
10. Kitagawa K, Okabe M, Yanagisawa S, Zhang XY, Nikaido T, Hayashi A. Use of a hyperdried cross linked amniotic membrane as initial therapy for corneal perforations. Jpn J Ophthalmol. 2011;55:16–21.
11. Tan DT, Chee SP, Dear KB, Lim AS. Effect of pterygium morphology on pterygium recurrence in a controlled trial comparing conjunctival autografting with bare sclera excision. Arch Ophthalmol. 1997;115:1235–40.
12. Tananuvat N, Martin T. The results of amniotic membrane transplantation for primary pterygium compared with conjunctival autograft. Cornea. 2004; (5):458–63.
13. Essex RW, Snibson GR, Daniell M, Tole DM. Amniotic membrane grafting in the surgical management of primary pterygium. Clin Exp Ophthalmol. 2004; 32:501–4.
14. Singh G, Wilson MR, Foster CS. Long-term follow-up study of mitomycin eye drops as adjunctive treatment of pterygia and its comparison with conjunctival autograft transplantation. Cornea. 1990;9:331–4.
15. Dadeya S, Kamlesh, Khurana C, Fatima S. Intraoperative daunorubicin versus conjunctival autograft in primary pterygium surgery. Cornea. 2002;21:766–9.
16. Barraquer JI, Binder PS, Buxton JN. Etiology and treatment of pterygium; symposium on medical and surgical diseases of the cornea. Transactions of the New Orleans academy of ophthalmology. St Louis: Mosby; 1980. p. 167–78.
17. Chen PP, Ariyasu RG, Kaza V, LaBree LD, McDonnell PJ. A randomized trial comparing mitomycin C and conjunctival autograft after excision of primary pterygium. Am J Ophthalmol. 1995;120:151–60.

18. Arvas S, Ozturk M, Toparlak T, Yolar M, Yetik H, Ozkan CS. Pterjiyumlu olgularda ultrastrukturel degerlendirme. T Oft Gaz. 2002;32:88–93.
19. Ti SE, Chee SP, Dear KB, Tan DT. Analysis of variation in success rates in conjunctival autografting for primary and recurrent pterygium. Br J Ophthalmol. 2002;84:385–9.
20. Dadeya S, Malik KP, Pterygiumsurgery GBP. conjunctival rotation autograft versus conjunctival autograft. Ophthalmic Surg Lasers. 2002;33:269–74.
21. Syam PP, Eleftheriadis H, Liu CSC. Inferior conjunctival autograft for primary pterygia. Ophthalmology. 2003;110:806–10.
22. Allen CL, Clare G, Stewart EA. Augmented dried versus cryopreserved amniotic membrane as an ocular surface dressing. PLoS One. 2013;8:e78441.
23. Libera RD, Melo GB, Lima Ade S, Haapalainen EF, Cristovam P, Gomes JA. Assessment of the use of cryopreserved x freeze-dried amniotic membrane (AM) for reconstruction of ocular surface in rabbit model. Arg Bras Oftalmol. 2008;71:669–73.
24. Luanratanakorn P, Ratanapakorn T, Suwanapichon O. Randomised controlled study of conjunctival autograft versus amniotic membrane graft in pterygium excision. Br J Ophthalmol. 2006;90:1476–80.
25. Ma DH, See LC, Liau SB. Amniotic membrane graft for primary pterygium: comparison with conjunctival autograft and topical mitomycin C treatment. Br J Ophthalmol. 2000;84:973–8.
26. Tananuvat N, Martin T. The results of amniotic membrane transplantation for primary pterygium compared with conjunctival autograft. Cornea. 2004; 23:458–63.
27. Hao Y, Ma DH, Hwang DG, Kim WS, Zhang F. Identification of antiangiogenic and anti-inflammatory proteins in human amniotic membrane. Cornea. 2000;19:348–52.
28. Bultmann S, You L, Spandau U. Amniotic membrane downregulates chemokine expression in human keratocytes. Investig Ophthalmol Vis Sci. 1999;40:S578.
29. Tseng SC, Li DQ, Ma X. Suppression of transforming growth factor-beta isoforms, TGF-beta receptor type II, and myofibroblast differentiation in cultured human corneal and limbal fibroblasts by amniotic membrane matrix. Journal of Cell Phys. 1999;179:325–35.
30. Kocamis O, Bilgec M. Evaluation of the recurrence rate for pterygium treated with conjunctival autograft. Graefes Arch Clin Exp Ophthalmol. 2014; 252:817–20.
31. Ye J, Kook KH, Yao K. Temporary amniotic membrane patch for the treatment of primary pterygium: mechanisms of reducing the recurrence rate. Graefes Arch Clin Exp Ophthalmol. 2006;244:583–8.
32. Kucukerdonmez C, Akova YA, Altinors DD. Comparison of conjunctival autograft with amniotic membrane transplantation for pterygium surgery: surgical and cosmetic outcome. Cornea. 2007;26:407–13.
33. Vrabec MP, Weisenthal RW, Elsing SH. Subconjunctival fibrosis after conjunctival autograft. Cornea. 1993;12:181–3.
34. Pirouzian A, Holz H, Merrill K, Sudesh R, Karlen K. Surgical management of pediatric limbal dermoids with sutureless amniotic membrane transplantation and augmentation. J Pediatr Ophthalmol Strabismus. 2012; 49:114–9.

3

Untreated Acute Posterior Multifocal Placoid Pigment Epitheliopathy (APMPPE): a case series

Olivia Xerri, Sawsen Salah[*] ⓘ, Dominique Monnet and Antoine P. Brézin

Abstract

Background: Acute Posterior Multifocal Placoid Pigment Epitheliopathy (APMPPE) is a rare inflammatory eye disease that affects the Retinal Pigment Epithelium and outer retina. The purpose of this study was to describe its presentations, as well as its prognosis in a series of untreated patients.

Methods: Records of patients seen in the department of Ophthalmology at Cochin University Hospital, Paris, between April 2002 and June 2015 were retrospectively studied. Patients were included if they presented with the typical findings of APMPPE characterized by whitish or yellowish bilateral placoid lesions, a typical pattern of early hypofluorescence and late hyperfluorescence on fluorescein angiography. Only untreated patients who had been followed for at least 1 month were included.

Results: Out of 22 patients' records with a diagnosis of APMPPE, 10 patients (9 women, 1 man), with a mean age of 24.5 ± 4.2 years, fulfilled the study criteria with a diagnosis of typical untreated APMPPE. Prodromal symptoms were reported in 7/10 patients. Macular lesions were observed in 18/20 eyes. Sub-retinal fluid was seen at presentation in 3 eyes. Initial mean BCVA was 0.56 ± 0.81 LogMAR [− 0.10 to 2.30]. In 9 out of 10 cases, the time interval between manifestations in the first affected eye and the fellow eye was less than 3 days. After 1 month, BCVA had improved to 0.05 ± 0.089 LogMAR [0–0.3], with a decimal BCVA ≥0.8 in 17/20 eyes.

Conclusions: In these 10 cases of untreated APMPPE, a favorable outcome was observed.

Keywords: Acute posterior multifocal placoid pigment epitheliopathy, Inflammatory disease, Posterior uveitis, Retina, Retinal pigment epithelium

Background

Acute posterior multifocal placoid pigment epitheliopathy (APMPPE) is a rare inflammatory disease that typically affects healthy young adults. Five decades after its first description, it remains debated whether the primary tissue involved is the choriocapillaris or the retinal pigment epithelium [1–4]. Patients typically present with a rapid onset of visual loss associated with central and paracentral scotomas. The disease is usually bilateral with both eyes involved within a week, but may be asymmetrical [5, 6]. Flu-like symptoms often precede the onset of the disease, but central nervous system (CNS) involvement ranging from headaches to diffuse cerebral vasculitis is also observed [7]. Cases following immunizations or infections have also been reported [8].

The observation of the fundus typically shows multifocal, yellowish-white, placoid lesions, varying in size, located from the posterior pole to the mid-periphery. On fluorescein angiograms, the lesions show early hypofluorescence and late hyperfluorescence ("blocks early, stains late"). Indocyanine green angiography reveals early and late hypofluorescence. The lesions fade gradually within weeks, to be replaced by varying degrees of hyperpigmentation and sometimes by retinal pigment epithelium (RPE) atrophy.

Optical Coherence Tomography (OCT) imaging and especially spectral domain Optical Coherence Tomography (SD-OCT) allowed the description of an aspect of

---
* Correspondence: sawsen.salah@gmail.com
Department of Ophthalmology, Hôpital Cochin, Assistance Publique Hôpitaux de Paris, Université Paris Descartes, Paris, France

heterogeneous sub-retinal-fluid (SRF) at the very early stages of the disease, evolving to outer nuclear layer (ONL) hyperreflectivity before thinning [9, 10]. Prior to the complete healing, a phase of disruption of the inner segment/ outer segment (IS/OS) layer with hyperreflectivity of the RPE can last until the third month [9].

The natural history of APMPPE was initially described as globally favourable, [11, 12] but some reports show that patients may experience an incomplete visual recovery [13–15]. Hence, whether to treat patients with APMPPE or not remains debated. Some authors have advocated systematic corticosteroid treatment, other limit the indications of therapy to cases with macular involvement [10, 16–18]. To our knowledge, there are no recent series using modern imaging techniques focused on untreated APMPPE patients. The purpose of our study was to assess the ocular and extra-ocular features, as well as the visual prognosis in a group of untreated patients.

Methods

This was a retrospective study of patients with a diagnosis of APMPPE seen between April 2002 and June 2015 in the department of Ophthalmology of the Cochin University Hospital, Paris. Patients were included if they demonstrated the typical fundus and fluorescein findings of APMPPE. Required features were multiple, geographic, deep white-yellowish lesions that were hypofluorescent at the early stages and hyperfluorescent at the late stages of the angiography. Only untreated patients with a follow-up of at least one-month were included. Patients with atypical features such as multifocal choroidal lesions and/or

atrophic punched-out lesions were excluded. Prodromal symptoms and/or concomitant extraocular manifestations were recorded. Our analyses included the following parameters assessed at entry and at the 1 month-follow-up: best-corrected-visual-acuity (BCVA), results of slit-lamp examination, Humphrey visual field testing and fundus imaging by fluorescein angiography. OCT imaging was performed using the Stratus (Carl Zeiss Meditec, Jena, Germany) from 2002 until 2011, then with the Spectralis (Heidelberg Engineering Inc., Heidelberg, Germany) tomographers. The study was approved by the Ethics Committee of the French Society of Ophthalmology and adhered to the Declaration of Helsinki for research involving human subjects.

Results

Out of 22 patients who had been diagnosed with APMPPE, 10 patients (1 man, 9 women) met our study criteria. The criteria for exclusion were atypical features in 3 cases: two with associated multifocal choroiditis and one with a systemic association of positive ANtineutrophil Cytoplasmic Antibodies (ANCAs). Seven cases were excluded for lack of follow-up and two treated patients were also excluded. Treatment in one of these cases was triggered by an episode of deafness with an onset 6 weeks after the ocular manifestations. In the second case, the treatment was triggered by an uncertain diagnosis with the possibility of Vogt-Koyanagi-Harada disease. Our patients' demographic data and their extraocular manifestations are summarized in Table 1.

The mean patients' age was 24.5 ± 4.2 years, with a female predominance: 9 women and 1 man. The mean

Table 1 Demographics, extra-ocular findings, BCVA at entry, and at 4 and 8 weeks

Patient #	Gender	Age	Prodromic symptoms (time interval prior to diagnosis)	Clinical signs of meningitis and CSF analysis		Initial BCVA (decimal)		BCVA at 4 weeks (decimal)		BCVA at 8 weeks (decimal)	
				Clinical signs	CSF analysis (cells/mm³)	RE	LE	RE	LE	RE	LE
1	F	20–30	Flu-like syndrome (1 week)	Headaches	Lymphocytic meningitis (121 cells)	HM	HM	0.8	0.6	1.0	0.9
2	F	20–30	Flu-like syndrome (3 weeks)	None	ND	FC	1.0	0.6	1.0	0.8	1.0
3	F	20–30	Gastro-enteritis and erythema nodosum (1 week)	None	Undetermined meningitis (11 cells)	1.2	1.2	0.9	1.0	1.0	1.0
4	F	10–20	None	None	ND	1.0	0.3	1.0	1.0	1.0	1.0
5	F	20–30	Flu-like syndrome	None	ND	0.9	0.8	0.9	0.8	1.0	1.0
6	M	20–30	Flu-like syndrome (1 week)	None	ND	0.8	0.25	1.0	0.8	1.0	0.8
7	F	10–20	None	None	ND	1.0	0.2	1.0	1.0	1.0	1.0
8	F	20–30	Fever and erythema nodosum (1 week)	None	ND	0.1	0.5	0.9	0.5	1.0	0.8
9	F	20–30	None	None	ND	1.0	0.8	1.0	1.0	1.0	1.0
10	F	30–40	Fever (10 days)	Headaches	ND	FC	1.0	1.0	1.0	NA	NA

F female, *M* Male, *BCVA* Best Corrected Visual Acuity, *RE* Right Eye, *LE* Left Eye, *ND* Not Done, *HM* Hand Motion vision, *FC* Finger Counting, *NA* Not Available

follow-up was 11.45 ± 14.84 months with a median of 5.5 months.

Prodromal flu-like manifestations were reported in 7 of 10 patients before the onset of visual loss. The time interval between the prodromal manifestations and the observation of fundus lesions ranged from 7 days to 3 weeks. Out of the 10 patients, 4 had no work-up and 6 had the following investigations which were negative or normal: complete blood count, C-reactive protein dosage, interferon production assay, Purified Protein Derivative (PPD) test, syphilitic serology (TPHA-VDRL), ANCA, angiotensin converting enzyme dosage, as well as radiological exams: Computed Tomography of the brain and chest radiography. Two patients had a lumbar puncture revealing meningitis, with 121 cells/mm^3 (100% lymphocytes) in one case and 11 cells/mm^3 in the other. At 4 weeks, all extra-ocular symptoms had subsided in all of our patients.

The mean LogMAR BCVA at presentation was 0.56 ± 0.81. Five of the 20 eyes had a decimal BCVA ≤ 0.1, while 11/20 eyes had a decimal BCVA ≥ 0.8 with a median of 0.8. Cells in the anterior chamber were observed in 9/20 eyes at onset and were $< 2+$ in all cases. The size of the whitish or yellowish placoid lesions ranged from 250 to 500 μm or more when merging, 13 eyes had more than 5 placoid lesions. The lesions were observed at the posterior pole in 19/20 eyes, as well as in the mid-periphery or in the periphery in 12/20 eyes. Figure 1 shows the imaging of a patient with a macular involvement. On OCT imaging, sub-retinal fluid was observed in 3 eyes, and alterations of the ellipsoid zone was seen in 7 eyes. At 4 weeks, the median decimal BCVA was 1.0 and the mean LogMAR acuity was 0.05 ± 0.089. At 8 weeks (9 patients), 16 eyes had a BCVA of 1.0, the median acuity was thus 1.0 and the mean acuity was 0.015 LogMar. Two eyes recovered a decimal BCVA of 1.0 after a follow-up longer than 8 weeks (at 10 months for one patient and at 5 months for the other one). The aspect of the lesions had evolved to a slight pigmentation at 4 weeks, except for 5 eyes for which the placoid lesions remained whitish-yellowish. The size of the lesions was unchanged or had decreased very moderately,

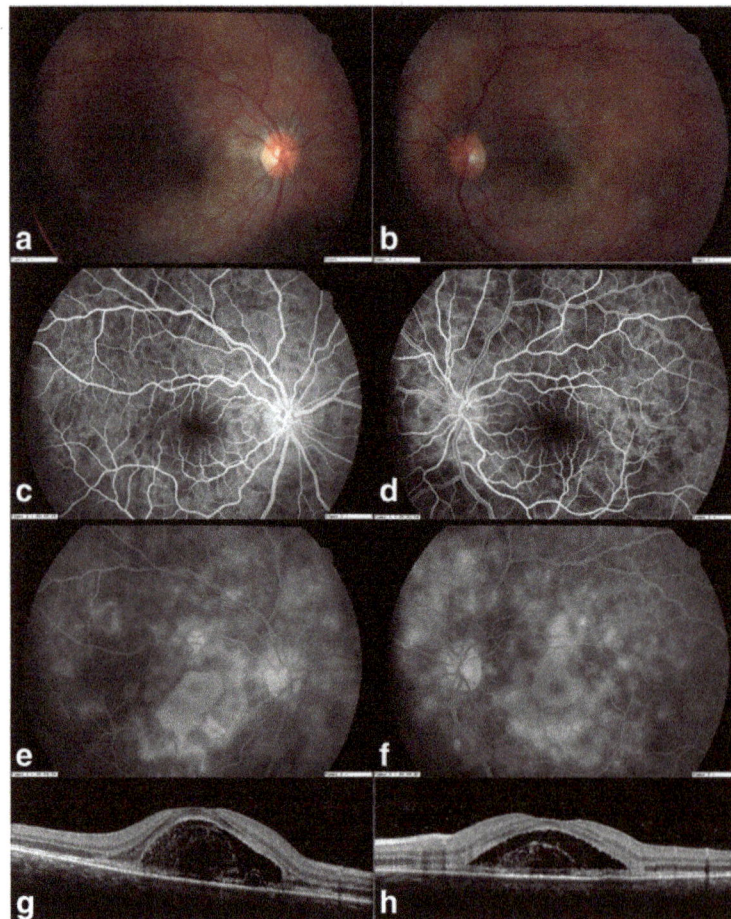

Fig. 1 Ocular findings at presentation. **a**, **b**. Color photographs. **c**, **d**. Early stage of the fluorescein angiography with hypofluorescent lesions. **e**, **f**. Late phase of the fluorescein angiography with hyperfluorescent lesions. **g**, **h**. SD-OCT imaging: Sub-Retinal Fluid

their location was unchanged. On OCT, the sub-retinal fluid had disappeared in all affected eyes, however alterations of the ellipsoid zone remained in 3 eyes on OCT imaging, with an hyperreflectivity of the outer nuclear layer. Figure 2 presents the follow-up of a patient with SD-OCT and compares the visual acuity with SD-OCT imaging and staging using Goldenberg's classification. At entry, subretinal fluid (SRF) was present, while acuity was limited to the detection of Hand Motion (HM). At 4 days, SRF had nearly disappeared and decimal BCVA improved to 0.3 OD and 0.1 OS. At 1 month, there was a persistent disruption of the ellipsoid zone and an hyperreflectivity of the Retinal Pigment Epithelium with a thinning of the Outer Nuclear Layer (ONL). BCVA had improved to decimal 0.8 and 0.6. At 4 months, BCVA was almost normal (OD:decimal 1.0 and OS: decimal 0.9). Finally, a complete recovery was observed at 10 months. OCT imaging showed a persistent thinning of the ONL and an irregularity of the ellipsoid zone, which might explain why some patients kept moderate visual consequences of their disease.

Discussion

The number of patients in published series of cases of APMPPE is limited and ours is the fourth largest within the past decade and the largest with untreated patients [13, 17, 18]. As in other series, the majority of cases affected patients in their third decade [18–20]. The 9:1 female predominance observed in our series was greater than in other reports, but that may just be a chance finding due to the relatively small number of patients in our series. All prodromal syndromes observed in our series have also been previously reported. In other series the cumulated frequency of these various manifestations ranged from 18 to 61% and were most often estimated around 30% [17, 18, 21]. We did not identify any particular link between extra-ocular symptoms and ocular findings.

In spite of early reports of favourable outcomes in untreated APMPPE, subsequent studies have frequently comprised both treated and untreated patients [17, 18]. In the literature, the following triggers for treatment have been reported: macular localization of lesions, subretinal fluid on OCT and/or severe visual loss. The most commonly used treatment method were corticosteroids with different dosages, including occasionally initial IV methylprednisolone pulses. Two series of 11 and 21 untreated patients had also observed a good recovery in terms of BCVA with final decimal BCVA of 0.94 and 0.86 respectively [11, 12].

Overall our observation of the favorable recovery of the visual acuity was within the spectrum or better than that of other reports. The two most recent series with treated patients also showed a very good recovery of visual acuity with mean final decimal acuities of 0.9 and 0.67 [9, 17].

We cannot rule out that the following biases could have influenced our observations: 2 treated patients were

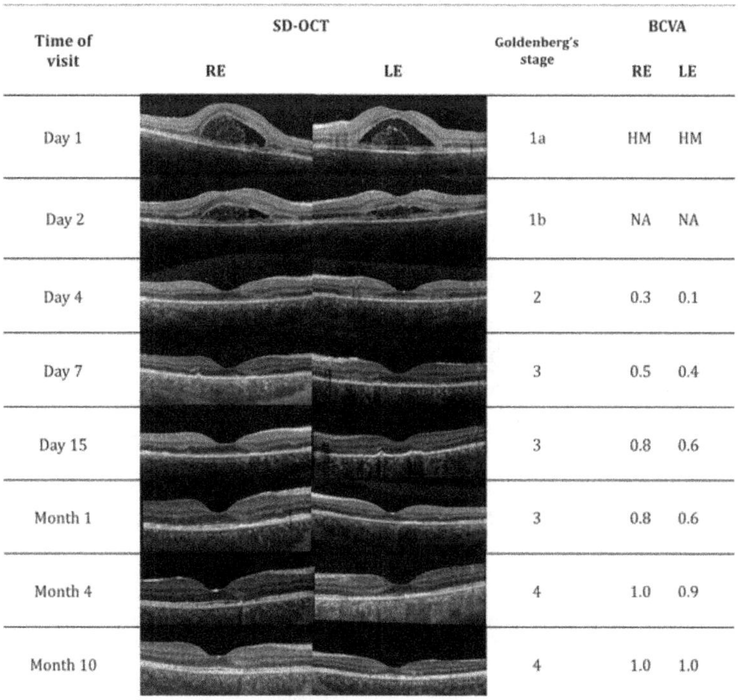

Time of visit	SD-OCT		Goldenberg's stage	BCVA	
	RE	LE		RE	LE
Day 1			1a	HM	HM
Day 2			1b	NA	NA
Day 4			2	0.3	0.1
Day 7			3	0.5	0.4
Day 15			3	0.8	0.6
Month 1			3	0.8	0.6
Month 4			4	1.0	0.9
Month 10			4	1.0	1.0

Fig. 2 Follow-up of visual acuity, SD-OCT imaging and Goldenberg's classification staging in a patient presenting with Sub-Retinal Fluid at entry

excluded and 7 patients were lost to follow-up. Although three-fourth of the eyes in our study had macular lesions, a good visual recovery was nevertheless also observed in those cases. Initial severe visual loss, subretinal fluid or hyperpigmentation of plaques during the patients' follow-up did not impede the recovery of a normal BCVA. Our study's outcome measure was focused on BCVA but persistent visual field alterations after APMPPE have been reported in up to 67.9% of patients [22]. Some patients may complain of an imperfect vision in the aftermath of their attack, in spite of a normal BCVA. In these cases, central visual field testing or microperimetry can be useful to identify visual defects at the site of healed atrophic or hyperpigmented plaques. In our study, the results of visual field testing was only available in 5 patients (data not shown). We cannot rule out treatment could favorably influence the outcome of visual field testing in subgroups of patients after their attack of APMPPE.

A classification of the OCT findings observed in APMPPE was suggested by Goldenberg et al. [9]. This included a first stage with sub-retinal fluid and later stages with outer nuclear layer (ONL) hyperreflectivity, thinning of the outer nuclear layer, disruption of the ellipsoid zone, hyperreflective bands of ellipsoid and RPE. Future studies entirely based on SD-OCT will allow to better understand the relation between BCVA and stages of APMPPE according to Goldenberg's classification. In some cases, the early stage of APMPPE may share features with the early stage of Vogt-Kayanagi-Harada disease [23]. Extraocular features reported in association with APMPPE have included neurological manifestations, yet in our series, headaches and/or lymphocytic meningitis were not a trigger for initiating treatment [24]. A case was reported, for which corticosteroids at a dosage of 80 mg per day did not prevent a stroke due to cerebral vasculitis [17].

Conclusions

Our series confirms that untreated patients with APMPPE can have a favourable outcome. Whether this applies to all cases of the disease remains unknown and there is no consensus regarding the factors that should trigger treatment in selected patients. As APMPPE is a rare disease, the assessment of the benefits of treatment would probably require an international trial to recruit enough patients for the gathering of evidence-based data. Until then, decisions to treat patients with APMPPE or not will remain rather empirical.

Abbreviations
ANCAs: ANtineutrophil cytoplasmic antibodies; APMPPE: Acute posterior multifocal placoid pigment epitheliopathy; BCVA: Best-corrected-visual-acuity; CNS: Central nervous system; IS: Inner segment; OCT: Optical coherence tomography; ONL: Outer nuclear layer; OS: Outer segment; PPD: Purified protein derivative; RPE: Retinal pigment epithelium; SD-OCT: Spectral domain optical coherence tomography; SRF: Sub-retinal-fluid

Funding
This research did not receive any specific grant from funding agencies in the public, commercial, or not-for-profit sectors.

Authors' contributions
OX and SS collected the data. OX and SS analyzed and interpreted the patient data under the supervision of AB and DM. AB and DM verified the analytical methods. All authors discussed the results and contributed to the final manuscript. OX and AB wrote the manuscript. All authors read and approved the final manuscript.

Competing interests
The authors declare that they have no competing interests.

References
1. Deutman AF, Oosterhuis JA, Boen-Tan TN, Aan de Kerk AL. Acute posterior multifocal placoid pigment epitheliopathy. Pigment epitheliopathy of choriocapillaritis? Br J Ophthalmol. 1972;56:863–74.
2. Chiquet C, Lumbroso L, Denis P, Papo T, Durieu I, Lehoang P. Acute posterior multifocal placoid pigment epitheliopathy associated with Wegener's granulomatosis. Retina. 1999;19:309–13.
3. Dolz-Marco R, Sarraf D, Giovinnazzo V, Freund KB. Optical coherence tomography angiography shows inner choroidal ischemia in acute posterior multifocal placoid pigment epitheliopathy. Retin Cases Brief Rep. 2016; 11(Suppl 1):S136–S143.
4. Salvatore S, Steeples LR, Ross AH, Bailey C, Lee RW, Carreno E. Multimodal imaging in acute posterior multifocal Placoid pigment Epitheliopathy demonstrating obstruction of the Choriocapillaris. Ophthalmic Surg Lasers Imaging Retina. 2016;47:677–81.
5. Jones NP. Acute posterior multifocal placoid pigment epitheliopathy. Br J Ophthalmol. 1995;79:384–9.
6. Quillen DA, Davis JB, Gottlieb JL, Blodi BA, Callanan DG, Chang TS, Equi RA. The white dot syndromes. Am J Ophthalmol. 2004;137:538–50.
7. O'Halloran HS, Berger JR, Lee WB, Robertson DM, Giovannini JA, Krohel GB, Meckler RJ, Selhorst JB, Lee AG, Nicolle DA, O'Day J. Acute multifocal placoid pigment epitheliopathy and central nervous system involvement: nine new cases and a review of the literature. Ophthalmology. 2001;108: 861–8.
8. Brezin AP, Massin-Korobelnik P, Boudin M, Gaudric A, LeHoang P. Acute posterior multifocal placoid pigment epitheliopathy after hepatitis B vaccine. Arch Ophthalmol. 1995;113:297–300.
9. Goldenberg D, Habot-Wilner Z, Loewenstein A, Goldstein M. Spectral domain optical coherence tomography classification of acute posterior multifocal placoid pigment epitheliopathy. Retina. 2012;32:1403–10.
10. Birnbaum AD, Blair MP, Tessler HH, Goldstein DA. Subretinal fluid in acute posterior multifocal placoid pigment epitheliopathy. Retina. 2010;30:810–4.
11. Williams DF, Mieler WF. Long-term follow-up of acute multifocal posterior placoid pigment epitheliopathy. Br J Ophthalmol. 1989;73:985–90.
12. Vianna R, van Egmond J, Priem H, Kestelyn P. Natural history and visual outcome in patients with APMPPE. Bull Soc Belge Ophtalmol. 1993;248:73–6.
13. Fiore T, Iaccheri B, Androudi S, Papadaki TG, Anzaar F, Brazitikos P, D'Amico DJ, Foster CS. Acute posterior multifocal placoid pigment epitheliopathy: outcome and visual prognosis. Retina. 2009;29:994–1001.
14. Saraux H, Pelosse B. Acute posterior multifocal placoid pigment epitheliopathy. A long-term follow-up. Ophthalmologica. 1987;194:161–3.
15. Taich A, Johnson MW. A syndrome resembling acute posterior multifocal placoid pigment epitheliopathy in older adults. Trans Am Ophthalmol Soc. 2008;106:56–62. discussion 62-53
16. Grkovic D, Oros A, Bedov T, Karadzic J, Gvozdenovic L, Jovanovic S. Acute posterior multifocal placoid pigment epitheliopathy-retinal "white dot syndrome". Med Glas. 2013;10:194–6.
17. Thomas BC, Jacobi C, Korporal M, Becker MD, Wildemann B, Mackensen F. Ocular outcome and frequency of neurological manifestations in patients with acute posterior multifocal placoid pigment epitheliopathy (APMPPE). J Ophthalmic Inflamm Infect. 2012;2:125–31.

18. Bures-Jelstrup A, Adan A, Casaroli-Marano R. Acute posterior multifocal placoid pigment epitheliopathy. Study of 16 cases. Arch Soc Esp Oftalmol. 2007;82:291–7.
19. Roberts TV, Mitchell P. Acute posterior multifocal placoid pigment epitheliopathy: a long-term study. Aust N Z J Ophthalmol. 1997;25:277–81.
20. Taich A, Johnson MW. A syndrome resembling acute posterior multifocal placoid pigment epitheliopathy in older adults. Retina. 2009;29:149–56.
21. Crawford CM, Igboeli O. A review of the inflammatory chorioretinopathies: the white dot syndromes. ISRN Inflamm. 2013;2013:783190.
22. Wolf MD, Alward WL, Folk JC. Long-term visual function in acute posterior multifocal placoid pigment epitheliopathy. Arch Ophthalmol. 1991;109:800–3.
23. Li B, Bentham RJ, Gonder JR. A case of unilateral and spontaneously resolving posterior uveitis with overlapping features of Vogt-Koyanagi-Harada disease and acute posterior multifocal placoid pigment epitheliopathy. Spring. 2016;5:1471.
24. Algahtani H, Alkhotani A, Shirah B. Neurological manifestations of acute posterior multifocal placoid pigment epitheliopathy. J Clin Neurol. 2016;12: 460–7.

4

The function and morphology of Meibomian glands in patients with thyroid eye disease

Chia-Yu Wang[1†], Ren-Wen Ho[2,3†], Po-Chiung Fang[2], Hun-Ju Yu[2], Chun-Chih Chien[4], Chang-Chun Hsiao[5] and Ming-Tse Kuo[2*] (iD)

Abstract

Background: To investigate function and morphology of the meibomian gland (MG) in patients with thyroid eye disease (TED).

Methods: In this prospective case series study, patients with unilateral or bilateral TED were consecutively enrolled. The diagnosis of TED was based on the typical orbital findings and/or radiographic evidence. The disease activity of TED was classified according to the clinical activity score (CAS). Degrees of lagophthalmos and exophthalmos, blinking rates, and results of the Schirmer test 1 were also recorded. All patients completed the SPEED questionnaire and underwent MG assessment, including lipid layer thickness (LLT), MG dropout (MGd), and MG expression.

Results: In total 31 eyes from 17 patients with unilateral or bilateral TED were included. Patients were divided into inactive TED (CAS 0–1; 20 eyes from 11 patients) and active TED (CAS 2–3, 11 eyes from 6 patients) groups. MGd was significantly more severe in the active TED than the inactive TED group [Median (Inter-quartile region): 3.0 (2.0–3.0) vs. 2.0 (1.0–2.0) degree, $P = 0.04$]. However, patients with active TED had thicker LLT than those with inactive TED (90.0 [80.0–100.0] vs. 65.0 [47.8–82.5] nm, $P = 0.02$), and LLT was positively correlated with lagophthalmos ($r = 0.37$, $P = 0.04$).

Conclusions: Patients with active TED had more severe MGd, but thicker LLT. Active TED may cause periglandular inflammation of MGs, leading to MGd, but compensatory secretion from residual MGs and lagophthalmos-induced forceful blinking might temporarily release more lipids over the tear film.

Keywords: Lipid layer thickness, Meibomian gland dysfunction, Thyroid eye diseases

Background

Thyroid eye disease (TED), also known as Graves' ophthalmopathy and thyroid-associated orbitopathy, is an ocular manifestation of a systemic autoimmune disorder. The orbit presents the same antigens as the thyroid gland, such as the thyroid-stimulating hormone receptor, thyrotropin receptor, and insulin-like receptor [1]. Consequently, for patients with immune-related thyroid dysfunction, the circulating autoantibodies may also attack the orbit by triggering a cytokine cascade and causing orbital fibroblast proliferation, adipose tissue expansion, and glycosaminoglycan secretion [2]. Finally, patients may develop lid edema, chemosis, lid retraction, exophthalmos, lagophthalmos, restrictive myopathy, and compressive optic neuropathy, and may complain of diplopia and decreased vision [3].

Dry eye disease (DED) is very common in patients with TED: the prevalence rate of DED in TED is up to 65.2% [4, 5]. Coulter et al. reported that 97% of patients with TED in a cohort study had dry eye symptoms [6]. Some underlying mechanisms have been proposed. First, lid retraction, exophthalmos, and lagophthalmos may cause ocular surface changes and blinking abnormalities

* Correspondence: mingtse@cgmh.org.tw

[†]Equal contributors

[2]Department of Ophthalmology, Kaohsiung Chang Gung Memorial Hospital and Chang Gung University College of Medicine, Kaohsiung, Taiwan

Full list of author information is available at the end of the article

[2, 7, 8], which increase the evaporation of tears and lead to DED in patients with TED [2, 9]. Second, lacrimal acinar cells physiologically express thyroid-stimulating hormone receptors [10]; thus, the antigen–antibody reaction of TED may impair the lacrimal gland and subsequently result in a decreased volume of reflex tearing [10, 11]. Third, TED may disturb the secretion of aqueous tears and make the tear film unstable, leading to shorter tear film breakup time and increased tear film osmolality [7, 10–12].

However, increasing evidence indicates that meibomian gland (MG) dysfunction is a major risk factor of DED [13, 14]. The International Dry Eye Work Shop have classified DED into aqueous tear deficiency (ATD) and evaporative dry eye (EDE) [15, 16], and recognized MG dysfunction as the primary cause of EDE [17]. Similar to patients with MG dysfunction, patients with TED usually also have dry eye symptoms. However, previous studies only focused on the ATD in patients with TED but neglected the MG dysfunction in these patients. MGs, which are special sebaceous glands in the eyelids, secrete lipids to stabilize the tear film, decrease the surface tension, and prevent the evaporation of aqueous tears [18]. MGs are arranged in parallel palisades throughout the tarsus plates of the eyelids, and the blinking motion serves as a pumping force that releases the meibomian lipids, which are formed by meibocytes within the acini, onto the lid margin [19, 20]. TED may cause eyelid inflammation, disturb the blinking motion, and gradually change the ocular surface environment as it progresses. Therefore, we hypothesized that TED may influence the performance of MGs, similar to many systemic inflammatory diseases, such as Sjögren syndrome, psoriasis, and rosacea [21–24], causing MG dysfunction. The aim of the present preliminarily study was to investigate the performance of MGs in patients with TED.

Methods
Subjects
This study was a prospective case series study, which formed part of an investigation of ocular adnexal microorganisms. All procedures involving human subjects adhered to the Declaration of Helsinki. Institutional Review Board (IRB)/Ethics Committee approval was obtained from the Committee of Medical Ethics and Human Experiments of Chang Gung Memorial Hospital (CGMH), Taiwan. Informed consent was obtained from each subject in the CGMH.

Patients with hyperthyroidism and unilateral or bilateral TED were included. All participants were asked not to instill topical eye drops for 4 h and ointment for 12 h before examination. Subjects with other systemic diseases (e.g., hypertension, diabetes mellitus, connective tissue diseases, etc.), had undergone previous eyelid and

ocular surgeries, or had super-active TED (clinical activity score [CAS] ≥ 4) [25] were excluded from this study. Seventeen age–sex–laterality-matched participants, who visited our clinics and met the same criteria, except for the absence of TED, were enrolled as a control group.

Diagnosis of thyroid eye disease
Diagnosis of TED was made on the basis of 2 of the following 3 criteria [26]. First, at least 1 immune-related thyroid dysfunction (Grave's hyperthyroidism, Hashimoto thyroiditis, circulating thyroid antibody) was present. Second, the imaging study revealed fusiform enlargement of at least 1 of the ocular muscles. Third, patients had at least 1 of the following typical orbital signs: upper eyelid retraction, exophthalmos, typical restrictive strabismus, fluctuating lid edema, or chemosis/caruncular edema [27].

Among the above ocular signs, the extent of exophthalmos was measured using Hertel's exophthalmometer, which measures the distance of the corneal apex from the level of the lateral orbital rim [28]. The amount of incomplete or defective closure of eyelids (lagophthalmos) was measured [29]. The duration of thyroid disease, from the onset of hyperthyroidism to receiving the ocular examination of this study, was recorded.

Classification of patients with thyroid eye disease by clinical activity score
The disease activity in patients with TED was scored according to the CAS clinical criteria proposed by Mourits et al. [25] This score contains 7 items including pain at rest, painful eye movement, red eyelid, red conjunctiva, swelling of the eyelid, chemosis, and swollen caruncle. Each item scores 1 point, so that each eye of a TED patient has a CAS score that can range from 0 to 7. For the purposes of our study, we defined inactive TED as CAS 0–1 and active TED as CAS 2–3 (Fig. 1). Super-active TED patients (CAS score ≥ 4) were excluded from this study, because the patients had unstable ocular conditions and received pulse corticosteroid therapy.

Measurement of blinking rates and eyelid patterns
The blinking motion of the eyelids was recorded and analyzed using a LipiView® II Ocular Surface Interferometer (TearScience, Inc., Morrisville, NC, USA) [30]. Blinks without complete closure were automatically distinguished from those with complete closure by this instrument. The partial blinking rate of each eye, the ratio of incomplete blinks to total blinks within 20 s, was recorded for analysis.

Assessment of amount of tears
Schirmer test 1 (ST-1) was used to evaluate the tear amount of each subject [31]. Without providing topical

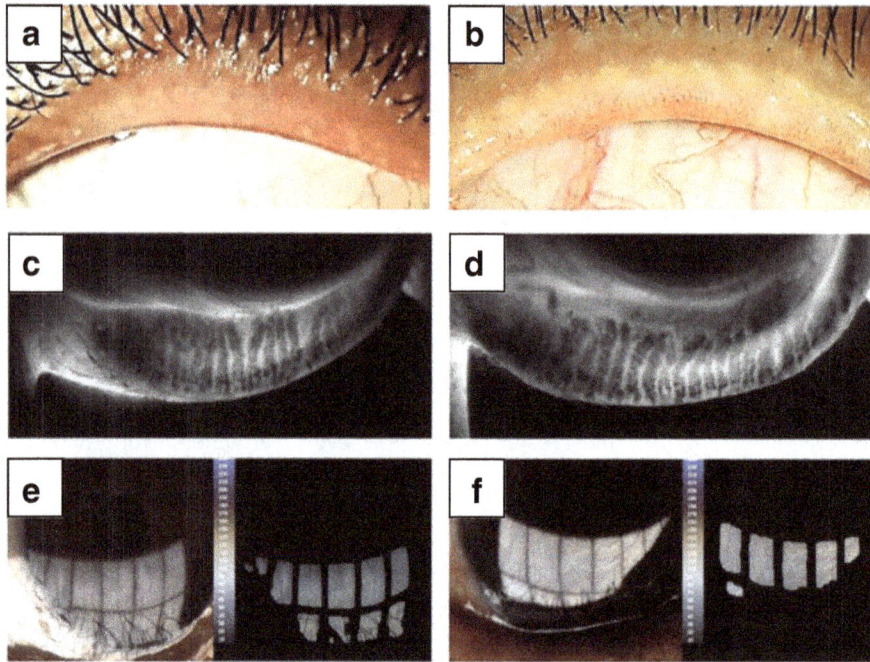

Fig. 1 Representative photos and LipidView® II images of inactive (**a**, **c**, **e**) and active (**b**, **d**, **f**) thyroid eye diseases. **a**, **b** External eye photos of upper lid margins (OS). **a**) A 37-year-old female with inactive thyroid eye disease (CAS 1). Upper lid margin showed no pouting or capping of meibomian gland orifices. Only mild telangiectasia was observed. **b**) A 49-year-old female with active thyroid eye disease (CAS 3). Upper lid margin showed pouting and plugging of meibomian gland orifices. Telangiectasia was also present. **c**, **d** Infrared images of meibomian gland of the left lower lid. **c**) Grade 1 meibomian gland dropout (0–25%). **d**) Grade 2 meibomian gland dropout (25–50%). **e**, **f** Image of lipid layer (OS). **e**) Average lipid layer thickness: 79 nm **f**) Average lipid layer thickness: 100^+ nm

anesthesia, the Schirmer strip was suspended on the inferior eyelid between the inner two-thirds and the outer one-third for 5 min. The length of the wetting part on the test strip was then recorded for each eye.

Standard patient evaluation of eye dryness questionnaire

The Standard Patient Evaluation of Eye Dryness (SPEED) questionnaire [32], designed for assessing the symptoms of dry eye, was used for these subjects. According to the frequency and severity of dry eye symptoms, the SPEED score ranges from 0 to 28, with asymptomatic patients scoring 0 and the most symptomatic patients scoring 28.

Eyelid signs representing meibomian gland dysfunction

Each eye of TED patients was carefully assessed for representative signs of MG dysfunction, including plugging of MG orifices, lid margin irregularities, thickening, vascular engorgement, and mucocutaneous junction shift (Fig. 1a, b) [33, 34]. Eyes with any of the above signs were designated as MG dysfunction sign-positive.

Grading of meibomian gland dropout

The structure of the MGs of each eye was assessed using meibography, a near-infrared (NIR) illumination captured using the LipiView® II Ocular Surface Interferometer (TearScience, Inc., Morrisville, NC). For standardization and minimization of invasiveness, only MGs in the lower eyelid were examined. The severity of MG dropout (MGd) was classified into degree 0 to degree 4 according to the meiboscale proposed by Pult et al. [35], in which the score increases by 1 degree for every 25% of MG loss (Fig. 1c, d).

Determination of meibum quality and meibomian gland expressibility

An MG evaluator (TearScience, Inc.), which can provide a stable pressure mimicking the pressure of the orbicularis oculi muscle on MGs during normal blinking was used to press the central lower eyelid for about 10–15 s for each patient [36]. Then, the meibum quality of each gland was scored from 0 to 3 points (0: clear liquid secretion; 1: cloudy liquid secretion; 2: cloudy particulate fluid; 3: inspissated, similar to toothpaste) [37]. MG expressibility (MGE) for each patient was recorded by counting the expressible glands (glands with scores of 0, 1, or 2) from the 8 glands of the central lower lid. Scores of 0, 1, and 2 indicates that ≥5 glands, 3–4 glands, and 1–2 glands are expressible, respectively; a score of 3 indicates that no gland is expressible. MGs yielding liquid secretion (MGYLS) were also recorded by counting the glands showing liquid secretion (glands with scores 0 or 1). Moreover, a total meibum quality score (TMQS) was defined by summing the scores from the 8 glands in the central lower lid.

Lipid layer thickness of tear film

The lipid layer thickness (LLT) of the tear film of each eye was measured and recorded using a Lipi-View® II Ocular Surface Interferometer (TearScience, Inc.) (Fig. 1e, f) [38]. An average interferometric color unit (ICU) (1 ICU = 1 nm) was used for quantification of LLT. Because the exact value of LLT cannot be estimated precisely or shown by this instrument if the value exceeds 100 nm, we set the LLT to 100 nm in cases where LLT ≥ 100 nm.

Order of testing procedures

First, after each participant had completed the informed consent form, we observed the participant's ocular surface by slit lamp, measuring the extent of exophthalmos and lagophthalmos, and recorded the SPEED questionnaire. Second, the blinking rate and LLT were simultaneously obtained by a LipiView® II Ocular Surface Interferometer, after which the structures of the MGs of the bilateral lower eyelids were sequentially assessed using the same instrument. Third, the Oxford staining score for each eye was recorded. Fourth, after each participant rested for about 30 min, ST-1 was carried out for 5 min. Finally, meibum quality and MG expressibility were determined using the MG evaluator.

Statistical analysis

Statistical analyses were performed in SPSS version 20.0 for Windows (IBM Corp, Armonk, NY). Wilcoxon signed-rank tests and Fisher's exact tests were used to compare the TED patients and non-TED participants. Wilcoxon's rank-sum test was used to compare the differences of parameters between the inactive and active TED groups. Spearman's rank correlation was used to examine the correlation between parameters. P-values < .05 were considered as statistically significant. Using a free power calculator (G*power; http://www.gpower.hhu.de), the sample size of at least 15 eyes was estimated based on the comparison of ST-1 and tear film break-up time between Graves' disease patients and normal subjects according to Bruscolini A et al. [39] under the power of 0.95.

Results

Participants

A total of 17 patients with TED (31 eyes) were collected consecutively from the Oculoplasty Clinic of CGMH between October 2015 and June 2016. Thirty-one age–sex–laterality-matched non-TED eyes were consecutively enrolled for comparison. The clinical profiles of these subjects are summarized in Table 1. When comparing the

TED with the non-TED group, the indices of TED complications, including degrees of exophthalmos and lagophthalmos, were significantly different between the groups. However, there was no statistically significant difference in partial blinking rate, tear volume, or SPEED score. Moreover, among the indices of MG performance, only MG dysfunction signs and MGYLS showed statistically significantly differences between TED and non-TED eyes.

Comparison between active and inactive TED from the indices of TED complications

When we compared the active and inactive TED eyes, the degrees of exophthalmos and lagophthalmos were significantly higher in active TED eyes ($P = .01$ and $P < .001$, respectively), while the partial blinking rate and ST-1 were not statistically significantly different ($P = .83$ and $P = .20$, respectively). Moreover, there was no significant difference in the SPEED score between the active and inactive TED patients ($P = .80$) (Table 2).

MG performance in active and inactive TED eyes

Among the parameters of MG performance, MGd and LLT were statistically significantly different between active and inactive TED eyes. MGd was significantly more severe in active TED eyes than in inactive TED eyes ($P = .03$). However, in conflict with the inference from the MGd result, active TED eyes had significantly thicker LLT than did those with inactive TED ($P = .02$). There were high proportions of TED patients with MG dysfunction signs. All active TED eyes and up to 80% of inactive TED eyes had signs of MG dysfunction, but there was no statistically significant difference between the 2 groups ($P = .27$). Moreover, the 2 groups did not show significant differences in MG expression, including MGE ($P = .15$), MGYLS ($P = .36$), and TMQS ($P = .48$) (Table 2 and Fig. 2).

Correlation between MG performance and TED complications

To investigate the impact of TED activity on MG performance, a correlation analysis between the parameters of MG performance and the indices of TED complications was performed. There was no significant association between MGd and TED complications, including exophthalmos, lagophthalmos, and partial blinking rate (Fig. 3). However, a significantly positive correlation was found between LLT and lagophthalmos ($r = 0.37$, $P = .04$), but no other parameters of TED complications correlated with LLT.

Discussion

The impact of MG dysfunction, the leading cause of DED, on patients with TED, has remained unclear. Interestingly,

Table 1 The clinical characteristics of the study subjects

	TED group (31 eyes of 17 patients)	Non-TED group (31 eyes of 17 controls)	P value[†]
Age (yr)	44.7 ± 11.0	44.7 ± 11.2	0.785
CAS	1.6 ± 0.7	–	–
Disease duration (months)	47.3 ± 63.5	–	–
Exophthalmos (mm)	20.4 ± 4.3	16.5 ± 1.1	< 0.001[*]
Lagophthalmos (mm)	0.9 ± 1.9	0.0 ± 0.0	0.015[*]
Partial blinking rate (%)	58.4 ± 34.7	55.1 ± 34.1	0.702
ST-1 (mm)	12.6 ± 9.0	13.0 ± 10.2	0.885
SPEED (score)	7.4 ± 4.1	6.8 ± 4.7	0.509
MG dysfunction signs[‡] (eyes)	27	1	< 0.001[*]
MGd (score)	2.1 ± 0.9	2.2 ± 0.9	0.555
MGE (score)	0.6 ± 1.1	0.8 ± 0.9	0.379
MGYLS (score)	4.7 ± 3.1	3.0 ± 2.5	0.014[*]
TMQS (score)	10.1 ± 8.0	8.5 ± 4.9	0.412
LLT (nm)	74.1 ± 21.7	72.0 ± 21.9	0.654

†Fisher's exact test was used to test the between-group differences in MG dysfunction signs, while the Wilcoxon signed-rank test was used to test other parameters
(*) Statistically significant (P < 0.05)
‡MG dysfunction signs, signs of meibomian gland (MG) dysfunction, including irregular lid margin, vascular engorgement, plugged meibomian gland orifices, and displacement of mucocutaneous junction
CAS Clinical activity score, ST-1 Schirmer test 1, SPEED Scores of SPEED questionnaire, MGd MG dropout, MGE MG expressibility, MGYLS MG yielding liquid secretion, TMQS Total meibum quality score, LLT Lipid layer thickness

Table 2 Comparison between active and inactive thyroid eye diseases

	Active TED[†] (11 eyes of 6 patients)	Inactive TED[‡] (20 eyes of 11 patients)	P value[§]
Age (yr)	45.2 ± 16.1	44.4 ± 7.3	0.679
Sex (female: male)	7: 4	11: 9	0.718
Disease duration (months)	80.8 ± 96.8	28.9 ± 20.5	0.264
Exophthalmos (mm)	23.1 ± 4.3	18.5 ± 3.3	0.005[*]
Lagophthalmos (mm)	2.13 ± 2.67	0.18 ± 0.59	< 0.001[*]
Partial blinking rate (%)	58.2 ± 29.9	58.5 ± 37.8	0.834
ST-1 (mm)	9.2 ± 5.6	14.5 ± 10.0	0.199
SPEED (score)	7.1 ± 4.6	7.6 ± 3.9	0.803
MG dysfunction signs[#] (no. of eyes; %)	11 (100%)	16 (80%)	0.269
MGd (score)	2.5 ± 0.9	1.8 ± 0.7	0.03[*]
MGE (score)	0.2 ± 0.4	0.9 ± 1.2	0.148
MGYLS (score)	5.4 ± 2.9	4.3 ± 3.1	0.362
TMQS (score)	8.2 ± 5.5	11.2 ± 9.0	0.482
LLT (nm)	86.3 ± 18.0	67.4 ± 21.0	0.024[*]

†,‡Patients with thyroid eye diseases (TED) were classified by the clinical activity score (CAS) as having active TED (CAS 2–3) or inactive TED (CAS 0–1); §Fisher's exact test was used to test the between-group differences in sex and MG dysfunction signs, while Wilcoxon's rank-sum test was used to test other parameters.
(*)Statistically significant (P < 0.05)
#MG dysfunction signs, signs of meibomian gland (MG) dysfunction, including irregular lid margin, vascular engorgement, plugged meibomian gland orifices, and displacement of mucocutaneous junction

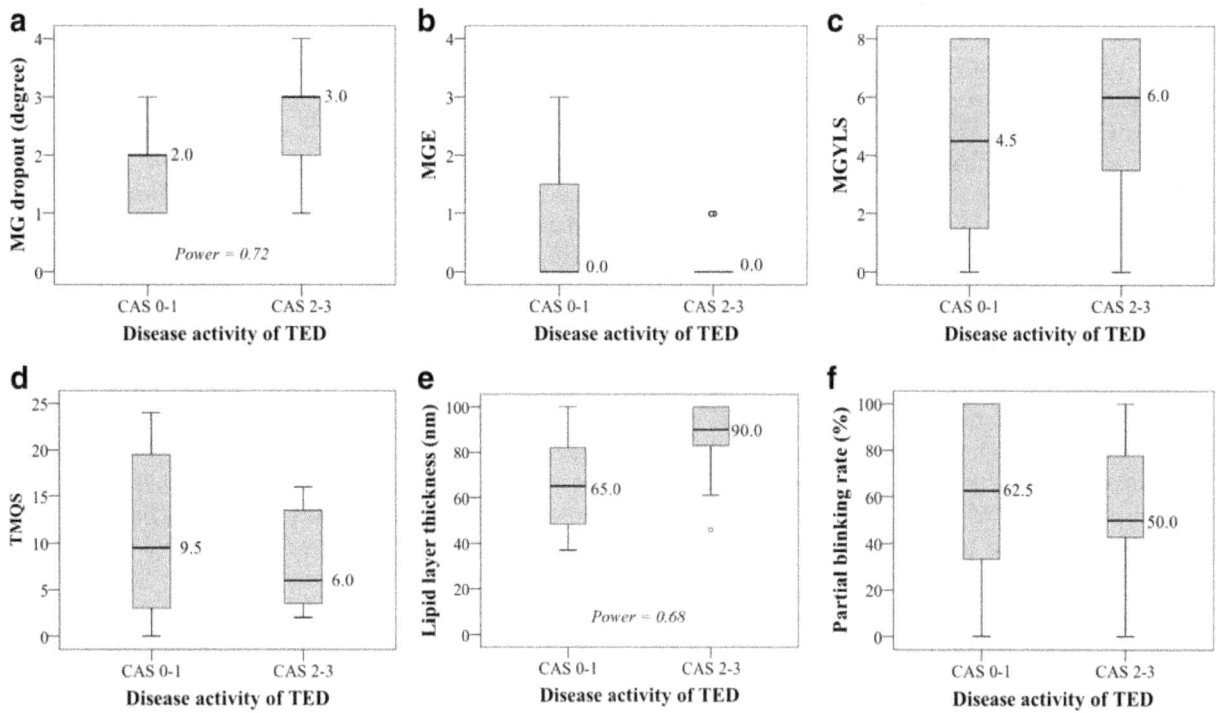

Fig. 2 Comparison between active and inactive thyroid eye diseases (TED) for meibomian gland dropout (MGd), meibomian gland expression, including meibomian gland expressibility (MGE), meibomian gland yielding liquid secretion (MGYLS), and total meibum quality score (TMQS), as well as lipid layer thickness (LLT), and partial blinking rate, by boxplot diagrams. The dot in Fig. 2b shows the 2 outliers of MGE in CAS 2–3. Box, 25th to 75th percentile; bold line in the box, median; bars, minimum and maximum values; dot, outliers

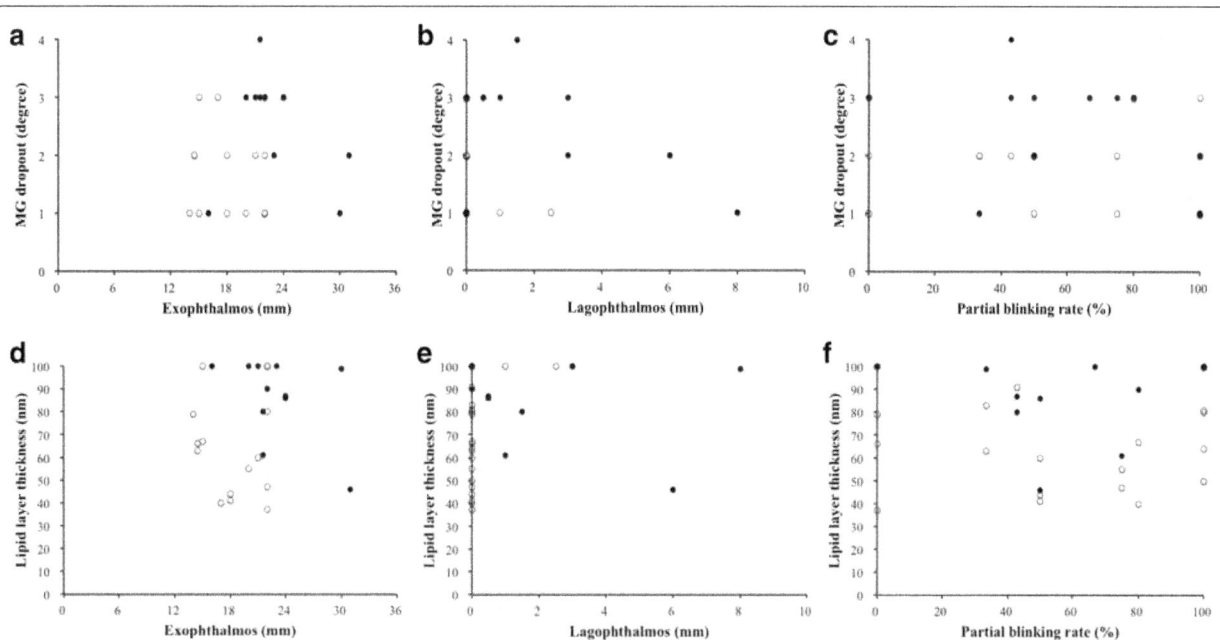

Fig. 3 Correlation between meibomian gland dropout (MGd) and exophthalmos, lagophthalmos, and blinking rate, respectively (**a–c**). Correlation between lipid layer thickness (LLT) and exophthalmos, lagophthalmos, and blinking rate, respectively (**d–f**). (○), inactive TED eye (CAS 0–1); (●), active TED eye (CAS 2–3)

27 eyes (87.1%) had signs of MG dysfunction, but the mean age of these TED patients was only 44.7 years (Table 1). We also found that active TED eyes (CAS 2–3) had a higher MGd, but thicker LLT, than inactive TED eyes (CAS 0–1) (Table 2 and Fig. 2). Although active TED eyes had more severe exophthalmos and lagophthalmos, only lagophthalmos was associated with a thicker LLT (Fig. 3). The finding of a thicker LLT, but higher MGd, in active TED suggests not only compensatory activity from the residual MGs, but also that lagophthalmos-mediated forceful blinking is involved. This could be a potential mechanism for decreasing ocular surface injury from the more severe lagophthalmos in active TED.

Active ocular inflammation may cause typical ocular surface changes in TED in patients with thyroid disease [2]. We hypothesized that active TED would further impede the performance of the MGs in these patients. Although the CAS score proposed by Mourits to reflect the inflammation status of TED ranged from 0 to 7 [25], only patients with a CAS of less than 4 were included in this study. All patients with CAS exceeding 3 received pulse-corticosteroid treatment, and they were excluded from this study to prevent a possible bias due to this treatment. A flair-up of TED may result in greater extraocular muscle enlargement, and this may be reflected in the greater exophthalmos and lagophthalmos of the active TED eyes in this study (Table 2).

In this study, the mean MGd of TED patients was 2.1 (Table 1), representing about 25–50% loss of MGs. Active TED eyes had significantly greater loss of MGs than inactive TED eyes (Table 2). However, loss of MGs was not associated with the target indices of TED complications (Figs. 3a, b, and c). Several studies have shown a strong association between MGd and inflammatory ocular surface diseases. Mathers et al. reported that patients with chronic blepharitis and giant papillary conjunctivitis demonstrated a greater loss of MGs [40, 41]. Shimazaki et al. reported that Sjögren syndrome was associated with MG dysfunction [22]. Knop et al. pointed out that inflammatory mediators could spread and lead to glandular dropout and potentially to acinar atrophy by way of the conjunctiva, through the tarsus and toward the MGs [42]. Thus, TED-associated ocular surface inflammation might cause periglandular inflammation, and subsequent loss of MGs.

A recent study proposed that a thinner LLT may predict a higher risk of MG dysfunction [43]. Eom et al. also found that greater loss of MGs is correlated with a thinner LLT [44]. It is reasonable that a stasis of lipid inside the MGs may increase pressure in the MGs, causing the ducts to dilate, and finally resulting in acinar atrophy [19]. However, in our study, the active TED eyes showed a greater loss of MGs, but thicker LLT, than the inactive TED eyes (Table 2 and Fig. 2). Additionally, we found a positive correlation between lagophthalmos and LLT (Fig. 3), and active TED eyes had greater lagophthalmos than inactive TED eyes (Table 2). Kim et al. reported that some MGs may be obstructive and atrophic, while other MGs may secrete lipids at normal or enhanced levels to compensate for MG dysfunction, whereby normal LLT is maintained [45]. Korb et al. found that forceful blinking could increase the LLT [46]. It is possible that active TED patients had more severe MGd, but thicker LLT, not only as a compensatory effect, but also as a stimulatory effect. The compensatory effect may be induced by MGd, based to some degree on a physiological response from residual MGs, but not on the over-production of lipids. However, patients with more severe lagophthalmos may show more severe punctate erosion on the ocular surface. Additionally, MG disease may increase corneal sensitivity [47]. Therefore, active TED patients with more severe lagophthalmos may have pathological lipid hypersecretion due to forceful blinks. Patients with TED might blink more forcefully, unconsciously, due to greater lagophthalmos. Although the active TED eyes demonstrated more severe MGd, the mixed compensatory and stimulatory effect may cause temporarily thicker LLT than that seen in inactive TED eyes.

In addition, the function of MGs may be maintained at a certain level, because the loss of MGs is partial (on average 25–50%) even in active TED eyes. Active TED eyes had greater exophthalmos than inactive TED eyes (Table 2 and Fig. 2). Exophthalmos could stretch the eyelid, inducing even higher lid tension and making it easier for the lipids in the MGs to be squeezed out. However, there was no significant correlation between exophthalmos and LLT (Fig. 3).

All but 1 of the patients with TED suffered from dry eye symptoms, as identified on the SPEED questionnaire. Despite the lack of statistically significant difference, lower aqueous tear secretion (ST-1) was found in patients with active TED (9.2 ± 5.6) than in patients with inactive TED and in the normal control group (14.5 ± 10.0 and 13.0 ± 10.2, respectively). These findings were compatible with those of Eckstein et al. [10], who concluded that ATD may be caused by diminished lacrimal gland function in active TED. The expression of inactive TED may be the same as proposed by Arita et al. [48], who pointed out that increased tear fluid is produced as a temporary compensatory response to loss of MGs.

There were some limitations in this preliminary study. The non-TED control group may be suitable for comparison with the TED group in our clinical practice, but this control group cannot truly represent a normal population. Some participants in the control group also had dry eye symptoms and inadequate MG performance. Both eyes of bilateral TED patients were pooled with the

3 eyes of the 3 unilateral TED patients. We had found similar results in the analyses of right eyes or left eyes. Although a trend for thicker LLT in active TED was noted, the wide range of standard deviation resulted in a non-significant difference. Thus, we classified both eyes of the same patient into the same CAS group, which might have caused a bias. However, all patients with active TED (CAS 2–3) in our study had ocular signs of similar severity, only 2 patients with inactive TED (CAS 0–1) had single eye involvement. One eye in the active TED group was excluded due to previous eyelid surgery. Furthermore, most patients routinely used eye ointment for lubrication at night. The usage of topical ointment should be more strictly limited to avoid its influence on LLT. The ingredients of an eye ointment might affect the tear film composition, yet all patients had ceased ointment application at least 12 h before examination. Moreover, we set LLT as 100 nm for the 5 eyes with LLT > 100 nm, which may have caused underestimation of the average value of LLT. Because the LipiView® II Ocular Surface Interferometer did not have a sensor to identify the blinking force, we cannot clearly prove the association between LLT and forceful blinks. A further study adopting simultaneous electromyography of the eyelid should be considered to verify this causality. Finally, the small sample size implies that our results should be interpreted with some caution. Subgroup analysis revealed that inactive TED eyes were not significantly different from non-TED eyes in terms of MG performance and LLT, but a trend for greater MGd and thicker LLT was observed between active TED eyes and non-TED eyes. Thus, a small proportion of active TED patients in our subjects might be the reason for the lack of statistically significant differences in many parameters between the TED group and the non-TED group. The performance of MGs in TED patients should be verified in a future study with a larger sample.

Conclusions

In conclusion, the results of this study indicated that patients with active TED had more severe MGd, but thicker LLT. Active TED may cause periglandular inflammation of MGs, leading to MGd, although lagophthalmos might induce a compensatory effect, involving increased lipid secretion from the residual MGs in an attempt to stabilize the tear film.

Abbreviations
ATD: Aqueous tear deficiency; CAS: Clinical activity score; DED: Dry eye disease; EDE: Evaporative dry eye; LLT: Lipid layer thickness; MG: Meibomian gland; MGd: Meibomian gland dropout; MGE: Meibomian gland expressibility; MGYLS: Meibomian gland yielding liquid secretion; SPEED: Standard patient evaluation of eye dryness; ST-1: Schirmer test 1; TED: Thyroid eye disease; TMQS: Total meibum quality score

Acknowledgments
The authors would like to thank all colleagues who contributed to this study. We are grateful to Prof. Sheng-Nan Lu, Prof. Hsueh-Wen Chang, Chih-Yun Lin, Shin-Yi Chien, and the Biostatistics and Bioinformatics Center, Kaohsiung Chang Gung Memorial Hospital for assistance with statistical analyses.

Funding
This work was supported by Chang Gung Research Proposal (CMRPG8C0762), and the Ministry of Science and Technology (Grant No. 104–2314-B-182A-101-MY3). The sponsors or funding organizations had no role in the design or conduct of this research.

Authors' contributions
CYW analyzed and interpreted the data, and was a major contributor in writing the manuscript. RWH designed and conducted the study, and a contributor in writing and reviewing the manuscript. CYW and RWH contributed to this manuscript equally. PCF designed the study and reviewed the manuscript. HJY reviewed the manuscript. CCC analyzed and interpreted the data. CCH reviewed the manuscript. MTK helped RWH to collect the patients' data and reviewed the manuscript. All authors read and approved the final manuscript.

Competing interests
The authors declare that they have no competing interests.

Author details
[1]Department of Ophthalmology, Taipei Tzu Chi Hospital, Buddhist Tzu Chi Medical Foundation, Taipei, Taiwan. [2]Department of Ophthalmology, Kaohsiung Chang Gung Memorial Hospital and Chang Gung University College of Medicine, Kaohsiung, Taiwan. [3]Graduate Institute of Clinical Medicine, College of Medicine, Kaohsiung Medical University, Kaohsiung, Taiwan. [4]Department of Laboratory Medicine, Kaohsiung Chang Gung Memorial Hospital and Chang Gung University College of Medicine, Kaohsiung, Taiwan. [5]Graduate Institute of Clinical Medical Sciences, Chang Gung University, Taoyuan City, Taiwan.

References
1. Bartalena L, Tanda ML. Clinical practice. Graves' ophthalmopathy. N Engl J Med. 2009;360(10):994–1001.
2. Sokol JA, Foulks GN, Haider A, Nunery WR. Ocular surface effects of thyroid disease. Ocul Surf. 2010;8(1):29–39.
3. Bartley GB, Fatourechi V, Kadrmas EF, Jacobsen SJ, Ilstrup DM, Garrity JA, Gorman CA. Clinical features of Graves' ophthalmopathy in an incidence cohort. Am J Ophthalmol. 1996;121(3):284–90.
4. Achtsidis V, Kozanidou E, Bournas P, Tentolouris N, Theodossiadis PG. Dry eye and clinical disease of tear film, diagnosis and management. Eur Ophthalmic Rev. 2014;8(1):17–22.
5. Ismailova DS, Fedorov AA, Grusha YO. Ocular surface changes in thyroid eye disease. Orbit. 2013;32(2):87–90.
6. Coulter I, Frewin S, Krassas GE, Perros P. Psychological implications of Graves' orbitopathy. Eur J Endocrinol. 2007;157(2):127–31.

7.   Gilbard JP, Farris RL. Ocular surface drying and tear film osmolarity in thyroid eye disease. Acta Ophthalmol. 1983;61(1):108–16.

8.   Cruz AA, Ribeiro SF, Garcia DM, Akaishi PM, Pinto CT. Graves upper eyelid retraction. Surv Ophthalmol. 2013;58(1):63–76.

9.   Schiffman RM, Christianson MD, Jacobsen G, Hirsch JD, Reis BL. Reliability and validity of the ocular surface disease index. Arch Ophthalmol. 2000; 118(5):615–21.

10. Eckstein AK, Finkenrath A, Heiligenhaus A, Renzing-Kohler K, Esser J, Kruger C, Quadbeck B, Steuhl KP, Gieseler RK. Dry eye syndrome in thyroid-associated ophthalmopathy: lacrimal expression of TSH receptor suggests involvement of TSHR-specific autoantibodies. Acta Ophthalmol Scand. 2004; 82(3 Pt 1):291–7.

11. Chang TC, Huang KM, Chang TJ, Lin SL. Correlation of orbital computed tomography and antibodies in patients with hyperthyroid Graves' disease. Clin Endocrinol. 1990;32(5):551–8.

12. Gupta A, Sadeghi PB, Akpek EK. Occult thyroid eye disease in patients presenting with dry eye symptoms. Am J Ophthalmol. 2009;147(5):919–23.

13. Viso E, Gude F, Rodriguez-Ares MT. The association of meibomian gland dysfunction and other common ocular diseases with dry eye: a population-based study in Spain. Cornea. 2011;30(1):1–6.

14. Tong L, Chaurasia SS, Mehta JS, Beuerman RW. Screening for meibomian gland disease: its relation to dry eye subtypes and symptoms in a tertiary referral clinic in Singapore. Invest Ophthalmol Vis Sci. 2010;51(7):3449–54.

15. Lemp MA. Report of the National eye Institute/Industry workshop on clinical trials in dry eyes. CLAO J. 1995;21(4):221–32.

16. Lemp MA: **The 1998** Castroviejo lecture. New strategies in the treatment of dry-eye states. Cornea 1999, 18(6):625–632.

17. Bron AJ, Tiffany JM. The contribution of meibomian disease to dry eye. Ocul Surf. 2004;2(2):149–65.

18. Bron AJ, Tiffany JM, Gouveia SM, Yokoi N, Voon LW. Functional aspects of the tear film lipid layer. Exp Eye Res. 2004;78(3):347–60.

19. Knop E, Knop N, Millar T, Obata H, Sullivan DA. The international workshop on meibomian gland dysfunction: report of the subcommittee on anatomy, physiology, and pathophysiology of the meibomian gland. Invest Ophthalmol Vis Sci. 2011;52(4):1938–78.

20. Knop N, Knop E. Meibomian glands. Part I: anatomy, embryology and histology of the Meibomian glands. Ophthalmologe. 2009;106(10):872–83.

21. Schaumberg DA, Nichols JJ, Papas EB, Tong L, Uchino M, Nichols KK. The international workshop on meibomian gland dysfunction: report of the subcommittee on the epidemiology of, and associated risk factors for, MGD. Invest Ophthalmol Vis Sci. 2011;52(4):1994–2005.

22. Shimazaki J, Goto E, Ono M, Shimmura S, Tsubota K. Meibomian gland dysfunction in patients with Sjogren syndrome. Ophthalmology. 1998; 105(8):1485–8.

23. Horwath-Winter J, Flogel I, Ramschak-Schwarzer S, Hofer A, Kroisel PM. Psoriasis and hypogonadism in chronic blepharokeratoconjunctivitis. A case report. Ophthalmologe. 2002;99(5):380–3.

24. Alvarenga LS, Mannis MJ. Ocular rosacea. Ocul Surf. 2005;3(1):41–58.

25. Mourits MP, Koornneef L, Wiersinga WM, Prummel MF, Berghout A, van der Gaag R. Clinical criteria for the assessment of disease activity in Graves' ophthalmopathy: a novel approach. Br J Ophthalmol. 1989;73(8):639–44.

26. Bartley GB, Gorman CA. Diagnostic criteria for Graves' ophthalmopathy. Am J Ophthalmol. 1995;119(6):792–5.

27. Bahn RS. Graves' Ophthalmopathy. N Engl J Med. 2010;362(8):726–38.

28. Onofrey BE, Skorin L, Holdeman NR. Ocular therapeutics handbook : a clinical manual. 3rd ed. Philadelphia: Wolters Kluwer/Lippincott Williams & Wilkins; 2012. p. 71–72

29. Pereira MV, Gloria AL. Lagophthalmos. Semin Ophthalmol. 2010;25(3):72–8.

30. Satjawatcharaphong P, Ge S, Lin MC. Clinical outcomes associated with thermal pulsation system treatment. Optom Vis Sci. 2015;92(9):e334–41.

31. American Academy of Ophthalmology. BCSC section 8. External disease and cornea. Sutphin JE ed. San Francisco: American Academy of Ophthalmology; 2009–2010. p. 62.

32. Ngo W, Situ P, Keir N, Korb D, Blackie C, Simpson T. Psychometric properties and validation of the standard patient evaluation of eye dryness questionnaire. Cornea. 2013;32(9):1204–10.

33. Driver PJ, Lemp MA. Meibomian gland dysfunction. Surv Ophthalmol. 1996; 40(5):343–67.

34. Bron AJ, Benjamin L, Snibson GR. Meibomian gland disease. Classification and grading of lid changes. Eye (Lond). 1991;5(Pt 4):395–411.

35. Pult H, Riede-Pult B. Comparison of subjective grading and objective assessment in meibography. Cont Lens Anterior Eye. 36(1):22–7.

36. Korb DR, Blackie CA. Meibomian gland diagnostic expressibility: correlation with dry eye symptoms and gland location. Cornea. 2008;27(10):1142–7.

37. Tomlinson A, Bron AJ, Korb DR, Amano S, Paugh JR, Pearce EI, Yee R, Yokoi N, Arita R, Dogru M. The international workshop on meibomian gland dysfunction: report of the diagnosis subcommittee. Invest Ophthalmol Vis Sci. 2011;52(4):2006–49.

38. Zhao Y, Tan CL, Tong L. Intra-observer and inter-observer repeatability of ocular surface interferometer in measuring lipid layer thickness. BMC Ophthalmol. 2015;15:53.

39. Bruscolini A, Abbouda A, Locuratolo N, Restivo L, Trimboli P, Romanelli F. Dry eye syndrome in non-exophthalmic Graves' disease. Semin Ophthalmol. 2015;30(5–6):372–6.

40. Mathers WD, Shields WJ, Sachdev MS, Petroll WM, Jester JV. Meibomian gland dysfunction in chronic blepharitis. Cornea. 1991;10(4):277–85.

41. Mathers WD, Billborough M. Meibomian gland function and giant papillary conjunctivitis. Am J Ophthalmol. 1992;114(2):188–92.

42. Knop E, Knop N. Meibomian glands : part IV. Functional interactions in the pathogenesis of meibomian gland dysfunction (MGD). Ophthalmologe. 2009;106(11):980–7.

43. Finis D, Pischel N, Schrader S, Geerling G. Evaluation of lipid layer thickness measurement of the tear film as a diagnostic tool for Meibomian gland dysfunction. Cornea. 2013;32(12):1549–53.

44. Eom Y, Lee JS, Kang SY, Kim HM, Song JS. Correlation between quantitative measurements of tear film lipid layer thickness and meibomian gland loss in patients with obstructive meibomian gland dysfunction and normal controls. Am J Ophthalmol. 2013;155(6):1104–10.

45. Kim HM, Eom Y, Song JS: The relationship between morphology and function of the meibomian glands. *Eye Contact Lens* 2016 [PMID: 27755288; Epub ahead of print].

46. Korb DR, Baron DF, Herman JP, Finnemore VM, Exford JM, Hermosa JL, Leahy CD, Glonek T, Greiner JV. Tear film lipid layer thickness as a function of blinking. Cornea. 1994;13(4):354–9.

47. Rahman EZ, Lam PK, Chu CK, Moore Q, Pflugfelder SC. Corneal sensitivity in tear dysfunction and its correlation with clinical parameters and blink rate. Am J Ophthalmol. 2015;160(5):858–66.

48. Arita R, Morishige N, Koh S, Shirakawa R, Kawashima M, Sakimoto T, Suzuki T, Tsubota K. Increased tear fluid production as a compensatory response to meibomian gland loss: a multicenter cross-sectional study. Ophthalmology. 2015;122(5):925–33.

Microbial keratitis-induced endophthalmitis: incidence, symptoms, therapy, visual prognosis and outcomes

Daniel Zapp [1†], Daria Loos[1], Nikolaus Feucht[1], Ramin Khoramnia[2], Tamer Tandogan[2], Lukas Reznicek[1] and Christian Mayer[1*†]

Abstract

Background: To evaluate symptoms, therapies and outcomes in rare microbial keratitis-induced endophthalmitis.

Methods: Retrospective study with 11 patients treated between 2009 and 2014. Clinical findings, corneal diseases, history of steroids and trauma, use of contact lenses, number and type of surgical interventions, determination of causative organisms and visual acuity (VA) were evaluated.

Results: The incidence of transformation from microbial keratitis to an endophthalmitis was 0.29% ($n = 11/3773$). In 90.9% ($n = 10/11$), there were pre-existent eyelid and corneal problems, in 45.5% ($n = 5/11$) rubeosis iridis with increased intraocular pressure and corneal decompensation, and in 18.2% ($n = 2/11$), ocular trauma. Specimens could be obtained in 10 of 11 samples: 33.3% of those 10 specimens were Gram-positive coagulase-negative Staphylococci ($n = 3/10$) or Gram-negative rods ($n = 3/10$) and 10.0% *Staphylococcus aureus* ($n = 1/10$). In 30% ($n = 3/10$), no pathogens were identifiable. 72.7% ($n = 8/11$) of all keratitis-induced endophthalmitis were treated with vitrectomy and 9.1% ($n = 1/11$) with amniotic-membrane transplantation. In 27.3% ($n = 3/11$) the infected eye had to be enucleated – 18.2% ($n = 2/11$) primarily, 9.1% ($n = 1/11$) secondarily. No patient suffered from sympathetic ophthalmia. The median initial VA was 2.1 logMAR ($n = 11/11$). At one month, median VA was 2.0 logMAR ($n = 7/11$), after three months 2.0 logMAR ($n = 6/11$), and after one year 2.05 logMAR ($n = 6/11$). The change in VA was not significant ($p > 0.99$). 36.4% ($n = 4/11$) of the cases resulted in blindness.

Conclusions: The overall outcome is poor. Enucleation should be weighed against the risk of local and systemic spread of the infection, prolonged rehabilitation and sympathetic ophthalmia.

Keywords: Endophthalmitis, Keratitis, Enucleation, Infection, Corneal ulcer

Background

Infectious endophthalmitis is a rare and severe inflammation of the intraocular tissues and fluids of the eye, involving the anterior and posterior eye segment and the adjacent sclera [1, 2]. Endophthalmitis of either form, exogenous or endogenous, can lead to a significant reduction of visual acuity and, at worst, result in a loss of the affected eye [3]. Exogenous endophthalmitis is caused by microbial pathogens that enter the eye after surgery or trauma, or infiltrate through the surface. Microbial keratitis-induced endophthalmitis is a sight-threatening disease, often bearing the worst possible visual outcome [4].

Microbial keratitis-induced endophthalmitis is uncommon (0.5% [5] to 6.1% [3, 6–9]), especially in an otherwise healthy eye [5, 8]. Different treatment options in severe keratitis exist, such as fortified local and/or systemic antibiotics, crosslinking and keratoplasty à chaud in contrast to intravitreal or vitrectomy in microbial keratitis-induced endophthalmitis. Literature shows a wide spread in prevalence rates, most probably due to the lack of a common definition of microbial keratitis cases, let alone microbial keratitis-induced endophthalmitis. Inconsistencies in

* Correspondence: Christian.mayer@mri.tum.de

†Equal contributors

[1]Department of Ophthalmology, Klinikum rechts der Isar, Technical University of Munich, Ismaninger Str. 22, 81675 Munich, Germany

Full list of author information is available at the end of the article

routinely taking swabs in cases of initially mild keratitis that later develop into endophthalmitis might further cloud a correct estimation of microbial association and detection rates.

In the majority of cases, endophthalmitis is diagnosed clinically, [7, 10] with typical symptoms of loss of vision, photophobia and pain (Fig. 1).

Clinical signs consist of conjunctival injection as well as infiltrates, oedema, opacities and endothelium precipitates on the cornea. Moreover, it might be possible to detect anterior chamber flare, cells, fibrin or hypopyon, altered pupil, vitreous infiltrates, periphlebitis, retinal haemorrhages, Roth's spots or reduced or even loss of fundus visualization [2, 11, 12]. Ultrasound can be of substantial aid in cases with reduced posterior visualization; however, it might also be misleading at times and its limited local availability should not lead to a delay in starting the treatment if sufficient clinical suspicion is raised. This is supported by the fact that the most common form of uncomplicated microbial keratitis holds a rather good prognosis when treated correctly and in a timely manner, contrary to endophthalmitis with a severely reduced visual prognosis of light-perception or worse [13, 14].

Pre-existing dry eye disease, blepharo-conjunctivitis, corneal perforation, recent trauma or surgery, immuno-suppression and local or systemic steroid therapy have all been identified as risk factors of progression to endophthalmitis in initially corneal infections [3, 5].

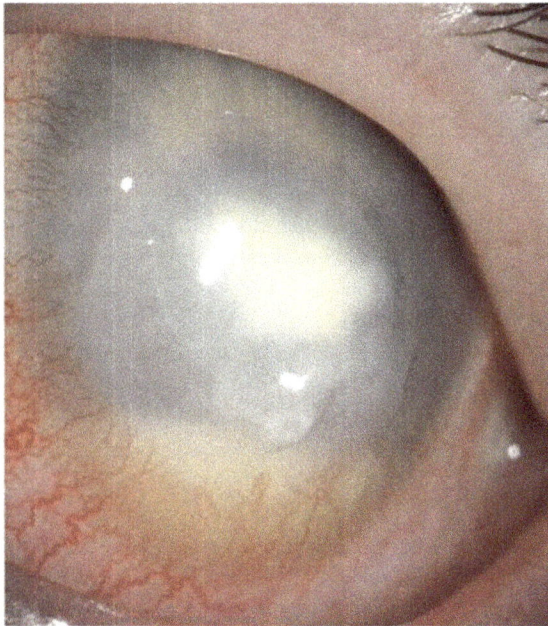

Fig. 1 Clinical image of microbial keratitis-induced endophthalmitis. The diagnosis is determined by clinical findings: visual acuity decrease, pain, hypopyon and vitreous body infiltration

Common forms of treatment include anti-inflammatory and antibiotic drugs, corneal scraping and vitrectomy [15, 16]. During surgery, samples may be taken for a microbiological or virological analysis followed by intravitreal antibiotic treatment.

The goal of this retrospective analysis was to evaluate symptoms, therapies and outcomes in rare but sight- and eye-threatening microbial keratitis-induced endophthalmitis in our department of ophthalmology.

Methods

In a retrospective analysis, all patients treated with endophthalmitis between December 2006 and December 2011 in the Department of Ophthalmology, Klinikum rechts der Isar, Technical University of Munich, Germany, were identified using the computer software program clinical information system I.S.H. med* (SAP* SE, Walldorf, Germany). From this collective, all cases of microbial keratitis-induced endophthalmitis were extracted, pseudonymized and included in this study. None of these patients had relevant ophthalmic preconditions to be excluded from the study. The following patient data was identified: age, gender, localisation, clinical findings and subjective symptoms, surgeries, trauma, prediagnosed corneal and eyelid diseases, history of steroids, previous history of trauma, and use of contact lenses. The study was conducted in accordance with the tenets of the Declaration of Helsinki and approved by the internal Institutional Review Board of Klinikum rechts der Isar, Technical University of Munich.

For all patients, the time interval between the onset of symptoms and diagnosis was analysed. In all cases, ultrasound examination was performed to confirm the clinical diagnosis of endophthalmitis. Corneal swabs were taken in all cases with diagnosed endophthalmitis upon intial presentation and directly processed by the on-site Microbiological Department by specimen cultivation. Broad-spectrum antibiotics were initiated according to the Magdeburg treatment regimen: [17] vancomycin (1 g bid intravenously) and ceftazidime (2 g tid intravenously) were administered to cover Gram-positive pathogens and Gram-negative pathogens respectively. Systemic steroids (prednisolone, 1-2 mg/kg) were added to the therapy one day after starting the antibiotic therapy to limit further tissue destruction by antigens and cytokines released from infiltrating leukocytes [2, 17]. Intensive topical moxifloxacin and a fixed combination of poly-myxin B, neomycin and gramicidin eye drops were administered initially ¼ to ½ hourly and tapered to hourly by day 2. Antibiotic therapy was adjusted after receiving the appropriate antibiogram [6].

Anterior chamber and vitreous sample aspiration were performed in eyes with increasing hypopyon and affected vitreous shown in ultrasound examination.

Following removal of the vitreous including gathering of microbial samples, an intravitreal and intracameral therapy with vancomycin (0.05 ml: 20 mg/ml) and ceftazidime (0.1 ml; 2.25 mg/ml) were applied. Postoperatively, subconjunctival and topical broad-spectrum antibiotics (gentamycin 40 mg/1 ml) and steroids (dexamethasone 4 mg/ml) were administered [17].

Amniotic membrane transplants were performed in cases of severe surface defects. Primary enucleation was only performed in cases of painful amaurosis with no light perception.

Best-corrected visual acuity (BCVA) was assessed on initial presentation (day 0), after one month (1 m), three months (3 m) and after one year (1y). Complications defined as retinal detachment, recurrence of infection, lack of improvement, enucleation and blindness were evaluated for a one-year follow-up time period.

A statistical comparison depending on the aetiology of keratitis-induced endophthalmitis (Kruskal-Wallis test), the clinical findings (Mann-Whitney U test) and the form of therapy (Kruskal-Wallis test) was performed. A p-value of < 0.05 was considered statistically significant.

Results

Altogether, 152 eyes of 149 individuals presented with endophthalmitis to the Department of Ophthalmology, Technical University of Munich, Germany between December 2006 and December 2011. In 74.3% ($n = 113/152$) of our cases, endophthalmitis originated from previous surgery, 5.3% ($n = 8/152$) had a history of recent trauma and in 13.2% ($n = 20/152$) an endogenous endophthalmitis was diagnosed. In 7.2% ($n = 11/152$), the endophthalmitis developed from an initial microbial keratitis (Fig. 2).

In that same time period, overall 3773 patients were recorded with diagnosed microbial keratitis who were treated at least with topical antibiotics. The transformation rate from microbial keratitis to an endophthalmitis in our collective was 0.29% ($n = 11/3773$).

In 90.9% ($n = 10/11$) of patients with keratitis-induced endophthalmitis, a pre-existence of eyelid and corneal problems was observed. Overall, 63.6% ($n = 7/11$) had a history of topical or systemic steroid therapy. Rubeosis iridis was present in 45.5% ($n = 5/11$), along with increased intraocular pressure (IOP) and corneal decompensation. In all of these cases, the IOP decompensation was caused by either retinal vein occlusion or diabetic retinopathy. In 18.2% ($n = 2/11$) of the microbial-induced endophthalmitis cases, patients had a history of a recent corneal trauma. None of the patients were contact-lens wearers.

The mean age of all patients with keratitis-induced endophthalmitis was 67 years (range 32-89), while the mean age of all patients with endophthalmitis was 70 years (range 17-89). About half of all patients with keratitis-induced endophthalmitis (45.5%, $n = 5/11$) were female. The right eye was affected more frequently (63.6%, $n = 7/11$) than the left. The timespan from first onset of patient reported complaints to diagnosis was four days (range 1-360 days). The patient with almost one year time to diagnosis had fluctuations in the severity of his symptoms and inflammation and was externally treated with antibiotics of varying extent and route before final exacerbation led to admission. All patients ($n = 11/11$) presented with a clinically "red eye", a reduction in visual acuity was initially present in 36.4% ($n = 4/11$). Pain was reported in 72.7% ($n = 8/11$), and a hypopyon could be detected in 90.9% (10/11). The fundus red reflex was lost in all cases ($n = 11/11$).

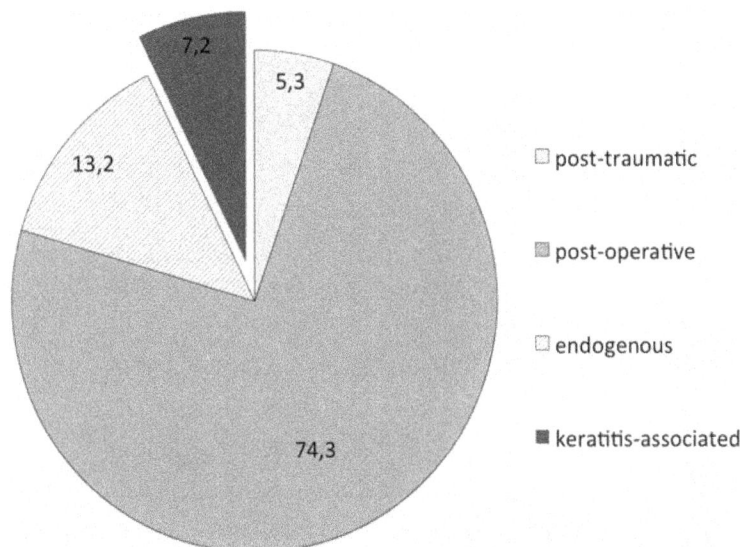

Fig. 2 Prevalence of microbial keratitis-induced endophthalmitis in comparison to all triggers of endophthalmitis (in %)

Microbiological samples could be obtained in 90.0% (n = 10/11) for causative organisms. Of those, 33.3% were Gram-positive coagulase-negative Staphylococci (n = 3/10) or Gram-negative rods (n = 3/10) respectively and 10.0% *Staphylococcus aureus* (n = 1/10). In 30% (n = 3/10), no pathogens were identifiable (Fig. 3).

Vitrectomy was performed in 72.7% (n = 8/11), primary enucleation in 18.2% (n = 2/11) and amniotic membrane transplantation in 9.1% (n = 1/11) of all keratitis-induced endophthalmitis cases.

The median initial BCVA was 2.1 logMAR (n = 11/11; range 2.0-2.2). At one month, the median BCVA was 2.0 logMAR (n = 7/11; range 2.0-2.2), after three months 2.0 logMAR (n = 6/11; range 2.0-2.2) and after one year 2.05 logMAR (n = 6/11; range 1.4-2.2). The change in BCVA from baseline was not significant over time (p > 0.99) (Fig. 4).

Overall, 90.9% (n = 10/11) of all patients in the keratitis-induced endophthalmitis group became legally blind in the affected eye and 36.4% (n = 4/11) resulted in amaurosis with no light perception.

The mean change in BCVA in the keratitis-induced endophthalmitis collective was − 0.1 logMAR, whereas the BCVA in the other endophthalmitis aetiologies were: − 0.6 logMAR in the post-operative, − 0.3 logMAR in the traumatic and ± 0 logMAR in the endogenous subgroup (p = 0.052; Fig. 5).

During the one-year follow-up, we did not observe any occurrences of retinal detachment. One patient (9.1%, n = 1/11) experienced a recurrence of endophthalmitis. Overall, 27.3% (n = 3/11) ended up in an enucleation (two of them were primary enucleations). No patient suffered from sympathetic ophthalmia. One patient died during the follow-up period from chronic cardiovascular disease, whereby a connection to keratitis-induced endophthalmitis remained unlikely.

Discussion

In our examined study population, patients suffering from microbial keratitis-induced endophthalmitis originating from initial lesions of the corneal surface constituted the third largest group of all endophthalmitis aetiologies. Accounting for 7.2% of all cases of endophthalmitis at our clinic, this group was substantial in comparison to published data [3, 7]. This may be partially due to the general focus of our clinic on the anterior segment as well as the fact that in the urban area of our university clinic setting, a high density of posterior segment surgeons are commonly available. Therefore, in our study the postoperative endophthalmitis group might have been underrepresented.

In a healthy eye, eyelid, tear-film, epithelium, stroma and an intact descemet membrane offer protection against intraocular infections. In our study population of keratitis-induced endophthalmitis, 18.2% of patients had a positive history of recent corneal surface trauma; chronic inflammatory eyelid or corneal alterations were pre-existent in 90.9% of the group. It would have been interesting to compare those patients to matching control groups with same pre-existing risk factors but no initial keratitis. However, an external infection progressing to endophthalmitis by bypassing the cornea would be is an even rarer disease aside from special anatomical exceptions like e.g. glaucoma tubes or severe scleritis.

We found a progress rate from microbial keratitis to an endophthalmitis in 0.29%. A review of currently available literature illustrates that, in general, 0.5% [5] up to 6.1% [9] of corneal ulcers seem to progress and end up in endophthalmitis.

In about 80% of these cases, local or systemic steroids had previously been used, posing a well-known risk factor for keratitis-induced endophthalmitis [5]. On the other hand, the Steroids for Corneal Ulcers Trial

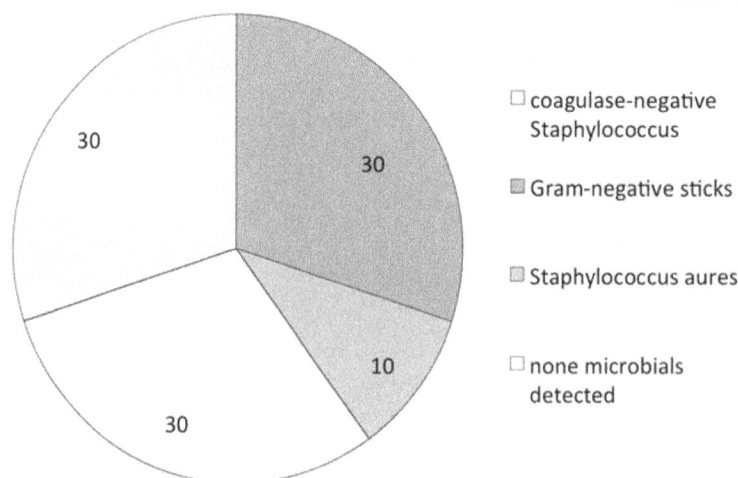

Fig. 3 Microbial detection in microbial keratitis-induced endophthalmitis (percentage and number). Seven of 11 specimens revealed microbials

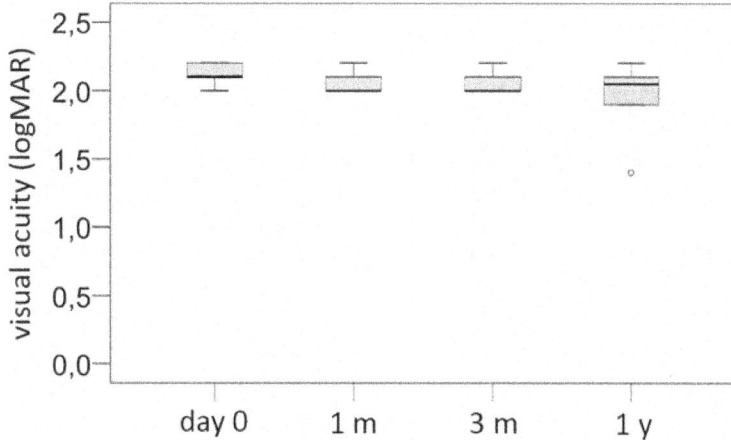

Fig. 4 Development of visual acuity (logMAR) in microbial keratitis-induced endophthalmitis: Day 0 = initial presentation, 1 m = 1 month, 3 m = 3 months, 1y = 1 year: at no time was there a statistically significant improvement in visual acuity (all $p > 0.05$ respectively)

(SCUT), a double-masked placebo controlled random-ized study, raised no safety concerns in its 500 cases of keratitis treated with or without topical steroids. None of the patients progressed to endophthalmitis proving the potential benefit of steroids under appropriate use and antibiotic coverage [18].

Immune dysfunction, fungal keratitis, keratitis next to a recent surgical wound and corneal penetration are also considered as potentially predisposing factors [5, 8]. Since none of these entities occurred in our study group, these risk factors could not be verified in our study. However, 45% of the patients had rubeosis iridis with secondary angle closure glaucoma causing corneal decompensation. Another study confirmed our findings and also reported a strong association of glaucoma and corneal oedema with secondary corneal ulcers in their patients [19]. Patho-physiologically, one might argue that elevated intraocular pressure levels and induced damage to the corneal

endothelial cells [20] lead to decompensation and second-ary oedema [21]. By decompensation and swelling of the cornea, tight junctions and microbiological barriers break down, allowing the keratitis to spread more easily and progress to a keratitis-induced endophthalmitis faster than in an uncompromised cornea.

In keratitis-induced endophthalmitis, the latency to definitive diagnosis can be expected to be higher than in other endophthalmitis entities [11]. This might be due to pre-existing minor visual loss and unremarkable pain caused by often associated chronic eyelid and corneal diseases. Therefore, patients are mostly accustomed to both to some extent, leading to a deferred consultation of an ophthalmologist.

On the other hand, keratitis-induced endophthalmitis could be rather difficult to diagnose: the frequent loss of the red-reflex may be related to intraocular inflamma-tion itself, but could also result from the underlying

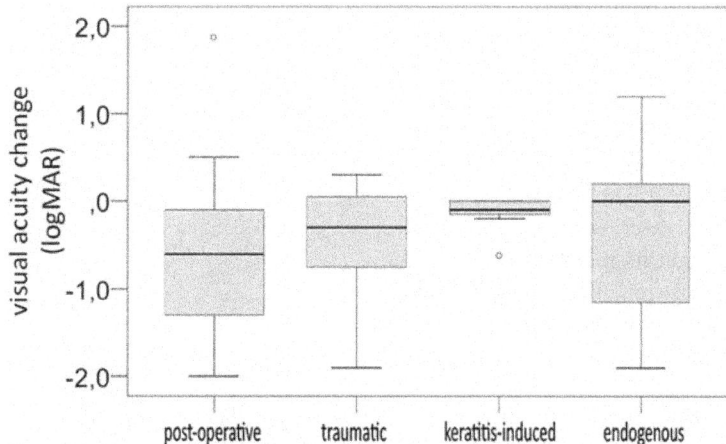

Fig. 5 Visual acuity change in logMAR in the four different endophthalmitis aetiologies: post-operative, traumatic, microbial keratitis-induced and endogenous

corneal diseases and the frequent incidence of a hypopyon since both factors reduce general insight into the eye.

The spectrum of causative organisms included Gram-positive coagulase-negative Staphylococci (30%) and Gram-negative rods (30%). Other studies also found fungi as frequent pathogens in keratitis-induced endophthalmitis [5, 8].

However, it remains unclear up to date whether the final outcome is more determined by the patient's comorbidities or the causative organisms. Fungi appear to show higher rates of progression to endophthalmitis and their prognosis is among the worst. Difficulties in cultivation, treatment availability and their ability to penetrate otherwise intact corneas potentially contribute to this [22]. In our study, we were unable to support these findings since we had no cases of proven fungal keratitis.

Patients with keratitis-induced endophthalmitis initially achieved a median visual acuity of 2.1 logMAR, which hardly improved to 2.05 logMAR within the first year. They therefore presented with a very poor visual outcome and prognosis. BCVA showed no significant changes at any of the follow-up intervals (all $p > 0.05$, median difference -0.1 logMAR). In 27.3% of our keratitis-induced endophthalmitis cases, the infected eye had to be primarily or secondarily enucleated. Other studies also show the typically reduced prognosis in keratitis-induced endophthalmitis, [5, 8] with high rates of enucleation or evisceration [19, 23, 24]. Predisposing chronic corneal pathology or advanced secondary glaucoma with further reduced prognosis and treatment success rates may be at least partially responsible for this association. In respect to this extremely low visual prognosis, a primary enucleation or evisceration especially in devastating cases with pre-existing ocular pathologies must be considered a valid option since it has been shown that the risk of sympathetic ophthalmia is increased in keratitis-induced endophthamitis [25].

Therefore, keratitis-induced endophthalmitis represents one of the severest ophthalmic entities. It often results in poor visual outcomes despite extensive treatment. While most cases of keratitis-induced endophthalmitis entail a positive history of predisposing ophthalmic risk factors, the range of established risk factors or comorbidities differs from the cases with keratitis alone [24]. Since severe isolated keratitis mostly presents with similar clinical features, at least initially, distinguishing it from the visually far more endangering posterior endophthalmitic form can be crucial if only to preserve the eye as such.

Conclusions

Microbial induced keratitis is a rare disease with variable presentation and course. Only 0,29% of initial keratitis

cases progressed to endophthalmitis. The overall outcome of microbial keratitis-induced endophthalmitis is very poor, including high rates of enucleation and evisceration. The decision for enucleation or evisceration should be considered carefully in order not to endanger patients' health by risk of systemic and local spread infection, prolonged rehabilitation and danger of sympathetic ophthalmia.

Abbreviations
BCVA: Best-corrected visual acuity; bid: Twice a day; IOP: Intraocular pressure; logMAR: Logarithm of the Minimum Angle of Resolution; m: Month; tid: Three times daily; y: Year

Authors' contributions
DZ and CM designed, set up and supervised the study. DL, LR and NF gathered the data and, when necessary, contacted the patients. DZ and CM drafted and revised the manuscript. RK and TT conducted the statistical analysis and provided critical input for the final version of the manuscript. All authors have read and approved the final version of the manuscript.

Competing interests
The authors declare that they have no competing interests.

Author details
[1]Department of Ophthalmology, Klinikum rechts der Isar, Technical University of Munich, Ismaninger Str. 22, 81675 Munich, Germany. [2]Department of Ophthalmology, University of Heidelberg, Heidelberg, Germany.

References
1. Forster RK, Zachary IG, Cottingham AJ Jr, Norton EW. Further observations on the diagnosis cause, and treatment of endophthalmitis. Am J Ophthalmol. 1976;81(1):52–6.
2. Meier P, Wiedemann P. Endophthalmitis–clinical picture, therapy and prevention. Klinische Monatsblatter fur Augenheilkunde. 1997;210(4):175–91.
3. Shrader SK, Band JD, Lauter CB, Murphy P. The clinical spectrum of endophthalmitis: incidence, predisposing factors, and features influencing outcome. J Infect Dis. 1990;162(1):115–20.
4. Otri AM, Fares U, Al-Aqaba MA, Miri A, Faraj LA, Said DG, Maharajan S, Dua HS. Profile of sight-threatening infectious keratitis: a prospective study. Acta Ophthalmol. 2013;91(7):643–51.
5. Henry CR, Flynn HW Jr, Miller D, Forster RK, Alfonso EC. Infectious keratitis progressing to endophthalmitis: a 15-year study of microbiology, associated factors, and clinical outcomes. Ophthalmology. 2012;119(12):2443–9.
6. Callegan MC, Engelbert M, Parke DW 2nd, Jett BD, Gilmore MS. Bacterial endophthalmitis: epidemiology, therapeutics, and bacterium-host interactions. Clin Microbiol Rev. 2002;15(1):111–24.
7. Essex RW, Yi Q, Charles PG, Allen PJ. Post-traumatic endophthalmitis. Ophthalmology. 2004;111(11):2015–22.
8. Scott IU, Flynn HW Jr, Feuer W, Pflugfelder SC, Alfonso EC, Forster RK, Miller D. Endophthalmitis associated with microbial keratitis. Ophthalmology. 1996;103(11):1864–70.

9. Ormerod LD. Causes and management of bacterial keratitis in the elderly. Can J Ophthalmol. 1989;24(3):112–6.
10. Kernt M, Kampik A. Endophthalmitis: pathogenesis, clinical presentation, management, and perspectives. Clin Ophthalmol. 2010;4:121–35.
11. Luther TT, Bartz-Schmidt KU. Endophthalmitis. Der Ophthalmologe : Zeitschrift der Deutschen Ophthalmologischen Gesellschaft. 1999;96(11):758–71.
12. Keynan Y, Finkelman Y, Lagace-Wiens P. The microbiology of endophthalmitis: global trends and a local perspective. Eur J Clin Microbiol Infect Dis. 2012;31(11):2879–86.
13. Cruz CS, Cohen EJ, Rapuano CJ, Laibson PR. Microbial keratitis resulting in loss of the eye. Ophthalmic Surg Lasers. 1998;29(10):803–7.
14. Margo CE. Eyes removed for primary ulcerative keratitis with endophthalmitis: microbial and histologic findings. Ophthalmic Surg Lasers. 1999;30(7):535–9.
15. Behrens-Baumann W. Endophthalmitis. Klinische Monatsblatter fur Augenheilkunde. 2008;225(11):917–8.
16. Baum J, Peyman GA, Barza M. Intravitreal administration of antibiotic in the treatment of bacterial endophthalmitis. III. Consensus. Surv Ophthalmol. 1982;26(4):204–6.
17. Behrens-Baumann W. Current therapy for postoperative endophthalmitis. Klinische Monatsblatter fur Augenheilkunde. 2008;225(11):919–23.
18. Srinivasan M, Mascarenhas J, Rajaraman R, Ravindran M, Lalitha P, Glidden DV, Ray KJ, Hong KC, Oldenburg CE, Lee SM, et al. Corticosteroids for bacterial keratitis: the steroids for corneal ulcers trial (SCUT). Arch Ophthalmol. 2012;130(2):143–50.
19. Kunimoto DY, Sharma S, Garg P, Gopinathan U, Miller D, Rao GN. Corneal ulceration in the elderly in Hyderabad, South India. Br J Ophthalmol. 2000; 84(1):54–9.
20. Higa A, Sakai H, Sawaguchi S, Iwase A, Tomidokoro A, Amano S, Araie M. Corneal endothelial cell density and associated factors in a population-based study in Japan: the Kumejima study. Am J Ophthalmol. 2010;149(5):794–9.
21. Schmedt T, Silva MM, Ziaei A, Jurkunas U. Molecular bases of corneal endothelial dystrophies. Exp Eye Res. 2012;95(1):24–34.
22. Dursun D, Fernandez V, Miller D, Alfonso EC. Advanced fusarium keratitis progressing to endophthalmitis. Cornea. 2003;22(4):300–3.
23. Kent DG. Endophthalmitis in Auckland 1983-1991. Aust N Z J Ophthalmol. 1993;21(4):227–36.
24. O'Neill EC, Yeoh J, Fabinyi DC, Cassidy D, Vajpayee RB, Allen P, Connell PP. Risk factors, microbial profiles and prognosis of microbial keratitis-associated endophthalmitis in high-risk eyes. Graefes Arch Clin Exp Ophthalmol. 2014; 252(9):1457–62.
25. Sisk RA, Davis JL, Dubovy SR, Smiddy WE. Sympathetic ophthalmia following vitrectomy for endophthalmitis after intravitreal bevacizumab. Ocul Immunol Inflamm. 2008;16(5):236–8.

6

Development of a new valid and reliable microsurgical skill assessment scale for ophthalmology residents

Zhihua Zhang[1,2,3†], Minwen Zhou[1,2,3†], Kun Liu[1,2,3†], Bijun Zhu[1,2,3], Haiyun Liu[1,2,3*], Xiaodong Sun[1,2,3] and Xun Xu[1,2,3]

Abstract

Background: More and more concerns have been arisen about the ability of new medical graduates to meet the demands of today's practice environment. In this study, we wanted to develop a valid, reliable and standardized assessment tool for evaluating the basic microsurgical skills of residents in a microsurgery laboratory, to get them well prepared before entering the surgical realm of ophthalmology.

Methods: Twenty-three experts who have teaching experience reviewed the assessment scale. Constructive comments were incorporated to ensure face and content validity. Twenty-one attendings from different specialties then graded eight corneal rupture suturing videos with the scale to investigate interrater reliability. Fourteen of them graded the same videos 3 months later to investigate intrarater reliability (repeatability).

Results: A total of 280 assessment scales were completed. All the ICC values of interrater reliability were greater than 0.8 with 75% data greater than 0.9 (range 0.860–0.976). All the ICC values of intrarater reliability (repeatability) were also greater than 0.8 with 63% data greater than 0.9 (range 0.833–0.954).

Conclusions: The assessment scale we developed is valid and reliable. This tool could be useful to ensure that junior residents achieve a certain level of microsurgical technique in a laboratory environment before training in the operation room. Hopefully, this tool will provide a structured template for other residency programs to assess their residents for basic microsurgical skills.

Keywords: Assessment scale, Cornea suturing, Medical education, Microsurgical skill

Background

Along with the development of ophthalmic medical education, the training of surgical skills has become a key part of it. More and more educators have realized the importance of residents' competence in the operating room; however, the traditional methods for assessing surgical skills are largely subjective. Those methods were lack of standardization, consistency and reliability. Moreover, for the student assessed, they didn't know the standards and goals of surgical training. In order to change the condition, educators worldwide had done a lot of work. A variety of surgical competency assessment tools had been developed by international ophthalmic educators, such as OASIS (Objective Assessment of Skills in Intraocular Surgery), GRASIS (Global Rating Assessment of Skills in Intraocular Surgery), OSACSS (Objective Structured Assessment of Cataract Surgical Skill) and OSCAR (Ophthalmology Surgical Competency Assessment Rubric), and the feedback from experts and application of those assessments showed excellent results [1–7]. By far, most of the assessments focus on the performance of residents during real-life operations, especially cataract surgeries.

China is a developing and industrialized country. Ocular rupture especially corneal rupture is a common and dangerous ophthalmic emergency, which usually is residents' first independent real-life surgery. Prompt and meticulous wound management may reduce severe

* Correspondence: tony373@163.com
†Equal contributors
[1]Shanghai Key Laboratory of Ocular Fundus Diseases, Shanghai, China
[2]Department of Ophthalmology, Shanghai General Hospital, Shanghai Jiao Tong University School of Medicine, 100 Haining Road, Shanghai 200080, China
Full list of author information is available at the end of the article

postoperative complications such as wound leak and endophthalmitis [8]. Thus, residents should be well prepared before they go into the operation room. What's more, suturing technique is a critical and fundamental part of microsurgery. Standardized and adept micromanipulation and suturing would pave the way for entering the surgical realm of ophthalmology. Therefore, in Shanghai, suturing corneal rupture on pig eyes is mandated to be one of the periodical exams of residency program. Appropriate evaluation of this procedure is essential because weaknesses in training and teaching are difficult to correct without factual data [9, 10]. Since no rating assessment for suturing corneal rupture has been created before, Chinese ophthalmic education workers need to develop a comprehensive assessment scale in response to the current demand. In this study, we aimed to establish an efficient and reliable assessment scale for suturing corneal rupture to ensure the basic surgical competency of residents.

Methods

This study was approved by the Ethics Committee of Shanghai General Hospital. All the operations were performed in a microsurgery laboratory using pig eyes (Fig. 1a). Each resident was given detailed information of what they were going to perform. The ruptures were "L" shaped involving the limbus. First, we made a full-thickness horizontal incision (about 6 mm) from 9 o'clock limbus to central cornea. The incision was then extended down for another 3 mm vertically (Fig. 1b). All necessary instruments, as well as distracter instruments, were laid out on the table. The whole process from gloves on to gloves off was videotaped and stored for later view. Senior attendings from different specialties were asked to watch those recorded videos and finish the assessment scales accordingly. The videotapes were chosen from residents at different rotating levels to include a range of surgical skills, and evaluators were blinded to the resident's level of training. What's more, 3 month later, each attending was asked to watch the same

videos and complete the scales again. In order to avoid the recall of the last scoring, the playing order of the videos was changed.

Validity of the assessment scale
A questionnaire was created (Fig. 2) to evaluate the scale's face validity (i.e., the extent to which the components address the vital aspects) and content validity (i.e., the extent to which the components assess resident competency and skill) [3, 7]. The questionnaire along with the assessment scale was sent to experts from several teaching and research offices including one member of the committee of Shanghai standardized residency program, and then the scale was revised according to their comments and suggestions.

Reliability and repeatability of the assessment scale
Senior attendings from different specialties were included in this evaluation to achieve a broad representation. The interrater reliability of different observers as well as the intrarater reliability of the same observer (repeatability) was tested using the intraclass correlation coefficient (ICC) [11]. The ICC is defined as the ratio of the between-subjects variance to the sum of the combined within-subjects and between-subjects variance [12]. ICC can very between 0 and 1, with 1 indicating perfect agreement. It should be greater than 0.7 in order for newly developed scales to be considered reliable [13–15]. We calculated the ICC using SPSS version 13.0 (Chicago, IL, USA). Considering the fact that we had a sample group of observers and cases, we used the Two-Way Random model. The Single Measures results were used to evaluate repeatability, and the Average Measures results were used for reliability. The significance level and confidence coefficients were set to 0.05 and 0.95, respectively.

Results
Validity of the assessment scale
Twenty-three experts completed the questionnaire, and the results of the questionnaire were noted in Table 1.

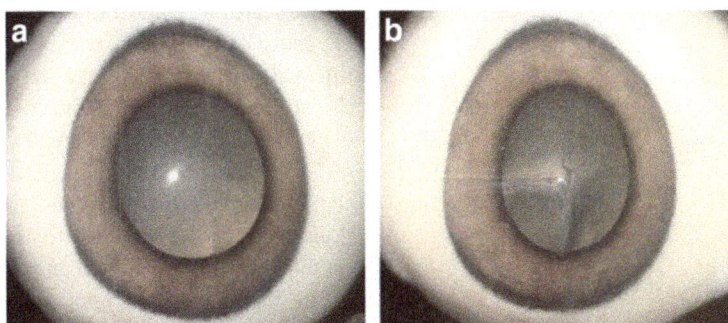

Fig. 1 Illustrations of fresh pig eye for microscopic suturing in wet lab. **a**. Fresh pig eye before incision was made; **b**. "L" shaped incision was made on pig eye

1. Are the instructions self-explanatory?   Yes_____ No_____
Comments_____

2. Is the rating scale appropriate?   Yes_____ No_____
Comments_____

3. Does the rating scale include all the factors
   essential to evaluate operative performance?   Yes_____ No_____
Comments_____

4. Is the "Microscope use" item appropriate?   Yes_____ No_____
Comments_____

5. Is the "Instrument handling" item appropriate?   Yes_____ No_____
Comments_____

6. Is the "Hands coordination" item appropriate?   Yes_____ No_____
Comments_____

7. Is the "Suturing order" item appropriate?   Yes_____ No_____
Comments_____

8. Is the "Stiches interval" item appropriate?   Yes_____ No_____
Comments_____

9. Is the "Stitches width " item appropriate?   Yes_____ No_____
Comments_____

10. Is the "Stitches depth" item appropriate?   Yes_____ No_____
Comments_____

11. Is the "Knotting" item appropriate?   Yes_____ No_____
Comments_____

12. Is the "Wound closure and anterior
    chamber formation" item appropriate?   Yes_____ No_____
Comments_____

13. Is the "Abnormal events management"
    item appropriate?   Yes_____ No_____
Comments_____

14. Is the "Overall performance" item appropriate?   Yes_____ No_____
Comments_____

15. Is there anything else that should be included
    in the assessment form (keeping in mind the
    goal of minimum time expenditure)?   Yes_____ No_____
Comments_____

Fig. 2 Survey sent to experts to determine the face and content validity of the assessment scale

Table 1 Results of the Content and Face Validity Survey

Are those items appropriate?	Percentage
Microscope use	21/23 (91%)
Instrument handling	21/23 (91%)
Hand coordination	23/23 (100%)
Suturing order	22/23 (96%)
Suturing interval	23/23 (100%)
Suturing width	23/23 (100%)
Suturing depth	23/23(100%)
Knotting	20/23 (87%)
Wound closure and anterior chamber formation	23/23 (100%)
Abnormal events management	18/23 (78%)
Overall performance	23/23(100%)

Reported as the fraction (percent) of respondents answering "Yes" to the question

Four experts recommended adding an assessment of "preoperative preparation and postoperative cleaning up" to the scale since the videotapes contained those parts and they were aspects of surgical skills. Two experts expressed that some of the descriptors were too explicit and burdensome to read and simplification may be better. Three experts suggested to use separated rating scales for "knotting", "knots tightness", and "knots exposure". One expert commented to add "Suturing" to the scale to assess the general suturing performance of the students such as needle load and needle entry. Five experts felt there was no need to include an assessment of "abnormal events management". All comments and suggestions were considered, and appropriate suggestions were incorporated into the assessment scale, thus establishing a level of face and content validity [6].

The finalized assessment scale was shown in Table 2. This assessment scale includes 6 measures of basic surgical skills (preoperative preparation, microscope use, instrument handling, hands coordination, postoperative

Table 2 Assessment Scale of Corneal Rupture Suturing

DATE _____ RESIDENT _____ EVALUATOR _____	1	2	3	4	5	Score
Preoperative preparation	Failed to wear hat, mask and gloves	Failed to wear two of the three	Failed to wear one of the three	Wearing hat, mask and gloves correctly	Wearing hat, mask and gloves smoothly	
Microscope use	Out of center and focus constantly	Out of center and focus frequently	Out of center and focus occasionally	Stay in center and focus constantly	Fluid moves with microscope	
Instrument handling	Constantly makes tentative and awkward moves with instruments by impropriate use	Frequently makes tentative and awkward moves with instruments	Fair use of instruments but occasionally stiff or awkward	Competent use of instruments	Fluid moves with instruments	
Hands coordination	Severely hands tremor and constantly instruments collision	Hands tremor and frequently instruments collision	Mild hands tremor and occasionally instrument collision	No hands tremor and instrument collision	Steady hands and perfect hands coordination	
Suturing	Sutures are done in an awkward, slow fashion with much difficulty. Bent needles	Sutures are done with difficulty	Sutures are done with little difficulty	Sutures are done properly. Loads needle 1/2 to 2/3 from tip. Approaches eye with flat portion of needle. Needle enters perpendicular to cornea	Smooth and perfect suturing. Always loads needle 1/2 to 2/3 from tip. Always approaches eye with flat portion of needle. Needle enters perpendicular to cornea	
Suturing order	Suture the rupture randomly	Suture the rupture in one direction	Selectively suture the rupture. Close the center first	Selectively suture the rupture. Close the angle first	Selectively suture the rupture. Surgical exploration of the limbus. Close the limbus first, then the angle	
Stitches interval	Awfully uneven	Uneven	Almost even	Even	Perfectly even, around 2 mm	
Stitches width	Awfully uneven	Uneven	Almost even	Even	Perfectly even, around 2 mm	
Stitches depth	Awfully uneven	Uneven	Almost even	Even	Perfectly even, around 2/3 of the cornea thickness	
Knotting	Knots are placed in an awkward, slow fashion with much difficulty	Knots are placed with difficulty	Knots are placed with little difficulty	Knots are placed properly with seldom breaking sutures	Knots are placed perfectly with no breaking sutures	
Knots tightness	Suture tightness is awfully uneven. Sutures are too tight or loose	Suture tightness is uneven. Sutures are tight or loose	Suture tightness is almost even. Sutures are a little bit tight or loose	Suture tightness is proper and even	Suture tightness is perfectly even. Sutures are placed tight enough to maintain the wound closed, but not too tight as to induce astigmatism	
Knots rotation	No suture rotation at all	Most of the sutures are not rotated	Parts of the sutures are not rotated	Most of the sutures are rotated	Complete suture rotation. No knots exposure	
Wound closure and anterior chamber formation	No wound closure and no anterior chamber formation	Part of wound closure and no anterior chamber formation	Questionable wound closure and anterior chamber formation	Complete wound closure and anterior chamber formation	Neat and watertight wound closure. Perfect anterior chamber formation with no anterior synechia of iris	
Postoperative clean up	Failed to clean up the pig eyes. Failed to settle the microscope and instruments. Failed to take off the hat, mask and gloves properly	Failed to do two of the three things	Failed to do one of the three things	Complete all the three things	Throw the pig eye in the yellow bag. Settle the microscope and instruments. Take off the hat, mask and gloves correctly	
Overall performance	Unable to finish the operation independently	Hesitant, frequent starts and stops. Finish the operation with difficulty	Occasional starts and stops. Finish the operation within 20mins	Competent, finish the operation within 15mins	Confident and fluid, finish the operation within 10mins	

clean up and overall performance) and 9 measures of the stages of suturing (suturing, suturing order, sutures interval, sutures width, sutures depth, knotting, knots tightness, knots exposure and wound leakage and anterior chamber formation), which are rated on a 5-point Likert scale, with each point anchored by explicit behavioral descriptors.

Reliability and repeatability of the assessment scale

Twenty-one attendings from different specialties finished 8-videotaped corneal suturing surgeries and completed the assessment scales accordingly for the first time. Specialties represented were cataract (4), glaucoma (3), cornea (3), strabismus (1), and retina (10). Only 14 attendings finished the scale again 3 month later. A total of 280 assessment scales were completed. All experts expressed that they could complete the scale within 5 min.

The interrater reliability of each surgical procedure step and overall score, considering 21 observers together, was summarized in Table 3. All the ICC values were greater than 0.8 with 75% data greater than 0.9. "Microscope use" Showed the highest reliability (0.976, 95%CI 0.942–0.994). The intrarater reliability (repeatability) of each step and overall score was listed in Table 4. All data were greater than 0.8, with 63% data greater than 0.9. "Suturing order" showed the highest repeatability (0.954, 95%CI 0.934–0.968).

Table 3 Interrater reliability of 23 observers for corneal rupture suturing assessing scale

	ICC	95% CI	
		Lower bound	Upper bound
Preoperative preparation	0.953***	0.888	0.989
Microscope use	0.976***	0.942	0.994
Instrument handling	0.940***	0.857	0.986
Hand coordination	0.963***	0.913	0.991
Suturing	0.866***	0.682	0.968
Suturing order	0.971***	0.932	0.993
Suturing interval	0.943***	0.863	0.986
Suturing width	0.939***	0.855	0.985
Suturing depth	0.860***	0.668	0.967
Knotting	0.922***	0.815	0.981
Knots tightness	0.886***	0.728	0.973
Knots rotation	0.913***	0.793	0.979
Wound closure and anterior chamber formation	0.892***	0.744	0.974
Postoperative clean up	0.920***	0.809	0.981
Overall performance	0.965***	0.917	0.992
Total score	0.959***	0.901	0.990

ICC intraclass correlation coefficient, CI confidential interval
***: P < 0.001

Table 4 Intrarater reliability (repeatability) for corneal rupture suturing assessing scale

Item	ICC	95% CI	
		Lower bound	Upper bound
Preoperative preparation	0.907***	0.867	0.935
Microscope use	0.934***	0.906	0.954
Instrument handling	0.866***	0.811	0.906
Hand coordination	0.904***	0.863	0.933
Suturing	0.865***	0.810	0.905
Suturing order	0.954***	0.934	0.968
Suturing interval	0.919***	0.884	0.943
Suturing width	0.901***	0.860	0.931
Suturing depth	0.885***	0.837	0.920
Knotting	0.916***	0.880	0.941
Knots tightness	0.833***	0.767	0.822
Knots rotation	0.843***	0.779	0.889
Wound closure and anterior chamber formation	0.901***	0.859	0.931
Postoperative clean up	0.893***	0.848	0.925
Overall performance	0.940***	0.915	0.959
Total score	0.946***	0.922	0.962

ICC intraclass correlation coefficient, CI confidential interval
***: P < 0.001

Discussion

Investigations suggested a trend towards enhanced acquisition of microsurgical skill in students allowed to practice microsurgery on all kinds of simulators and/or in the wet laboratory [16–18]. Nevertheless, in the early twenty-first century, the ophthalmic education of residents in China was unstructured and of variable quality. There were more and more concerns arising about the ability of new medical graduates to meet the demands of today's practice environment. Thus, China started the residency program about 10 years ago and Shanghai was one of the pilot cities. Up to now, each city is still responsible for its own resident training and examination. In Shanghai, the committee of ophthalmic resident training standardized the program as 3 years of ophthalmology education, and every year they will attend an annual ophthalmology residency-in-training examination. The major purpose of those examinations is to evaluate residents' competence in 4 aspects: (1) medical knowledge, (2) patient care and communication skills, (3) case-based learning and analyzing, and (4) surgical skills. Suturing technique is a critical and fundamental part of microsurgery. Standardized and adept micromanipulation and suturing would pave the way for entering the surgical realm of ophthalmology. Therefore, the surgical skills of junior residents are assessed by performance on suturing corneal rupture on pig eyes. This kind of examination has been held for 5 years and the ophthalmic educators found out that the traditional scoring method might be unreliable due to grade inflation and overt subjective assessments [10, 19, 20]. Residency examination is supposed to enable competence in all aspects by collecting performance data that reliably and accurately reflects the resident's real ability. Thus, a valid and reliable assessment tool is desperately needed.

To our knowledge, this is the first throughout assessment scale for corneal rupture suturing in wet laboratory. Fisher et al. [1] developed a phacoemulsification/ wound construction and suturing technique assessment scale for ophthalmology residents, but suturing technique assessment was only part of the scale containing 8 general items. The scale was simple and only had 2 choices (not done/incorrect and done correctly). There was no behavioral or skill-based rubric for the observers to use when assessing the resident's performance. Feldman et al. [21] used a corneal laceration repair assessment to evaluate microsurgical skill improvement after training on the simulator. However, the assessment was totally objective and only measured suture depth, bite size and suture spacing. In this study, we created a comprehensive, globally applicable assessment scale to evaluate the key components of corneal rupture suturing. This assessment scale breaks down to 15 essential items including 6 measures of basic surgical skills and 9 measures of the stages of suturing, with basic skill measures similar to that employed in GRASIS and OSCAR. Moreover, the scale is rated on a 5-point Likert scale with behavioral anchors for each level in each step of the surgical procedure.

The reliability and repeatability of the assessment tools mentioned above were seldom detected. In this study, we investigated validity, reliability and repeatability of our assessment scale. For validity, we asked 23 experts from different teaching and research offices, and all the comments were considered and appropriate suggestions were incorporated into the assessment scale. Therefore, a level of face and content validity was established. Considering the reliability for the entire group of 21 observers, the ICC values were higher than 0.8 (range 0.860–0.976) in all 15 individual categories as well as the overall score, indicating reliability of the tool as a whole. What's more, the assessment scale yielded very good repeatability, with ICC values ranging from 0.833 to 0.954. An assessment scale is considered to give almost perfect outcomes when ICC value is 0.75 and above [13, 15, 22].

Drawbacks of the assessment scale are that it is relatively simple and it cannot provide information about resident's judgment and handling of complications on real operations. However, it is a standardized tool that can be used to determine whether a resident is adequately prepared, in terms of their basic microsurgical skills, to enter the operating room. The "passing" threshold could be set at a score of > 3 for each item on the 5-point Likert scale. In addition, process in the wet laboratory can be standardized so that each resident is assessed under comparable circumstances, and ophthalmic educators can easily track their improvements or adjust the complexity to train residents of different rotating levels by changing the rupture (straight/ "Y" shaped rupture, with/without limbus).

Conclusions

In this study, we aimed to create a standardized tool to assess basic surgical skills and to improve overall process of early surgical education. In summary, the assessment scale we developed is valid and reliable. It is an analytical scoring system that contains observable and measurable components of surgical performance. It will help educators to reduce the subjectivity of the assessment and clearly express to the residents what is expected to obtain competence. Hopefully, this tool will provide a structured template for other residency programs to assess their residents for basic surgical skills.

Abbreviations
GRASIS: Global rating assessment of skills in intraocular surgery; ICC: Intraclass correlation coefficient; OASIS: Objective assessment of skills in intraocular surgery; OSACSS: Objective structured assessment of cataract surgical skill; OSCAR: Ophthalmology surgical competency assessment rubric

Acknowledgements
Not applicable

Funding
This work was supported by National Natural Science Foundation of China (81600704), Interdisciplinary Program of Shanghai Jiao Tong University (YG2015QN19), and Shanghai Ophthalmology Practical Training Platform Construction Grant. The grants had no role in the design or conduct of this research.

Authors' contributions
All authors conceived of and designed the experimental protocol. ZHZ, MWZ and KL collected the data. All authors were involved in the analysis and interpretation of the data. ZHZ and KL wrote the first draft of the manuscript. MWZ, HYL, BJZ, XX and XDS reviewed and revised the manuscript and produced the final version. All authors read and approved the final manuscript.

Competing interests
The authors declare that they have no competing interests.

Author details
[1]Shanghai Key Laboratory of Ocular Fundus Diseases, Shanghai, China.
[2]Department of Ophthalmology, Shanghai General Hospital, Shanghai Jiao
Tong University School of Medicine, 100 Haining Road, Shanghai 200080, China.
[3]Shanghai Engineering Center for Visual Science and Photomedicine, Shanghai,
China.

References
1. Fisher JB, Binenbaum G, Tapino P, Volpe NJ. Development and face and content validity of an eye surgical skills assessment test for ophthalmology residents. Ophthalmology. 2006;113:2364–70.
2. Cremers SL, Ciolino JB, Ferrufino-Ponce ZK, Henderson BA. Objective assessment of skills in intraocular surgery (OASIS). Ophthalmology. 2005;112:1236–41.
3. Cremers SL, Lora AN, Ferrufino-Ponce ZK. Global rating assessment of skills in intraocular surgery (GRASIS). Ophthalmology. 2005;112:1655–60.
4. Feldman BH, Geist CE. Assessing residents in phacoemulsification. Ophthalmology. 2007;114:1586.
5. Saleh GM, Gauba V, Mitra A, Litwin AS, Chung AK, Benjamin L. Objective structured assessment of cataract surgical skill. Arch Ophthalmol. 2007;125:363–6.
6. Golnik KC, Beaver H, Gauba V, Lee AG, Mayorga E, Palis G, et al. Cataract surgical skill assessment. Ophthalmology. 2011;118:427. e1-5
7. Golnik KC, Haripriya A, Beaver H, Gauba V, Lee AG, Mayorga E, et al. Cataract surgical skill assessment. Ophthalmology. 2011;118:2094–e2.
8. Kong GY, Henderson RH, Sandhu SS, Essex RW, Allen PJ, Campbell WG. Wound-related complications and clinical outcomes following open globe injury repair. Clin Exp Ophthalmol. 2015;43:508–13.
9. Scott DJ, Valentine RJ, Bergen PC, Rege RV, Laycock R, Tesfay ST, et al. Evaluating surgical competency with the American Board of Surgery in-Training Examination, skill testing, and intraoperative assessment. Surgery. 2000;128:613–22.
10. Moorthy K, Munz Y, Sarker SK, Darzi A. Objective assessment of technical skills in surgery. BMJ. 2003;327:1032–7.
11. Koch GG. Intraclass correlation coefficient; in Kotz S, Johnson NL (eds): encyclopedia of statistical sciences 4. New York: Wiley; 1982. p. 213–7.
12. Meyer JJ, Gokul A, Vellara HR, Prime Z, McGhee CN. Repeatability and agreement of Orbscan II, Pentacam HR, and Galilei tomography Systems in Corneas with Keratoconus. Am J Ophthalmol. 2017;175:122–8.
13. Zaki R, Bulgiba A, Nordin N, Azina IN. A systematic review of statistical methods used to test for reliability of medical instruments measuring continuous variables. Iran J Basic Med Sci. 2013;16:803–7.
14. Cronbach LJ, Shavelson RJ. My current thoughts on coefficient alpha and successor procedures. Educ Psychol Meas. 2004;64:391–418.
15. Barraquer RI, Pinilla Cortés L, Allende MJ, Montenegro GA, Ivankovic B, D'Antin JC, et al. Validation of the nuclear cataract grading system BCN 10. Ophthalmic Res. 2017;57:247–51.
16. Thomsen AS, Subhi Y, Kiilgaard JF, la Cour M, Konge L. Update on simulation-based surgical training and assessment in ophthalmology: a systematic review. Ophthalmology. 2015;122:1111–30. e1
17. Bourcier T, Chammas J, Becmeur PH, Sauer A, Gaucher D, Liverneaux P, et al. Robot-assisted simulated cataract surgery. J Cataract Refract Surg. 2017;43:552–7.
18. Thomsen AS, Bach-Holm D, Kjærbo H, Højgaard-Olsen K, Subhi Y, Saleh GM, et al. Operating room performance improves after proficiency-based virtual reality cataract surgery training. Ophthalmology. 2017;124:524–31.
19. Lee AG, Carter KD. Managing the new mandate in resident education: a blueprint for translating a national mandate into local compliance. Ophthalmology. 2004;111:1807–12.
20. Mills RP, Mannis MJ. American Board of Ophthalmology Program Directors' task force on competencies. Report of the American Board of Ophthalmology Task Force on the competencies. Ophthalmology. 2004;111:1267–8.
21. Feldman BH, Ake JM, Geist CE. Virtual reality simulation. Ophthalmology. 2007;114:828. e1-4
22. Dong J, Jia YD, Wu Q, Zhang S, Jia Y, Huang D, et al. Interchangeability and reliability of macular perfusion parameter measurements using optical coherence tomography angiography. Br J Ophthalmol. 2017;101:1542–9.

7

Association between glaucoma severity and driving cessation in subjects with primary open-angle glaucoma

Aya Takahashi, Kenya Yuki *🄳, Sachiko Awano-Tanabe, Takeshi Ono, Daisuke Shiba and Kazuo Tsubota

Abstract

Background: The aim of this study, which included a baseline cross-sectional study and a 3-year follow-up prospective study, was to investigate the association between glaucomatous visual field damage and driving cessation in subjects with primary open-angle glaucoma (POAG).

Methods: A total of 211 POAG subjects divided into 3 groups according to POAG severity (mild, moderate, or severe) in the better eye were enrolled along with 148 control subjects; subjects were asked about changes in their driving status. In the 3-year follow-up study, 185 of the POAG subjects and 80 of the controls annually reported their driving status. Adjusted odds ratios and 95% confidence intervals for the prevalence and incidence of driving cessation were estimated with a multiple logistic regression model.

Results: In the original cross-sectional study, 11/148 (7%) members of the control group reported having given up driving over the previous 5 years; the corresponding figures for the mild POAG, moderate POAG, and severe POAG groups were 9/173 (5%), 0/22 (0%), and 5/16 (31%), respectively ($p = 0.001$, Fisher's exact test), with severe POAG found to be associated with driving cessation after adjustment for age, gender, systemic hypertension, and diabetes mellitus (odds ratio 11.52 [95% CI 2.87-46.35], ref. control, $p = 0.001$). In the follow-up study, the proportions of subjects who ceased driving were 1/80 (1.3%) in the control group, 8/152 (5.3%) in the mild POAG group, 5/22 (22.7%) in the moderate POAG group, and 2/11 (18.2%) in the severe POAG group ($p = 0.001$, Fisher's exact test). Moderate POAG and severe POAG in the better eye were found to be associated with driving cessation after adjustment for age, gender, systemic hypertension, and diabetes mellitus (moderate POAG in the better eye: odds ratio 37.7 [95% CI 3.7-383.8], ref. control, $p = 0.002$, and severe POAG in the better eye: odds ratio 52.8 [95% CI 3.5-797.0], ref. control, $p = 0.004$).

Conclusion: Moderate and Severe POAG in the better eye is associated with driving cessation.

Background

Driving cessation is associated with a number of adverse outcomes, including depression [1, 2], declines in physical and social function [3], admission to long-term care [4], and mortality [5].

Glaucoma is the second leading cause of blindness in the world [6]. In glaucomatous optic neuropathy, retinal ganglion cells are slowly and progressively destroyed, with a concomitant loss of peripheral and central vision. Age is a significant risk factor for glaucoma [7], so the number of elderly drivers with glaucoma can be expected to increase in the future. Several reports have shown that subjects with glaucoma are likely to stop driving [8–10]. However, little is known about the association between glaucoma and driving cessation, and most previous studies have had cross-sectional designs. The aim of our study was to investigate the association between glaucomatous VF damage and driving cessation in subjects with POAG in both a cross-sectional and a prospective study. Our hypothesis was that severe glaucoma in the better eye is associated with driving cessation.

Subjects and methods

The procedures followed in this study conformed to the tenets of the Declaration of Helsinki and to national (Japanese) and institutional (Keio University School of Medicine) regulations. The study was approved by the

---
* Correspondence: yukikenya114@gmail.com
Department of Ophthalmology, Keio University School of Medicine, Shinanomachi 35, Shinjyuku-ku, Tokyo, Japan

Ethics Committee of Keio University School of Medicine (#2010293). All study subjects gave informed, written consent prior to enrolment.

Study design and subject enrolment

This study consisted of a baseline cross-sectional study and a 3-year follow-up prospective cohort study. Descriptive research design, baseline evaluation of subjects with glaucoma, diagnostic criteria for POAG, and exclusion criteria were shown in our previous paper [11, 12]. This is a sub-analysis of our two previous reports.

Baseline question on driving status

All study subjects answered the following question (translated from the original Japanese) at the baseline ophthalmic examination:

(1) Do you have a driver's license? (Yes/No/Previously)

Subjects who answered "previously" were included in the prevalence of driving cessation data.

Demographic information recorded for all subjects included age, sex, height, weight, alcohol intake (yes/no), smoking (yes/no/previous), and current and previous illnesses (e.g., systemic hypertension, diabetes mellitus, depression, brain infarction).

Follow-up question on driving status

All study subjects were asked the same question about whether they had a driver's license every 12 months (± 1 month) for 3 years after they answered it at baseline. Those who answered "yes" at baseline and "previously" during follow-up were included in the incidence of driving cessation data.

Glaucoma severity grading

For the purposes of this study, we defined mild POAG as a VF defect corresponding to a mean deviation (MD) of − 6 dB or better in the better eye, moderate POAG as corresponding to an MD of > − 6 dB to − 12 dB in the better eye, and severe POAG as an MD of > − 12 dB or worse in the better eye [13]. The eye with the better VF was defined as the eye with the higher (i.e., less negative) MD.

Statistical analysis

The one-way ANOVA and Fisher's exact test were used to calculate statistics for the demographic, medical, and visual-function variables between subjects among the control, mild, moderate, and severe POAG group. Age, visual acuity, and MD were analyzed with ANOVA test. Scheffé post hoc tests were also performed after one-way ANOVA. Gender, prevalence of diabetes mellitus, and prevalence of systemic hypertension were analyzed with Fisher's exact test. Adjusted odds ratios and 95% confidence intervals for the prevalence and incidence of driving cessation were estimated with a multiple logistic regression model to examine the effects of the following (possible confounding) factors on unadjusted results (forced-entry method): age, sex, prevalence of diabetes mellitus, and prevalence of systemic hypertension. A p-value less than 0.05 was considered statistically significant. Decimal visual acuity was converted to LogMAR visual acuity for analysis. All analyses were performed with Stata 11.2 (Stata Co. Texas. USA) software.

Results
Results of the cross-sectional study

A total of 211 POAG subjects divided into 3 groups according to MD in the better eye (143 men, 68 women; age: 65.5 ± 10.7 years) and 148 control subjects (77 men, 71 women; age: 67.6 ± 11.1 years) were evaluated in this study. All subjects were Japanese, and their demographic characteristics are summarized in Table 1. There were

Table 1 Demographics and characteristics of the control and POAG groups (Baseline)

Glaucoma severity	Control	Mild glaucoma	Moderate glaucoma	Severe glaucoma	P value
Number	148	173	22	16	
Age (years)	72.2 ± 6.3	69.4 ± 6.1	70.4 ± 5.9	70.9 ± 6.9	0.002
Gender (male/female)	77/71 (52.0%/48.0%)	115/58 (66.5%/33.5%)	14/8 (63.6%/36.4%)	14/2 (87.5%/12.5%)	0.007
VA in the better eye (LogMar)	0.006 ± 0.03	0.003 ± 0.02	0.009 ± 0.03	0.006 ± 0.02	0.93
VA in the worse eye (LogMar)	0.02 ± 0.05	0.02 ± 0.04	0.02 ± 0.05	0.02 ± 0.05	0.95
MD in the better eye (dB)	–	−1.5 ± 1.7 [+ 2.2–6.0]	−8.2 ± 1.4 [− 6.2–11.9]	−18.2 ± 5.1 [− 12.6–29.0]	0.0001
MD in the worse eye (dB)	–	−6.3 ± 5.9 [+ 0.24–31.0]	− 14.7 ± 5.2 [− 6.2–27.4]	−21.6 ± 5.0 [− 12.7–30.4]	0.0001
Diabetes mellitus (Yes)	16/148 (10.8%)	32/173 (18.5%)	4/22 (18.2%)	3/16 (18.8%)	0.27
Systemic hypertension (Yes)	68/148 (45.9%)	65/173 (37.6%)	6/22 (27.3%)	4/16 (25.0%)	0.13

Glaucoma severity was determined on the basis of visual field in the better eye
Mean ± standard deviation [range]. Age, visual acuity, and MD were analyzed with ANOVA test. Gender, prevalence of diabetes mellitus, and prevalence of systemic hypertension with Fisher's exact test
Abbreviations: POAG primary open-angle glaucoma, VA visual acuity, MD mean deviation, dB decibel

statistically significant differences in age and sex among the 4 groups; the control group had a significantly higher average age than the POAG groups ($p < 0.001$, Scheffé post hoc test). No significant differences in BCVA in the better or worse eye were observed among the groups.

The proportion of subjects who had ceased driving in the control group was 11/148 (7%); the corresponding figures for the mild POAG, moderate POAG, and severe POAG groups were 9/173 (5%), 0/22 (0%), and 5/16 (31%), respectively ($p = 0.001$, Fisher's exact test) (Fig. 1).

The association between POAG severity and driving cessation was analyzed with a logistic regression model. Severe POAG in the better eye (odds ratio 11.52 [95% CI 2.87-46.35], ref. control, $p = 0.001$) is associated with driving cessation after adjustment for age, gender, systemic hypertension and diabetes mellitus. Socio-demographic factors associated with driving cessation were age (odds ratio 1.16 [95% CI 1.08-1.23] years, $p = 0.001$) and female gender (odds ratio 2.83 [95% CI 1.12-7.18], ref. male gender, $p = 0.028$).

Results of the prospective study

Of the 211 POAG subjects and 129 controls who agreed to participate in the follow-up study (19 control subjects declined), 185 POAG subjects (26/211 [12.3%] were lost to follow-up) and 80 controls (49/129 [38.0%] were lost to follow-up) answered questions annually over a period of 3 years about the possession of a driver's license. The POAG subjects were divided into 3 groups according to their MD value in the better eye. Their demographic

characteristics are summarized in Table 2. Statistically significant differences in age and prevalence of systemic hypertension were observed among the 4 groups. The control group was significantly older than the POAG groups ($p < 0.001$, Scheffé post hoc test). There were no significant differences in BCVA in the better or worse eye.

Among these 185 subjects and 80 controls, 16 of the subjects ceased driving in the 3-year follow-up, or 1.8% per year: 4/265 (1.5%) in the first year, 2/265 (0.8%) in the second, and 10/265 (3.8%) in the third. The proportions of subjects who ceased driving were 1/80 (1.3%) in the control group, 8/152 (5.3%) in the mild POAG group, 5/22 (22.7%) in the moderate POAG group, and 2/11 (18.2%) in the severe POAG group ($p = 0.001$, Fisher's exact test; Fig. 2).

Significant predictor of driving cessation in this prospective study was moderate POAG in the better eye: odds ratio 37.7 [95% CI 3.7-383.8], ref. control, $p = 0.002$, and severe POAG in the better eye: odds ratio 52.8 [95% CI 3.5-797.0], ref. control, $p = 0.004$) after adjustment for age, gender, for systemic hypertension, and for diabetes mellitus. Socio-demographic factors associated with driving cessation were age (odds ratio 1.17 [95% CI 1.06-1.28] years, $p = 0.001$) and female gender (odds ratio 11.99 [95% CI 2.99-48.13], ref. male gender, $p = 0.001$).

Discussion

This study shows that moderate and severe glaucoma in the better visual field eye is associated with driving cessation.

In the Blue Mountain Eye Study, the subjects with POAG were found to be 2.2 times more likely to stop driving (95% CI 1.3-3.9) than the controls [10]. In the Salisbury Eye Study, among the 1135 drivers (including 70 with unilateral glaucoma and 68 with bilateral glaucoma), multivariable regression analysis showed that the subjects with bilateral glaucoma were more likely to have given up driving (odds ratio 2.6, $p = 0.002$ vs. odds ratio 1.5, $p = 0.3$) than the subjects without glaucoma [8]. Van Landingham et al. also reported a higher probability of driving cessation among the glaucoma subjects than among the controls (odds ratio 4.0 [95% CI 1.1-14.7], $p = 0.03$) after multivariable adjustment. In this study, the odds of driving cessation doubled with each 5-dB decrement in MD in the better-eye (odds ratio 2.0 [95% CI 1.4-2.9], $p < 0.001$) [9]. As with our study, these previous studies suggest that severe glaucoma is associated with driving cessation. It is possible that subjects with severe glaucoma in the better eye find driving more difficult than those with unilateral glaucoma. Therefore, subjects with severe glaucoma in the better eye may be more likely to cease driving.

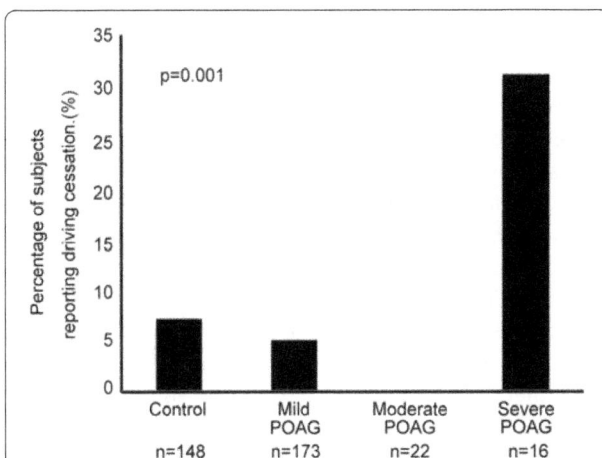

Fig. 1 Percentage of subjects found to have given up driving in the baseline cross-sectional study. The proportions and percentages were 11/148 (7%) in the control group, 9/173 (5%) in the mild POAG group, 0/22 (0%) in the moderate POAG group, and 5/16 (31%) in the severe POAG group ($p = 0.001$, Fisher's exact test). We defined mild POAG as a visual field defect corresponding to an MD of −6 dB or better in the better eye, moderate POAG as an MD of > −6 dB to −12 dB in the better eye, and severe POAG as an MD of > −12 dB or worse in the better eye

Table 2 Demographics and characteristics of the control and POAG groups (Follow-up)

Glaucoma severity[a]	Control	Mild glaucoma	Moderate glaucoma	Severe glaucoma	P value
Number	80	152	22	11	
Percentage of subjects reporting driving cessation	1 (1.3%)	8 (5.3%)	5 (22.7%)	2 (18.2%)	0.001
Age (years)	72.6 ± 6.0	69.0 ± 5.9	70.5 ± 5.9	69.5 ± 4.9	0.0002
Gender (male/female)	46/34 (57.5%/42.5%)	101/51 (66.4%/33.6%)	14/8 (63.6%/36.4%)	9/2 (81.8%/18.2%)	0.36
VA in the better eye (LogMar)	0.005 ± 0.03	0.003 ± 0.02	0.009 ± 0.03	0.009 ± 0.03	0.59
VA in the worse eye (LogMar)	0.02 ± 0.04	0.02 ± 0.04	0.02 ± 0.05	0.03 ± 0.05	0.62
MD in the better eye (dB)	–	− 1.5 ± 1.8 [+ 2.2 - -6.0]	− 8.2 ± 1.4 [− 6.2 - -11.9]	−16.9 ± 5.1 [− 12.6 - -29.0]	0.0001
MD in the worse eye (dB)	–	− 6.1 ± 5.5 [+ 0.24 - -26.8]	−14.7 ± 5.2 [− 6.2 - -27.4]	−20.4 ± 4.8 [− 12.7 - -29.0]	0.0001
Diabetes mellitus (Yes)	6/80 (7.5%)	29/152 (19.1%)	4/22 (18.2%)	2/11 (18.2%)	0.09
Systemic hypertension (Yes)	42/80 (52.5%)	57/152 (37.5%)	6/22 (27.3%)	2/11 (18.2%)	0.03

Mean ± standard deviation [range]. Age, visual acuity, and MD were analyzed with ANOVA test. Gender, prevalence of diabetes mellitus, and prevalence of systemic hypertension with Fisher's exact test
Abbreviations: POAG primary open-angle glaucoma, VA visual acuity, MD mean deviation, dB decibel
[a]Glaucoma severity was determined on the basis of visual field in the better eye

Ours is the first study to show an association between glaucoma severity and driving cessation in a Japanese population: previous studies showing such an association were carried out in Western countries [8–10]. In Japan, the visual standard for driver's licensing is 0.7 (0.15 LogMar) or greater with both eye, and 0.3 or greater (0.5 LogMar) in each eye. In most of Western countries, the visual standard for driver's licensing is 20/40 or greater with both eyes. (http://lowvision.preventblindness.org/daily-living-2/state-vision-screening-and-standards-for--license-to-drive/). Japan's standard for vision is more restrict than western countries. Therefore, severe glaucoma subjects were more likely to fail to renew driver's license in Japan.

Our study also showed that age and female gender were associated with driving cessation, and the Salisbury Eye Study revealed that age and female gender were risk factors for not driving [8]. The Blue Mountain Eye Study showed increasing odds of driving cessation with each decade increase in age (odds ratio 2.4 [95% CI 2.1-2.7]). Female gender was also associated with driving cessation (odds ratio 3.2 [95% CI 2.5-3.9]) in the Blue Mountain eye study [10]. These results are compatible with ours.

We acknowledge several limitations in our study. First, the main outcome relied on self-reported receipt of a driver's license, so the results could have been affected by recall bias. Second, the number of subjects who reported driving cessation was relatively small. However, an association between worsened VF in the better eye and driving cessation was shown in both the baseline cross-sectional study and the follow-up prospective study, which suggests that the results are robust. A third weakness is that data on other possible risk factors for driving cessation, including depressive symptoms, marital status, place of residence, and economic status, were not collected, which could have led to some bias in our analysis. Fourth, it is not possible to determine if POAG was the cause of driving cessation in this study. Fifth, we acknowledge that there are intermediate steps between the first signs of functional loss and driving cessation: since severe glaucoma is associated with depressive symptoms [14], functional loss could indirectly lead to driving cessation by causing depressive symptoms. Sixth, we classified driving cessation on the basis of giving up a driver's license, but we recognize that in fact, many older adults who stop driving voluntarily continue to hold a

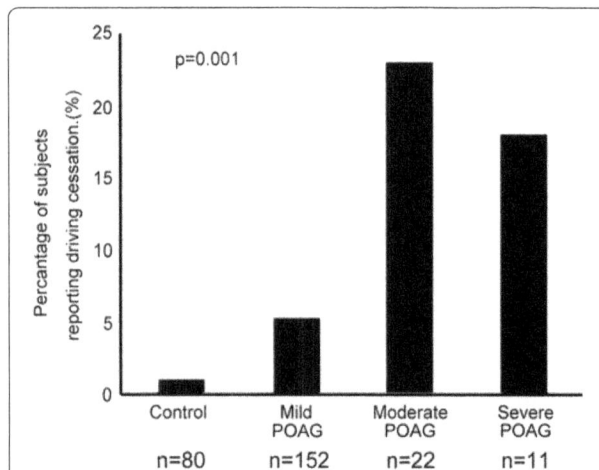

Fig. 2 Percentage of subjects found to have given up driving in the 3-year follow-up prospective study. The proportions and percentages were 1/80 (1.3%) in the control group, 8/152 (5.3%) in the mild POAG group, and 5/22 (22.7%) in the moderate POAG group, and 2/11 (18.2%) in the severe POAG group (p = 0.001, Fisher's exact test). We defined mild POAG as a visual field defect corresponding to an MD of − 6 dB or better in the better eye, moderate POAG as corresponding to an MD of > − 6 dB to − 12 dB in the better eye, and severe POAG as an MD of > − 12 dB or worse in the better eye

license; account of this should be taken in future studies. Seventh, the 95% confidence interval presented in the result section is very wide, this may be because the number of subjects who gave up driving is relatively small.

Conclusion

Moderate and Severe glaucoma in the eye with the better visual field is associated with driving cessation, and may be a clinical predictor of driving cessation.

Acknowledgements

The authors are grateful to Dr. Masaru Shimoyama, Dr. Kazumi Fukagawa, Dr. Naoki Ozeki, Dr. Joji Tanabe, and Dr. Naohiko Tanabe for their help with data collection.

Authors' contributions

AT, SH, TO, ST, DS, KT, and KY have made substantial contributions to conception and design, and interpretation of data; KY, TO, ST, have made substantial contribution to acquisition of data; AT, SH, TO, ST, KT, and KY have been involved in drafting the manuscript or revising it critically for important intellectual content; KY performed statistical analysis; and all authors read and approved the final manuscript.

Competing interests

The authors declare that they have no competing interests.

References

1. Marottoli RA, Mendes de Leon CF, Glass TA, Williams CS, Cooney LM Jr, Berkman LF, et al. Driving cessation and increased depressive symptoms: prospective evidence from the New Haven EPESE. Established Populations for Epidemiologic Studies of the Elderly. J Am Geriatr Soc. 1997;45:202–6.
2. Ragland DR, Satariano WA, MacLeod KE. Driving cessation and increased depressive symptoms. J Gerontol A Biol Sci Med Sci. 2005;60:399–403.
3. Edwards JD, Lunsman M, Perkins M, Rebok GW, Roth DL. Driving cessation and health trajectories in older adults. J Gerontol A Biol Sci Med Sci. 2009; 64:1290–5.
4. Freeman EE, Gange SJ, Munoz B, West SK. Driving status and risk of entry into long-term care in older adults. Am J Public Health. 2006;96:1254–9.
5. Edwards JD, Perkins M, Ross LA, Reynolds SL. Driving status and three-year mortality among community-dwelling older adults. J Gerontol A Biol Sci Med Sci. 2009;64:300–5.
6. Tham YC, Li X, Wong TY, Quigley HA, Aung T, Cheng CY. Global prevalence of glaucoma and projections of glaucoma burden through 2040: a systematic review and meta-analysis. Ophthalmology. 2014;121:2081–90.
7. Coleman AL, Miglior S. Risk factors for glaucoma onset and progression. Surv Ophthalmol. 2008;53:S3–10.
8. Ramulu PY, West SK, Munoz B, Jampel HD, Friedman DS. Driving cessation and driving limitation in glaucoma: the Salisbury Eye Evaluation Project. Ophthalmology. 2009;116:1846–53.
9. van Landingham SW, Hochberg C, Massof RW, Chan E, Friedman DS, Ramulu PY. Driving patterns in older adults with glaucoma. BMC Ophthalmol. 2013;13:4.
10. Gilhotra JS, Mitchell P, Ivers R, Cumming RG. Impaired vision and other factors associated with driving cessation in the elderly: the Blue Mountains Eye Study. Clin Exp Ophthalmol. 2001;29:104–7.
11. Yuki K, Awano-Tanabe S, Ono T, Shiba D, Murata H, et al. Risk factors for motor vehicle collisions in patients with primary open-angle glaucoma: a multicenter prospective cohort study. PlosOne. 2016;11:e0166943.
12. Tanabe S, Yuki K, Ozeki N, Shiba D, Abe T, et al. The association between primary open-angle glaucoma and motor vehicle collisions. Invest Ophthalmol Vis Sci. 2011;52:4143–50.
13. Mills RP, Budenz DL, Lee PP, Noecker RJ, Walt JG, et al. Categorizing the stage of glaucoma from pre-diagnosis to end-stage disease. Am J Ophthalmol. 2006;141:24–30.
14. Mabuchi F, Yoshimura K, Kashiwagi K, Yamagata Z, Kanba S, et al. Risk factors for anxiety and depression in patients with glaucoma. Br J Ophthalmol. 2012; 96:821–5.

8

The effect of fenofibrate on early retinal nerve fiber layer loss in type 2 diabetic patients: a case-control study

Rui Shi[1*], Lei Zhao[2] and Yun Qi[3]

Abstract

Background: Previous studies suggested that use of fenofibrate could significantly reduce the rate of progression into diabetic retinopathy (DR), and that retinal nerve fiber layer (RNFL) loss, which has been considered an important indicator for retinal neurodegeneration, might precede microvascular changes. The aim of this study was to assess the effect(s) of fenofibrate on RNFL thickness at early stage of DR in patients with type 2 diabetes mellitus (DM).

Methods: In this retrospective matched case-control study we included a cohort of 89 patients with type 2 DM, aged 40 or above, between Jan 1, 2017 and March 31, 2017. Among the subjects, 48 patients received fenofibrate therapy and the other 41 patients did not receive fenofibrate treatment. We defined use of fenofibrate as the presence of any prescription for fenofibrate within 1 year before or any time after the diagnosis of DM, and all the patients had either no DR or non-proliferative diabetic retinopathy (NPDR). The fibrate users were well matched with non-fenofibrate users for gender, age and axial length. The RNFL thickness in all quadrants of both eyes was examined with spectral domain optical coherence tomography (SD-OCT). The multiple linear regression analysis was used to assess the association of RNFL thickness with potential risk factors of DR other than fenofibrate use.

Results: The non-fenofibrate users had significantly reduced RNFL thickness of the superior quadrant of the right eye compared to the fenofibrate users ($t = 2.384$, $P = 0.019$). On the contrary, BMI ($p = 0.034$) and ACR ($p = 0.024$) were both negatively correlated to the RNFL thickness of the right eye.

Conclusion: Oral administration of fenofibrate was suggestively associated with thicker RNFL in superior quadrant of the right eye of patents with early DR.

Keywords: Diabetic retinopathy, Fenofibrate, Retinal nerve fiber layer, Optical coherence tomography

Background

Diabetic retinopathy (DR) is the leading cause of blindness in patients with diabetes mellitus (DM) and considered as a microvascular retinal disease [1]. Previous studies have reported that increased serum cholesterol and triglyceride concentrations were associated with the development and severity of DR [2, 3]. Fibrates are peroxisome proliferator-activated receptor alpha (PPARα) agonists, which have been reported to effectively delay the progression of DR [4–6]. However, this benefit did not persist [7], and the potential mechanism of early DR remains unclear.

The most up-to-date studies have indicated that retinal neurodegeneration preceded microangiopathy of the retina and occurred at the earliest stage of DR [8–10]. Neuronal apoptosis and reduction in thickness of the inner retinal layers have been considered to cause defects in dark adaptation and contrast sensitivity, disturbances in color vision and abnormal microperimetry [11]. Topical administration of statins, the most widely used type of lipid-lowering reagents, has been proven to have a potent effect on preventing retinal neurodegeneration induced by DM [12]. The effect(s) of fibrates, another type of commonly used lipid-lowering drugs, on early retinal neurodegeneration still need further investigation.

* Correspondence: vivianlio@163.com
[1]Department of Ophthalmology, Shaanxi Provincial People's Hospital, No.256 Youyi west Road, Xi'an 710068, Shaanxi Province, China
Full list of author information is available at the end of the article

The introduction of optical coherence tomography (OCT) has provided a useful tool for performing high-resolution imaging of the retina and subsequently measuring the thickness of the retinal nerve fiber layer (RNFL). The decreased RNFL thickness has been considered an important indicator for retinal neurodegeneration [13]. By using OCT several research groups have found that retinal thickness was decreased in diabetic patients without DR or with minimal DR compared to normal controls [14–17], and this decrease was associated with some risk factors, such as glycemic variability and vitamin D deficiency [13, 18]. However, the exact role(s) of these systemic risk factors in the development of retinal neurodegenerative lesions in DR remains largely unknown due to limited data. In the present study, we aimed to investigate the effect of fenofibrate on RNFL loss at early stage of DR and to explore the possible mechanism(s).

Methods

Participants and grouping

A total of 89 patients diagnosed with type 2 diabetes at age 40 or above were recruited from the Department of Endocrinology at Shaanxi provincial peoples' hospital between Jan 1, 2017 and March 31, 2017, among whom were 48 fibrate users and 41 non-fibrate users. Use of fibrates was defined as regular or intermittent administration of fenofibrate for at least 1 year at any dosage. We also retrieved their medication history of taking sulfonylurea and insulin. We included patients who used fenofibrate before or after their diagnosis of diabetes; they either did not have DR or just had non-proliferative diabetic retinopathy (NPDR), but none of them had proliferative diabetic retinopathy. The fenofibrate users were well-matched with those who did not use fenofibrate for gender, age and axial length. We excluded patients younger than 40 years because they were unlikely to receive lipid-lowering reagents [19]. We also excluded patients who had one of the following situation: glaucoma, a positive family history of glaucoma, a refractive error of more than SE + 5 or SE − 3 diopters [13], AL > 25 mm in at least one eye [20], previous refractive surgeries, intraocular surgery, significant media opacity, a history of uveitis or retinal disease and neuro-ophthalmic disease. The patients who had received statins or any other type of lipid-lowering agents regularly were also excluded.

Ophthalmological examinations

We identified all patients with careful examinations of both eyes by ophthalmologists. A detailed review of medical and ocular histories was also carried out for each patient. The fundus was examined with a handheld lens (90D Volk Optical) before the slit-lamp test. DR was graded blindly based on the Early Treatment Diabetic Retinopathy Study (ETDRS). Peripapillary RNFL (pRNFL) thickness was measured with 3D scan OCT imaging (6.0 × 6.0 mm, 512 × 128, 3D OCT-1, ver.8.30, Topcon Corporation, Tokyo, Japan) after pupillary dilation. Only the well-focused and well-centered images with quality strength of 25 or more and without eye movement were analyzed. The superior, inferior, nasal, temporal and average RNFL thickness was measured and then subjected to further analysis. The axial length was measured for three times with Zeiss IOLMaster 500 (Germany). The intraocular pressure (IOP) of all participants was measured with a non-contact tonometer (Tomey FT1000, Japan) for three times. Before each use, the tonometer was calibrated in accordance to the user's manual and only the measurements with errors < 5% were used for data analysis.

Laboratory tests

All included participants were diagnosed with type 2 DM according to the following criteria: a fasting plasma glucose level of 7.0 mmol/L or above or symptoms of diabetes plus a casual blood glucose level of 11.1 mmol/L or above [21]. Oral fenofibrate dosage and duration were collected from both medical records and questionnaires performed by ophthalmologists to ensure the accuracy of data. We defined regular fenofibrate use as a prescription obtained within 1 year after the date of diagnosis. Irregular use was any other use of fenofibrate for at least 1 year. The serum lipid profiles, including total cholesterol (TC), triglycerides (TG), high density lipoprotein cholesterol (HDL-C), low density lipoprotein cholesterol (LDL-C), glycated hemoglobin (HbA1c) and albumin/creatinine ratio (ACR) were collected from patients' medical records.

Statistical analysis

Statistical analyses were performed using GraphPad Prism 7 (GraphPad Software Inc., USA) and SPSS for Windows version 21.0 (SPSS, Inc., Chicago, IL, USA). Data were presented as mean ± standard deviation (SD) of each group. The independent-sample t-test was carried out to compare the means of two groups. The multiple linear regressions analysis was performed to identify factors potentially related to the RNFL loss; in this assay the RNFL thickness in superior quadrant of the right eye was the dependent variable, and the independent variables included age, gender, DR status, diabetes duration, serum lipids, ACR, AL, IOP and the duration of fenofibrate use. A p value < 0.05 was defined as statistically significant.

Results

Basic characteristics of the subjects

According to the inclusion and exclusion criteria, a total of 89 participants (178 eyes) with type 2 DM, aged 40 or above, were included in this study, among whom were 48 fibrate users and 41 non-fibrate users. At baseline, compared to the non-fibrate users, patients who had received fenofibrate treatment had a longer diabetic duration, higher BMI, increased blood TC and TG and lower HDL levels. No significant differences were discovered between the two groups in term of age, gender, AL, IOP, DR status, ACR and medication for DM treatment. The basic clinical and laboratory characteristics of all participants were summarized in (Table 1).

The RNFL thickness

The RNFL thickness of the superior quadrant of the right retina of the non-fibrate users was significantly thinner ($t = -2.384$, $P = 0.019$) than that of the fenofibrate users, which can be seen in the pictures of SD-OCT (Fig. 1a and b). However, no significant differences were discovered in the RNFL thickness of the superior quadrant of the left eye and in the average, inferior, temporal and nasal RNFL thickness of both eyes between the two groups (Table 2).

The potential risk factors for loss of RNFL thickness

To determine whether other risk factors, in particular blood lipids levels, were involved in the thinning of the right eye RNFL, a multiple linear regression analysis was employed and the results were shown in Table 3. Fenofibrate use was positively associated with the RNFL thickness of the superior quadrant of the right eye ($p = 0.042$). On the contrary, BMI ($p = 0.034$) and ACR ($p = 0.024$) were both found negatively correlated with the RNFL thickness of the right eye. However, no relationship between blood lipids levels and RNFL thickness was established in the analysis.

Discussion

The present study investigated the thickness of RNFL at early stage of DR in diabetic patients whom were treated with or without fenofibrate. The results demonstrated that patients who did not use fenofibrate

Table 1 Basic characteristics of the participants

Characteristics	Non-fibrate user	Fibrate user	t/x^2	p
Subjects (N)	41	48	N/A	N/A
Age (yrs)	58.80 ± 12.68	57.71 ± 12.90	0.396	0.693
Women (%)	46.4	37.7	0.646	0.421
Diabetes duration (yrs)	10.39 ± 6.91	7.16 ± 4.92	2.514	*0.014
AL of the right eye (mm)	23.32 ± 0.40	23.45 ± 0.52	1.304	0.195
AL of the left eye (mm)	23.44 ± .056	23.61 ± 0.64	1.322	0.189
IOP of the right eye (mmHg)	19.11 ± 3.32	18.47 ± 4.01	0.811	0.419
IOP of the left eye (mmHg)	18.77 ± 3.99	18.34 ± 4.17	0.494	0.622
BMI(kg/m^2)	24.63 ± 2.62	25.74 ± 2.43	−2.044	*0.044
Laboratory findings				
HbA1c (%)	8.52 ± 0.29	8.46 ± 0.28	0.991	0.324
Total cholesterol (mmol/l)	4.43 ± 0.21	4.75 ± 0.16	−8.148	*0.000
Triglyceride (mmol/l)	2.20 ± 0.28	3.02 ± 0.21	−15.76	*0.000
LDL (mmol/l)	2.74 ± 0.14	2.81 ± 0.12	−1.817	0.072
HDL (mmol/l)	1.27 ± 0.04	1.21 ± 0.05	6.177	*0.000
ACR (μg/mg creatinine)	23.15 ± 35.72	27.49 ± 44.64	−0.500	0.618
DR status (%)				
No DR	34.1	35.5	2.335	0.311
Mild NPDR	48.7	57.7		
Moderate NPDR	17	6.6		
Diabetes treatment (%)				
Sulfonylurea	62.5	58.3	0.035	0.852
Insulin	12.5	16.6	0.065	0.798

Each participant who used fenofibrate was exactly matched with a non-fibrates user for gender, age and DR status. *BMI* body mass index, *DR* diabetic retinopathy, *HbA1c* glycated hemoglobin, *HDL* high-density lipoprotein, *LDL* low-density lipoprotein, *RNFL* retinal nerve fiber layer, *AL* axial length, and *IOP* intraocular pressure. Data represented the mean ± standard deviation (SD) of each group. * $p < 0.05$. $p < 0.05$ was considered statistically significant. Diabetes duration, BMI, total cholesterol, triglyceride, HDL were found significant difference between groups

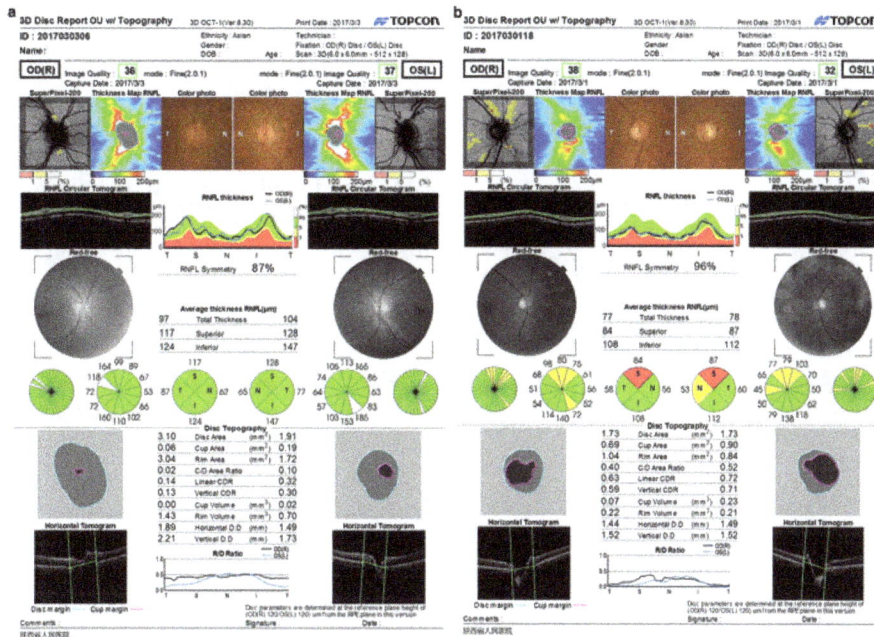

Fig. 1 a and **b**. Representative images of the OCT test for both eyes in two matched patients. (**a**) The OCT image of a patient who use fenofibrate regularly. (**b**) The OCT image of a matched non-fenofibrate user. In both images, green, yellow and red colors represented within normal range, threshold thickness and occurrence of RNFL thinning, respectively

had a thinner superior quadrant RNFL thickness than fenofibrate user, when the results were adjusted for age, gender, AL, IOP, DR status, ACR and medication for DM treatment. Regarding the potential risk factors for RNFL loss, we found that the effect of fenofibrate on RNFL loss was not likely related to its lipid-lowering effect, but might be associated with its ability to regulate vascular endothelial function. This notion, however, needs to be examined by further studies.

DR is considered to be manifested by neurodegenerative changes at early stage before vascular abnormality occurs. Accumulating clinical and experimental studies have shown that neuronal abnormalities and apoptosis of different types of neuronal cells appeared in all retinal layers at early stages of DR [22, 23], and RNFL thinning was considered to be an important changes in diabetic retinal neurodegeneration and related to the severity of DR [24] . Early intervention was the only effective way to delay irreversible vision loss [25]. As one type of the

Table 2 The peripapillary RNFL thickness of fibrate user and non-fibrate user

Eyes	Non-fibrate users ($n = 41$)	Fibrate users ($n = 48$)	t	p
Right eye				
Superior quadrant	111.8 ± 3.596	123.0 ± 3.083	−2.384	*0.019
Inferior quadrant	120.4 ± 3.148	130.0 ± 3.925	−1.863	0.066
Nasal quadrant	70.95 ± 3.065	69.94 ± 2.252	0.271	0.787
Temporal quadrant	78.12 ± 3.021	76.02 ± 1.844	0.605	0.547
Average	95.89 ± 2.611	99.08 ± 2.192	0.940	0.351
Left eye				
Superior quadrant	116.7 ± 3.701	125.5 ± 3.262	−1.788	0.077
Inferior quadrant	124.7 ± 3.397	132.4 ± 3.985	−1.072	0.286
Nasal quadrant	72.51 ± 2.547	69.10 ± 2.127	1.035	0.303
Temporal quadrant	73.32 ± 1.59	72.38 ± 1.504	0.429	0.668
Average	96.95 ± 2.386	99.90 ± 2.089	−0.932	0.353

RNFL retinal nerve fiber layer. Data was presented as means ± SD of each group. *$P < 0.05$. $P < 0.05$ was considered statistically significant between the fibrate user and non-fibrate user group

Table 3 Association between fenofibrate use and the RNFL thickness of the right eye in patients with type 2 diabetes

Risk factors	B	S.E.	Sig.	95%CI for OR	
				upper	lower
Fenofibrate	3.225	1.605	*0.042	0.027	6.424
BMI	−3.475	1.611	*0.034	−6.678	−0.271
ACR	−0.650	0.281	*0.024	−1.210	−0.090
TC	−5.584	−0.269	0.538	−23.58	12.41
TG	−0.779	2.745	0.777	−6.248	4.689
HDL	9.329	13.320	0.486	17.211	35.869
LDL	6.834	10.310	0.510	13.710	27.378
HbA1c	1.382	1.703	0.420	−2.012	4.776
Diabetic duration	−0.337	0.484	0.488	−1.300	0.627
AL	−1.318	0.720	0.061	0.809	15.013
IOP	−0.547	0.550	0.310	0.126	1.573

BMI body mass index, *DR* diabetic retinopathy, *HbA1c* glycated hemoglobin, *HDL* high-density lipoprotein, *LDL* low-density lipoprotein, *TC* Total cholesterol, *TG* Triglyceride, *ACR* urinary albumin-to-creatinine ratio, *RNFL* retinal nerve fiber layer. *S.E.*standard error. *Sig.* significant. *CI* Confidence Interval, *OR* Odds Ratios. The multiple liner regression models were adjusted by age, gender, diabetic duration. * $p < 0.05$. A p value < 0.05 was defined as statistically significant

most widely used lipid-lowering agents, fibrates have been reported to prevent DR progression and to reduce the need for laser treatment [4, 6] [26–29]. However, the correlation between fenofibrate use and retinal neurodegeneration in diabetic patients has not been reported yet. The present study therefore investigated the relationship between use of fenofibrate and the reduction in risk for RNFL loss at early stage of type 2 DM. We found that oral administration of fenofibrate could prevent RNFL loss in the superior quadrant of the right eye in diabetic patients without DR or with NPDR. Patients who never used fibrates had reduced RNFL thickness than those who were administrated with fenofibrate. Choi et al. [30] reported that RNFL defects in type 2 DM occurred more frequently on the superior side of retina (75.6% and 71.0% in right and left eyes, respectively). Lopes et al. [31] also reported that RNFL thickness of the superior segment became significantly thinner in patients with type 1 diabetes without DR than in normal population. Therefore, the superior quadrant of RNFL might represent the earliest and most significantly affected region in the retina; decrease in thickness of this area could be detected with SD-OCT and be used as an important indicator for assessing the effects of fenofibrate.

Fibrates are orally administered fibric acid derivatives that are conventionally used alone or as an adjunct to statins in treating dyslipidemia [32]. To assess whether the effect of fenofibrate on RNFL loss was related to its lipid-lowering effect, we performed a linear regressions analysis for the association between RNFL thickness and

blood lipids levels. However, no significant difference was found between the level of any type of blood lipid and the superior quadrant RNFL thickness of the right eye. The results suggested that lowering the serum lipids levels might not represent the mechanism accounting for fenofibrate's effect on RNFL loss. On the contrary, BMI was found negatively correlated with the superior RNFL thickness of the right eye, therefore, we suggested that restrict control of body weight might be another protective factor for delaying diabetic retinal neurodegeneration in DM patients.

Concerning other factors that might have an effect on RNFL thickness and were not well-matched between two groups, we found that ACR was negatively related to the superior RNFL thickness. ACR was regarded as an indirect indicator of endothelial function [33–35]. Some researchers considered that diabetic retinal neurodegeneration was partially associated with endothelial dysfunction by decreasing blood supply to the optic nerve head [30] [36]. A vascular insufficient optic nerve head might result in RNFL thinning in the optic disc on the superior side because of the gravitational influence. Therefore, vascular endothelial dysfunction represented the main pathophysiology of diabetes and was closely related to the severity of DR and retinal neurodegeneration [37]. We presumed that the effect of fenofibrate on RNFL loss might be partially related to endothelial dysfunction in patients with type 2 DM. However, the specific mechanism still need further study with animal experiments.

Several studies have shown that fibrates could affect signaling pathways involved in inflammation [38], angiogenesis [39] and cell survival [40], such as AMPK pathway [41] that plays important roles in diabetic vascular dysfunction and neurodegeneration. Therefore, we hypothesized that oral administration of fenofibrate might prevent RNFL loss through adjusting the endothelial dysfunction in retina; this could improve blood flow in vessels and reduce vascular leakage [42], and therefore increase the blood supply of the optic disc to avoid cell death. In addition, we also hypothesized that fibrates might delay neuron death and glial cell reactivation through its anti-inflammation and anti-apoptosis properties [43], which needs to be proved by further clinical and experimental studies. However, due to the limitations of observational study, we couldn't assess the direct relationship between fenofibrate administration and ACR fluctuation, which might be completed by a well-matched prospective cohort study in future.

There were several limitations in the present study. Firstly, this was a case-control study, which mainly explored the association between use of fibrates and diabetic RNFL loss but did not take into account the dose of fibrates. Secondly, we didn't perform subgroup analyses to compare the patients who used fibrates regularly and irregularly. Thirdly, we couldn't collect the multi-focal electroretinogram data of all the subjects, which was considered another effective method to assess neurodegeneration in retina [44], because patients at early stage of DR were not requested to do this examination.

Conclusions
Oral administration of fenofibrate was suggestively associated with thicker RNFL in superior quadrant of the right eye of patents with early DR.

Abbreviations
AL: Axial length; BMI: body mass index; DM: Diabetic mellitus; DR: diabetic retinopathy; DR: Diabetic retinopathy; HbA1c: Glycated hemoglobin; HDL: High-density lipoprotein; IOP: Intraocular pressure; LDL: Low-density lipoprotein; RNFL: Retinal nerve fiber layer

Acknowledgements
We thank all patients and their families for kindly participating in the study.

Funding
This work was supported by a grant Science & Technology project for Social development of Shaanxi Province in China (No. 2017SF-249) to Rui Shi. The funders had no role in study design, data collection and analysis, decision to publish, or preparation of the manuscript.

Author contributions
SR designed the study, collected clinical data and performed the analyses; QY operated OCT. SR and ZL drafted and revised the manuscript. All authors read and approved the final version of the manuscript.

Competing interests
All authors declare that they have no competing interests.

Author details
[1]Department of Ophthalmology, Shaanxi Provincial People's Hospital, No.256 Youyi west Road, Xi'an 710068, Shaanxi Province, China. [2]Department of Molecular Physiology and Biophysics, Holden Comprehensive Cancer Center, University of Iowa Carver College of Medicine, Iowa City, IA 52242, USA. [3]Department of Ophthalmology, the First Affiliated Hospital of Xi'an Jiaotong University, Xi'an 710061, Shaanxi Province, China.

References
1. Cheung AK, Fung MK, Lo AC, Lam TT, So KF, Chung SS, Chung SK. Aldose reductase deficiency prevents diabetes-induced blood-retinal barrier breakdown, apoptosis, and glial reactivation in the retina of db/db mice. Diabetes. 2005;54(11):3119–25.
2. Chew EY, Klein ML, Ferris FR, Remaley NA, Murphy RP, Chantry K, Hoogwerf BJ, Miller D. Association of elevated serum lipid levels with retinal hard exudate in diabetic retinopathy. Early treatment diabetic retinopathy study (ETDRS) report 22. Arch Ophthalmol. 1996;114(9):1079–84.
3. Davis MD, Fisher MR, Gangnon RE, Barton F, Aiello LM, Chew EY, Ferris FR, Knatterud GL. Risk factors for high-risk proliferative diabetic retinopathy and severe visual loss: early treatment diabetic retinopathy study report #18. Invest Ophthalmol Vis Sci. 1998;39(2):233–52.
4. Chew EY, Ambrosius WT, Davis MD, Danis RP, Gangaputra S, Greven CM, Hubbard L, Esser BA, Lovato JF, Perdue LH, et al. Effects of medical therapies on retinopathy progression in type 2 diabetes. N Engl J Med. 2010;363(3):233–44.
5. Firth J. Fenofibrate and diabetic retinopathy. Lancet. 2008;371(9614):722, 722.
6. Keech AC, Mitchell P, Summanen PA, O'Day J, Davis TM, Moffitt MS, Taskinen MR, Simes RJ, Tse D, Williamson E, et al. Effect of fenofibrate on the need for laser treatment for diabetic retinopathy (FIELD study): a randomised controlled trial. Lancet. 2007;370(9600):1687–97.
7. Persistent Effects of Intensive Glycemic Control on Retinopathy in Type 2 Diabetes in the Action to Control Cardiovascular Risk in Diabetes (ACCORD) Follow-On Study. Diabetes Care. 2016;39(7):1089–100.
8. Chihara E, Matsuoka T, Ogura Y, Matsumura M. Retinal nerve fiber layer defect as an early manifestation of diabetic retinopathy. Ophthalmology. 1993;100(8):1147–51.
9. Sohn EH, van Dijk HW, Jiao C, Kok PH, Jeong W, Demirkaya N, Garmager A, Wit F, Kucukevcilioglu M, van Velthoven ME, et al. Retinal neurodegeneration may precede microvascular changes characteristic of diabetic retinopathy in diabetes mellitus. Proc Natl Acad Sci U S A. 2016;113(19):E2655–64.
10. Jindal V. Neurodegeneration as a primary change and role of neuroprotection in diabetic retinopathy. Mol Neurobiol. 2015;51(3):878–84.
11. de Moraes G, Layton CJ. Therapeutic targeting of diabetic retinal neuropathy as a strategy in preventing diabetic retinopathy. Clin Exp Ophthalmol. 2016;44(9):838–52.
12. Hernandez C, Garcia-Ramirez M, Corraliza L, Fernandez-Carneado J, Farrera-Sinfreu J, Ponsati B, Gonzalez-Rodriguez A, Valverde AM, Simo R. Topical administration of somatostatin prevents retinal neurodegeneration in experimental diabetes. Diabetes. 2013;62(7):2569–78.
13. Gungor A, Ates O, Bilen H, Kocer I. Retinal nerve Fiber layer thickness in early-stage diabetic retinopathy with vitamin D deficiency. Invest Ophthalmol Vis Sci. 2015;56(11):6433–7.
14. Mizutani T, Fowler BJ, Kim Y, Yasuma R, Krueger LA, Gelfand BD, Ambati J. Nucleoside reverse transcriptase inhibitors suppress laser-induced choroidal neovascularization in mice. Invest Ophthalmol Vis Sci. 2015;56(12):7122–9.
15. Biallosterski C, van Velthoven ME, Michels RP, Schlingemann RO, DeVries JH, Verbraak FD. Decreased optical coherence tomography-measured pericentral retinal thickness in patients with diabetes mellitus type 1 with minimal diabetic retinopathy. Br J Ophthalmol. 2007;91(9):1135–8.
16. Nilsson M, von Wendt G, Wanger P, Martin L. Early detection of macular changes in patients with diabetes using rarebit fovea test and optical coherence tomography. Br J Ophthalmol. 2007;91(12):1596–8.
17. Toprak I, Yildirim C, Yaylali V. Optic disc topographic analysis in diabetic patients. Int Ophthalmol. 2012;32(6):559–64.
18. Picconi F, Parravano M, Ylli D, Pasqualetti P, Coluzzi S, Giordani I, Malandrucco I, Lauro D, Scarinci F, Giorno P, et al. Retinal neurodegeneration in patients with type 1 diabetes mellitus: the role of glycemic variability. Acta Diabetol. 2017;
19. Sugai T, Suzuki Y, Yamazaki M, Shimoda K, Mori T, Ozeki Y, Matsuda H, Sugawara N, Yasui-Furukori N, Minami Y, et al. High prevalence of obesity, hypertension, hyperlipidemia, and diabetes mellitus in Japanese outpatients with schizophrenia: a Nationwide survey. PLoS One. 2016;11(11):e166429.
20. Peng PH, Hsu SY, Wang WS, Ko ML. Age and axial length on peripapillary retinal nerve fiber layer thickness measured by optical coherence tomography in nonglaucomatous Taiwanese participants. PLoS One. 2017;12(6):e179320.
21. Basevi V, Di Mario S, Morciano C, Nonino F, Magrini N. Comment on: American Diabetes Association. Standards of medical care in diabetes–2011. Diabetes care 2011;34(Suppl. 1):S11-S61. DIABETES CARE. 2011;34(5):e53–4.
22. Abu-El-Asrar AM, Dralands L, Missotten L, Al-Jadaan IA, Geboes K. Expression of apoptosis markers in the retinas of human subjects with diabetes. Invest Ophthalmol Vis Sci. 2004;45(8):2760–6.
23. Curtis TM, Hamilton R, Yong PH, McVicar CM, Berner A, Pringle R, Uchida K, Nagai R, Brockbank S, Stitt AW. Muller glial dysfunction during diabetic

retinopathy in rats is linked to accumulation of advanced glycation end-products and advanced lipoxidation end-products. Diabetologia. 2011;54(3): 690–8.

24. Takahashi H, Goto T, Shoji T, Tanito M, Park M, Chihara E. Diabetes-associated retinal nerve fiber damage evaluated with scanning laser polarimetry. Am J Ophthalmol. 2006;142(1):88–94.

25. Stitt AW, Curtis TM, Chen M, Medina RJ, McKay GJ, Jenkins A, Gardiner TA, Lyons TJ, Hammes HP, Simo R, et al. The progress in understanding and treatment of diabetic retinopathy. Prog Retin Eye Res. 2016;51:156–86.

26. Sacks FM. After the Fenofibrate intervention and event lowering in diabetes (FIELD) study: implications for fenofibrate. Am J Cardiol. 2008;102(12A):34L–40L.

27. Massin P, Peto T, Ansquer JC, Aubonnet P, MacuFEN SIF. Effects of fenofibric acid on diabetic macular edema: the MacuFen study. Ophthalmic Epidemiol. 2014;21(5):307–17.

28. Chew EY, Davis MD, Danis RP, Lovato JF, Perdue LH, Greven C, Genuth S, Goff DC, Leiter LA, Ismail-Beigi F, et al. The effects of medical management on the progression of diabetic retinopathy in persons with type 2 diabetes: the action to control cardiovascular risk in diabetes (ACCORD) eye study. Ophthalmology. 2014;121(12):2443–51.

29. Bogdanov P, Hernandez C, Corraliza L, Carvalho AR, Simo R. Effect of fenofibrate on retinal neurodegeneration in an experimental model of type 2 diabetes. Acta Diabetol. 2015;52(1):113–22.

30. Choi JA, Ko SH, Park YR, Jee DH, Ko SH, Park CK. Retinal nerve fiber layer loss is associated with urinary albumin excretion in patients with type 2 diabetes. Ophthalmology. 2015;122(5):976–81.

31. Lopes DFJ, Russ H, Costa VP. Retinal nerve fibre layer loss in patients with type 1 diabetes mellitus without retinopathy. Br J Ophthalmol. 2002;86(7): 725–8.

32. Sharma N, Ooi JL, Ong J, Newman D. The use of fenofibrate in the management of patients with diabetic retinopathy: an evidence-based review. Aust Fam Physician. 2015;44(6):367–70.

33. Jacobsen LM, Winsvold BS, Romundstad S, Pripp AH, Holmen J, Zwart JA. Urinary albumin excretion as a marker of endothelial dysfunction in migraine sufferers: the HUNT study, Norway. BMJ Open. 2013;3(8)

34. Vlachou E, Gosling P, Moiemen NS. Microalbuminuria: a marker of endothelial dysfunction in thermal injury. Burns. 2006;32(8):1009–16.

35. Yan Y, Chang Q, Li Q, Li L, Wang S, Du R, Hu X. Identification of plasma vascular endothelia-cadherin as a biomarker for coronary artery disease in type 2 diabetes mellitus patients. Int J Clin Exp Med. 2015;8(10):19466–70.

36. Ozdek S, Lonneville YH, Onol M, Yetkin I, Hasanreisoglu BB. Assessment of nerve fiber layer in diabetic patients with scanning laser polarimetry. Eye (Lond). 2002;16(6):761–5.

37. Mazereeuw G, Herrmann N, Bennett SA, Swardfager W, Xu H, Valenzuela N, Fai S, Lanctot KL. Platelet activating factors in depression and coronary artery disease: a potential biomarker related to inflammatory mechanisms and neurodegeneration. Neurosci Biobehav Rev. 2013;37(8):1611–21.

38. Chen Y, Hu Y, Lin M, Jenkins AJ, Keech AC, Mott R, Lyons TJ, Ma JX. Therapeutic effects of PPARalpha agonists on diabetic retinopathy in type 1 diabetes models. Diabetes. 2013;62(1):261–72.

39. Panigrahy D, Kaipainen A, Huang S, Butterfield CE, Barnes CM, Fannon M, Laforme AM, Chaponis DM, Folkman J, Kieran MW. PPARalpha agonist fenofibrate suppresses tumor growth through direct and indirect angiogenesis inhibition. Proc Natl Acad Sci U S A. 2008;105(3):985–90.

40. Tomizawa A, Hattori Y, Inoue T, Hattori S, Kasai K. Fenofibrate suppresses microvascular inflammation and apoptosis through adenosine monophosphate-activated protein kinase activation. Metabolism. 2011;60(4):513–22.

41. Kim J, Ahn JH, Kim JH, Yu YS, Kim HS, Ha J, Shinn SH, Oh YS. Fenofibrate regulates retinal endothelial cell survival through the AMPK signal transduction pathway. Exp Eye Res. 2007;84(5):886–93.

42. Hu Y, Chen Y, Ding L, He X, Takahashi Y, Gao Y, Shen W, Cheng R, Chen Q, Qi X, et al. Pathogenic role of diabetes-induced PPAR-alpha down-regulation in microvascular dysfunction. Proc Natl Acad Sci U S A. 2013; 110(38):15401–6.

43. Ouk T, Amr G, Azzaoui R, Delassus L, Fossaert E, Tailleux A, Bordet R, Modine T. Lipid-lowering drugs prevent neurovascular and cognitive consequences of cardiopulmonary bypass. Vasc Pharmacol. 2016;80:59–66.

44. Raz-Prag D, Grimes WN, Fariss RN, Vijayasarathy C, Campos MM, Bush RA, Diamond JS, Sieving PA. Probing potassium channel function in vivo by intracellular delivery of antibodies in a rat model of retinal neurodegeneration. Proc Natl Acad Sci U S A. 2010;107(28):12710–5.

9

Safety and satisfaction of myopic small-incision lenticule extraction combined with monovision

Dan Fu[1†], Li Zeng[1†], Jing Zhao[1], Hua-mao Miao[1], Zhi-qiang Yu[1,2] and Xing-tao Zhou[1,2*]

Abstract

Background: To investigate the safety and optical quality of small-incision lenticule extraction (SMILE) combined with monovision, and patient satisfaction with the procedure.

Methods: The present study assessed a non-random case series involving 60 eyes of 30 patients (mean age 45.53 ± 3.20 years [range 41 to 52 years]) treated bilaterally using the VisuMax 500 system (Carl Zeiss Meditec, Jena, Germany) between January and July 2016. The target refraction was plano for the distance eye, and between − 0.5 and − 1.75 diopters (D) for the near eye. Visual acuity, refraction errors, ocular aberrations, and satisfaction questionnaire scores were calculated 1 year after surgery.

Results: All surgeries were uneventful, with a mean safety index of 1.03 and 1.04 in dominant and nondominant eyes, respectively. Binocular uncorrected distance visual acuity of all patients was ≥20/32, while binocular uncorrected near visual acuity was ≥20/40 1 year postoperatively. Higher-order aberration (0.45 ± 0.14, 0.51 ± 0.15 μm), spherical (0.18 ± 0.15, 0.21 ± 0.14 μm) and coma aberration (0.31 ± 0.16, 0.27 ± 0.17 μm) were identical between dominant and nondominant eyes after surgery. The overall satisfaction rate was 86.7% (26/30), with large contributions from age (OR = 1.76 95% CI: 1.03–2.53; $P = 0.036$). Binocular uncorrected distance visual acuity was related to preoperative spherical diopter ($r = − 0.500$; $P = 0.005$).

Conclusions: Monovision appears to be a safe and effective option for myopia patients with presbyopia who are considering the SMILE procedure. Patients with younger age were more satisfied with the procedure.

Keywords: Monovision, SMILE, Presbyopia, Safety, Satisfaction

Background

Presbyopia refers to an impairment of near vision that is common among adults > 40 years of age, resulting from declined amplitude of accommodation [1]. Currently, several surgical methods are used to correct presbyopia, including the excimer laser procedure, conductive keratoplasty, intrastromal femtosecond ring incisions, and pseudophakic multifocal intraocular lens [2]. Each procedure has advantages and disadvantages; nevertheless, surgical correction of presbyopia remains a major challenge for refractive surgeons. In recent years, refractive surgeries combined with monovision have emerged as an alternative for compensation of presbyopia, and was proven to be effective in conductive keratoplasty and laser in situ keratomileusis [3, 4]. This strategy aims to give patients both near and distance vision without glasses. It is not as invasive as multifocal intraocular changes [3], and more convenient than contact lens correction. However, reduced contrast sensitivity, reduced stereopsis, and small-angle esotropic shift associated with monovision correction were reported to be compromises after surgery [5].

With advances in refractive surgery technology, small incision lenticule extraction (SMILE) is becoming more prevalent due to its excellent safety, efficiency, and good preservation of corneal biomechanics [6, 7]. To the best

* Correspondence: doctzhouxingtao@163.com

Dan Fu and Li Zeng as equal first authors.

[†]Dan Fu and Li Zeng are contributed equally to this work.

[1]Department of Ophthalmology, Eye and ENT Hospital, Fudan University, Shanghai, China

[2]NHC Key Laboratory of Myopia (Fudan University), No. 83 FenYang Road, Shanghai 200031, People's Republic of China

of our knowledge, however, few reports have described visual outcomes of monovision induced by SMILE in myopic patients with presbyopia [8]. Accordingly, we examined monovision combined with SMILE to investigate its efficacy, safety, and patient satisfaction over a long-term follow-up period.

Methods

The present study was a non-comparative case series, and was approved by the Ethics Committee of the Eye and ENT Hospital of Fudan University (Shanghai, China) and a written informed consent from each patient was obtained before surgery as a standard protocol preoperatively. All procedures were adhered to Declaration of Helsinki. Patients who underwent bilateral SMILE (performed by the same surgeon [ZX]) between January and July 2016, with available 1-year follow-up data, were reviewed. A total of 30 patients (10 male; mean age 45.53 ± 3.20 years [range, 41 to 52 years]) were enrolled. The cohort had a mean preoperative spherical diopter (D) of − 6.12 ± 2.39 D (− 1.5 to − 10 D), cylinder of − 0.79 ± 0.62 D (− 3.0 to 0 D), binocular uncorrected near visual acuity ranging from 20/32 to 20/20, and add 0.85 ± 0.56 D (0 to 2.25 D).

Inclusion criteria were as follows: ≥40 years of age; best corrected visual acuity ≥20/20 in either eye; spherical diopter ≤ − 10.0 D; add > 0 D; and cylinder ≤ − 3.0D. Exclusion criteria included severe eye comorbidities such as diabetic retinopathy, age-related macular degeneration, cataract causing visual impairment, or glaucoma with significant field loss, and a history of severe amblyopia or strabismus.

Regular preoperative examinations, including cycloplegic refraction, corrected visual acuity, slit-lamp examination, corneal topography (Pentacam, Oculus Optikgerate, Wetzlar, Germany), ocular aberration (WASCA wavefront analyzer, Carl Zeiss Meditec, Jena, Germany), and fundus examination were performed. The dominant eye was determined using the "hole test" [9]. Patient was asked to align a dot 4 m away through a 1″ diameter hole in a A4 sheet of paper, held at arm length. Two eyes were covered in turn, and the eye with which the dot appeared most centered was regarded as the dominant eye. The procedures above repeated at least 3 times until the result was the same for at least 2 times consecutively.

The 1-year examinations typically included manifest refraction, assessments of monocular and binocular uncorrected distance visual acuity (UDVA) (at 4 m), uncorrected neat visual acuity (UNVA) (at 33 cm) and corrected distance visual acuity (CDVA) under the same illumination. In addition, we constructed a questionnaire considering patient satisfaction including spectacle dependence for daily activities, halo, glare, visual fatigue, dry eye, and overall satisfaction [6]. Each question was graded on 4 levels: 0 indicated no discomfort whatsoever; 1 indicated discomfort occasionally occurred but did not influence life; 2 indicated discomfort, and usually influenced daily life; and 3 indicated discomfort that was too serious to tolerate. At the end of the questionnaire, patients were asked to grade overall satisfaction on a scale between 0 and 10, in which 0 indicated not satisfied at all and 10 indicated extremely satisfied.

The surgical procedure was similar to the standard SMILE treatments described by the authors in a previous study [6]. The dominant eye was corrected for distance and the nondominant eye for near, with target ranging from − 0.5 D to − 1.75 D,. Preoperatively, we used glasses to simulate target refractive status, with binocular distance visual acuity ≥20/32(the residual myopia in the nondominant eye is −X for instance). If X ≥ adding power (A), then residual myopia is set to be −A; if X ≤ A, then residual myopia is set to be −X. The overall purpose of this design was to ensure good postoperative UDVA with increasing near visual acuity as much as possible. Thus, we considered preoperative presbyopia degree only and no preventive amount of residual myopia was added into design. This principle is derived from years of surgical l experience, though individual cases will be adjusted according to the needs of life.

Statistical analysis was performed using SPSS version 22.0 (IBM Corporation, Armonk, NY, USA), and all data are presented as mean ± SD. Visual acuity data are in LogMAR units. The paired t test was performed to compare root mean square (RMS) differences in ocular aberration, and the Wilcoxon signed-rank test was performed to compare safety indexes, which were nonlinear values between the dominant and nondominant eye. For satisfaction was subjectively graded on 4 ordered levels, orderly regression analysis was used to detect factors affecting satisfaction. Factors included in this analysis are age, sex, and preoperative spherical equivalent, which are independent variables.Spearman's test was used to determine relationships between visual acuity and other parameters; $P < 0.05$ was considered to be statistically significant.

Results

All surgeries were uneventful, with no intraoperative or postoperative complications. The mean safety index was 1.03 and 1.04 ($P > 0.05$) in the dominant and nondominant eye, respectively. In the dominant eyes, the percentage of UDVA ≥20/32 were 96.7%; in the nondominant eyes, the percentage of UDVA ≥20/40 was 76.7%. Predictability and accuracy are presented in Fig. 1.

As shown in Figs. 2, 93.3% of the nondominant eyes achieved UNVA ≥20/40, while 76.7% of the dominant eyes achieved UNVA ≥20/40. Binocular near visual acuity ≥20/40 was achieved in all patients.

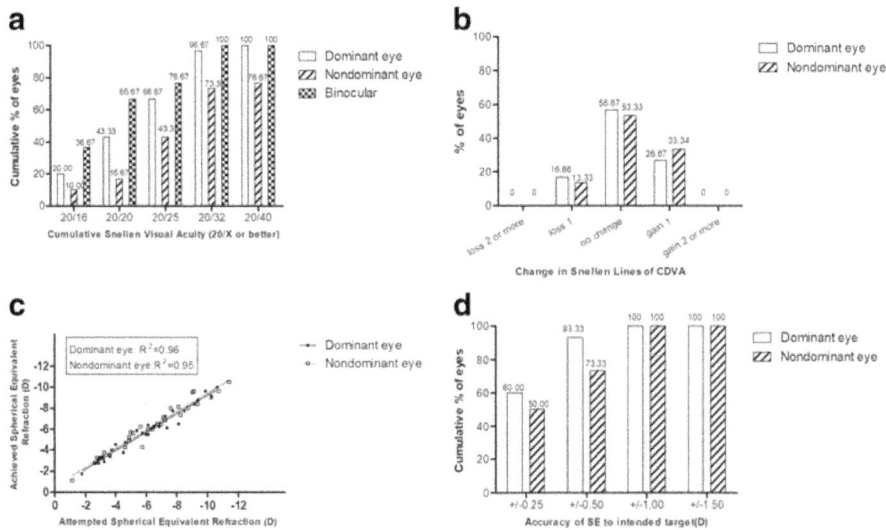

Fig. 1 Refractive outcomes after small incision lenticule extraction combined with monovision. **a** Uncorrected Distance Visual Acuity. **b** Changes in Corrected Distance Visual Acuity. **c** Spherical Equivalent Attempted vs Achieved. **d** Spherical Equivalent Refractive vs Accuracy

Ocular aberrations in both eyes are summarized in Table 1. Compared with preoperative values, the RMS of total high-order aberration (HOA) and spherical aberration were not different postoperatively. Coma increased significantly after surgery (0.17 ± 0.10, 0.29 ± 0.17; $P < 0.001$) (60 eyes).

Results of the satisfaction survey revealed that 63.3, 6.7, and 3.3% patients experienced mild, moderate, and severe halo, respectively; 86.7% patients complained of dry eye, of which 69.2% was mild dry eye. Three patients still required reading glasses occasionally, and 6 required glasses when driving. The completely "glasses-off" rate was 76.7%. The mean satisfaction score was 8.32 ± 1.27 (range 5 to 10).

In orderly regression analysis, age, and sex constitutes a significant mode ($P = 0.02$). On that premise, age (OR = 1.76; 95% CI: 1.03–2.53; $P = 0.036$) was

related to the satisfaction, while sex ($P = 0.67$) was not significant.

Spearman's test revealed that preoperative spherical D was related to postoperative binocular UDVA ($r = -0.500$; $P = 0.005$).

Discussion

Monovision excimer laser correction has a considerable history in photorefractive keratectomy and laser-assisted in situ keratomileusis (LASIK), although various degrees of satisfaction have been reported in previous studies [9, 10]. With the advantages of SMILE highlighted, making use of SMILE combined with monovision has become a new treatment option for individuals with presbyopia. However, few studies have investigated the results of SMILE combined with monovision.

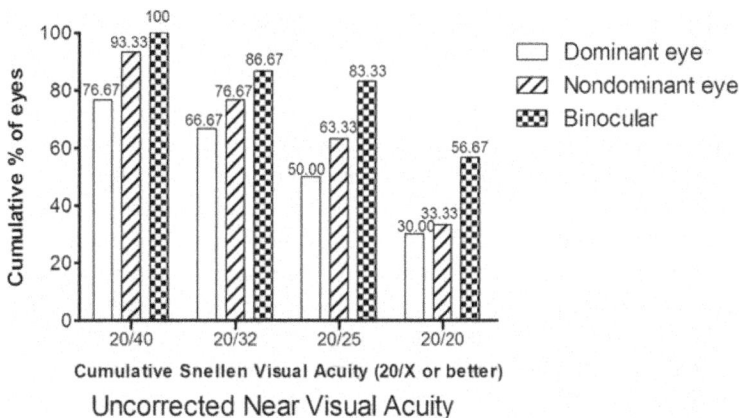

Fig. 2 Near visual acuity after small lenticule extraction combined with monovision

Table 1 Ocular aberration in dominant and nondominant eyes before and after surgery (μm)

	Preoperative (6 mm)			Postoperative (6 mm)			P[a]
	Dominant	Nondominant	P	Dominant	Nondominant	P	
HOA	0.39 ± 0.11	0.41 ± 0.33	0.896	0.45 ± 0.14	0.51 ± 0.15	0.079	0.542
SA	0.15 ± 0.07	0.12 ± 0.07	0.468	0.18 ± 0.15	0.21 ± 0.14	0.092	0.231
Coma	0.17 ± 0.10	0.13 ± 0.11	0.149	0.31 ± 0.16	0.27 ± 0.17	0.317	< 0.001

HOA higher-order aberration, *SA* spherical aberration
[a]Paired *t* test between preoperative and postoperative values

In our study, the mean safety index was 1.04 and 1.03 in the dominant and nondominant eye, respectively, with no statistically significant differences found between eyes. The percentage of remaining or gained BCVA was 83.3 and 86.7% in the dominant and nondominant eyes, respectively. This result is consistent with previous SMILE results [7, 11]. Levinger et al. [10] studied patients ≥40 years of age, and found that BCVA was unchanged at the 1-year follow-up. Both LAISIK and SMILE were demonstrated efficient in presbyopia treatment, though less studies about SMILE monovision are reported [8]. SMILE owes the advantage of smaller incision and less flap-related complication [12]. Accordingly, the visual quality was reported better after SMILE than LASIK, such as ocular aberration and contrast sensitivity [13]. The difference between surgeries may partly account for the various postoperative results and subjective feelings, however, direct comparison is unavailable for different criteria.

All patients in this study achieved a binocular UDVA ≥20/32, and the percentage of binocular UDVA ≥20/25 was 76.7%, which was a significant improvement from preoperative values. In terms of binocular UNVA, 100% of patients achieved UNVA ≥20/40, and the percentage of patients with UNVA ≥20/25 was 83.3%. Accordingly, SMILE combined with monovision was effective in both far and near vision. Similar results were also found in the study by Goldberg et al. [14], in which 79% of patients achieved UDVA ≥20/25, and 87.7% of patients achieved UNVA of J1 or better. However, a retreatment rate of 13.2% was reported in their study, and 5 nondominant eyes were retreated to enhance distance visual acuity. Although no patient requested retreatment in our study, distance vision loss remains a forfeit in most cases with monovision. Garcia-Gonzalez et al. [15] reported a loss in UDVA after LASIK-induced monovision. One patient in our study was dissatisfied with this surgery due to difficulty with night driving [16]. We speculate that interocular blur suppression is less effective at night and this may be a source of postoperative dissatisfaction.

Spherical aberration and HOA were unchanged after surgery, while coma increased significantly. Ocular was usually associated with postoperative glare and halo. It has been reported that SMILE-induced aberration can be restored over a long period [17]. Therefore, unchanged

HOA and spherical aberration may result over a long period. Differences between the dominant and nondominant eyes were not found. A previous study reported that higher myopia errors possibly led to an increase in postoperative coma [18]. Regardless of target myopia in the nondominant eye, we found that the minor monovision would not induce unbalanced ocular aberration in both eyes, which may have contributed to postoperative satisfaction.

The satisfaction rate in this study was 86.7%, which is different from that of contact lens with monovision, which ranged from 60 to 80% in a previous study, [19] and also different from the 96% satisfaction with LASIK-induced monovision reported in the study by Goldberg et al. [14]. Further questioning of the unsatisfied patients revealed the following reasons for dissatisfaction: difficulty with night driving; visual fatigue when reading; and reduction in distance acuity. Unlike LASIK monovision, SMILE lacks the induction of spherical aberration to enhance depth of field. Though near vision is acceptable in current study, the improvement of near vison is not so obvious as the improvement of distance vision for myopic patients. Besides, the target refraction for the nondominant eye ranges from − 0.5 D to − 1.75 D, considering anisometropia tolerance for most patients. Consistent with the recommendation offered by Wright et al. [20] we are cautious about target refractions > − 2.0 D to avoid integration difficulties. Barisic et al. [3] found that − 0.5 D to − 1.25 D was suitable for presbyopic individuals < 50 years of age. Although most individuals are satisfied with this surgery, patient selection and information are critical to optimize monovision designs and warrant further study.

Although age has been considered to be unrelated to the success of monovision, [21] we found that younger individuals in the present study expressed higher satisfaction after surgery. Correspondingly, patients with early presbyopia were more satisfied. Relatively abundant accommodation reserve is helpful in acceptable UNVA. Given less surgery-induced anisometropia, patients with less severe presbyopia may have better optical quality based on a previous study [20]. Patients with higher preoperative spherical diopters tended to experience worse binocular UDVA postoperatively. Kim et al. [22] compared the efficacy of SMILE between subjects with high and mild-moderate myopia, and reported that a lower percentage of patients achieved UDVA ≥20/20 in the high-myopia group 1-year postoperatively. Coincidentally, worse predictability, efficacy and spherical aberration were found in highly myopic patients in the study by Jin et al. [23].

One limitation of the present study was the lack of a control group and, given the relatively small sample size, it was difficult to make comparisons between subgroups. Further comparison between groups stratified according to different target refraction or sex would be interesting areas of investigation. Furthermore, we only analyzed data 1-year postoperatively, and consecutive observation would be helpful to further understand the adaption period of these patients.

Conclusions

In conclusion, SMILE combined with monovision appeared to be safe and effective in a population of presbyopic patients. Patients with younger agewere more satisfied with the procedure.

Abbreviations
CDVA: Corrected distance visual acuity; LASIK: Laser-assisted in situ keratomileusis; SMILE: Small incision lenticule extraction; UDVA: Uncorrected distance visual acuity; UNVA: Uncorrected near visual acuity

Funding
National Natural Science Foundation of China (Grant No. 81570879). Natural Science Foundation of Shanghai (Grant No. 17140902900). National Natural Science Foundation of China for Young Scholars (Grant No. 81600762).

Authors' contributions
FD and ZL drafted the manuscript and performed the literature. ZJ participated in information gathering and editing. MHM, YZQ and ZXT conceived the idea and supervised writing of this paper/ All authors read and approved the final manuscript.

Competing interests
The authors declare that they have no competing interests.

References
1. Patel I, West SK. Presbyopia: prevalence, impact, and interventions. Community Eye Health. 2007;20(63):40–1.
2. Gil-Cazorla R, Shah S, Naroo SA. A review of the surgical options for the correction of presbyopia. Br J Ophthalmol. 2016;100(1):62–70.
3. Barisic A, Gabric N, Dekaris I, Romac I, Bohac M, Juric B. Comparison of different presbyopia treatments: refractive lens exchange with multifocal intraocular lens implantation versus LASIK monovision. Coll Antropol. 2010; 34(Suppl 2):95–8.
4. Wyzinski P. Why are refractive surgeons still wearing glasses? Ophthalmic Surg. 1987;18(5):349–51.
5. Hayashi K, Ogawa S, Manabe S, Yoshimura K. Binocular visual function of modified pseudophakic monovision. Am J Ophthalmol. 2015;159(2):232–40.
6. Miao H, Tian M, Xu Y, Chen Y, Zhou X. Visual outcomes and optical quality after femtosecond laser small incision Lenticule extraction: an 18-month prospective study. J Refract Surg. 2015;31(11):726–31.
7. Vestergaard AH, Grauslund J, Ivarsen AR, Hjortdal JO. Efficacy, safety, predictability, contrast sensitivity, and aberrations after femtosecond laser lenticule extraction. J Cataract Refract Surg. 2014;40(3):403–11.
8. Luft N, Siedlecki J, Sekundo W, Wertheimer C, Kreutzer TC, Mayer WJ, Priglinger SG, Dirisamer M. Small incision lenticule extraction (SMILE) monovision for presbyopia correction. Eur J Ophthalmol. 2018;28(3):287–93.
9. Reinstein DZ, Archer TJ, Gobbe M. LASIK for myopic astigmatism and presbyopia using non-linear aspheric micro-Monovision with the Carl Zeiss Meditec MEL 80 platform. J Refract Surg. 2011;27(1):23–37.
10. Levinger E, Trivizki O, Pokroy R, Levartovsky S, Sholohov G, Levinger S. Monovision surgery in myopic presbyopes: visual function and satisfaction. Optom Vis Sci. 2013;90(10):1092–7.
11. Xu Y, Yang Y. Small-incision lenticule extraction for myopia: results of a 12-month prospective study. Optom Vis Sci. 2015;92(1):123–31.
12. Arba-Mosquera S, de Ortueta D. Geometrical analysis of the loss of ablation efficiency at non-normal incidence. Opt Express. 2008;16(6):3877–95.
13. Fau GS, Gupta R. Comparison of visual and refractive outcomes following femtosecond laser- assisted lasik with smile in patients with myopia or myopic astigmatism. J Refrac Surg. 2014;30(9):590–6.
14. Goldberg DB. Laser in situ keratomileusis monovision. J Cataract Refract Surg. 2001;27(9):1449–55.
15. Garcia-Gonzalez M, Teus MA, Hernandez-Verdejo JL. Visual outcomes of LASIK-induced monovision in myopic patients with presbyopia. Am J Ophthalmol. 2010;150(3):381–6.
16. Chu BS, Wood JM, Collins MJ. Effect of presbyopic vision corrections on perceptions of driving difficulty. Eye Contact Lens. 2009;35(3):133–43.
17. Pedersen IB, Ivarsen A, Hjortdal J. Three-year results of small incision lenticule extraction for high myopia: refractive outcomes and aberrations. J Refract Surg. 2015;31(11):719–24.
18. de Castro LE, Sandoval HP, Bartholomew LR, Vroman DT, Solomon KD. High-order aberrations and preoperative associated factors. Acta Ophthalmol Scand. 2007;85(1):106–10.
19. Jain S, Arora I, Azar DT. Success of monovision in presbyopes: review of the literature and potential applications to refractive surgery. Surv Ophthalmol. 1996;40(6):491–9.
20. Wright KW, Guemes A, Kapadia MS, Wilson SE. Binocular function and patient satisfaction after monovision induced by myopic photorefractive keratectomy. J Cataract Refract Surg. 1999;25(2):177–82.
21. Jain S, Ou R, Azar DT. Monovision outcomes in presbyopic individuals after refractive surgery. Ophthalmology. 2001;108(8):1430–3.
22. Kim JR, Kim BK, Mun SJ, Chung YT, Kim HS. One-year outcomes of small-incision lenticule extraction (SMILE): mild to moderate myopia vs. high myopia. BMC Ophthalmol. 2015;15:59.
23. Jin HY, Wan T, Wu F, Yao K. Comparison of visual results and higher-order aberrations after small incision lenticule extraction (SMILE): high myopia vs. mild to moderate myopia. BMC Ophthalmol. 2017;17(1):118.

10

The prevalence and systemic risk factors of diabetic macular edema

Durgul Acan[1]*, Mehmet Calan[2], Duygu Er[1], Tugba Arkan[2], Nilufer Kocak[1], Firat Bayraktar[2] and Suleyman Kaynak[1]

Abstract

Background: The aim of this study was to evaluate the prevalence of diabetic macular edema (DME) utilizing optical coherence tomography (OCT), and to clarify the effects of the systemic findings and risk factors on the development of DME.

Methods: This cross-sectional study was conducted in the departments of ophthalmology and endocrinology at the Dokuz Eylul University School of Medicine in Izmir, Turkey. The demographics, type and duration of diabetes mellitus, treatment modality, smoking and alcohol consumption habits, as well as the systemic blood pressure, renal functional tests, hemoglobulin A1c level, serum lipid profile, and 24-h urine albumin level were noted and statistically analyzed. The relationships between the systemic findings and DME were studied.

Results: Four-hundred and thirteen eyes of 413 diabetic patients who were examined between January 2011 and July 2012 were enrolled in this study. The prevalence of DME was 15.3% among the patients. The males exhibited DME significantly more frequently than the females ($p = 0.031$), and the duration of diabetes was significantly longer in those patients with DME ($p < 0.001$). Those patients without DME frequently used antihyperlipidemic drugs and had a higher level of high density lipoprotein cholesterol ($p = 0.040$ and $p = 0.046$, respectively). The patient's alcohol consumption, nephropathy, neuropathy, previous cataract surgery, severity of diabetic retinopathy, and insulin usage were statistically significant factors with regard to the DME prevalence.

Conclusions: This study demonstrated the prevalence of DME in Turkey by utilizing OCT. The development of DME can be avoided or limited and the response to treatment may be improved by the regulation of the DME risk factors.

Keywords: Diabetic macular edema, Optical coherence tomography, Prevalence

Background

Since 1980, the adult population living with diabetes has increased four-fold to approximately 422 million according to the most recent World Health Organization's *Global Report on Diabetes*. This sharp rise can be attributed to overweight and obesity, which have resulted in an increase in type 2 diabetes [1]. The prevalence of diabetes in Turkey has recently been reported as 13.2% [2].

The most common reason for vision loss in diabetic patients is diabetic macular edema (DME). Unfortunately, the absolute prevalence of DME may be increasing due to the overall increase in the prevalence of diabetes in industrialized nations [3]. Population-based studies have reported the prevalence of DME in type 1 diabetic patients as 4.2–7.9%, while the rate for type 2 diabetes patients ranges from 1.4–12.8% [4–27]. In a Cochrane review of the DME prevalence evaluated using optical coherence tomography (OCT), the prevalence rates covered a wide range (19%–65%) [28].

In recent years, the use of OCT has become more widespread for the objective measurement of retinal thickness and the other elements of macular edema [29–31]. The Diabetic Retinopathy Clinical Research network (DRCR. net) has adopted standard OCT DME assessments in multicenter studies of diabetic retinopathy (DR). Since this assessment is quantitative with the use of OCT, rather than

* Correspondence: durgul2029@hotmail.com
[1]Department of Ophthalmology, Dokuz Eylul University School of Medicine, Izmir, Turkey
Full list of author information is available at the end of the article

qualitative when applying photography or biomicroscopy, this is considered to be a significant advantage.

The epidemiology and disease burden have not yet been fully elucidated, and there is limited information on the current state of DME in Turkey. Therefore, the aim of this study was to evaluate the prevalence, demographic characteristics of the patients, and systemic associations of DME utilizing OCT in Izmir, Turkey.

Methods

This cross-sectional study was conducted in the departments of ophthalmology and endocrinology at the Dokuz Eylul University School of Medicine in Izmir. A total of 413 eyes of 413 diabetic patients who were followed up in the clinics between January 2011 and July 2012 were enrolled. The demographic data, diabetes type, diabetic age, treatment modality, smoking and alcohol consumption habits, as well as the systemic blood pressure, renal functional test results, hemoglobulin A1c (HbA1c) level, serum lipid profile, 24-h urine albumin level, and the existence of neuropathy were noted and statistically analyzed. The ophthalmological evaluation of each participant included the best corrected visual acuity (BCVA), slit-lamp biomicroscopy, intraocular pressure (IOP) measurement, and dilated fundoscopy. Fluorescein angiography and a central macular thickness (CMT) analysis with OCT were also performed. The relationships between the systemic findings and the prevalence of DME were studied.

Those patients ≥18 years old with type 1 or 2 diabetes diagnosed by an endocrinologist at the Dokuz Eylul University Hospital Endocrinology Clinic between January 2011 and July 2012, who were then referred to the Ophthalmology Department Retina Unit for DME and DR screenings, were included in this study.

The exclusion criteria were as follows: eyes with an ocular abnormality other than DME (vitreomacular traction, epiretinal membrane, etc.) and media opacities interfering with the reliability of OCT imaging (dense cataract, uveitis, etc.), and those patients with insufficient data for the study protocol.

Ophthalmological examination

The BCVA was evaluated using the Bailey-Lovie chart after correcting for refractive errors. An anterior segment examination was conducted using slit-lamp biomicroscopy and dilated fundoscopy. The IOP was obtained with a Goldmann applanation tonometer, and Heidelberg retinal angiography (HRA) and OCT were performed using the Spectralis HRA-OCT II (Heidelberg, Germany). After obtaining a fixation point for the patient, 6 OCT shots were lined up with the radial line scan and each other at an angle of 30°. The eyes were evaluated for clinically significant macular edema

(CSME) as defined by the Early Treatment Diabetic Retinopathy Study (ETDRS) and with a central macular thickness (CMT) (mean thickness at the point of the intersection of 6 radial scans) via OCT ≥ 250 μm attributable to DME [32].

Statistical analysis

The data from all of the subjects who fulfilled the inclusion/exclusion criteria were analyzed using SPSS 16.0 software. For the descriptive analysis, the mean, standard deviation, and percentage were used. The chi-squared test, Fisher's exact test, and t-test were applied for the univariate analysis. A p value < 0.05 was considered to be statistically significant.

Results

Of the 425 patients who met the study criteria, 413 were included for evaluation. DME was detected in 15.3% (63) of the patients and DR was determined in 32% (132) of the patients. Moreover, DME was found in 14.8% (4) of the patients with type 1 diabetes and in 15.3% (59) of the patients with type 2 diabetes ($p = 0.604$). Of the 63 DME patients, 15 received previous focal/grid laser treatments, 8 received previous intravitreal anti-vascular endothelial growth factor (VEGF) or steroid treatments, and 5 received previous combined focal/grid laser and anti-VEGF/steroid treatments. In addition, 9 patients without DME received previous focal/grid treatments and one patient underwent a vitrectomy.

The demographic and laboratory characteristics of the patients are summarized in Table 1. DME was significantly more prevalent in the males than the females ($p = 0.031$), and the male subjects had higher HbA1c levels than the female subjects ($8.30 \pm 2.25\%$ and $7.89 \pm 2.13\%$, respectively) ($p = 0.054$). Although there was no direct statistical correlation between the HbA1c levels and DME, a significant increase in the frequency of DME was observed particularly in those subjects with HbA1c values of 7.0% or more ($p = 0.037$). While the type of diabetes did not have an effect on DME, the duration of diabetes was significantly longer in the DME patients, particularly in those diagnosed between 10 and 20 years previously ($p < 0.001$). Those patients without DME were determined to have a significantly higher rate of antihyperlipidemic drug usage and a higher level of high density lipoprotein cholesterol (HDL-C) ($p = 0.040$ and $p = 0.046$, respectively). The mean serum creatinine levels in those patients with and without DME were 1.13 ± 0.81 mg/dL and 0.87 ± 0.63 mg/dL, respectively, and this difference was statistically significant ($p = 0.021$).

In the comparison of the normoalbuminuric, microalbuminuric, and macroalbuminuric patients in terms of the DME frequency, a statistically significant difference was seen between the 3 groups ($p < 0.001$). While 11.0%

Table 1 Comparison of the demographic and laboratory characteristics of the patients with and without DME

Characteristics	Patients with DME (n = 63, 15.3%)	Patients without DME (n = 350, 84.7%)	P value
Age (years)	58.86 ± 11.27	56.03 ± 11.95	0.082
Gender (female/male)	26/37	196/154	0.031*
BMI (kg/m^2)	29.25 ± 5.78	29.46 ± 5.80	0.797
Type of diabetes (1/2)	4/59	23/327	0.604
Duration of diabetes (years)	16.77 ± 8.16	7.64 ± 7.12	< 0.001*
DR (n)			
Mild-moderate DR	18 (28.6%)	52 (14.9%)	< 0.001*
Severe-very severe	10 (15.9%)	6 (1.7%)	
PDR	35 (55.5%)	11 (3.1%)	
Smoking (n = 97, 23.5%)	12 (19%)	85 (24.2%)	0.367
Alcohol (n = 10, 2.4%)	5 (7.9%)	5 (1.4%)	0.010*
Hypertension (n = 242, 58.5%)	42 (66.6%)	200 (57.1%)	0.158
Systolic blood pressure (mmHg)	130.37 ± 20.15	128.56 ± 17.86	0.469
Diastolic blood pressure (mmHg)	79.25 ± 8.87	79.05 ± 9.91	0.881
Anti-hyperlipidemic drug usage (n = 109, 26.4%)	10 (15.9%)	99 (28.3%)	0.040*
CVD (n = 78, 18.9%)	16 (25.4%)	62 (17.7%)	0.152
Peripheral neuropathy (n = 209, 50.6%)	42 (66.6%)	167 (47.7%)	0.006*
Nephropathy (n = 99, 24.0%)	28 (44.4%)	71(20.3%)	< 0.001*
Normoalbuminuria (n = 314, 76%)	35 (55.5%)	279 (79.7%)	< 0.001*
Microalbuminuria (n = 69, 16.7%)	20 (31.7%)	49 (14%)	
Macroalbuminuria (n = 30, 7.3%)	8 (12.7%)	22 (6.2%)	
HbA1c (%)	8.39 ± 1.97	8.02 ± 2.23	0.226
FBG (mg/dL)	164.50 ± 57.86	157.50 ± 65.84	0.523
Creatinine (mg/dL)	1.13 ± 0.81	0.87 ± 0.63	0.021*
GFR (mL/min/1.73 m^2)	76.21 ± 28.82	88.25 ± 22.35	0.002*
Total cholesterol (mg/dL)	187.95 ± 41.75	194.00 ± 50.72	0.372
LDL-C (mg/dL)	114.44 ± 33.76	117.85 ± 36.72	0.494
HDL-C (mg/dL)	40.19 ± 11.87	43.45 ± 11.92	0.046*
Triglyceride (mg/dL)	165.24 ± 86.87	158.52 ± 113.69	0.656

Results are given as the mean ± SD. A p value of < 0.05 was considered to be significant (*). *BMI* body mass index, *CVD* cardiovascular disease, *CMT* central macular thickness, *DR* diabetic retinopathy, *HbA1* hemoglobin A1c, *GFR* glomerular filtration rate, *FBG* fasting blood glucose, *HDL-C* high density lipoprotein cholesterol, *LDL-C* low density lipoprotein cholesterol, *PDR* proliferative diabetic retinopathy

of the patients without nephropathy had DME, 29.0% of patients with microalbuminuria and 26.7% of the patients with macroalbuminuria had DME ($p < 0.001$). Peripheral neuropathy was also significantly frequent in those patients with DME ($p = 0.006$). The mean BCVAs of the eyes with and without DME were 0.55 ± 0.59 logMAR and 0.04 ± 0.10 logMAR, respectively ($p < 0.001$). The mean IOPs of the eyes with and without DME were 14.91 ± 2.45 mmHg and 15.12 ± 2.64 mmHg, respectively, and no statistical difference was seen ($p = 0.562$).

The prevalence of DME was 28.6% in those patients with mild to moderate non-proliferative diabetic retinopathy (NPDR) and 72.6% in those patients with severe NPDR to proliferative diabetic retinopathy (PDR) ($p < 0.001$). The DME prevalences in the phakic and pseudophakic eyes were 12.9% (49) and 43.7% (14), respectively ($p < 0.001$). Assuming the possible effects of cataract surgery on DME and evaluating only the phakic patients showed that the duration of diabetes, nephropathy, neuropathy, and antihyperlipidemic drug use significantly affected the DME in similar ways ($p < 0.001$, $p = 0.020$, $p = 0.012$, and $p = 0.038$, respectively). However, in the phakic patients, the gender, creatinine level, and HDL-C level did not have statistically significant effects on the DME ($p = 0.610$, $p = 0.227$, and $p = 0.233$, respectively).

Discussion

There is a known increasing worldwide prevalence of DME. Correspondingly, an increase in diabetes-related complications is expected with the increase in diabetes mellitus cases in Turkey. In one study from Turkey, the prevalence of DME was found to be 14.2% in the pre-OCT era [33]. Most studies have used non-stereoscopic fundus photography; therefore, the accuracy of the DME assessment is in doubt. The use of stereoscopic slit-lamp biomicroscopy alone may also lead to both the underdiagnosis and overdiagnosis of DME. Macular edema was defined using the CSME criteria in approximately one-half of the previous studies, and thus, only covered the more severe DME spectrum. The clinical use of OCT has enabled the detection of DME that was previously overlooked in a stereoscopic fundus examination. When compared to a clinical examination, the OCT detection and assessment of DME is more objective and reproducible, ensuring greater uniformity in the interventions applied and the treatment outcomes when compared to the pre-OCT era [34, 35]. According to DRCR.net, for DME trial inclusion and retreatment eligibility, the central subfield mean thickness on a Stratus OCT must be ≥250 μm. The current study used the Spectralis HRA-OCT II, which produces high resolution histological macular images, and the prevalence of DME was found to be 15.3%. This ratio was higher than the prevalence in a previous study conducted in 2006, and thus supports the sensitivity of the OCT.

The DME prevalence is related to the disease duration. In the present study, the prevalence of DME was 2.8% within 5 years of the diabetes diagnosis and 22.0% 5 years after the diagnosis ($p < 0.001$). After 10 years, the prevalence rose prominently. In a study by Aiello et al. [36], the prevalence was 5% within the first 5 years after the diagnosis and 15% at 15 years.

The males in this study exhibited DME more frequently than the females, and the odds ratio (OR) for the males was 1.811 (95% CI: $1.051 < OR < 3.121$) ($p = 0.031$). In addition, the HbA1c levels were significantly higher in the males than the females; therefore, and it can be suggested that not only gender, but also worse diabetic control in male patients can indicate a higher prevalence of DME. The HbA1c level in the patients with DME ($8.39 \pm 1.97\%$) was slightly higher than that in the patients without DME ($8.02 \pm 2.23\%$), but this difference was not statistically significant ($p = 0.226$). The prevalences of DME in those patients with HbA1c levels $< 7.0\%$ and $\geq 7.0\%$ were 10.62% and 18.18%, respectively ($p = 0.037$). In the Diabetes Control and Complications Trial (DCCT), it was shown that the strict control of blood glucose in type 1 diabetes patients led to a 29% decrease in the cumulative incidence of macular edema at the 9-year follow-up, and halved the application of focal laser treatment for DME [37, 38]. Even if

there is a deterioration in control later in life, the effects of improved glycemic control sustained over many years have been shown to persist. In the Epidemiology of Diabetes Interventions and Complications (EDIC) study, which was an extension of the DCCT in which the level of glycemic control of the former intensive and conventional control groups converged, it was reported that the former intensive control group continued to fare better than the former conventional control group. Four years after the end of the DCCT, the CSME incidence was 2% in the former intensive control group, compared to the 8% rate in the former conventional control group ($p < 0.001$) [39].

In the UK Prospective Diabetes Study, an analogous, randomized clinical trial of type 2 diabetes patients, it was reported that strict blood glucose control resulted in a 29% reduction in laser treatment in a follow-up period of 10 years; of the laser treatments required, 78% were for DME [40]. In the current study, the prevalence of DME was conspicuously higher in the insulin-taking patients ($p < 0.000$). In previous studies, taking insulin has been reported to trigger the development of DME in the acute period. In this period, the hypoxia-inducible factor connects to the VEGF promotor region, and the VEGF transcription increases. Subsequently, the blood-retina barrier breaks down and permeability increases with the activation of protein kinase C. In the chronic period, insulin shows anti-inflammatory and anti-apoptotic effects and reduces oxidative stress [41]. The high prevalence of DME in the insulin-taking patients in the present study may be the result of the poor glycemic control in these patients.

The UK Prospective Diabetes Study also reported that the mean systolic blood pressure was reduced by 10 mmHg and the diastolic blood pressure was reduced by 5 mmHg in a median follow-up period of 8.4 years, which resulted in a 35% decrease in the retinal laser treatments, 78% of which were for DME [42]. In addition, the Wisconsin Epidemiologic Study of Diabetic Retinopathy determined that systemic hypertension increased the prevalence of DME 3-fold. It has been suggested that not only is hypertension a risk factor for macular edema development, but the treatment may have important benefits in patients with uncontrolled hypertension [43]. In the current study, the prevalences of DME in those patients with and without systemic hypertension were 17.4% and 12.3%, respectively ($p = 0.158$). In addition, there was no statistically significant difference with respect to the systolic and diastolic blood pressure levels between those patients with and without DME. However, anti-hypertensive medications may affect these results. The beneficial effects of anti-hypertensive medications that target the renin-angiotensin-aldosterone system (RAAS) in DR and DME have been evaluated in several clinical trials, such as the

Diabetic Retinopathy Candesartan Trials (DIRECT) and Renin-Angiotensin System Study (RASS).

A recent meta-analysis revealed that patients with DME or PDR were more likely to have incident cardiovascular disease (CVD) and fatal CVD when compared to those without DME or PDR in type 2 diabetes mellitus [44]. It is accepted that fluid retention due to cardiac failure, or another CVD can exacerbate DME and may be an important concern when managing it [45]. In the present study, DME was detected in 20.5% (16) of the patients with type 2 diabetes and CVD and in 14.0% (43) of those without CVD, but the difference was not statistically significant ($p = 0.151$). However, the patients were not examined by a cardiologist, the subclinical findings may not have been noticed, and/or the patients may not have been aware of their CVD.

The prevalence of DME was significantly higher in those patients who consumed alcohol (50%) ($p = 0.010$). In the advanced analysis, alcohol consumption was seen to increase the odds-relative risk 5.95-fold (95% CI: $1.67 < OR < 21.19$). This could be due to the deleterious effects of alcohol on glycemic control or because of the compromised treatment compliance in patients who drink regularly. However, in a previous study from Turkey, there was no significant correlation between alcohol consumption and the prevalence of DME [33].

Dyslipidemia has been implicated as an independent risk factor for vision loss and DME [46–48]; however, no single lipid measure has been found to be consistently associated with DR or DME [49]. Of the recent studies, only the Madrid Diabetes Study determined an association between low density lipoprotein cholesterol (LDL-C) and DR incidence [50]. In the current study, the HDL-C was significantly lower in the patients with DME ($p = 0.046$). Moreover, the prevalences of DME in the patients who were and were not using antihyperlipidemic drugs were 9.2% and 17.4%, respectively ($p = 0.040$). Of the 109 patients using antihyperlipidemic drugs, 106 were taking statins. In a 2004 study, it was reported that the atorvastatin in statins reduced the severity of hard exudates and the migration of subfoveal lipids in CSME in dyslipidemic type 2 diabetic patients [51]. In another study from Greece, the use of atorvastatin reduced the severity of hard exudates and fluorescein leakage in diabetic maculopathy in dyslipidemic diabetic patients [52]. In DME-associated lipid exudates, there will generally be a spontaneous resolution over 2 years or longer [53]. Macrophages clear the exudates by phagocytosis [54], and the clearance of lipid exudates in DME can be independently accelerated by serum lipid control and by focal/grid photocoagulation [51]. With decreasing serum lipid levels, statins are also thought to reduce inflammation and secondary microvascular leukocytosis [54]. In contrast, one meta-analysis reported the dose-dependent

relationship between statin use and an increased risk of diabetes [55]. This led to the belief that statins might influence glucose homeostasis by decreasing insulin production or increasing insulin resistance, or both [56]. Consequently, the effects of statins on diabetes and DME remain controversial.

The mean serum creatinine levels in patients with and without DME were 1.13 ± 0.81 mg/dl and 0.87 ± 0.63 mg/dl, respectively, and this difference was statistically significant ($p = 0.021$). While 11% of the patients without nephropathy had DME, 29.0% of the patients with microalbuminuria and 26.7% of patients with macroalbuminuria did ($p < 0.001$). In a 15-year follow-up study, the development of macroalbuminuria was found to be associated with the development of DME in type 1 diabetes [57]. In this study, not only macroalbuminuria, but also microalbuminuria was associated with DME.

The major ocular risk factor associated with DME is DR severity. Although DME can be seen at any level of DR, an increasing DR severity has been associated with an increasing prevalence of DME [58–62]. In one study, the 14-year incidence of DME increased from 25% to 37% as the baseline retinopathy severity increased from mild to moderate NPDR [60]. In addition, point estimates of 4% and 15% for the prevalence of subclinical DME in mild to moderate NPDR and severe NPDR to PDR, respectively, have been reported. In this study, the DME prevalence rate was 28.6% in those patients with mild-moderate NPDR, while it was 72.6% in those patients with severe NPDR to PDR ($p < 0.001$).

Starling's law explains the balance between intravascular and extravascular liquid passage. Based on this, a study published decades ago advocated the idea that high IOP levels protect against the development of exudates [62]. However, there has not yet been enough research done in this regard. In this study, the mean IOPs in those eyes with and without DME were 14.91 ± 2.45 mmHg and 15.12 ± 2.64 mmHg, respectively, but the difference was not statistically significant ($p = 0.562$). Although the findings are inconsistent, diabetes has been found to be a risk factor for developing primary glaucoma in some population-based studies [63]. For instance, the Singapore Malay Eye Study found an association between ocular hypertension and diabetes, but not glaucoma [64].

Diabetes is associated with the early and rapid development of cataracts, and cataract surgery, other types of intraocular surgery, and ocular inflammatory disease may produce inflammatory and angiogenic mediators that can produce macular edema in eyes with or without DR [65–69]. In accordance with this, in the present study, the DME prevalences in the phakic and pseudophakic eyes were 12.9% (49) and 43.7% (14), respectively ($p < 0.001$).

Conclusions

In 2010, the prevalence of diabetes in Turkey was 13.7% as reported in the Turkish Diabetes Epidemiology II (TURDEP-II) study. In the USA, DR is the leading cause of blindness in individuals aged < 60 years old, and DME is the most common cause of visual loss in those with DR [56, 66]. Fortunately, permanent vision loss can be prevented by the early diagnosis and treatment of DME. The DME prevalence has been reported at a wide range of rates in numerous studies in the literature, but there have been no previous studies in Turkey on this topic. The development of DME may be avoided or limited and the response to treatment may be improved by the regulation of the DME risk factors. In this study, the prevalence of DME was associated with male gender, diabetes duration, HbA1c ≥ 7.0%, insulin usage, alcohol consumption, low HDL-C levels, nephropathy, neuropathy, severity of DR, and previous cataract surgery. However, antihyperlipidemic drugs may be protective against DME. The cross-sectional design could be considered a limitation of this study; therefore, longitudinal studies with more subjects are needed.

Abbreviations

BCVA: Best corrected visual acuity; CMT: Central macular thickness; CSME: Clinically significant macular edema; DCCT: Diabetes Control and Complications Trial; DIRECT: Diabetic Retinopathy Candesartan Trials; DME: Diabetic macular edema; DR: Diabetic retinopathy; DRCR.net: Diabetic Retinopathy Clinical Research network; EDIC: Epidemiology of Diabetes Interventions and Complications; HbA1c: Hemoglobin A1c; HDL-C: High density lipoprotein cholesterol; IOP: Intraocular pressure; LDL-C: Low density lipoprotein cholesterol; NPDR: Non-proliferative diabetic retinopathy; OCT: Optical coherence tomography; PDR: Proliferative diabetic retinopathy; RAAS: Renin-angiotensin-aldosterone system; RASS: Renin-Angiotensin System Study; VEGF: Vascular endothelial growth factor

Acknowledgements
None.

Funding
None.

Authors' contributions
DA: 1st author, conception and design, data collection, analysis and interpretation, writing the manuscript, critical revision of the manuscript, and statistical expertise. MC, DE, and TA: data collection. NK and SK: analysis and interpretation, writing the manuscript, and critical revision of the manuscript. FB: conception and design. All authors read and approved the final manuscript.

Competing interests
The authors declare that they have no competing interests.

Author details
[1]Department of Ophthalmology, Dokuz Eylul University School of Medicine, Izmir, Turkey. [2]Department of Endocrinology and Metabolism, Dokuz Eylul University School of Medicine, Izmir, Turkey.

References

1. Global report on diabetes. World Health Organization, Geneva. 2016. http://www.who.int/diabetes/global-report/en/.
2. Diabetes country profiles. World Health Organization, Geneva. 2016. http://www.who.int/diabetes/country-profiles/en/.
3. Cugati S, Kifley A, Mitchell P, Wang JJ. Temporal trends in the age-specific prevalence of diabetes and diabetic retinopathy in older persons: population-based survey findings. Diabetes Res Clin Pract. 2006;74:301–8.
4. Pedro RA, Ramon SA, Marc BB, Juan FB, Isabel MM. Prevalence and relationship between diabetic retinopathy and nephropathy, and its risk factors in the north-east of Spain, a population-based study. Ophthalmic Epidemiol. 2010;17:251–65.
5. Bertelsen G, Peto T, Lindekleiv H, Schirmer H, Solbu MD, Toft I, Sjølie AK, Njølstad I. Tromsø eye study: prevalence and risk factors of diabetic retinopathy. Acta Ophthalmol. 2013;91:716–21.
6. Knudsen LL, Lervang HH, Lundbye-Christensen S, Gorst-Rasmussen A. The north Jutland county diabetic retinopathy study: population characteristics. Br J Ophthalmol. 2006;90:1404–9.
7. Roy MS, Klein R, O'Colmain BJ, Klein BE, Moss SE, Kempen JH. The prevalence of diabetic retinopathy among adult type 1 diabetic persons in the United States. Arch Ophthalmol. 2004;122:546–51.
8. Kempen JH, O'Colmain BJ, Leske MC, Haffner SM, Klein R, Moss SE, Taylor HR, Hamman RF, Eye Diseases Prevalence Research Group. The prevalence of diabetic retinopathy among adults in the United States. Arch Ophthalmol. 2004;122:552–63.
9. Zhang X, Saaddine JB, Chou CF, Cotch MF, Cheng YJ, Geiss LS, Gregg EW, Albright AL, Klein BE, Klein R. Prevalence of diabetic retinopathy in the United States, 2005–2008. JAMA. 2010;304:649–56.
10. Jee D, Lee WK, Kang S. Prevalence and risk factors for diabetic retinopathy: the Korea National Health and nutrition examination survey 2008–2011. Invest Ophthalmol Vis Sci. 2013;54:6827–33.
11. Raman R, Rani PK, Reddi Rachepalle S, Gnanamoorthy P, Uthra S, Kumaramanickavel G, Sharma T. Prevalence of diabetic retinopathy in India: Sankara Nethralaya diabetic retinopathy epidemiology and molecular genetics study report 2. Ophthalmology. 2009;116:311–8.
12. Zheng Y, Lamoureux EL, Lavanya R, Wu R, Ikram MK, Wang JJ, Mitchell P, Cheung N, Aung T, Saw SM, Wong TY. Prevalence and risk factors of diabetic retinopathy in migrant Indians in an urbanized society in Asia: the Singapore Indian eye study. Ophthalmology. 2012;119:2119–24.
13. Al Ghamdi AH, Rabiu M, Hajar S, Yorston D, Kuper H, Polack S. Rapid assessment of avoidable blindness and diabetic retinopathy in Taif, Saudi Arabia. Br J Ophthalmol. 2012;96:1168–72.
14. Dehghan MH, Katibeh M, Ahmadieh H, Nourinia R, Yaseri M. Prevalence and risk factors for diabetic retinopathy in the 40 to 80 year-old population in Yazd, Iran: the Yazd eye study. J Diabetes. 2015;7:139–41.
15. Thapa R, Joshi DM, Rizyal A, Maharjan N, Joshi RD. Prevalence, risk factors and awareness of diabetic retinopathy among admitted diabetic patients at a tertiary level hospital in Kathmandu. Nepal J Ophthalmol 2014;6:24–30.
16. Kahloun R, Jelliti B, Zaouali S, Attia S, Ben Yahia S, Resnikoff S, Khairallah M. Prevalence and causes of visual impairment in diabetic patients in Tunisia, North Africa. Eye. 2014;28:986–91.
17. Mathenge W, Bastawrous A, Peto T, Leung I, Yorston D, Foster A, Kuper H. Prevalence and correlates of diabetic retinopathy in a population-based survey of older people in Nakuru, Kenya. Ophthalmic Epidemiol. 2014;21:169–77.
18. Sharew G, Ilako DR, Kimani K, Gelaw Y. Prevalence of diabetic retinopathy in Jimma University Hospital, Southwest Ethiopia. Ethiop Med J. 2013;51:105–13.
19. Wong TY, Cheung N, Tay WT, Wang JJ, Aung T, Saw SM, Lim SC, Tai ES, Mitchell P. Prevalence and risk factors for diabetic retinopathy: the Singapore Malay eye study. Ophthalmology. 2008;115:1869–75.
20. Al-Rubeaan K, Abu El-Asrar AM, Youssef AM, Subhani SN, Ahmad NA, Al-Sharqawi AH, Alquwaihes A, Alotaibi MS, Al-Ghamdi A, Ibrahim HM. Diabetic retinopathy and its risk factors in a society with a type 2 diabetes epidemic: a Saudi National Diabetes Registry-based study. Acta Ophthalmol. 2015;93:e140–7.
21. Pugliese G, Solini A, Zoppini G, Fondelli C, Zerbini G, Vedovato M, Cavalot F, Lamacchia O, Buzzetti R, Morano S, Nicolucci A, Penno G, Renal Insufficiency and Cardiovascular Events (RIACE) Study Group. High prevalence of advanced retinopathy in patients with type 2 diabetes from the renal insufficiency and cardiovascular events (RIACE) Italian multicenter study. Diabetes Res Clin Pract. 2012;98:329–37.

22. Dutra Medeiros M, Mesquita E, Papoila AL, Genro V, Raposo JF. First diabetic retinopathy prevalence study in Portugal: RETINODIAB study-evaluation of the screening programme for Lisbon and Tagus Valley region. Br J Ophthalmol. 2015;99:1328–33.

23. Nathoo N, Ng M, Rudnisky CJ, Tennant MT. The prevalence of diabetic retinopathy as identified by teleophthalmology in rural Alberta. Can J Ophthalmol. 2010;45:28–32.

24. Esteves JF, Kramer CK, Azevedo MJ, Stolz AP, Roggia MF, Larangeira A, Miozzo SA, Rosa C, Lambert JH, Pecis M, Rodriques TC, Canani LH. Prevalence of diabetic retinopathy in patients with type 1 diabetes mellitus. Rev Assoc Med Bras. 2009;55:268–73.

25. Villena JE, Yoshiyama CA, Sanchez JE, Hilario NL, Merin LM. Prevalence of diabetic retinopathy in Peruvian patients with type 2 diabetes: results of a hospital-based retinal telescreening program. Rev Panam Salud Publica. 2011;30:408–14.

26. Thomas RL, Distiller L, Luzio SD, Chowdhury SR, Melville VJ, Kramer B, Owens DR. Ethnic differences in the prevalence of diabetic retinopathy in persons with diabetes when first presenting at a diabetes clinic in South Africa. Diabetes Care. 2013;36:336–41.

27. Kaidonis G, Mills RA, Landers J, Lake SR, Burdon KP, Craig JE. Review of the prevalence of diabetic retinopathy in indigenous Australians. Clin Exp Ophthalmol. 2014;42:875–82.

28. Virgili G, Menchini F, Murro V, Peluso E, Rosa F, Casazza G. Optical coherence tomography (OCT) for detection of macular oedema in patients with diabetic retinopathy. Cochrane Database Syst Rev. 2011;7:CD008081.

29. Koozekanani D, Roberts C, Katz SE, Herderick EE. Intersession repeatability of macular thickness measurements with the Humphrey 2000 OCT. Invest Ophthalmol Vis Sci. 2000;41:1486–91.

30. Hee MR, Puliafito CA, Wong C, et al. Quantitative assessment of macular edema with optical coherence tomography. Arch Ophthalmol. 1995;113:1019–29.

31. Hee MR, Puliafito CA, Duker JS, Reichel E, Coker JG, Wilkins JR, Schuman JS, Swanson EA, Fujimoto JG. Topography of diabetic macular edema with optical coherence tomography. Ophthalmology. 1998;105:360–70.

32. Early Treatment Diabetic Retinopathy Study Research Group. Photocoagulation for diabetic macular edema. Early treatment diabetic retinopathy study report number 1. Arch Ophthalmol. 1985;103:1796–806.

33. Taş A, Bayraktar MZ, Erdem Ü, Sobacı G, Açıkel C, Durukan AH, Karagül S. Diyabetik hastalarda retinopati gelişimine etki eden risk faktörlerinin değerlendirilmesi: çok merkezli çalışma (Türkiye'de Diyabetik Retinopati Epidemiyolojisi Araştırma Grubu). Gülhane Tıp Dergisi. 2006;48:94–100.

34. Browning DJ, McOwen MD, Bowen RM Jr, O'Marah TL. Comparison of the clinical diagnosis of diabetic macular edema with diagnosis by optical coherence tomography. Ophthalmology. 2004;111:712–5.

35. Brown JC, Solomon SD, Bressler SB, Schachat AP, DiBernardo C, Bressler NM. Detection of diabetic foveal edema; contact lens biomicroscopy compared with optical coherence tomography. Arch Ophthalmol. 2004;122:330–5.

36. Aiello LP, Gardner TW, King GL, Blankenship G, Cavallerano JD, Ferris FL III. Diabetic retinopathy. Diabetes Care. 1998;21:143–56.

37. Diabetes Control and Complications Trial Research Group. Progression of retinopathy with intensive versus conventional treatment in the diabetes control and complications trial. Ophthalmology. 1995;102:647–61.

38. Diabetes Control and Complications Trial Research Group. Early worsening of diabetic retinopathy in the diabetes control and complications trial. Arch Ophthalmol. 1998;116:874–86.

39. The writing team for the diabetes control and complications trial/ epidemiology of diabetes interventions and complications research group. Effect of intensive therapy on the microvascular complications of type 1 diabetes mellitus. JAMA. 2002;287:2563–9.

40. UK Prospective Diabetes Study (UKPDS) Group. Intensive blood-glucose control with sulphonylureas or insulin compared with conventional treatment and risk of complications in patients with type 2 diabetes (UKPDS 33). Lancet. 1998;352:837–53.

41. Jacot JL, Vinik AI. Diabetic retinopathy: unraveling the paradoxical effects of intensive insulin treatment. Insulin. 2006;2(1):4–11.

42. UK Prospective Diabetes Study Group. Tight blood pressure control and risk of macrovascular and microvascular complications in type 2 diabetes: UKPDS 38. BMJ. 1998;317:703–14.

43. Bresnick GH. Diabetic macular edema. A review. Ophthalmology. 1986;93:989–97.

44. Xie J, Ikram MK, Cotch MF, Klein B, Varma R, Shaw JE, Klein R, Mitchell P, Lamoureux EL, Wong TY. Association of diabetic macular edema and proliferative diabetic retinopathy with cardiovascular disease: a systematic review and meta-analysis. JAMA Ophthalmol. 2017;135(6):586–93.

45. Early Treatment Diabetic Retinopathy Study Research Group. Treatment techniques and clinical guidelines for photocoagulation of diabetic macular edema. Early treatment diabetic retinopathy study report number 2. Ophthalmology. 1987;94:761–74.

46. Miljanovic B, Glynn RJ, Nathan DM, et al. A prospective study of serum lipids and risk of diabetic macular edema in type 1 diabetes. Diabetes. 2004;53:2883–92.

47. The DCCT Research Group. Effects of intensive diabetes therapy on neuropsychological function in adults in the diabetes control and complications trial. Ann Intern Med. 1996;124:379–88.

48. Ferris FL 3rd, Chew EY, Hoogwerf BJ. Serum lipids and diabetic retinopathy. Early treatment diabetic retinopathy study research group. Diabetes Care. 1996;19:1291–3.

49. Ding J, Wong TY. Current epidemiology of diabetic retinopathy and diabetic macular edema. Curr Diab Rep. 2012;12:346–54.

50. Salinero-Fort MA, San Andres-Rebollo FJ, de Burgos-Lunar C, Arrieta-Blanco FJ, Gomez-Campelo P. MADIABETES group. Four-year incidence of diabetic retinopathy in a Spanish cohort: the MADIABETES study. PLoS One. 2013;8:e76417.

51. Gupta A, Gupta V, Thapar S, Bhansali A. Lipid-lowering drug atorvastatin as an adjunct in the management of diabetic macular edema. Am J Ophthalmol. 2004;137:675–82.

52. Panagiotoglou TD, Ganotakis ES, Kymionis GD, Moschandreas JA, Fanti GN, Charisis SK, Malliaraki NE, Tsilimbaris MK. Atorvastatin for diabetic macular edema in patients with diabetes mellitus and elevated serum cholesterol. Ophthalmic Surg Lasers Imaging. 2010;41:316–22.

53. King RC, Dobree JH, Kok D, Foulds WS, Dangerfield WG. Exudative diabetic retinopaty. Spontaneous changes and effects of a corn oil diet. Br J Ophthalmol. 1963;47:666–72.

54. Cusick M, Chew EY, Chan CC, Kruth HS, Murphy RP, Ferris FL 3rd. Histopathology and regression of retinal hard exudates in diabetic retinopathy after reduction of elevated serum lipid levels. Ophthalmology. 2003;110:2126–33.

55. Preiss D, Seshasai SR, Welsh P, Murphy SA, Ho JE, Waters DD, DeMicco DA, Barter P, Cannon CP, Sabatine MS, Braunwald E, Kastelein JJ, de Lemos JA, Blazing MA, Pedersen TR, Tikkanen MJ, Sattar N, Ray KK. Risk of incident diabetes with intensive-dose compared with moderate-dose statin therapy: a meta-analysis. JAMA. 2011;305:2556–64.

56. Sheely D, Jialal I. Strategies to lower low-density lipoprotein cholesterol in metabolic syndrome: averting the diabetes risk. Metab Syndr Relat Disord. 2013;11:149–51.

57. Romero P, Baget M, Mendez I, Fernández J, Salvat M, Martinez I. Diabetic macular edema and its relationship to renal microangiopathy: a sample of type I diabetes mellitus patients in a 15-year follow-up study. J Diabetes Complicat. 2007;21:172–80.

58. Mohamed Q, Gillies MC, Wong TY. Management of diabetic retinopathy. A systematic review. JAMA. 2007;298:902–16.

59. Klein R, Knudtson MD, Lee KE, Gangnon R, Klein BEK. The Wisconsin epidemiologic study of diabetic retinopathy XXIII. The twenty-five year incidence of macular edema in persons with type 1 diabetes. Ophthalmology. 2009;116:497–503.

60. Klein R, Klein BEK, Moss SE, Cruickshanks KJ. The 14-year incidence and progression of diabetic retinopathy and associated risk factors in type 1 diabetes. Ophthalmology. 1998;105:1801–15.

61. Lattanzio R, Brancato R, Pierro L, Bandello F, Iaccheri B, Fiore T, Maestranzi G. Macular thickness measured by optical coherence tomography (OCT) in diabetic patients. Eur J Ophthalmol. 2002;12:482–7.

62. Browning DJ, Fraser CM, Clark S. The relationship of macular thickness to clinically graded diabetic retinopathy severity in eyes without clinically detected diabetic macular edema. Ophthalmology. 2007;115:533–9.

63. Igersheimer J. Intraocular pressure and its relation to retinal extravasation. Arch Ophthalmol. 1944;32:50–5.

64. Jeganathan VS, Wang JJ, Wong TY. Ocular associations of diabetes other than diabetic retinopathy. Diabetes Care. 2008;31:1905–12.

65. Chiang PP, Lamoureux EL, Zheng Y, Tay WT, Mitchell P, Wang JJ, Wong TY. Frequency and risk factors of non-retinopathy ocular conditions in people with diabetes: the Singapore Malay eye study. Diabet Med. 2013;30:e32–40.

66. Fineman MS, Benson WE, Scott IU. Cataract management in diabetes. In: Scott IU, Flynn HW, Smiddy WE, editors. Diabetes and ocular disease: past, present and future therapies. Second edition. Oxford University Press; 2010. p.301–319.

11

Uteroglobin and FLRG concentrations in aqueous humor are associated with age in primary open angle glaucoma patients

Esther L. Ashworth Briggs[1], Tze'Yo Toh[2], Rajaraman Eri[1], Alex W. Hewitt[1,3] and Anthony L. Cook[1,4*]

Abstract

Background: The pathophysiological changes occurring in the trabecular meshwork in primary open angle glaucoma are poorly understood, but are thought to include increased extracellular matrix deposition, trabecular meshwork cell apoptosis, inflammation, trabecular meshwork calcification and altered protein composition of the aqueous humor. Although many proteins are present in aqueous humor, relatively few have been studied extensively, and their potential roles in primary open angle glaucoma are unknown.

Methods: Analyte concentrations in aqueous humor from 19 primary open angle glaucoma and 18 cataract patients were measured using a multiplex immunoassay. Fisher's exact test was used to assess statistical significance between groups, and correlations of analyte concentrations with age, intraocular pressure, pattern standard deviation, mean deviation, cup-to-disc ratio and disease duration since commencing treatment were tested by Spearman's method.

Results: CHI3L1, FLRG, HGF, MIF, P-selectin and Uteroglobin were detected in more than 50% of samples of one or both patient groups, some of which have not previously been quantified in aqueous humor. In the glaucoma but not the cataract group, significant correlations were determined with age for Uteroglobin/SCGB1A1 ($r_s = 0.805$, $p < 0.0001$) and FLRG ($r_s = 0.706$, $p = 0.0007$). Furthermore, HGF correlated significantly with disease duration ($r_s = -0.723$, $p = 0.0007$). There were no differences in analyte concentrations between groups, and no other significant associations with clinical descriptors that passed correction for multiple testing.

Conclusions: The correlations of uteroglobin and FLRG with age in primary open angle glaucoma but not cataract may suggest a heightened requirement for anti-inflammatory (uteroglobin) or anti-calcification (FLRG) activity in the ageing glaucomatous trabecular meshwork.

Keywords: Primary open angle glaucoma, Trabecular meshwork, Aqueous humor, Uteroglobin/SCGB1A1, FLRG

Background

Aqueous humor is a clear fluid that circulates throughout the anterior chamber of the eye to provide nutrients to and remove metabolic waste products from the tissues it contacts, and thus contributes to the maintenance of normal eye function [1]. The majority of aqueous humor drains from the eye via the trabecular meshwork (TM), a specialised porous tissue responsible for the regulation of intraocular pressure (IOP) [2]. In primary open angle glaucoma (POAG), decreased drainage of aqueous humor through a compromised TM leads to elevated IOP [1], causing optic nerve degeneration and thus a progressive loss of peripheral vision unless treated. Elevated IOP is the only modifiable risk factor for the development of glaucoma, and all current treatments for POAG are aimed at reducing IOP [2].

The molecular and cellular changes that contribute to TM dysfunction and elevated IOP in POAG are poorly understood. Several processes, including altered extracellular matrix (ECM) turnover [3], oxidative stress [4], inflammation [5], reduced TM cellularity [6], increased TM stiffness [7] and TM calcification [8] are all potential contributors to the pathological changes occurring in the TM during POAG. Many clinical studies of glaucomatous

* Correspondence: anthony.cook@utas.edu.au
[1]School of Health Sciences, University of Tasmania, Launceston, Australia
[4]Wicking Dementia Research and Education Centre, University of Tasmania, Hobart 7001, Australia
Full list of author information is available at the end of the article

aqueous humor samples have reported alterations of multiple inflammatory mediators, including TGF- β2 [9–11], IL-8 [12], IL12, IFNγ and CXCL9 [13, 14] compared to controls, and a pro-inflammatory environment of the aqueous humor has been reported for an animal model of glaucoma [15]. Furthermore, inflammation can cause TM cell apoptosis and lead to a dysfunctional trabecular meshwork, thus contributing to an elevated IOP [5].

Whilst many proteins have been detected in aqueous humor using discovery-based proteomics approaches [16–22], no detailed studies have been performed with regards to these proteins, and thus any potential role in eye physiology or diseases such as glaucoma remains undetermined. Increased knowledge of the proteins present in aqueous humor from POAG patients may provide clues to improve our understanding of the disease processes involved and how they interact with each other. Accordingly, the aims of this study were to compare the concentrations of selected proteins from these studies, including several not previously analysed in eye diseases, in aqueous humor samples obtained from a well-defined cohort of 19 POAG patients against 18 non-glaucomatous cataract samples. Subsequently, we sought to determine the extent of correlation between each of these proteins and relevant clinical descriptors including age, IOP, field of vision (quantified by Humphrey's visual field pattern standard deviation (PSD) score and mean deviation (MD)), optic cup/disc ratio (CDR) and disease duration since commencing treatment. Here, we report the concentrations of six aqueous humor proteins, and identify significant correlations of age with Uteroglobin and FLRG specific to the POAG group, as well as a correlation of HGF with POAG disease duration.

Methods

Patient eligibility and recruitment: This study was approved by the Health and Medical Human Research Ethics Committee Tasmania (H0013264), and executed in adherence to the tenets of the Declaration of Helsinki. All participants were recruited through Tze'Yo Toh at the Launceston Eye Institute and gave written consent with regards to donation and use of aqueous humor samples. POAG was diagnosed based on characteristic optic disc cupping, corresponding visual field loss, and retinal nerve fibre layer thinning, regardless of the presenting IOP. The anatomy of the drainage angle was assessed by gonioscopic examination. Non-glaucomatous cataract patients (referred to herein as the cataract group) were recruited to serve as a control for this study. POAG patients who had previously had a trabeculectomy or vitrectomy were excluded from this study. Furthermore, POAG and cataract subjects were excluded if they had other retinal (such as diabetic retinopathy or age-related macular degeneration) or neurological disease.

Clinical descriptors including age, IOP and CDR were recorded for both patient groups. IOP was measured in all patients using a calibrated Goldmann Applanation tonometer. For POAG patients, only the latest treated IOP measurement taken during the consultation prior to the surgery was used for this study. Vertical CDR was estimated by one observer (Tze'Yo Toh), using a 60D lens during indirect slit lamp fundoscopy and further confirmed with an optic disc profile scan using Ocular Coherence Tomography. MD and PSD were included as measures for vision loss, but were not available for all patients (MD was recorded for 13/19 POAG and 5/18 cataract patients, PSD for 19/19 POAG and 6/18 cataract patients). Furthermore, disease duration since commencing treatment was noted for POAG patients at the time AH samples were collected.

All POAG patients recruited were receiving IOP-lowering eye drops, in the form of monotherapy, or a combination of up to four of the following compounds: Timolol (beta-blocker), Bimatoprost, Tafluprost, Latanoprost, Travoprost (prostaglandin derivatives), Brimonidine (alpha 2 agonist) and Brinzolamide (carbonic anhydrase inhibitor).

Aqueous humor collection: Aqueous humor samples (50–100 μL) were collected from 19 patients with POAG during routine cataract surgery. Aqueous humor was also collected from 18 non-glaucomatous patients undergoing routine cataract surgery to serve as a control for this study [16, 23]. For all samples, aqueous humor was collected from the centre of the anterior chamber by paracentesis at the beginning of surgery, immediately frozen at − 20 °C, and transferred to − 80 °C within 48 h, where they were stored for analysis.

Multiplex immunoassay: We used discovery-based proteomic studies of AH in combination with other relevant scientific literature to select 30 proteins for inclusion in a custom magnetic bead-based multiplex immunoassay (R&D Systems, Inc., Minneapolis, MN) to enable simultaneous measurement of each protein in aqueous humor samples. The 30 proteins included were: Angiopoietin-1, Angiopoietin-2, BMP-2, BMP-4, BMP-9, CCL27/CTACK, CHI3L1/YKL-40, Collagen IV alpha 1, Cripto-1, DcR3, EGF, Endoglin/CD105, Endothelin-1, Epo, FLRG, Follistatin, Growth Hormone, HGF, IGFBP-1, IGFBP-3, IL-6, IL-9, LIF, MFG-E8, MIF, P-Selectin, Thrombospondin-2, Uteroglobin, VCAM-1 and vWF-A2. Some of these proteins (endothelin-1, HGF, EPO, MIF) have previously been shown to be present in aqueous humor using immunoassay techniques, but there are scant or no subsequent studies reporting correlation to clinical descriptors [12, 24–28]. Others (e.g. thromobospondin-2, follistatin) have been shown to be altered in animal [29] or cell culture-based [30] models of glaucoma, but there are no reports of their levels in aqueous humor. We also selected several proteins (e.g.

CHI3L1, CTACK, Cripto-1, DcR3, Endoglin, uteroglobin, FLRG, MFG-E8, P-selectin) that have been identified as being present in aqueous humor, but for which there is a paucity of studies characterising their involvement in glaucoma.

The assay was performed in accordance with manufacturer's instructions on a Bio-Plex 200 System (Bio-Rad Laboratories, Inc., Hercules, CA). Aqueous humor dilutions with assay diluent were kept to a minimum, with dilution factors ranging from 1.5–5.5, sufficient to allow loading of 50 μl of diluted sample per assay well. Fluorescence intensity (FI) was measured and analysed using Bio-Plex Manager 6.0. The majority of concentrations out of range were below the detection limit for the relevant analyte, with the exception of MIF, which resulted in FIs above the highest standard for two cataract and three POAG samples. Readings out of range of the standard curve were excluded from all subsequent analyses. The concentration ranges of the standard curves and the number of samples in range for each analyte tested are given in Additional file 1: Table S1.

Normalisation to total protein concentration: Total aqueous humor protein concentration was measured using a BCA protein assay (Thermo Fisher Scientific, Waltham, MA). Aqueous humor samples were diluted 6-fold in ultrapure water and assessed as described in the manufacturer's protocol. Individual analyte concentrations were normalised to total protein concentration for each sample prior to calculation of correlations as described below.

Statistical analyses: All statistical analyses were conducted with Prism 7 (GraphPad Software, San Diego, CA), using unpaired two-tailed tests with a significance threshold of $p = 0.05$. Differences in age, IOP, CDR and total protein concentration were assessed using unpaired T-tests, MD and PSD were evaluated with Mann-Whitney U tests due to non-Gaussian data distribution, and gender was tested using Fisher's exact test. Analyte concentrations measured for POAG and cataract samples were grouped and the number of samples within range versus out of range of the standard curve were compared using Fisher's exact test. Due to the non-normal distributions obtained for some analyte data sets, correlations with clinical descriptors were calculated using the non-parametric Spearman's method (r_s: Spearman's correlation coefficient). To minimise identification of false associations in our data, Bonferroni's method was used to correct for multiple testing of the analyte concentration data set across different analyses, resulting in an adjusted significance threshold of $p = 0.0017$ (conventional threshold of 0.05/30 protein analytes = adjusted threshold of $p = 0.0017$).

Results
In this study, aqueous humor samples from 19 POAG and 18 non-glaucomatous cataract patients were analysed using a multiplex assay, to quantify the concentrations of 30 proteins reported to be present in aqueous humor [16, 17]. Clinical descriptors including age, IOP and CDR were collected for all patients and are presented in Table 1. MD and PSD were included as measures of vision loss; however, MD data was only available for 13 POAG and 5 cataract patients, and PSD for 6 cataract patients (Table 1). In addition, disease duration since commencing treatment was recorded for the POAG group (Table 1). There were no significant differences between cataract and POAG groups with regards to age ($p = 0.335$), gender ($p = 0.313$), IOP ($p = 0.783$) or total aqueous protein concentration ($p = 0.077$). Whilst the differences in MD and PSD were also non-significant ($p = 0.846$ and $p = 0.0818$, respectively), this is likely due to the lack of data for the majority of cataract patients. The difference in CDR was statistically significant, with a mean CDR of 0.78 in POAG compared to 0.40 in the cataract group ($p < 0.0001$). All patients in the POAG cohort were receiving IOP-lowering medication, with 63% (12/19) on a monotherapy regime of one prostaglandin derivative. The remaining patients received a combination of up to four compounds. All POAG patients were treated with a prostaglandin derivative, and 32% (6/19) were simultaneously prescribed with Timolol (β-blocker). A small percentage of patients received an α2-agonist (1/19) and/or a carbonic anhydrase inhibitor (2/19) in addition to the prostaglandin derivative and β-blocker. In this initial study, we have not attempted to assess differences in analyte concentrations due to specific medication regimes.

Out of the 30 proteins tested, 6 were detectable in ≥50% of samples in one or both groups: CHI3L1, FLRG, HGF, MIF, P-selectin and Uteroglobin (Table 2). The remaining 24 analytes were either not detected, or detected in only a small number of samples, and were therefore excluded from all subsequent analyses (see Additional file 1: Table S1). Of those proteins analysed further, CHI3L1 was present at the highest levels, with median concentrations above 65 ng/ml. FLRG and MIF were detected at intermediate levels, with median concentrations ranging from 3.6 to 6 ng/ml, whereas HGF, P-selectin and Uteroglobin were all quantified at median concentrations below 1 ng/ml.

The number of samples in range versus below the range of the standard curve were compared for each analyte using Fisher's exact test. Whilst analysis revealed a difference for HGF ($p = 0.003$) between cataract (9/18 in range) and POAG (18/19 in range), the result did not pass correction for multiple testing (adjusted p-value threshold = 0.0017). In addition, no sample was consistently below the 5th or above the 95th percentile for all analytes reported.

Significant correlation of FLRG and uteroglobin with age in POAG but not cataract
Prior to calculating correlations, analyte concentrations were normalised using total aqueous humor protein

Table 1 Clinical data for non-glaucomatous cataract and POAG patients

Parameters	Cataract	POAG	p-value
Age (years; Mean ± SD)	66.5 ± 7.0	68.9 ± 7.9	0.335
Sample number (M/F)	18 (5/13)	19 (9/10)	0.313
IOP (Mean, ± SD)	17.9 ± 3.5	17.6 ± 3.4	0.783
MD (Median, IQR)	−3.1, −4.8 to − 0.9	− 3.6, − 4.8 to −2.0	0.846
PSD (Median, IQR)	1.63, 1.40–2.95	2.11, 1.69–5.26	0.082
CDR (Mean ± SD)	0.40, 0.22	0.78, 0.09	**< 0.0001**
Disease duration (years; Mean ± SD)	N/A	2.59, 2.15	N/A
AH total protein (mg/ml; Mean ± SD)	3.21 ± 0.88	3.77 ± 0.97	0.077

POAG: Primary open angle glaucoma; SD: standard deviation; M: male; F: female; IOP: intraocular pressure in mmHg; MD: mean deviation; IQR: interquartile range; PSD: Humphrey's visual field pattern standard deviation; CDR: optic cup/disc ratio; N/A: not applicable; AH: aqueous humor. Statistical significance was assessed using Fischer's exact test (gender), unpaired T-test (age, IOP, CDR, total protein) and Mann-Whitney U-test (MD, PSD) with $p < 0.05$ considered significant (highlighted in bold)

concentration. The total protein concentrations determined for POAG and cataract samples (mean concentrations of 3.77 and 3.21 mg/ml, respectively) did not differ significantly between groups ($p = 0.077$). Similarly, normalised analyte concentrations did not differ significantly between the POAG and cataract group (Fig. 1).

Correlations between normalised analyte concentrations and age were assessed for both patient groups (Table 3). Significant positive correlations were obtained with FLRG ($r_s = 0.706$, $p = 0.0007$) and Uteroglobin ($r_s = 0.805$, $p < 0.0001$) for POAG but not the cataract group ($r_s = 0.475$, $p = 0.065$ and $r_s = 0.555$, $p = 0.022$, respectively). Whilst further correlations were determined for CHI3L1 ($r_s = 0.566$, $p = 0.012$) and HGF ($r_s = 0.642$, $p = 0.004$) in POAG, these did not pass correction for multiple testing. No significant correlations were obtained between age and other analytes (all $p \geq 0.05$).

HGF correlated significantly with POAG disease duration since commencing treatment

Analyte concentrations were also assessed for correlations with CDR, IOP, PSD and MD for both patient groups, and with disease duration since commencing treatment in POAG only (Table 4 and Additional file 1: Tables S2-S5). A significant correlation was determined between HGF and disease duration ($r_s = - 0.723$, $p = 0.0007$, Table 4).

Further correlations with disease duration were determined for CHI3L1 and FLRG ($r_s = - 0.555$, $p = 0.014$ and $r_s = - 0.673$, $p < 0.002$, respectively, Table 4), and CHI3L1 correlated with CDR in cataract ($r_s = - 0.539$, $p = 0.021$, Additional file 1: Table S3), however, they did not pass correction for multiple testing (adjusted p-value threshold = 0.0017). No correlations were obtained between IOP (Additional file 1: Table S2), MD (Additional file 1: Table S4) or PSD (Additional file 1: Table S5) and any analyte for either patient group.

Discussion

In this present study, aqueous humor samples were collected and analysed from 19 POAG and 18 non-glaucomatous cataract patients as controls. Out of the 30 analytes measured, 6 were quantified in sufficient samples to allow for further analysis (CHI3L1, FLRG, HGF, MIF, P-selectin and Uteroglobin), some of which have not previously been assessed with regards to eye physiology or disease. The concentrations obtained for HGF and MIF are consistent with existing literature [12, 26, 31] and to the best of our knowledge, no quantitative measures of CHI3L1, FLRG, P-selectin or Uteroglobin have been reported in aqueous humor. Four of these proteins are directly linked to inflammation: P-selectin and MIF are both pro-inflammatory mediators, with P-selectin mediating

Table 2 Aqueous humor analyte concentrations in non-glaucomatous cataract versus POAG

Analyte	Cataract			POAG			p-value
	Median	IQR	In range	Median	IQR	In range	
CHI3L1	65,171	53,191–91,124	18/18	83,122	65,958–95,018	19/19	1.000
FLRG	3614	2857–4412	16/18	4303	3679–5323	19/19	0.230
HGF	171.2	114–227	9/18	170.7	133–222	18/19	0.003
MIF	5592	4061–10,039	15/18	4809	3697–5830	15/19	1.000
P-selectin	791	691–874	9/18	927	803–1193	15/19	0.091
Uteroglobin	335	198–463	17/18	253	174–477	18/19	1.000

Median and interquartile range (IQR) calculated for data in range, reported as pg/ml. Significance was tested using the Fisher's exact test for comparison of number of detected vs. undetected samples in each group. Following correction for multiple testing using Bonferroni's method, a p-value of < 0.0017 was considered significant

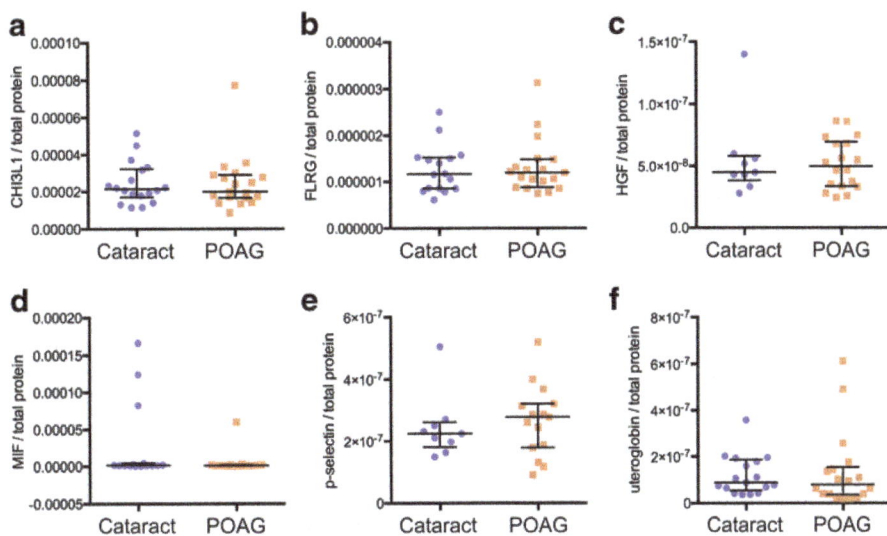

Fig. 1 Normalised analyte distributions in cataract and primary open angle glaucoma (POAG) samples. Distribution of CHI3L1 (**a**), FLRG (**b**), HGF (**c**), MIF (**d**), P-selectin (**e**) and Uteroglobin (**f**) concentrations in aqueous humor normalised to total aqueous humor protein concentration from non-glaucomatous cataract (blue) and POAG (orange). Median and interquartile range are indicated

leukocyte-endothelium adhesion [32], and MIF suppressing the anti-inflammatory and immunosuppressive effects of glucocorticoids [33]. CHI3L1 exerts its pro-inflammatory effects at least in part by inhibiting apoptosis of T-cells, macrophages and eosinophils [34]. In contrast, uteroglobin has anti-inflammatory effects [35, 36]. Furthermore, HGF is involved in tissue repair [26] and FLRG acts as an inhibitor to members of the TGFβ superfamily [37]. Whilst no significant differences were found between normalised analyte concentrations, significant correlations of specific analytes with disease descriptors were obtained, which are discussed below.

A positive correlation was determined for Uteroglobin with age in POAG but not cataract samples, which may indicate an increased need for anti-inflammatory activity in the ageing glaucomatous TM. Uteroglobin is primarily known for its association with various allergic and

inflammatory lung diseases [38], where it exerts an anti-inflammatory effect by supressing various inflammatory mediators, including INFγ, PLA2 and TNFα [35, 36]. In addition, Uteroglobin plays a protective role against oxidative stress [39]. In eosinophilic chronic rhinosinusitis, uteroglobin suppresses the expression of pro-inflammatory CHI3L1 [40]. CHI3L1 is a commonly used TM cell marker [41–43], although it is only expressed by TM cells in the most anterior and posterior regions of the TM tissue [42], which may reflect areas subject to the greatest levels of tissue remodelling within the TM. Interestingly, in this study, uteroglobin and CHI3L1 correlated in the POAG group but not in the cataract group (POAG $p = 0.006$, $r_s = 0.624$; cataract $p = 0.126$, $r_s = 0.387$), which may suggest that a similar mechanism could be occurring in POAG, however, this correlation did not pass correction for multiple testing.

Table 3 Correlation of measured analytes to age for non-glaucomatous cataract and POAG samples

Analyte	Cataract			POAG		
	r_s	p-value	N	r_s	p-value	N
CHI3L1	−0.066	0.794	18	0.566	0.012	19
FLRG	0.475	0.065	16	0.706	**0.0007**	19
HGF	0.170	0.662	9	0.642	0.004	18
MIF	0.404	0.135	15	0.159	0.570	15
P-selectin	−0.756	0.835	9	0.500	0.060	15
Uteroglobin	0.555	0.022	17	0.805	**< 0.0001**	18

Correlations of normalised analyte concentrations to age were determined using Spearman's rank correlation. Following correction for multiple testing using Bonferroni's method, a p-value of < 0.0017 was considered significant (highlighted in bold). r_s: Spearman correlation coefficient. N: number of correlation pairs

Table 4 Correlation of measured analytes to disease duration for POAG samples

Analyte	Disease duration*		
	r_s	p-value	N
CHI3L1	−0.555	0.014	19
FLRG	−0.673	0.002	19
HGF	−0.723	**0.0007**	18
MIF	−0.306	0.246	15
P-selectin	−0.312	0.226	15
Uteroglobin	−0.377	0.123	18

Correlations of normalised analyte concentrations to disease duration (*in years since commencing treatment) were determined using Spearman's rank correlation. Following correction for multiple testing using Bonferroni's method, a p-value of < 0.0017 was considered significant (highlighted in bold). r_s: Spearman correlation coefficient. N: number of correlation pairs

HGF levels were negatively associated with disease duration since commencing treatment in POAG samples, indicating a reduction of HGF over time, which may be linked to or independent from treatment for hypertension. HGF plays a role in tissue repair, and is therefore closely linked to inflammation [26]. HGF stimulates proliferation, migration and differentiation of many cell types, including TM cells [44], and can stimulate MMP activity in endothelial cells [45]. In this study, the number of samples where HGF was above a set threshold of detection was analysed between the POAG and cataract group (Table 2, $p = 0.003$); whilst this comparison did not pass correction for multiple testing, the result is in line with published literature, showing a significant increase in HGF in glaucomatous aqueous humor in relation to cataract samples [26]. It has been suggested that elevated HGF levels in glaucomatous aqueous humor may play a compensatory role, by increasing aqueous humor outflow, or aiding in repairing TM damage [26]. The correlation suggests that this compensation may be lost over time.

Similar to uteroglobin, FLRG correlated positively with age in POAG but not cataract. FLRG is a secreted glycoprotein highly homologous to follistatin [46] that binds to and thereby inactivates members of the TGFβ superfamily, including activin A and BMP2, by disabling their ability to interact with cell surface receptors [37]. Interestingly, whilst FLRG was measurable, follistatin was not detected in any of the samples analysed in this study. Within the anterior segment, FLRG may be involved in the regulation of BMP2-induced calcification of the trabecular ECM, which has been suggested to occur with age and to be more prominent in glaucomatous TM [8]. The correlation of FLRG with age may indicate a greater need for BMP-2 inhibition, due to increased calcification. BMP2-induced calcification of the TM has been shown to directly lead to elevated IOP in a POAG rat model [8] and also agrees with existing reports of increased TM stiffness in POAG [7].

Whilst several correlations were determined between analytes and disease descriptors at a significance threshold of $p = 0.05$, six out of nine did not pass correction for multiple testing (adjusted $p = 0.0017$), but may do so in other appropriately powered studies. Although this study did not include a replication cohort, each analyte measured was selected from either discovery-based proteomic studies or immunoassay-based results reported by other groups [12, 16, 24–28]. Despite this, we were unable to detect many of the proteins included in this study at levels above the lower limit of our standard curves. Aside from technical limitations of our chosen multiplex immunoassay, contributing factors many include the variation in proteins identified across multiple proteomic studies [16, 20], as well as the wide spread of specific analyte concentrations observed between aqueous humor samples from different individuals, as reported in some studies [47].

It is important to note that some topical treatments commonly used to treat ocular hypertension, such as latanoprost and brimonidine, may contribute to aqueous inflammation [48, 49]. Whilst the potential effects of such medication on the protein concentrations discussed here are not specifically known, altered aqueous humor concentrations of other proteins have been reported [50]. Although there were no differences between the normalised analyte concentrations measured in POAG and cataract for the 6 analytes studied here, the potential contributions from patient medications to the associations reported here cannot be excluded.

Conclusion

In conclusion, this study has expanded our knowledge of aqueous humor composition by providing quantitative measures for four proteins previously undetermined for aqueous humor. The correlations of Uteroglobin and FLRG with age in POAG may suggest an increased need for compensation of inflammatory and calcifying activity in the ageing glaucomatous TM to maintain functionality, but at present it is unclear whether these proteins play a causative or compensatory role. If any or all of these proteins are to have clinical utility, be it as a diagnostic biomarker or therapeutic target, further research is needed to define their contributions to TM cell physiology, particularly in respect to aqueous humor inflammation and TM outflow resistance, and to determine if these proteins have roles in the onset and progression of POAG.

Abbreviations

CDR: Cup-to-disk ratio; ECM: Extracellular matrix; FI: Fluorescence intensity; IOP: Intraocular pressure; MD: Mean deviation; POAG: Primary open angle glaucoma; PSD: Humphrey's visual field pattern standard deviation; TM: Trabecular meshwork

Acknowledgements

The authors thank the Clifford Craig Medical Research Trust Tasmania (Grant Number 121) and the Ophthalmic Research Institute of Australia for funding this work, and the University of Tasmania for supporting ELAB with an APA scholarship. We are grateful to the study participants for their generosity, to Sally Baxter for assistance with sample collection, to Aidan Bindoff for guidance with statistical analysis and to Laura Danderian and Courtney Brusamarello for technical assistance.

Funding

The Clifford Craig Medical Research Trust Tasmania (Grant Number 121) and the Ophthalmic Research Institute of Australia provided funding this work, and the University of Tasmania supported ELAB with an APA scholarship. Neither organisation played any role in the design of the study, data collection, analysis or interpretation, or in writing the manuscript.

Authors' contributions

ELAB performed the laboratory data collection, analysis and interpretation and drafted the majority of the manuscript. TYT recruited all study participants, recorded clinical data and performed sample collection during surgery. RE made substantial contributions to the study conception and design. AWH was involved in the study conception and design as well as data interpretation, especially with regards to clinical aspects of the manuscript. ALC conceived and designed the study, assisted with data analysis and interpretation and made substantial contributions to drafting and revising the manuscript for publication. All authors were involved in drafting the manuscript or revision of its content, and all authors gave final approval of the work.

Competing interests

The authors declare that they have no competing interests.

Author details

[1]School of Health Sciences, University of Tasmania, Launceston, Australia. [2]Launceston Eye Institute and Launceston Eye Doctors, Launceston, Australia. [3]Centre for Eye Research Australia, University of Melbourne, Melbourne, Australia. [4]Wicking Dementia Research and Education Centre, University of Tasmania, Hobart 7001, Australia.

References

1. Kwon YH, Fingert JH, Kuehn MH, Alward WL. Primary open-angle glaucoma. N Engl J Med. 2009;360:1113–24.
2. Roy Chowdhury U, Hann CR, Stamer WD, Fautsch MP. Aqueous humor outflow: dynamics and disease. Invest Ophthalmol Vis Sci. 2015;56:2993–3003.
3. Gabelt BT, Kaufman PL. Changes in aqueous humor dynamics with age and glaucoma. Prog Retin Eye Res. 2005;24:612–37.
4. Izzotti A, Sacca SC, Cartiglia C, De Flora S. Oxidative deoxyribonucleic acid damage in the eyes of glaucoma patients. Am J Med. 2003;114:638–46.
5. Saccà SC, Gandolfi S, Bagnis A, Manni G, Damonte G, Traverso CE, et al. From DNA damage to functional changes of the trabecular meshwork in aging and glaucoma. Ageing Res Rev. 2016;29:26–41.
6. Alvarado J, Murphy C, Juster R. Trabecular meshwork cellularity in primary open-angle glaucoma and nonglaucomatous normals. Ophthalmology. 1984;91:564–79.
7. Last JA, Pan T, Ding Y, Reilly CM, Keller K, Acott TS, et al. Elastic modulus determination of normal and glaucomatous human trabecular meshwork. Invest Ophthalmol Vis Sci. 2011;52:2147–52.
8. Buie LK, Karim MZ, Smith MH, Borras T. Development of a model of elevated intraocular pressure in rats by gene transfer of bone morphogenetic protein 2. Invest Ophthalmol Vis Sci. 2013;54:5441–55.
9. Inatani M, Tanihara H, Katsuta H, Honjo M, Kido N, Honda Y. Transforming growth factor-beta 2 levels in aqueous humor of glaucomatous eyes. Graefes Arch Clin Exp Ophthalmol. 2001;239:109–13.
10. Ozcan AA, Ozdemir N, Canataroglu A. The aqueous levels of TGF-beta2 in patients with glaucoma. Int Ophthalmol. 2004;25:19–22.
11. Tripathi RC, Li J, Chan WF, Tripathi BJ. Aqueous humor in glaucomatous eyes contains an increased level of TGF-beta 2. Exp Eye Res. 1994;59:723–7.
12. Takai Y, Tanito M, Ohira A. Multiplex cytokine analysis of aqueous humor in eyes with primary open-angle glaucoma, exfoliation glaucoma, and cataract. Invest Ophthalmol Vis Sci. 2012;53:241–7.
13. Chua J, Vania M, Cheung CM, Ang M, Chee SP, Yang H, et al. Expression profile of inflammatory cytokines in aqueous from glaucomatous eyes. Mol Vis. 2012;18:431–8.
14. Engel LA, Muether PS, Fauser S, Hueber A. The effect of previous surgery and topical eye drops for primary open-angle glaucoma on cytokine expression in aqueous humor. Graefes Arch Clin Exp Ophthalmol. 2014;252:791–9.
15. Zhou X, Li F, Kong L, Tomita H, Li C, Cao W. Involvement of inflammation, degradation, and apoptosis in a mouse model of glaucoma. J Biol Chem. 2005;280:31240–8.
16. Chowdhury UR, Madden BJ, Charlesworth MC, Fautsch MP. Proteome analysis of human aqueous humor. Invest Ophthalmol Vis Sci. 2010;51:4921–31.
17. Izzotti A, Longobardi M, Cartiglia C, Saccà SC. Proteome alterations in primary open angle glaucoma aqueous humor. J Proteome Res. 2010;9:4831 8.
18. Richardson MR, Price MO, Price FW, Pardo JC, Grandin JC, You J, et al. Proteomic analysis of human aqueous humor using multidimensional protein identification technology. Mol Vis. 2009;15:2740–50.
19. Bouhenni RA, Al Shahwan S, Morales J, Wakim BT, Chomyk AM, Alkuraya FS, et al. Identification of differentially expressed proteins in the aqueous humor of primary congenital glaucoma. Exp Eye Res. 2011;92:67–75.
20. Kim TW, Kang JW, Ahn J, Lee EK, Cho KC, Han BN, et al. Proteomic analysis of the aqueous humor in age-related macular degeneration (AMD) patients. J Proteome Res. 2012;11:4034–43.
21. Pollreisz A, Funk M, Breitwieser FP, Parapatics K, Sacu S, Georgopoulos M, et al. Quantitative proteomics of aqueous and vitreous fluid from patients with idiopathic epiretinal membranes. Exp Eye Res. 2013;108:48–58.
22. Richardson MR, Segu ZM, Price MO, Lai X, Witzmann FA, Mechref Y, et al. Alterations in the aqueous humor proteome in patients with Fuchs endothelial corneal dystrophy. Mol Vis. 2010;16:2376–83.
23. Ashworth Briggs EL, Toh TY, Eri R, Hewitt AW, Cook AL. TIMP1, TIMP2, and TIMP4 are increased in aqueous humor from primary open angle glaucoma patients. Mol Vis. 2015;21:1162–72.
24. Choritz L, Machert M, Thieme H. Correlation of endothelin-1 concentration in aqueous humor with intraocular pressure in primary open angle and pseudoexfoliation glaucoma. Invest Ophthalmol Vis Sci. 2012;53:7336–42.
25. Lopez-Riquelme N, Villalba C, Tormo C, Belmonte A, Fernandez C, Torralba G, et al. Endothelin-1 levels and biomarkers of oxidative stress in glaucoma patients. Int Ophthalmol. 2015;35:527–32.
26. Hu DN, Ritch R. Hepatocyte growth factor is increased in the aqueous humor of glaucomatous eyes. J Glaucoma. 2001;10:152–7.
27. Nassiri N, Nassiri N, Majdi M, Mehrjardi HZ, Shakiba Y, Haghnegahdar M, et al. Erythropoietin levels in aqueous humor of patients with glaucoma. Mol Vis. 2012;18:1991–5.
28. Wang ZY, Zhao KK, Zhao PQ. Erythropoietin is increased in aqueous humor of glaucomatous eyes. Curr Eye Res. 2010;35:680–4.
29. Haddadin RI, Oh DJ, Kang MH, Villarreal G Jr, Kang JH, Jin R, et al. Thrombospondin-1 (TSP1)-null and TSP2-null mice exhibit lower intraocular pressures. Invest Ophthalmol Vis Sci. 2012;53:6708–17.
30. Fitzgerald AM, Benz C, Clark AF, Wordinger RJ. The effects of transforming growth factor-beta2 on the expression of follistatin and activin a in normal and glaucomatous human trabecular meshwork cells and tissues. Invest Ophthalmol Vis Sci. 2012;53:7358–69.
31. Alexander JP, Samples JR, Acott TS. Growth factor and cytokine modulation of trabecular meshwork matrix metalloproteinase and TIMP expression. Curr Eye Res. 1998;17:276–85.
32. McEver RP. Selectins: initiators of leucocyte adhesion and signalling at the vascular wall. Cardiovasc Res. 2015;107:331–9.
33. Lolis E, Bucala R. Macrophage migration inhibitory factor. Expert Opin Ther Targets. 2003;7:153–64.
34. Lee CG, Da Silva CA, Dela Cruz CS, Ahangari F, Ma B, Kang MJ, et al. Role of chitin and chitinase/chitinase-like proteins in inflammation, tissue remodeling, and injury. Annu Rev Physiol. 2011;73:479–501.
35. Wang H, Liu Y, Liu Z. Clara cell 10-kD protein in inflammatory upper airway diseases. Curr Opin Allergy Clin Immunol. 2013;13:25–30.
36. Dierynck I, Bernard A, Roels H, De Ley M. Potent inhibition of both human interferon-gamma production and biologic activity by the Clara cell protein CC16. Am J Respir Cell Mol Biol. 1995;12:205–10.
37. Tsuchida K, Arai KY, Kuramoto Y, Yamakawa N, Hasegawa Y, Sugino H. Identification and characterization of a novel follistatin-like protein as a binding protein for the TGF-beta family. J Biol Chem. 2000;275:40788–96.
38. Shijubo N, Kawabata I, Sato N, Itoh Y. Clinical aspects of Clara cell 10-kDa protein/ uteroglobin (secretoglobin 1A1). Curr Pharm Des. 2003;9:1139–49.
39. Broeckaert F, Bernard A. Clara cell secretory protein (CC16): characteristics and perspectives as lung peripheral biomarker. Clin Exp Allergy. 2000;30:469–75.
40. Wang H, Long XB, Cao PP, Wang N, Liu Y, Cui YH, et al. Clara cell 10-kD protein suppresses chitinase 3-like 1 expression associated with eosinophilic chronic rhinosinusitis. Am J Respir Crit Care Med. 2010;181:908–16.
41. Du Y, Yun H, Yang E, Schuman JS. Stem cells from trabecular meshwork home to TM tissue in vivo. Invest Ophthalmol Vis Sci. 2013;54:1450–9.
42. Liton PB, Liu X, Stamer WD, Challa P, Epstein DL, Gonzalez P. Specific targeting of gene expression to a subset of human trabecular meshwork cells using the chitinase 3-like 1 promoter. Invest Ophthalmol Vis Sci. 2005;46:183–90.
43. Abu-Hassan DW, Li X, Ryan EI, Acott TS, Kelley MJ. Induced pluripotent stem cells restore function in a human cell loss model of open-angle glaucoma. Stem Cells. 2015;33:751–61.

44. Wordinger RJ, Clark AF, Agarwal R, Lambert W, McNatt L, Wilson SE, et al. Cultured human trabecular meshwork cells express functional growth factor receptors. Invest Ophthalmol Vis Sci. 1998;39:1575–89.

45. Wang H, Keiser JA. Hepatocyte growth factor enhances MMP activity in human endothelial cells. Biochem Biophys Res Commun. 2000;272:900–5.

46. Forissier S, Razanajaona D, Ay AS, Martel S, Bartholin L, Rimokh R. AF10-dependent transcription is enhanced by its interaction with FLRG. Biol Cell. 2007;99:563–71.

47. Ohira S, Inoue T, Iwao K, Takahashi E, Tanihara H. Factors influencing aqueous Proinflammatory cytokines and growth factors in Uveitic glaucoma. PLoS One. 2016;11:e0147080.

48. Fechtner RD, Khouri AS, Zimmerman TJ, Bullock J, Feldman R, Kulkarni P, et al. Anterior uveitis associated with latanoprost. Am J Ophthalmol. 1998;126:37–41.

49. Byles DB, Frith P, Salmon JF. Anterior uveitis as a side effect of topical brimonidine. Am J Ophthalmol. 2000;130:287–91.

50. Konstas AG, Koliakos GG, Karabatsas CH, Liakos P, Schlotzer-Schrehardt U, Georgiadis N, et al. Latanoprost therapy reduces the levels of TGF beta 1 and gelatinases in the aqueous humour of patients with exfoliative glaucoma. Exp Eye Res. 2006;82:319–22.

12

The effects of local administration of mesenchymal stem cells on rat corneal allograft rejection

Zhe Jia[†], Fei Li[†], Xiaoyu Zeng, Ying Lv and Shaozhen Zhao[*]

Abstract

Background: Mesenchymal stem cells (MSCs) have been reported to promote long-term cellular and organ transplant acceptance due to their immunotherapeutic characteristics. Previous work from our lab using a rat allograft model has shown that systemic infusion of MSCs inhibited corneal allograft rejection and prolonged graft survival. Here, we further investigated the effects of local MSCs administration in the same animal model.

Methods: Donor-derived MSCs were isolated and cultured while corneal grafts obtained from Wistar rats were transplanted into Lewis rat hosts. Hosts were then randomly separated into four groups and treated with previously cultured MSCs at different times and doses. Graft survival was clinically assessed using slit-lamp biomicroscopy and the median survival time (MST) was calculated. Grafts were examined histologically using hematoxylin-eosin (H-E) staining and immunohistochemically using antibodies against CD4. A comprehensive graft analysis of IL-2, IL-4, IL-10, and IFN-γ expression was also conducted using both real-time polymerase chain reaction (PCR) and enzyme-linked immunosorbent assay (ELISA).

Results: Postoperative MSCs injection prolonged graft survival time when compared with controls (MST 9.8 ± 1.2 days). Injection twice of MSCs (MST 12.6 ± 1.4 days) was more effective than a single injection (MST 10.8 ± 1.3 days). MSCs-treated groups also showed suppression of inflammatory cell as well as CD4 + T cell infiltration in the allograft region. IL-4 and IL-10 levels were significantly increased in grafts obtained from postoperative twice MSCs-treated rats when compared with controls. There were no significant differences in IL-2 or IFN-γ expression across groups.

Conclusions: Subconjunctival injection of MSCs in rats was effective in prolonging corneal allograft survival. This effect was mediated by inhibition of inflammatory and immune responses, indicating an anti-inflammatory shift in the balance of T helper (Th)1 to T helper(Th) 2.

Keywords: Mesenchymal stem cells, Local administration, Cell-based immunomodulatory therapy, Corneal allograft rejection

Background

Corneal transplantation is currently the most effective method for visual rehabilitation once deterioration or disease has affected corneal clarity [1]. Although it is also the most successful transplant method, host rejection due to immune responses remains the predominant reason for graft failure [2]. To prevent rejection, current approaches use systemic corticosteroids and immuno-suppressants (e.g. cyclosporine A) to prolong corneal graft survival [3]. However, this systemic immunosuppressive approach comes with the attendant risk of drug toxicity and the potential for life-threatening complications. Given this risk, new therapies to ensure the viability of corneal transplantation are in need.

Several studies have demonstrated that mesenchymal stem cells (MSCs) have potent immunomodulatory properties, including immunosuppressive effects that have been shown both in vitro and in vivo [4–6].

* Correspondence: doctorzsz@yeah.net
[†]Zhe Jia and Fei Li contributed equally to this work.
Tianjin Medical University Eye Hospital, Tianjin Medical University Eye Institute & Tianjin Medical University School of Optometry and Ophthalmology, No. 251, Fukang R., Nankai Dist, Tianjin, China

Mechanistically, MSCs modulate adaptive immunity by suppressing T cell proliferation and cytokine secretion as well as B cell maturation. In addition, MSCs can also influence innate immunity by inhibiting dendritic cell (DC) maturation and activation as well as natural killer cell (NK) cytotoxicity [7]. In both cases, the governing factors for MSCs' effects on immunity are through direct cell-to-cell interactions and soluble factor secretion [8].

Given the effects of MSCs on immunity, previous work from our lab sought to understand the effects of MSCs in a rat model of allograft rejection. This work found that MSCs were able to significantly reduce the rate of allograft rejection, with systemic delivery being an effective delivery routine for their administration [9]. The current work presented here sought to improve upon these therapeutic results by extending MSCs efficacy duration and reducing therapeutic dose. We further investigated the effect of local administration of MSCs on corneal allograft rejection in lieu of a systemic approach. Our results indicate that subconjunctival injection of MSCs can prolong corneal allograft survival. Mechanistic results indicated that this effect was due to the inhibition of the inflammatory response and an up-regulation of Th2 cytokines. Taken together, these findings indicate that local MSCs application is a promising, alternative method for the prevention and treatment of immune rejection after corneal transplantation.

Methods
Animals
Female Wistar rats (180–220 g) were used to harvest donor corneal grafts. Corneal transplantation was performed on the right eyes of recipient female Lewis (180–220 g) rats. All Wistar and Lewis rats were purchased from the Experimental Animal Center of Academy of Military Medical Sciences (Beijing, China). All animals were maintained at 25 ± 1 °C with relative humidity of $40 \pm 5\%$ under 12 h light-dark illumination cycles (8 am to 8 pm). The animals were fed with food and water ad lib.

The experimental protocol was approved by the Ethical Committee of Tianjin Medical University. All animal procedures and protocols were approved by the Laboratory Animal Care and Use Committee of the Tianjin Medical University and handled in accordance with the ARVO Statement for the Use of Animals in Ophthalmic and Vision Research.

Corneal transplantation animal model
Donor and recipient rats were anesthetized with chloral hydrate (intraperitoneal, i.p., 3 mg/kg). Recipient pupils were completely dilated using 0.5% tropicamide. Donor corneas were obtained from the central corneal region (3.5 mm diameter) using a 3.5 mm trephine and recipient corneal graft beds were simultaneously readied by making a 3 mm diameter button. Donor corneal grafts were then secured onto recipient beds with eight, interrupted 10–0 nylon sutures.

Mesenchymal stem cell (MSCs) preparation
Wistar rats were used for all MSCs derivation and were isolated and maintained as previously described [10]. Briefly, primary MSCs were cultivated in flasks with complete culture medium consisting of DMEM/F12 (Gibco, New York) supplemented with 10% fetal calf serum (FCS, Gibco, New York), 1% L-glutamine (Gibco, New York), 100 U/ml penicillin (Gibco, New York), and 50 mg/ml streptomycin (Gibco, New York). Cultures were maintained at 37 °C in 5% CO_2 and the medium was changed every three days. When cultures reached 80–90% confluence, adherent cells were harvested and re-plated in new flasks. MSCs were subsequently collected and characterized as to their differentiation in vitro (Additional file 1: Figure S1) under the appropriate culture conditions. Later expression analysis revealed that MSCs were positive for CD90, Sca-1, CD73, and CD44 expression, but negative for CD45, CD34, and CD11b. MSCs from passages 3–5 were used for all later experiments.

MSCs administration
Recipient rats were randomly divided into one of four groups. Groups B-D were all administered subconjunctival injections (100 μl) 2×10^6 MSCs in phosphate buffered saline (PBS). Group B subjects received one injection before transplantation (day – 3), Group C immediately after transplantation (day 0), and Group D received two injections (a) immediately after transplantation and (b) three days post-op (days 0 and 3). The dose was selected based on previously published work [11], which has been proved to be safety (Additional file 2: Figure S2). Group A subjects were controls and were administered postoperatively with the same volume of PBS.

Preparation of subconjunctival MSCs administration of 0.1 ml PBS containing 2×10^6 MSCs. MSCs from passages 3–5 were collected and suspected in 1 ml phosphate phosphate buffered saline (PBS). Counted the cell numbers and diluted with PBS. The diluted MSCs were used for later experiments. GFP (green fluorescent protein) labeled MSCs (Cyagen Biosciences Co. Ltd., Suzhou, China) were used for tracking experiments.

Clinical assessment
Clinical evaluations of all grafts were performed using a slit lamp. They were scored daily for corneal transplant rejection for three weeks post-op. Graft rejection was defined according to the criteria presented in Larkin [12]. Specifically, rejection was determined based on the day when graft opacity, edema, and vascularization was

moderate to severe as defined by an opacity score ≥ 3 and a total rejection score ≥ 5. Any subject with surgical complications was excluded from the study and replaced with a new recipient rat.

Histopathological and immunohistochemistry staining

Histopathological evaluation was conducted on day 10 post-transplantation. Briefly, three rats were randomly selected from Groups A and D, euthanized, and their eyeballs removed for evaluation. Tissue was fixed in 10% neutral formalin for 24 h under room temperature, paraffin-embedded, and then sliced into 4 μm sections. Paraffin sections were then stained using a standard hematoxylin&eosin (H&E) protocol [13].

For immunohistochemical assessment, corneal sections were selected and incubated for 30 min with rabbit anti-rat CD4+ polyclonal antibody (Santa Cruz, USA) or CD68+ polyclonal antibody (Santa Cruz, USA). Slices were then incubated with a biotinylated rabbit anti-goat immunoglobulin (ZSGB-Bio, Beijing, China). Slices were rinsed and allowed to react with horseradish peroxidase (HRP) (ZSGB-Bio) at room temperature for 30 min. All slices were counterstained with hematoxylin.

We use ImageJ software (available in the public domain at http://rsb.info.nih.gov) semi-automatically for quantification of positive cells from immunohistochemistry section. Two independent observers who were masked to the conditions of this study counted the staining. The stained sections were pictured under the bright field by a BX51 microscope (Olympus Optical Co. Ltd., Tokyo, Japan). 3 sections from the comparable positions of cornea were selected and the stained cells were counted.

MSCs tracking observation

For immunofluorescence staining, freshly excised eyeballs were snap frozen in Tissue-Tek optimum cutting temperature compound (Sakura Finetechnical, Tokyo, Japan) and frozen sections of 6 um thick were fixed by 4% paraformaldehyde for 15 min, permeabilized with 0.1% Triton X-100 for 5 min and blocked with normal serum for 1 h. The samples were stained with Alexa Fluor 488-conjugated anti-GFP (Life Technologies) overnight at 4 °C and subsequently with fluorescein-conjugated secondary antibodies at room temperature for 1 h. All staining was examined by the cellSens Standard electronic system (Olympus Optical Co. Ltd., Tokyo, Japan) under the fluorescence microscope (BX51, Olympus Optical Co. Ltd., Tokyo, Japan) after counterstaining with 4',6-Diamidino-2-Phenylindole (DAPI)(Vectashield; Vector Laboratories, Burlingame, CA, USA).

Graft Th1 and Th2 cytokine expression

Transcript levels of corneal graft pro- (IFN-γ and IL-2) and anti-inflammatory cytokines (IL-4 and IL-10) were assessed with real-time polymerase chain reaction (real-time PCR). On days 7 and 10 post-op, six rats were euthanized and one cornea from each was harvested. Two corneas collected from two rats in the same group were pooling together as one sample. The collected corneas were thoroughly digested with proteinase K, and total RNA was extracted using TRIzol method according to manufacturer's instruction. And cDNA was subsequently generated in a 20 μl reaction volume using commercially available reverse transcription PCR (RT-PCR) reagents (Thermo, USA). Generated cDNA was then used with inflammatory cytokine primers to assess relative levels. Forward and reverse primer sequences are as follows:

IFN-γ: F: 5' -CACGCCGCGTCTTGGT-3', R: 5' -GAGT GTGCCTTGGCAGTAACAG-3';

IL-2: F: 5' -GCATGCAGCTCGCATCCT-3', R: 5' -TTGA AGTGGGTGCGCTGTT-3';

IL-4: F: 5'- AGGGTGCTTCGCAAATTTTACT-3', R: 5' -CCGAGAACCCCAGACTTGTTC-3'; IL-10: F: 5'- CCCT GGGAGAGAAGCTGAAGA-3', R: 5'- CACTGCCTT GCTTTTATTCTCACA-3';

GAPDH: F: 5' - ACAAGGCTGCCCCGACTAC-3', R: 5' -CTCCTGGTATGAAATGGCAAATC-3'.

Forward and reverse primers for GAPDH were used as an internal control (see above). Thermalcycling parameters consisted of the following steps: Denaturation for 2 min at 50 °C and 10 min 95 °C followed by 40 cycles of 15 s at 95 °C and 1 min at 60 °C. For each sample, threshold cycle (CT) value of IL-4 was normalized using the formula $\Delta CT = CT_{IL-4} - CT_{GAPDH}$. Mean$\Delta CT$ was determined and relative IL-4 mRNA expression was calculated using the $2^{\Delta CT}$ method. This same approach for relative expression was used to evaluate IL-2, IFN-γ, and IL-10 transcript levels.

Enzyme-linked immunosorbent assay (ELISA)

Six rats were selected from group A and D and their corneas were harvested. The total protein from each corneal graft was harvested using the commercially available Tissue Protein Extraction Kit (CWBIO, Beijing, China) according to the manufacturer's instructions. Commercially available ELISA kits (R&D Systems, USA) were used to measure IL-4 and IL-10 concentrations.

Statistical analysis

Penetrating keratoplasty (PKP) clinical scores were assessed with a Kaplan-Meier analysis for survival time. A one-way ANOVA was used to measure transcript levels of IL-2, IFN-γ, IL-10, and IL-4. All data were analyzed using the statistical package SPSS (version 19.0; SPSS, Inc). Data are expressed as mean ± SD and $p < 0.05$ was considered statistically significant.

Results

Rat MSCs characterization

MSCs were harvested from rat bone marrow and subsequently purified by their adherence to plastic culture flasks [10]. Analysis revealed that adherent MSCs had a spindle-shaped, fibroblast morphology. MSCs have the potential to differentiate into multiple cell types, including adipocytes and chondrocytes, depending on the media provided. Phenotypic analysis of MSCs using flow cytometry showed that bone marrow MSCs were positive for CD90 and CD29, but lacked expression for CD45 and CD34 [10].

Corneal grafts survival

To understand the effect of MSCs on corneal transplantation, graft survival in each group was assessed (Fig. 1) and compared. In the control group (Group A), mean graft survival time (MST) was 9.8 ± 1.2 days (Fig. 1a, Table 1). Preoperative MSCs therapy (Group B) accelerated immune rejection with a MST of 8.0 ± 0.9 days. This effect was significant ($p = 0.007$) when compared with control allografts. Group C (single post-op MSCs injection) did not significantly prolong graft survival time when compared with controls (10.8 ± 1.3 days, $p > 0.05$). However, Group D (dual post-op MSCs injection) had significantly prolonged graft survival time when compared with control allografts (12.6 ± 1.4 days, $p = 0.002$) (Fig. 2) (Table 1).

MSCs treatment suppresses inflammatory and CD4 + T cell infiltration

At day 10 after transplantation, corneal allograft rejection was observed in the control group (Group A),

Table 1 Corneal allograft survival time(d, $x \pm s$)

Group	Graft survival time (days)	n	Mean ± SD
A	$8 \times 4,9 \times 6,10 \times 6,11 \times 6,12 \times 2$	24	9.8 ± 1.2
B	$7 \times 4,8 \times 4,9 \times 4$	12	8.0 ± 0.9^a
C	$9 \times 2,10 \times 2,11 \times 6,13 \times 2$	12	10.8 ± 1.3^b
D	$10 \times 2,11 \times 2,12 \times 8,13 \times 4,14 \times 6,15 \times 2$	24	12.6 ± 1.4^a

$^a p < 0.05$ vs Group A; $^b p > 0.05$ vs Group A

Group B, and C; but not in the Group D, which received the MSC subconjunctivally injections on Day 0 and 3. Therefore, the control group without any treatment and group D, the MSC injection group with the optimal effects on allograft survival, were selected for histological analyses at this time point. Epithelial vacuolization and disordered lamellar structure of the stromal collagen were present in the rejected grafts from controls (Group A). H&E staining also revealed extensive infiltration of inflammatory cells (Fig. 3a). In contrast, inflammatory infiltration was markedly decreased in corneal grafts of rats given high MSCs doses (Group D, Fig. 3b). Histologically, such graft had ordered lamellar structure of stromal collagen, indicating reduced inflammation and inhibited rejection. Immunohistochemical results for CD4+ T cells were similar, with extensive infiltration of CD4+ T cells in rejected grafts from Group A (Fig.4a) and only mild infiltration in grafts from Group D (Fig. 4b). Inflammatory cells number (Fig. 3c), CD4 + T cells number (Fig. 4e) as well as CD68+ cell number (Fig. 5) of Group A and Group D were calculated by Image J.

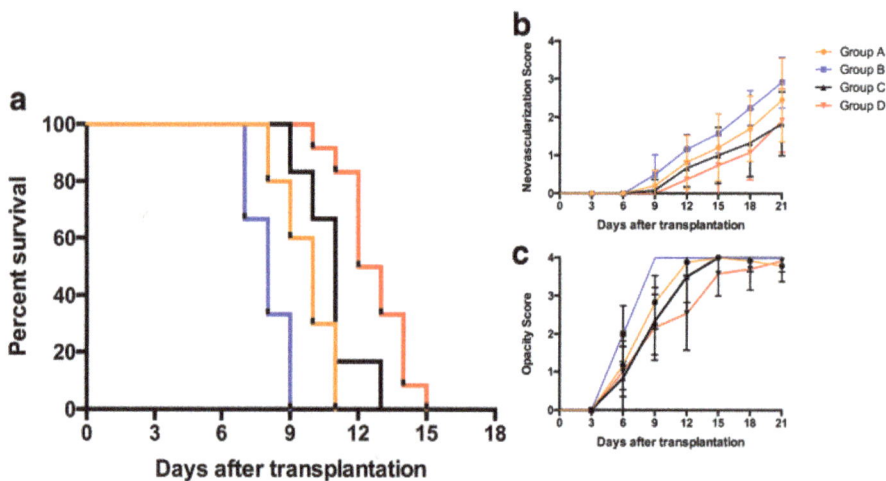

Fig. 1 Group survival time The Kaplan–Meier survival plot of corneal allografts in mesenchymal stem cell (MSCs)-treated and untreated rat (**a**). When compared with vehicle-treated rats (Group A) (9.8 ± 1.2 days), rats receiving postoperative, dual injections of MSCs (Group D) (12.6 ± 1.4 days, $p = 0.002$) had significantly prolonged graft survival time. A single MSCs injection (Group C) (10.8 ± 1.3) did not result in statistically significant changes in graft survival time. However, preoperative MSCs (Group B) (8.0 ± 0.9 days, $p = 0.007$) accelerated graft rejection time when compared with controls. The scores of neovascularization (**b**) and opacity (**c**) are shown over time

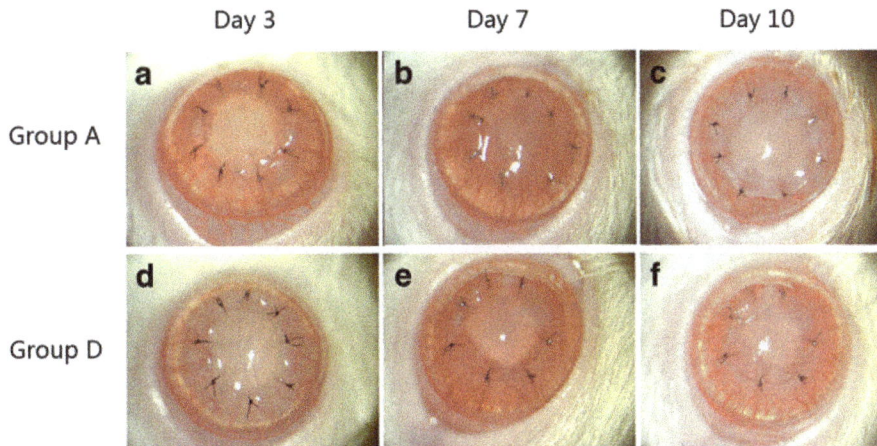

Fig. 2 Clinical assessment of grafts. Three days post-op, corneal grafts were transparent in Groups A (**a**) and D (**d**). Corneal neovascularization began to grow into the cornea from the limbus. At day 7 and when compared to controls (**b**), both corneal edema and neovascularization of Group D were mitigated (**e**). By day 10, corneal edema was severe in controls (**c**). The rejected grafts were opaque and a large number of new vessels had grown into the central portion of the grafts. In MSCs-treated groups (**f**), the cornea was still transparent with a pupil and new vessels were not near the peripheral portion of the grafts

MSCs effect on Th1/Th2 balance

To examine the possible mechanisms behind the effectiveness of local MSCs therapy, we next analyzed corneal grafts for the time course of inflammation- and immune-related transcript levels. To this end, IFN-γ, IL-2, IL-10 and IL-4 were examined at days 7 and 10 post-op using quantitative real-time PCR (Fig. 6).

At day 7, clinical scores of grafts were not reached rejection from control group (Group A). However, IL-4 and IL-10 mRNA expression in MSCs twice injection group (Group D) were significantly higher than in controls. MSCs treatment also resulted in reduced IFN-γ mRNA expression (Table 2). As a result, the Th1/Th2 ratio was also significantly reduced. At day 10, mRNA expression levels of IFN-γ, IL-2, IL-4, and IL-10 were all significantly increased. The grafts of MSCs twice treated group showed a trend towards higher IL-4 and IL-10 mRNA expression, but lower IFN-γ and IL-2 mRNA

expression. However, these trends were not statistically different (Table 3). The Th1/Th2 ratio remained reduced in MSCs-treated grafts. Taken together, these results suggest that MSCs shift the balance in our corneal allograft rejection model between Th1 and Th2 towards the latter. This is especially true for Th2 cytokines.

We next sought to examine whether MSCs could alter Th2 cytokine levels in corneal allografts. ELISA results indicated that both IL-4 and IL-10 were detected in the grafts. On day 10, the level of anti-inflammatory Th2-type cytokine IL-10 was significantly increased in corneal grafts from MSCs-treated groups when compared with controls ($p = 0.002$, Fig. 6e). IL-4 levels were too low in two groups to be detected (data not showed).

Tracking of MSCs

We use GFP and DAPI co-labeled MSCs to investigate the trace of MSCs after subconjunctival injection. The

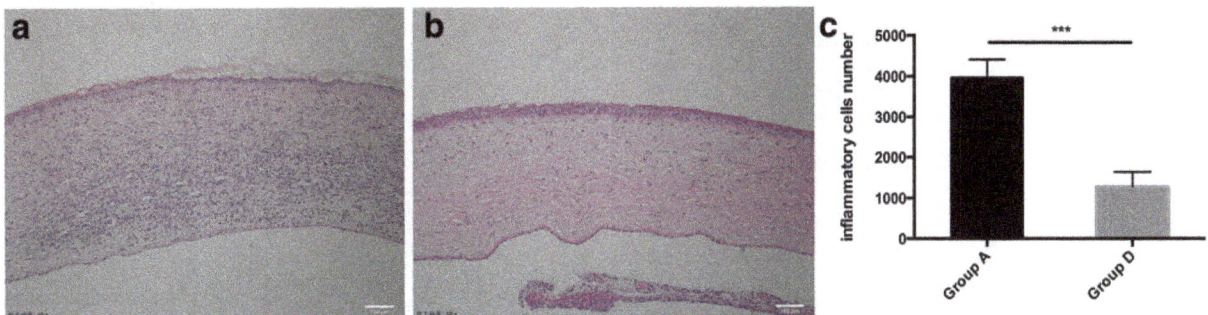

Fig. 3 H&E staining. H&E staining in control (Group A) and double injection groups (Group D). H&E corneal graft staining at day 10 showed heavy infiltration of inflammatory cells in the rejected allografts of controls (**a**) and much less inflammatory cell infiltration in the Group D allografts (**b**). ***$p < 0.001$

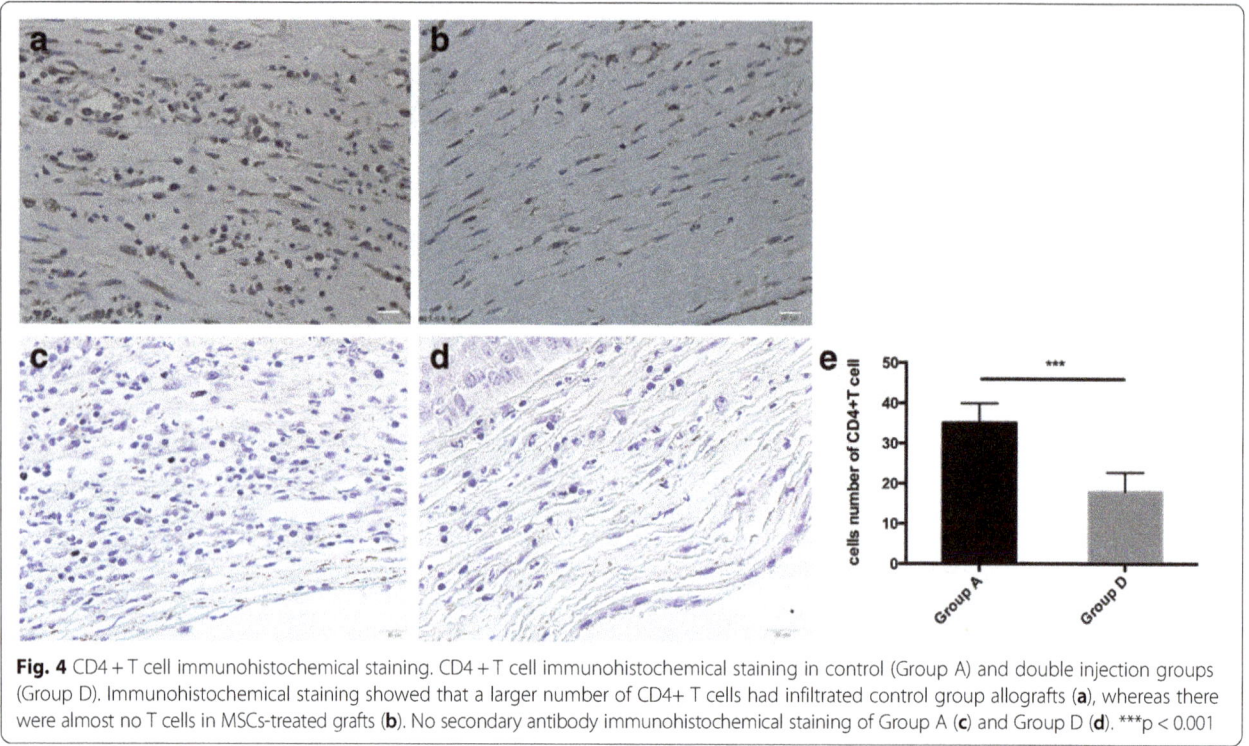

Fig. 4 CD4 + T cell immunohistochemical staining. CD4 + T cell immunohistochemical staining in control (Group A) and double injection groups (Group D). Immunohistochemical staining showed that a larger number of CD4+ T cells had infiltrated control group allografts (**a**), whereas there were almost no T cells in MSCs-treated grafts (**b**). No secondary antibody immunohistochemical staining of Group A (**c**) and Group D (**d**). ***p < 0.001

labeled MSCs were detected via confocal laser scanning microscopy (Fig. 7). After double injection of MSCs (Day0, Day 3), there is a large quantity of MSCs can be detected on Day 7 as well as 7 days after (Day 14). (Operation Day is considered as Day 0).

Discussion

MSCs have been shown to be effective in a series of studies examining a variety of transplant types. These studies have included both preclinical, experimental work as well as clinical trials. From this work, it became clear that MSCs could effectively modulate immune response. Critically, this could delay immune

rejection and prolong graft survival time in heart, kidney, islet, liver, and other organs [14–19]. MSCs have also shown promise in corneal allograft rejection models [9, 20–23]. However, systemic injections of MSCs has obvious disadvantages, including their intrinsic tumorigenic potential and differentiation capabilities [24]. It has also been confirmed that MSCs occur less frequently in sites with tissue damage [22]. After systemic intravenous injection, most cells become trapped in the lungs and other non-target organs, such as the liver, kidney, and spleen [25]. Due to these limitations, local delivery of MSCs has been considered. This would allow MSCs to overcome these

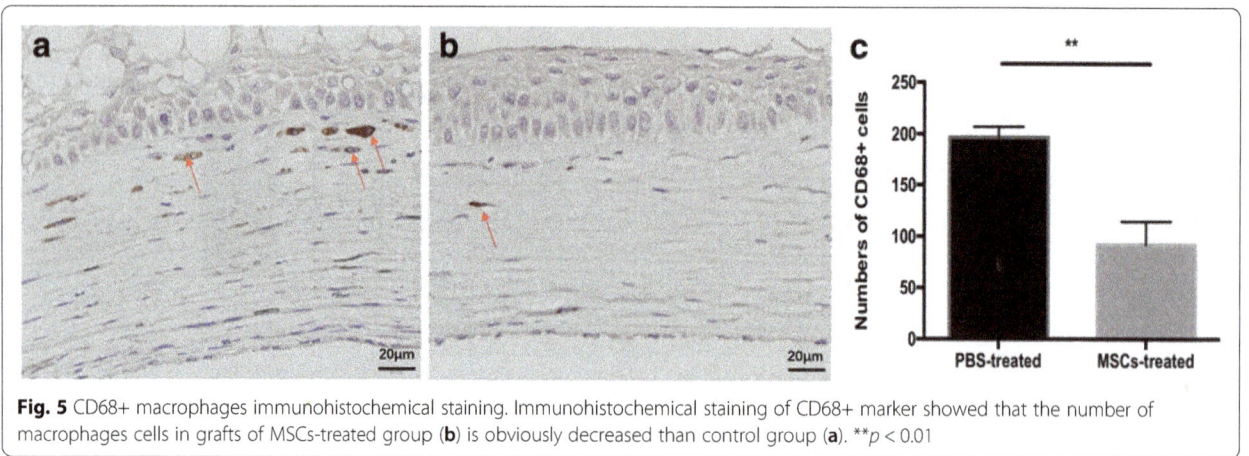

Fig. 5 CD68+ macrophages immunohistochemical staining. Immunohistochemical staining of CD68+ marker showed that the number of macrophages cells in grafts of MSCs-treated group (**b**) is obviously decreased than control group (**a**). **p < 0.01

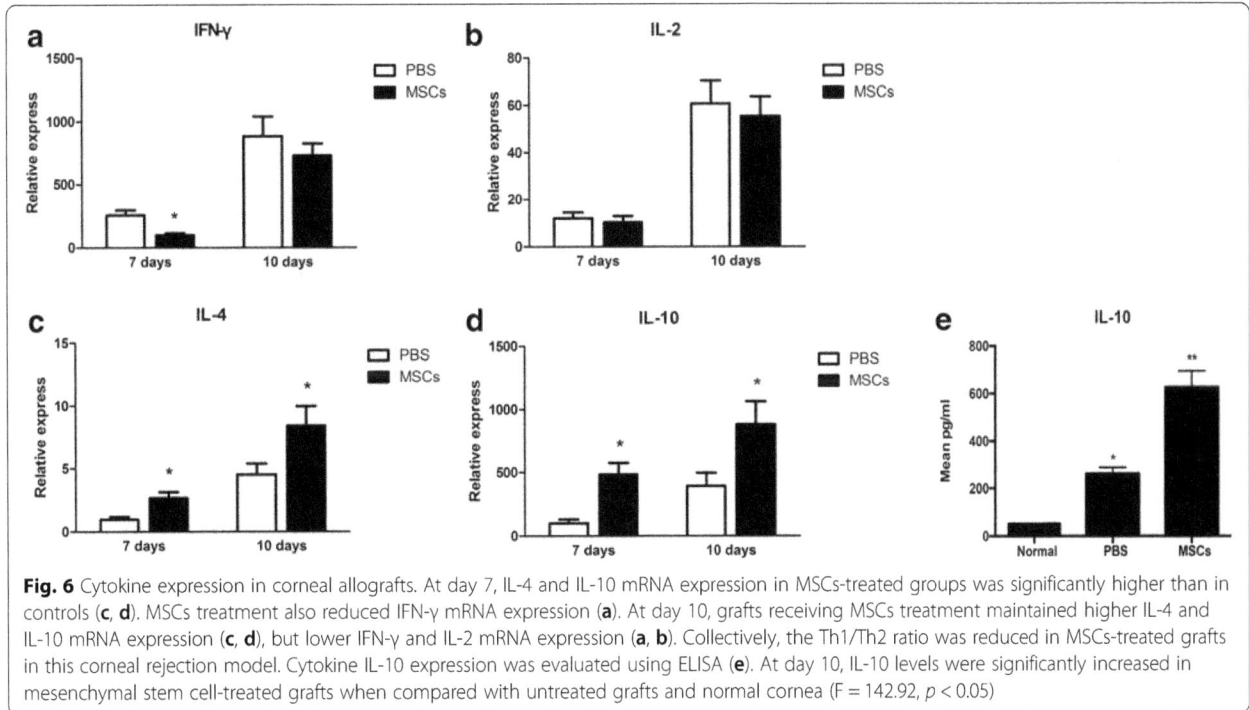

Fig. 6 Cytokine expression in corneal allografts. At day 7, IL-4 and IL-10 mRNA expression in MSCs-treated groups was significantly higher than in controls (**c, d**). MSCs treatment also reduced IFN-γ mRNA expression (**a**). At day 10, grafts receiving MSCs treatment maintained higher IL-4 and IL-10 mRNA expression (**c, d**), but lower IFN-γ and IL-2 mRNA expression (**a, b**). Collectively, the Th1/Th2 ratio was reduced in MSCs-treated grafts in this corneal rejection model. Cytokine IL-10 expression was evaluated using ELISA (**e**). At day 10, IL-10 levels were significantly increased in mesenchymal stem cell-treated grafts when compared with untreated grafts and normal cornea (F = 142.92, $p < 0.05$)

biological barriers, thereby modifying their potency, efficiency, and safety [25–28].

The cornea is located on the ocular surface and has a unique immune microenvironment [29]. Local drug administration is a common treatment approach for a variety of ocular surface diseases [30]. To this end, the effectiveness of subconjunctival injection of MSCs has already been validated [11, 31]. For instance, topical MSCs application suppresses inflammation and angiogenesis, in addition to protecting injured corneal cells. Recent studies shows that MSCs provide therapeutic effects through both cell-membrane contact and soluble factors. Local MSCs administration during the acute stage of a rat corneal chemical burn has been shown to facilitate corneal wound repair by the secretion of soluble factors [32]. According to Yao [11], a suspension of 2×10^6 MSCs in 0.1 ml PBS were administrated via subconjunctival injection on days 0 and 3 after a corneal alkali burn. After seven days, a large number of MSCs still remained in subconjunctival sac. However, only few MSCs could found in the wounded cornea tissue. We also speculated that soluble factors secreted by the

MSCs rather than cell-membrane contact played a role in subconjuctival injection route. This injection route is thought to improve MSCs concentration as well as soluble factors in the surrounding cornea. We have also shown in the current work that local, subconjunctival MSCs injection is a useful treatment route to delay corneal allograft rejection and prolong corneal graft survival time.

MSCs need to be activated to have an effect. The activation requires an inflammatory microenvironment and stimulation by pro-inflammatory cytokines, either through IFN-γ and TNF-α that are produced from effector T cells or some other connection with immune cells [33]. In previous work, pre-operative injections resulted in longer organ transplant survival times [34, 35]. These studies verified that an intravenous, pre-operative MSCs infusion could modulate regulatory T cell (Treg) expansion early and induce immune tolerance prior to the start of inflammation and the immune response. However, in our study, local MSCs injection prolonged corneal allograft survival only when administered after the operation. Preoperative infusion was shown to

Table 2 Immune-related cytokine mRNA expression in rat corneal allografts (day 7) ($\bar{x} \pm s, 2^{-\Delta\Delta Ct}$)

Group	n	IFN-γ mRNA	IL-2 mRNA	IL-4 mRNA	IL-10 mRNA
Normal	6	0.000	0.80 ± 0.13	0.54 ± 0.16	1.54 ± 0.43
A (PBS)	6	254.71 ± 40.33[ac]	11.95 ± 2.56[bc]	0.97 ± 0.22[ac]	100.37 ± 31.11[a,c]
D (MSCs)	6	98.35 ± 15.91[c]	10.21 ± 2.71[c]	2.67 ± 0.45[c]	283.68 ± 67.40[c]

When compared with group A, [a]$P<0.05$, [b]$P>0.05$; when compared with control, [c]$P<0.05$ (one-way ANOVA, Bonferroni correction)

Table 3 Immune cytokine mRNA expression in rat corneal allografts (day 10) ($\bar{x} \pm s, 2^{-\Delta\Delta Ct}$)

Group	N	IFN-γ mRNA	IL-2 mRNA	IL-4 mRNA	IL-10 mRNA
Normal	6	0.000	0.80 ± 0.13	0.54 ± 0.16	1.54 ± 0.43
A (PBS)	6	883.33 ± 155.55[b,c]	60.70 ± 9.69[b,c]	4.51 ± 0.87[a,c]	392.14 ± 103.83[a,c]
D (MSCs)	6	730.833 ± 94.51[c]	55.33 ± 8.40[c]	8.41 ± 1.56[c]	880.90 ± 181.68[c]

When compared with group A, [a]P<0.05,[b]P>0.05; when compared with control, [c]P<0.05 (one-way ANOVA, Bonferroni-correction)

accelerate immune rejection. It is possible that preoperative MSCs infusion requires inflammation factors "activated" or "permitted" to play a role in immunological rejection in a microenvironment. Without, they will not effect on immunomodulation. A large number of MSCs that have gathered in the narrow, conjunctival sac might change the microenvironment around the cornea before corneal transplantation. The cornea is an immune privileged tissue and is situated in a special, immune microenvironment that triggers delayed-type hypersensitivity [36]. Although these MSCs did not destroy this status of the cornea, a change of the local corneal microenvironment might be a risk factor for corneal graft rejection. Therefore, as demonstrated here, the postoperative administration of MSCs might be more effective at prolonging graft survival time. Moreover, these results also indicate that MSCs therapy is not always beneficial, and might actually exacerbate disease under certain circumstances.

MSCs dose is another element that influences cell therapeutic effects. During mixed lymphocyte reactions in vitro, MSCs can inhibit T lymphocyte proliferation, but this depends on the graded number of MSCs. In our study, we selected a concentration of suspension of 2×10^6 MSCs in 0.1 ml PBS to inject based on the previous reference which showed to be safe and effective. Our research showed that MSCs administration improved corneal graft survival, but that survival depended on MSCs dose. More specifically, dual injections were more effective than a single injection.

Corneal allograft rejection is mainly mediated by T cells [37] and T helper (Th) cells play the most important role in the immune response. Th1 cells produce pro-inflammatory cytokines IL-2 and IFN-γand are closely associated with graft rejection. Th2 cells secrete IL-4 and IL-10 and can cross-regulate Th1 cytokines, thus contributing to immune tolerance [38, 39]. In general, the balance between Th1 and Th2 is maintained at a relatively stable level, resulting in normal cellular and humoral immune function. In most of transplantation studies, MSCs were able to induce T cell immune tolerance by inhibiting the Th1 response [19, 38]. Here, we found that local application of donor-derived MSCs suppressed the infiltration of inflammatory and CD4+ T

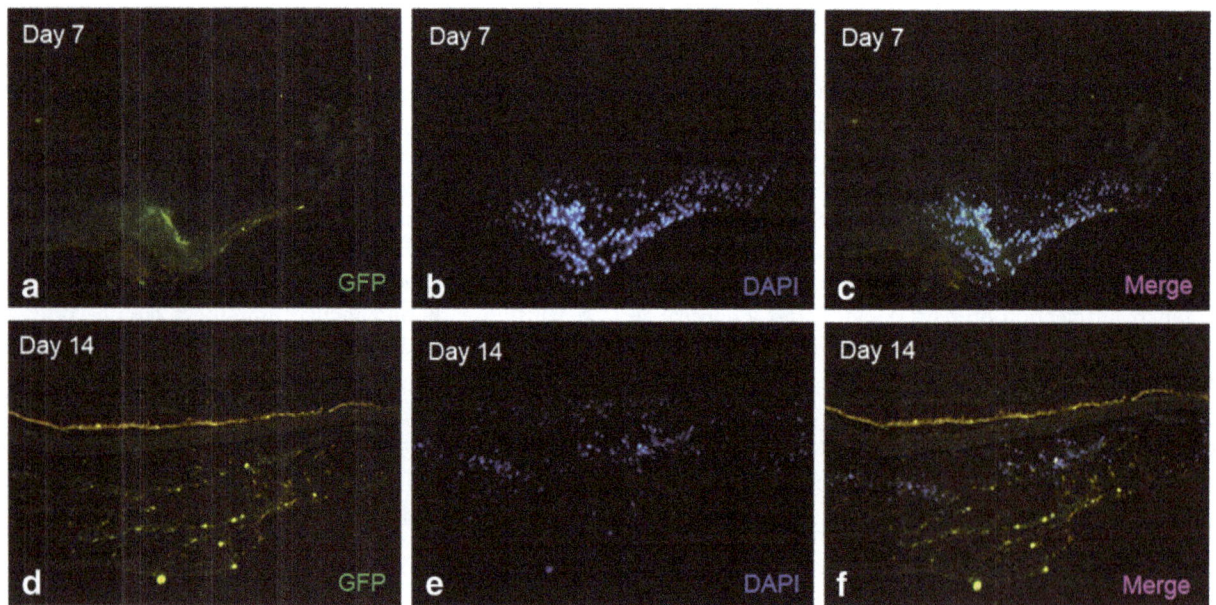

Fig. 7 MSCs tracking. GFP and DAPI co-labeled MSCs were used in tracking MSCs in subconjunctival sac. GFP-fluorescence (**a**), DAPI nuclear stain (**b**, **e**) and merged (**c**, **f**) images are shown. After double injection of MSCs (Day 0, Day 3), there is a large quantity of MSCs can be detected on Day 7 (**c**). There are still some MSCs can be checked on Day 14 (**f**)

cells in grafts. This shifted the Th1/Th2 balance towards a Th2-type response, yielding a significant up-regulation of Th2-response cytokines.

The results presented here suggest that local MSCs injection exerts an immunoregulatory role in corneal transplantation. Moreover, that MSCs-derived therapy is an effective therapeutic strategy to prolong corneal grafts survivial time. However, corneal graft survival time is still not ideal. On the one hand, in vivo MSCs application alone for immune regulation is not sufficient. The application of MSCs combined with a sub-therapeutic dose of an immunosuppressive agent not only exerts a synergistic function in suppressing the immune response [40], but also reduces the side effects caused by large-doses of immunomodulators administered alone. One the other hand, Th1 cells are dominant in graft rejections. Although Th2 cytokines were notably up-regulated in our study, the shift in balance between Th1 and Th2 was not critical enough to prolong corneal allograft survival.

Conclusions

In conclusion, we demonstrated that subconjunctival MSCs injection suppressed corneal allograft rejection to some extent. Postoperative MSCs injection prolonged graft survival time, with dual MSCs injections being more effective than a single injection. This effect was mediated by inhibition of inflammatory and immune responses, indicated by an anti-inflammatory shift in the Th1/Th2 balance. Although the survival time was not nearly long enough, these findings may offer some value regarding treatment strategies in using MSCs for corneal transplantation.

Abbreviations
DAPI: 4′,6-Diamidino-2-Phenylindole; DCs: Dendritic cells; ELISA: Enzyme-linked Immunosorbent Assay; FCS: Fetal calf serum; GFP: Green fluorescent protein; H&E: Hematoxylin&eosin; MSCs: Mesenchymal stem cells; MST: Median survival time; NKs: Natural killer cells; PCR: Polymerase chain reaction; PKP: Penetrating keratoplasty

Funding
This work was supported by grants from Tianjin Municipal Science and Technology Commission Youth Project (16JQNJC12500).

Authors' contributions
SZ designed the study while ZJ and FL analyzed the data and wrote the manuscript. XZ and YL made critical revisions and suggestions to the article. ZJ and FL contributed equally to the research and are considered co-first authors. The corresponding author for this manuscript is SZ (email: doctorzsz @yeah.net). All authors read and approved of the final manuscript.

Competing interests
The authors declare that they have no competing interests.

References
1. Tan DT, Dart JK, Holland EJ, Kinoshita S. Corneal transplantation. Lancet. 2012;379(9827):1749–61.
2. Wilson SE, Kaufman HE. Graft failure after penetrating keratoplasty. Surv Ophthalmol. 1990;34(5):325–56.
3. Yu T, Rajendran V, Griffith M, Forrester JV, Kuffova L. High-risk corneal allografts: a therapeutic challenge. World J Transplant. 2016;6(1):10–27.
4. Hoogduijn MJ, Popp F, Verbeek R, Masoodi M, Nicolaou A, Baan C, Dahlke MH. The immunomodulatory properties of mesenchymal stem cells and their use for immunotherapy. Int Immunopharmacol. 2010;10(12):1496–500.
5. De Miguel MP, Fuentes-Julian S, Blazquez-Martinez A, Pascual CY, Aller MA, Arias J, Arnalich-Montiel F. Immunosuppressive properties of mesenchymal stem cells: advances and applications. Curr Mol Med. 2012;12(5):574–91.
6. English K. Mechanisms of mesenchymal stromal cell immunomodulation. Immunol Cell Biol. 2013;91(1):19–26.
7. Crop M, Baan C, Weimar W, Hoogduijn M. Potential of mesenchymal stem cells as immune therapy in solid-organ transplantation. Transpl Int. 2009; 22(4):365–76.
8. Shi Y, Su J, Roberts AI, Shou P, Rabson AB, Ren G. How mesenchymal stem cells interact with tissue immune responses. Trends Immunol. 2012;33(3): 136–43.
9. Jia Z, Jiao C, Zhao S, Li X, Ren X, Zhang L, Han ZC, Zhang X. Immunomodulatory effects of mesenchymal stem cells in a rat corneal allograft rejection model. Exp Eye Res. 2012;102:44–9.
10. Zhang X, Ren X, Li G, Jiao C, Zhang L, Zhao S, Wang J, Han ZC, Li X. Mesenchymal stem cells ameliorate experimental autoimmune uveoretinitis by comprehensive modulation of systemic autoimmunity. Invest Ophthalmol Vis Sci. 2011;52(6):3143–52.
11. Yao L, Li ZR, Su WR, Li YP, Lin ML, Zhang WX, Liu Y, Wan Q, Liang D. Role of mesenchymal stem cells on cornea wound healing induced by acute alkali burn. PLoS One. 2012;7(2):e30842.
12. Larkin DF, Calder VL, Lightman SL. Identification and characterization of cells infiltrating the graft and aqueous humour in rat corneal allograft rejection. Clin Exp Immunol. 1997;107(2):381–91.
13. Feldman AT, Wolfe D. Tissue processing and hematoxylin and eosin staining. Methods Mol Biol. 2014;1180:31–43.
14. Ma T, Wang X, Jiang D. Immune tolerance of mesenchymal stem cells and induction of skin allograft tolerance. Curr Stem Cell Res Ther. 2017;12(5): 409–15.
15. Chambers DC, Enever D, Lawrence S, Sturm MJ, Herrmann R, Yerkovich S, Musk M, Hopkins PM. Mesenchymal stromal cell therapy for chronic lung allograft dysfunction: results of a first-in-man study. Stem Cells Transl Med. 2017;6(4):1152–7.
16. English K. Mesenchymal stem cells to promote islet transplant survival. Curr Opin Organ Transplant. 2016;21(6):568–73.
17. Casiraghi F, Perico N, Cortinovis M, Remuzzi G. Mesenchymal stromal cells in renal transplantation: opportunities and challenges. Nat Rev Nephrol. 2016; 12(4):241–53.
18. Argani H. Cell therapy in solid-organ transplant. Experimental Clin Transplant Official J Middle East Society for Organ Transplant. 2016;14(3):6–13.
19. Reinders ME, Rabelink TJ, de Fijter JW. The role of mesenchymal stromal cells in chronic transplant rejection after solid organ transplantation. Curr Opin Organ Transplant. 2013;18(1):44–50.
20. Murphy N, Lynch K, Lohan P, Treacy O, Ritter T. Mesenchymal stem cell therapy to promote corneal allograft survival: current status and pathway to clinical translation. Curr Opin Organ Transplant. 2016;21(6):559–67.
21. Zhang L, Coulson-Thomas VJ, Ferreira TG, Kao WW. Mesenchymal stem cells for treating ocular surface diseases. BMC Ophthalmol. 2015;15(1):155.
22. Oh JY, Lee RH, Yu JM, Ko JH, Lee HJ, Ko AY, Roddy GW, Prockop DJ. Intravenous mesenchymal stem cells prevented rejection of allogeneic corneal transplants by aborting the early inflammatory response. Mol Ther J Am Society Gene Ther. 2012;20(11):2143–52.
23. Lan Y, Kodati S, Lee HS, Omoto M, Jin Y, Chauhan SK. Kinetics and function of mesenchymal stem cells in corneal injury. Invest Ophthalmol Vis Sci. 2012;53(7):3638–44.
24. Phinney DG, Prockop DJ. Concise review: mesenchymal stem/multipotent stromal cells: the state of transdifferentiation and modes of tissue repair–current views. Stem Cells. 2007;25(11):2896–902.
25. Gao J, Dennis JE, Muzic RF, Lundberg M, Caplan AI. The dynamic in vivo distribution of bone marrow-derived mesenchymal stem cells after infusion. Cells Tissues Organs. 2001;169(1):12–20.

26. Salama M, Sobh M, Emam M, Abdalla A, Sabry D, El-Gamal M, Lotfy A, El-
    Husseiny M, Sobh M, Shalash A, et al. Effect of intranasal stem cell
    administration on the nigrostriatal system in a mouse model of Parkinson's
    disease. Exp Ther Med. 2017;13(3):976–82.
27. Wang M, Liang C, Hu H, Zhou L, Xu B, Wang X, Han Y, Nie Y, Jia S, Liang J,
    et al. Intraperitoneal injection (IP), intravenous injection (IV) or anal injection
    (AI)? Best way for mesenchymal stem cells transplantation for colitis. Sci
    Rep. 2016;6:30696.
28. Tracy CJ, Sanders DN, Bryan JN, Jensen CA, Castaner LJ, Kirk MD, Katz ML.
    Intravitreal implantation of genetically modified autologous bone marrow-
    derived stem cells for treating retinal disorders. Adv Exp Med Biol. 2016;854:
    571–7.
29. Niederkorn JY. Cornea: window to ocular immunology. Curr Immunol Rev.
    2011;7(3):328–35.
30. Miller TR. Principles of therapeutics. The Veterinary clinics of North America
    Equine practice. 1992;8(3):479–97.
31. Ma Y, Xu Y, Xiao Z, Yang W, Zhang C, Song E, Du Y, Li L. Reconstruction of
    chemically burned rat corneal surface by bone marrow-derived human
    mesenchymal stem cells. Stem Cells. 2006;24(2):315–21.
32. Oh JY, Kim MK, Shin MS, Lee HJ, Ko JH, Wee WR, Lee JH. The anti-
    inflammatory and anti-angiogenic role of mesenchymal stem cells in
    corneal wound healing following chemical injury. Stem Cells. 2008;26(4):
    1047–55.
33. Ren G, Su J, Zhang L, Zhao X, Ling W, L'Huillie A, Zhang J, Lu Y, Roberts AI,
    Ji W, et al. Species variation in the mechanisms of mesenchymal stem cell-
    mediated immunosuppression. Stem Cells. 2009;27(8):1954–62.
34. Casiraghi F, Azzollini N, Todeschini M, Cavinato RA, Cassis P, Solini S, Rota C,
    Morigi M, Introna M, Maranta R, et al. Localization of mesenchymal stromal
    cells dictates their immune or proinflammatory effects in kidney
    transplantation. Am J Transplant Off J Am Soc Transplant Am Soc
    Transplant Surg. 2012;12(9):2373–83.
35. Casiraghi F, Azzollini N, Cassis P, Imberti B, Morigi M, Cugini D, Cavinato RA,
    Todeschini M, Solini S, Sonzogni A, et al. Pretransplant infusion of
    mesenchymal stem cells prolongs the survival of a semiallogeneic heart
    transplant through the generation of regulatory T cells. J Immunol. 2008;
    181(6):3933–46.
36. Niederkorn JY. Corneal transplantation and immune privilege. Int Rev
    Immunol. 2013;32(1):57–67.
37. Niederkorn JY. Immune mechanisms of corneal allograft rejection. Curr Eye
    Res. 2007;32(12):1005–16.
38. Schweizer R, Gorantla VS, Plock JA. Premise and promise of mesenchymal
    stem cell-based therapies in clinical vascularized composite
    allotransplantation. Curr Opin Organ Transplant. 2015;20(6):608–14.
39. Cunnusamy K, Chen PW, Niederkorn JY. Paradigm shifts in the role of CD4+
    T cells in keratoplasty. Discov Med. 2010;10(54):452–61.
40. Eggenhofer E, Renner P, Soeder Y, Popp FC, Hoogduijn MJ, Geissler EK,
    Schlitt HJ, Dahlke MH. Features of synergism between mesenchymal stem
    cells and immunosuppressive drugs in a murine heart transplantation
    model. Transpl Immunol. 2011;25(2–3):141–7.

13

A rabbit model of corneal Ectasia generated by treatment with collagenase type II

Jing Qiao, Haili Li, Yun Tang, Wenjing Song, Bei Rong, Songlin Yang, Yuan Wu and Xiaoming Yan[*]

Abstract

Background: To investigate use of collagenase type II for generating a rabbit model of corneal ectasia.

Methods: Ten New Zealand white rabbits were used with right eyes treated as the experimental group and left eyes treated as the control group. After epithelial debridement, a collagenase type II solution (200 μL of 5 mg/mL) was applied in the experimental group at room temperature (24 °C) for 30 min, and a 200 μL solution without collagenase was applied in the control group. Slit-lamp microscopy, the mean keratometry (Km), and central cornea thickness (CCT) were examined before and after the procedure. Corneas were obtained on day 14 for biomechanical evaluation.

Results: No obvious inflammatory reaction was observed in all eyes after the procedure. A statistically significant increase in Km (1.54 ± 1.29D vs -0.82 ± 0.44D at day7 and 0.89 ± 0.89D vs -2.11 ± 1.02D at day14) and a statistically significant decrease in CCT (-23.10 ± 12.17 μm vs 6.20 ± 16.51 μm at day7 and -16.10 ± 10.46 μm vs 11.60 ± 0.88 μm at day14) were observed in the experimental group compared with the control group. The mean stresses and elastic modulus at 5%, 10%, 15%, and 20% deformities in the experimental group decreased and the differences in elastic modulus between the two groups were statistically significant at 10% and 15% deformities.

Conclusions: Collagenase type II treatment results in mimic KC with increased corneal keratometry and corneal thinning and a lower elastic modulus. An animal model for corneal ectasia can be generated by treatment with collagenase type II.

Keywords: Keratoconus, Corneal ectasia, Collagenase type II, Animal model

Background

Keratoconus (KC) is a non-inflammatory, progressive ectatic disorder, which is usually bilateral, characterized by corneal thinning, scarring, and apical protrusion of the cornea and irregular corneal topography [1, 2]. KC is a common clinical disorder throughout the world, with a reported incidence of approximately 1 per 2000, with no sex or race predilection [3]. This disorder usually begins as a teenager, and often progresses until middle age. KC usually results in progressive visual impairment due to myopia and astigmatism. It is the most common disorder for corneal transplantation in developed countries [4]. Thus, KC has become the focus of extensive clinical

and basic research in ophthalmology. The exact etiology of KC is still unknown, although it may involve both genetic and environmental factors [5, 6].

Therapeutic treatments for KC include contact lenses, rigid gas permeable lenses, corneal collagen crosslinking, intracorneal ring segment insertion, and corneal transplantation [7]. Understanding processes involved in disease occurrence and progression can assist in detecting the etiology and treatment of KC. As a valuable and indispensable tool for basic research, in vivo animal models could enable researchers to better understand the pathophysiology of KC and to verify hypotheses of pathogenesis, as well as to evaluate potential treatments. However, no suitable animal model of KC is available, which may be due to its complex and unknown etiology. As a result, there is a need for an animal model that can

---

* Correspondence: yanxiaoming7908@163.com
Department of Ophthalmology, Peking University First Hospital, Beijing 100034, China

reproduce the pathophysiological features of this disorder.

KC is the most common corneal ectatic disorder, so it is important to establish a corneal ectasia model to mimic KC. Corneal ectasia can be iatrogenic, which can be a complication of corneal laser refractive procedures [8, 9]. Corneal refractive surgeries remove corneal tissue, disrupt cornea biomechanics, and decrease the collagen tensile strength [10]. Laser in situ keratomileusis (LASIK) on animal corneas, especially rabbits, to develop ectasia has been the most common corneal ectasia animal model [11]. However, post-LASIK ectasia and KC may differ in histopathology and ultrastructure [12]; thus, the post-LASIK ectasia model is not an ideal keratoconic animal model.

An imbalance between degradative enzymes such as acid esterase, acid phosphatase, and cathepsins B and G, and their inhibitors such as corneal inhibitors and macroglobulin is believed to be involved in KC [13–15]. Moreover, studies have reported a reduction in collagen content in the stroma during this disorder [16, 17]. Laboratory studies have reported that collagenase activities increase in organ-cultured KC corneas [16], leading to the possibility that topical collagenase application could be used to generate a corneal ectasia model. Hong et al. reported a significant increase in corneal curvature in human donor corneas after topical collagenase application [18]. In a pilot study, we also observed increased corneal curvature in postmortem collagenase-treated rabbit corneas. However, the supply of collagenase-treated donor corneas is limited. As a result, in the following study, we investigated the use of collagenase type II for generating a rabbit model of corneal ectasia.

Methods
Animals and preparation of collagenase type II
Ten female New Zealand white rabbits weighing 3.0–3.5 kg were used in this study. The animals were obtained from Beijing FYY Laboratory Animal Co., Ltd. (Beijing, China) (SCXK 2014–0012). The experimental protocol was approved by the Ethical Committee of Peking University First Hospital. Rabbits were housed in a controlled environment with a 12 h-light/12 h-dark cycle. Food and water were available ad libitum. Continuous clinical care (24 h per day/7 days per week) was provided throughout the study to ensure prompt intervention when needed. Animals were anesthetized intravenously with 0.6 mL/kg of 5% sodium pentobarbital, and 0.4% oxybuprocaine hydrochloride eye drops were used for topical anesthesia during the surgery, as well as pre- and postoperative eye examinations. All of the animals in this study were treated in accordance with the NIH statement for the use of Animals in Research. Collagenase type II (Worthington, Lakewood, NJ,

USA) was obtained in powder form and dissolved in balanced salt solution with 15% dextran to a final concentration of 5 mg/mL.

Surgery
Twenty eyes of 10 rabbits were divided into two groups. The right eyes were treated as the experimental group and the left eyes were treated as the control group. Rabbits were anesthetized intravenously with 0.6 mL/kg of 5% sodium pentobarbital. Topical anesthesia using 0.4% oxybuprocaine hydrochloride eye drops was applied to the eyes. After epithelial debridement, corneal trephines were placed on the corneas. In the experimental group, 200 μL of 5 mg/mL collagenase type II solution was transferred into the corneal trephines, and corneas were immersed in collagenase type II solution at room temperature (24 °C) for 30 min. The solution was then removed by cotton swabs and the corneas were rinsed with 0.9% sodium chloride solution. The control eyes were subjected to the same protocol, but lacking collagenase type II in the applied solution.

Ophthalmological examinations
Before surgery, the rabbit eyes underwent slit-lamp examinations for the evidence of conjunctival injection, corneal infiltration and cornea stromal inflammation, which were repeated every day during the 14-day study.

Corneal keratometry
Corneal keratometry was performed on the day before the surgery and 7 and 14 days after the surgery, using a handheld keratometer (Suowei; Tianjin Suowei, Tianjin, China). Eight measurements were taken at each time point and the mean keratometry (Km) and the changes of Km (ΔKm) were recorded in diopters (D).

Corneal pachymetry
Central cornea thickness (CCT) was recorded on the day before the surgery and 7 and 14 days after the surgery, using a handheld pachymeter (PachPen; Acctome Ultrasound, Malvern, PA, USA) under topical anesthesia. Six measurements were taken at each time point and the mean CCT and the changes of CCT (ΔCCT) were recorded.

Biomechanical measurements
Rabbits were euthanized with an intravenous overdose of sodium pentobarbital on day 14. The entire cornea with the adjacent sclera (2.0 mm wide) was obtained from each eye. A 4 mm-wide central corneal strip, including 2.0 mm sclera on both ends, was cut by a double-bladed scalpel along the vertical direction (12:00–6:00 o'clock). Corneal strips were fixed in the clamps of a microcomputer-controlled

testing machine (Instron 5848 Micro Tester; Instron, Norwood, MA, USA) with a force of 5 N. The corneal strips were stretched at a speed of 3.0 mm/min. Load and deformation were recorded. Elastic modulus is defined as the ratio of tensile stress (amount of force causing deformation per unit trans-sectional area of corneal strips) to the tensile strain (percentage change of the length caused by the stress).

Histology

The remaining cornea samples were fixed in 4% paraformaldehyde for 3 days and embedded in paraffin. Then they were vertically sliced into sections 8 μm thick, used for hematoxylin-eosin staining.

Statistical analyses

All results are expressed as the mean ± standard error (SE). Comparisons of changes of Km and CCT between two groups were performed using two-way ANOVA. A two-tailed paired t-test was used in the statistical analyses to examine the elastic modulus between two groups. Analyses were performed using SPSS Statistics, version 17.0 (SPSS, Chicago, IL, USA). A value of $P < 0.05$ was considered to be statistically significant.

Results

Ophthalmological examinations

After the surgery, daily slit-lamp examinations showed no conjunctival injection, corneal infiltration and cornea stromal inflammation throughout the follow-ups. Fluorescein stain examinations showed complete corneal epithelial healing at approximately 5 days after the surgery.

Corneal keratometry

Before the surgery, there was no significant difference in the Km between the two groups ($P > 0.05$). After the surgery, there was an increase in Km in the experimental group and a decrease in Km in the control group. Km in the experimental group increased significantly by 1.54 ± 1.29D and 0.89 ± 0.89D at day 7 and 14 ($P < 0.05$). The changes of Km were significant at both time points (day 7 and 14) compared with the control group ($P < 0.05$) (Fig. 1).

Corneal pachymetry

Before the operation there was no significant difference in the CCT between the two groups ($P > 0.05$). CCT in the experimental group decreased significantly by – 23. 10 ± 12.17 μm and – 16.10 ± 10.46 μm at day 7 and 14 ($P < 0.05$). The changes of CCT were significant at both time points (day 7 and 14) compared with the control group ($P < 0.05$) (Fig. 2).

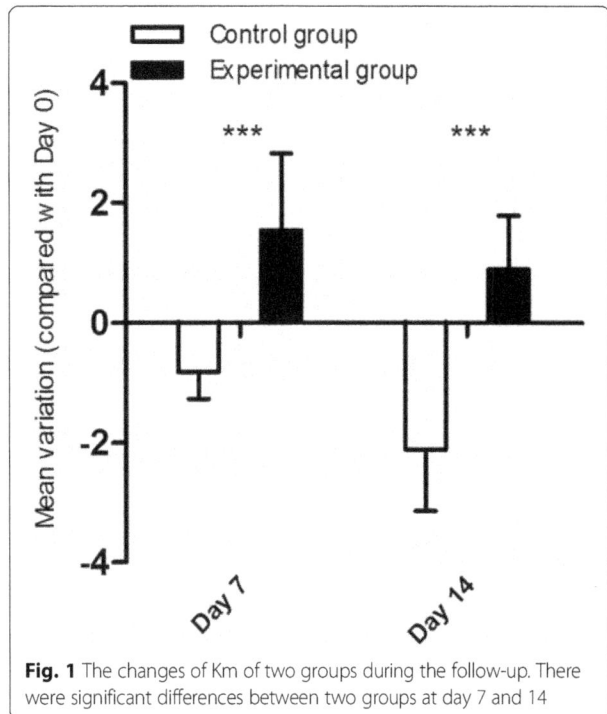

Fig. 1 The changes of Km of two groups during the follow-up. There were significant differences between two groups at day 7 and 14

Biomechanical measurements

The stress–strain measurements showed a decrease in the stiffness of the corneas exposed to collagenase. The mean stresses at 5%, 10%, 15%, and 20% deformities were 0.40 ± 0.18 MPa, 1.06 ± 0.32 MPa, 1.69 ± 0.23 MPa, and 2.23 ± 0.20 MPa for the control corneas, and 0.35 ±

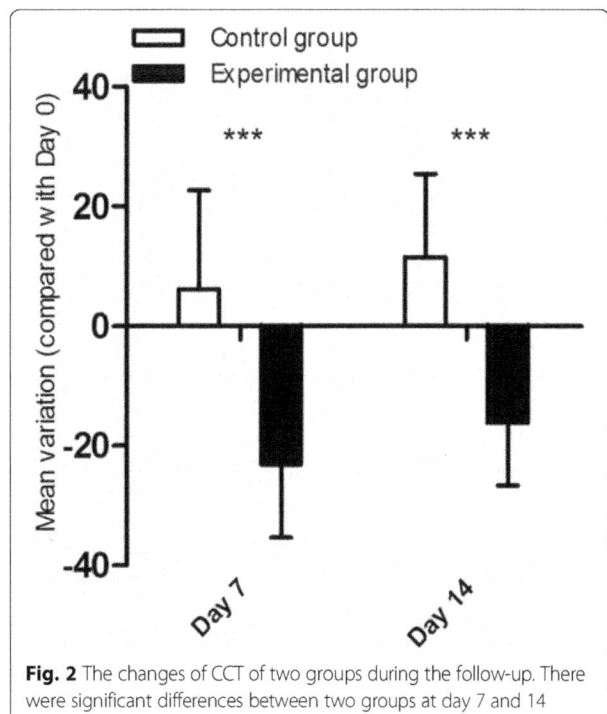

Fig. 2 The changes of CCT of two groups during the follow-up. There were significant differences between two groups at day 7 and 14

0.17 MPa, 0.91 ± 0.25 MPa, 1.43 ± 0.20 MPa, and 1.77 ± 0.20 MPa for the treated corneas, respectively, with a decrease of 11.64%, 14.74%, 15.37%, and 17.95%, respectively. The differences between the two groups were not significant (all, $P > 0.05$) (Fig. 3). After collagenase treatment, the elastic modulus of the corneas was significantly lower. The elastic modulus of the treated corneas at 5%, 10%, 15%, and 20% deformities were lower than that of control corneas, and the differences between the two groups were statistically significant at 10% and 15% deformities ($P < 0.05$) (Table 1).

Histology

Compared to the control group (Fig. 4a), collagen fibers in the experimental group appeared more loosely arranged and interlamellar clefts were observed (Fig. 4b).

Discussion

KC is a corneal ectatic disease of unknown etiology characterized by irregular corneal topography and progressive thinning and steeping of the cornea. However, progresses in basic research and clinical treatments have been limited by the lack of a suitable animal model for this disorder. It has been postulated that weakening of the cornea induced by abnormal structure and/or composition play an important role in the development of KC [3]. Decreased collagen lamellae, abnormal organization of the collagen fiber network, and loss of collagen fibrils in the stroma are observed in keratoconic corneas. These processes may be related to the abnormal regulation of collagenase, protease, and inhibitors of matrix metalloproteinase (MMP)-1 and MMP-3 in the degradative pathway of collagen [19–21]. It has been reported that abnormal corneal structure and composition

Table 1 Comparison of the elastic modulus in collagenase-treated and control corneas

Strain	Elastic modulus (Mpa)		P
	Experimental group	Control group	
5%	10.23 ± 4.50	11.43 ± 5.00	0.614
10%	11.18 ± 1.56	13.99 ± 1.52	0.048*
15%	9.46 ± 4.68	12.22 ± 4.66	0.015*
20%	7.02 ± 1.79	9.09 ± 0.86	0.125

*$P < 0.05$

also contribute to the biomechanical failure that characterizes the pathological process of KC. It is therefore possible that a keratoconic model can be generated by degrading collagens. Collagenase is a member of the MMP family of enzymes that degrade collagen [22]. Collagenase type II preferentially degrades collagen I, which is the main collagen component of cornea; thus, it is possible that exposure to collagenase can generate a corneal ectasia model.

Previous studies have used an animal model of corneal ectasia involving removal of excess corneal stroma, to produce a postsurgical corneal ectasia [23]. Ectasia after LASIK surgery is thought to be caused by failure of structural integrity due to excess tissue removal or to the presence of subclinical KC [24]. As previously mentioned, abnormal structure, abnormal composition, and biomechanical weakness due to the abnormal degradative pathway of collagen may play a major role in KC. The pathogenesis of ectasia after LASIK surgery may therefore differ from KC. Furthermore, previous studies have reported histopathological and ultrastructural differences between ectasia after LASIK surgery and KC [12]. Although ectasia after LASIK surgery and KC both have fewer and thinner lamellae, the lamellae only exist in the residual stromal bed in ectasia after LASIK surgery, but are more widely present in KC. In addition, corneal thinning during ectasia after LASIK surgery is mainly due to tissue removal, which does not occur in KC. Ectasia after LASIK surgery therefore cannot be regarded as a suitable model for KC.

In the present study, collagenase treatment induced a significant increase in Km (1.54D and 0.89D) and a significant decrease in CCT (23.1 μm and 16.1 μm) at day 7 and 14, respectively, which is consistent with the clinical characteristics of irregular corneal topography and progressive corneal thinning. Other studies have shown the similar findings ex vivo. Hong CW et al. reported that collagenase treatment resulted in a significant increase in corneal curvature in human donor corneas by 6.6 ± 1.1D [18]. Wang X et al. demonstrated that rabbit corneas exposed to collagenase ex vivo showed a significant decrease in CCT [25]. Interestingly we found time also had a significant influence in Km in two-way

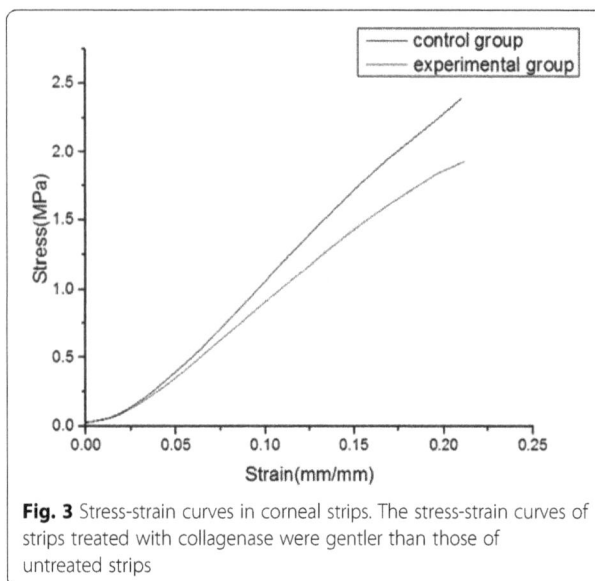

Fig. 3 Stress-strain curves in corneal strips. The stress-strain curves of strips treated with collagenase were gentler than those of untreated strips

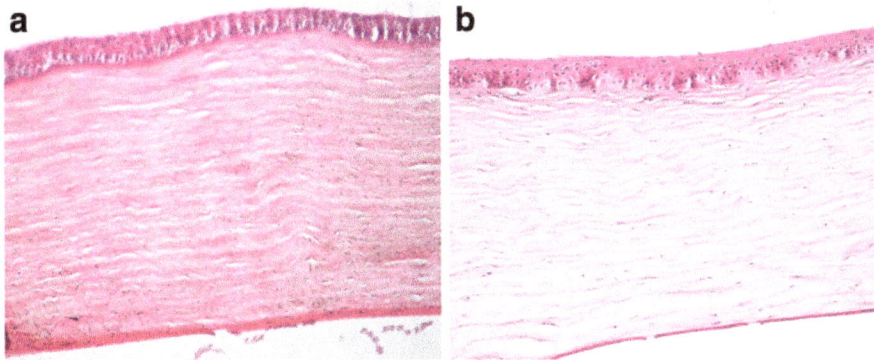

Fig. 4 Hematoxylin-eosin stained corneal sections. Compared to the control group (**a**), collagen fibers in the experimental group (**b**) appeared more loosely arranged and interlamellar clefts appeared

ANOVA analyses. Some studies also focus on the relationship between the corneal keratometry and time. Angunawela RI et al. reported that normal rabbit corneas flattened and had a reduction in the mean keratometry of − 1.9 ± 1.0D over 56 days [26]. Kompa S et al. also demonstrated a continuous decrease of refractive power in rabbits by about 2D in 26 days [27]. Doughty MJ et al. explained that this decrease of refractive power was a natural aging phenomenon caused by the growth of rabbit's globe [28]. Our study also revealed similar decrease of Km in the control group. When considering the natural flattening of the cornea and the reduction in keratometry in both eyes, the total keratometry of the experimental eyes increased by more than 2D. Moreover, the increase in keratometry and decrease in CCT after collagenase exposure lasted for 2 weeks, suggesting that the rabbit model of corneal ectasia generated by collagenase treatment support good short-time feasibility for the future evaluation of novel therapies of KC.

As previously mentioned, biomechanical failure plays a major role in pathogenesis of KC. Numerous studies comparing biomechanical properties between keratoconic and normal corneas reported lower rigidity, increased stress, increased strain, and increased energy absorption in keratoconic corneas [14, 29]. As an indicator of material stiffness, the elastic modulus is usually used to evaluate the biomechanical properties of keratoconic corneas. Relative to normal corneas, some studies have reported reductions in the elastic modulus in keratoconic corneas [29–31]. The finite element model of KC has been considered a tool for theoretical analyses of the geometry and optical responses to biomechanical alterations and corneal thinning. Gefen et al. reported that corneal thinning combined with a lower elastic modulus, but not corneal thinning alone, could produce forward displacement and peak dioptric values consistent with clinical cases of KC in a finite element model of KC [32]. They concluded that corneal thinning and reduction in

the elastic modulus are both involved in the pathogenesis of KC. Histopathology revealed more loosely arranged collagen fibers and interlamellar clefts after collagenase treatment.

In the present study, tensile testing of corneal strips showed that the elastic modulus of corneas exposed to collagenase were significantly lower compared with that of the controls, resulting in both corneal thinning and reduced tensile strength. Furthermore, no obvious inflammatory reactions were observed in the eyes throughout the follow-ups, indicating that treatment with collagenase does not result in inflammation.

Our study did not examine the long-term effects of this novel corneal ectasia model, which is the main limitation. First of all, this 2-week observation may be too short for a comprehensive understanding of this enzymatic degradation model, although in the present study it had shown a significant increase in Km and significant decreases in CCT and elastic modulus in 2 weeks. Besides, long-time observation is necessary for further identification the changes of Km, CCT and tensile strength, which could confirm the sustainability of this novel model. Additional studies with long-time observation are warranted to better investigate the feasibility and efficacy of this rabbit model of corneal ectasia in vivo. The development of novel acute animal model has a great potential for assessing the experimental therapies for KC. Fourteen days may be sufficient for an acute cornea ectasia model to preliminarily evaluate novel treatments for KC after careful review of other studies that develop novel in vivo corneal models [33, 34]. Our findings obtained in 2 weeks showed that collagenase treatment may provide a successful model of corneal ectasia.

Conclusions

Our study described a rabbit model of corneal ectasia involving collagenase treatment, which simulated KC in corneal topography, corneal thinning, and a lower elastic modulus. The model can be used to further investigate the pathogenesis of KC and to evaluate novel treatments for this disorder.

Abbreviations

CCT: Central cornea thickness; KC: Keratoconus; Km: Mean keratometry; LASIK: Laser in situ keratomileusis

Funding

This study was supported by National Natural Science Foundation of China (Grant No.11372011), Beijing Natural Science Foundation (Grant No.7142159). The funding organizations had no role in the design or conduct of this research.

Authors' contributions

Design of the Study (JQ, HLL, XMY); Conduct of the study (JQ, HLL, YT, WJS, BR); Collection, management, analysis, and interpretation of the data (JQ, SLY, WY); Preparation, review and approval of manuscript (JQ, HLL, XMY, YT, WJS, BR, SLY, WY). All authors read and approved the final manuscript.

Competing interests

The authors declare that they have no competing interests.

References

1. Katsoulos C, Karageorgiadis L, Vasileiou N, Mousafeiropoulos T, Asimellis G. Customized hydrogel contact lenses for keratoconus incorporating correction for vertical coma aberration. Ophthalmic Physiol Opt. 2009;29 (3):321–9.
2. Krachmer JH, Feder RS, Belin MW. Keratoconus and related noninflammatory corneal thinning disorders. Surv Ophthalmol. 1984;28 (4):293–322.
3. Ambekar R, Toussaint KC Jr, Wagoner Johnson A. The effect of keratoconus on the structural, mechanical, and optical properties of the cornea. J Mech Behav Biomed Mater. 2011;4(3):223–36.
4. Rabinowitz YS. Keratoconus. Surv Ophthalmol. 1998;42(4):297–319.
5. Abu-Amero KK, Al-Muammar AM, Kondkar AA: Genetics of keratoconus: where do we stand? J Ophthalmol 2014, 2014:641708.
6. Nielsen K, Hjortdal J, Pihlmann M, Corydon TJ. Update on the keratoconus genetics. Acta Ophthalmol. 2013;91(2):106–13.
7. Espandar L, Meyer J. Keratoconus: overview and update on treatment. Middle East Afr J Ophthalmol. 2010;17(1):15–20.
8. Seiler T, Koufala K, Richter G. Iatrogenic keratectasia after laser in situ keratomileusis. J Refract Surg. 1998;14(3):312–7.
9. Tervo TM. Iatrogenic keratectasia after laser in situ keratomileusis. J Cataract Refract Surg. 2001;27(4):490–1.
10. Binder PS. Analysis of ectasia after laser in situ keratomileusis: risk factors. J Cataract Refract Surg. 2007;33(9):1530–8.
11. Liu YC, Konstantopoulos A, Riau AK, Bhayani R, Lwin NC, Teo EP, Yam GH, Mehta JS. Repeatability and reproducibility of corneal biometric measurements using the Visante Omni and a rabbit experimental model of post-surgical corneal Ectasia. Trans Vis Sci Technol. 2015;4(2):16.
12. Dawson DG, Grossniklaus HE, McCarey BE, Edelhauser HF. Biomechanical and wound healing characteristics of corneas after excimer laser keratorefractive surgery: is there a difference between advanced surface ablation and sub-Bowman's keratomileusis? J Refract Surg. 2008;24(1):S90–6.
13. Collier SA. Is the corneal degradation in keratoconus caused by matrix-metalloproteinases? Clin Exp Ophthalmol. 2001;29(6):340–4.
14. Kenney MC, Brown DJ, Rajeev B. Everett Kinsey lecture. The elusive causes of keratoconus: a working hypothesis. CLAO J. 2000;26(1):10–3.
15. Collier SA, Madigan MC, Penfold PL. Expression of membrane-type 1 matrix metalloproteinase (MT1-MMP) and MMP-2 in normal and keratoconus corneas. Curr Eye Res. 2000;21(2):662–8.
16. Kao WW, Vergnes JP, Ebert J, Sundar-Raj CV, Brown SI. Increased collagenase and gelatinase activities in keratoconus. Biochem Biophys Res Commun. 1982;107(3):929–36.
17. Mackiewicz Z, Maatta M, Stenman M, Konttinen L, Tervo T, Konttinen YT. Collagenolytic proteinases in keratoconus. Cornea. 2006;25(5):603–10.
18. Hong CW, Sinha-Roy A, Schoenfield L, McMahon JT, Dupps WJ Jr. Collagenase-mediated tissue modeling of corneal ectasia and collagen cross-linking treatments. Invest Ophthalmol Vis Sci. 2012;53(4):2321–7.
19. Sawaguchi S, Yue BY, Chang I, Sugar J, Robin J. Proteoglycan molecules in keratoconus corneas. Invest Ophthalmol Vis Sci. 1991;32(6):1846–53.
20. Meek KM, Tuft SJ, Huang Y, Gill PS, Hayes S, Newton RH, Bron AJ. Changes in collagen orientation and distribution in keratoconus corneas. Invest Ophthalmol Vis Sci. 2005;46(6):1948–56.
21. Sawaguchi S, Yue BY, Sugar J, Gilboy JE. Lysosomal enzyme abnormalities in keratoconus. Arch Ophthalmol. 1989;107(10):1507–10.
22. Overall CM, Lopez-Otin C. Strategies for MMP inhibition in cancer: innovations for the post-trial era. Nat Rev Cancer. 2002;2(9):657–72.
23. Riau AK, Liu YC, Lwin NC, Ang HP, Tan NY, Yam GH, Tan DT, Mehta JS. Comparative study of nJ- and muJ-energy level femtosecond lasers: evaluation of flap adhesion strength, stromal bed quality, and tissue responses. Invest Ophthalmol Vis Sci. 2014;55(5):3186–94.
24. Roberts CJ, Dupps WJ Jr. Biomechanics of corneal ectasia and biomechanical treatments. J Cataract Refract Surg. 2014;40(6):991–8.
25. Wang X, Huang Y, Jastaneiah S, Majumdar S, Kang JU, Yiu SC, Stark W, Elisseeff JH. Protective effects of soluble collagen during ultraviolet-a crosslinking on enzyme-mediated corneal Ectatic models. PLoS One. 2015; 10(9):e0136999.
26. Angunawela RI, Riau AK, Chaurasia SS, Tan DT, Mehta JS. Refractive lenticule re-implantation after myopic ReLEx: a feasibility study of stromal restoration after refractive surgery in a rabbit model. Invest Ophthalmol Vis Sci. 2012; 53(8):4975–85.
27. Kompa S, Ehlert E, Reim M, Schrage NF. Microbiopsy in healthy rabbit corneas. A long-term study. Acta Ophthalmol Scand. 2000;78(4):411–5.
28. Doughty MJ. The cornea and corneal endothelium in the aged rabbit. Optom Vis Sci. 1994;71(12):809–18.
29. Andreassen TT, Simonsen AH, Oxlund H. Biomechanical properties of keratoconus and normal corneas. Exp Eye Res. 1980;31(4):435–41.
30. Edmund C. Corneal topography and elasticity in normal and keratoconic eyes. A methodological study concerning the pathogenesis of keratoconus. Acta Ophthalmol Suppl. 1989;193:1–36.
31. Nash IS, Greene PR, Foster CS. Comparison of mechanical properties of keratoconus and normal corneas. Exp Eye Res. 1982;35(5):413–24.
32. Gefen A, Shalom R, Elad D, Mandel Y. Biomechanical analysis of the keratoconic cornea. J Mech Behav Biomed Mater. 2009;2(3):224–36.
33. Mello GR, Pizzolatti ML, Wasilewski D, Santhiago MR, Budel V, Moreira H. The effect of subconjunctival bevacizumab on corneal neovascularization, inflammation and re-epithelization in a rabbit model. Clinics. 2011;66 (8):1443–50.
34. Gronkiewicz KM, Giuliano EA, Kuroki K, Bunyak F, Sharma A, Teixeira LB, Hamm CW, Mohan RR. Development of a novel in vivo corneal fibrosis model in the dog. Exp Eye Res. 2016;143:75–88.

14

One-year follow-up of accelerated transepithelial corneal collagen cross-linking for progressive pediatric keratoconus

Mi Tian, Weijun Jian, Ling Sun, Yang Shen, Xiaoyu Zhang and Xingtao Zhou[*]

Abstract

Background: Keratoconus typically presents in the teenage years and is more advanced in younger patients when compared with adults. In the present study, we aimed to assess the safety and efficacy of accelerated transepithelial corneal collagen cross-linking (ATE-CXL) in children with progressive keratoconus.

Methods: In this retrospective consecutive study, 18 eyes were enrolled from 17 pediatric patients (15 boys and 2 girls) with a mean age of 14.44 ± 1.98 years. Manifest refraction, best-corrected visual acuity (BCVA), steepest meridian keratometry (K1), flattest meridian keratometry (K2), maximum keratometry (Kmax), thinnest corneal thickness (TCT), posterior central elevation (PCE), and posterior mean elevation (PME) were measured before and after ATE-CXL. The patients were followed-up at 1, 6, and 12 months. Repeated measures analysis of variance was used for statistical analysis. $P < 0.05$ was considered statistically significant.

Results: There were no complications in any case during or after ATE-CXL. BCVA improved from 0.64 ± 0.32 preoperatively to 0.69 ± 0.32 at 1-year postoperatively. The Kmax value was 56.67 ± 9.60 D before the treatment and 56.19 ± 8.55 D, 56.08 ± 8.85 D, and 55.94 ± 8.46 D at 1, 6, and 12 months postoperatively, respectively. No statistically significant differences were present in K1, K2, Kmax, PCE, and TCT before and after ATE-CXL during the 12-month follow-up ($P > 0.05$).

Conclusions: ATE-CXL is a safe and effective treatment in pediatric progressive keratoconus patients. The long-term effects need further observation.

Keywords: Accelerated transepithelial corneal collagen cross-linking, Keratoconus, Pediatrics

Background

Keratoconus is a bilateral, noninflammatory, progressive corneal ectasia. The clinical characteristics of keratoconus are progressive thinning and steepening of the cornea, leading to irregular astigmatism and loss of visual acuity [1]. Keratoconus typically presents in the teenage years and progresses until the third or fourth decade [2]. The disease typically is more advanced in younger patients and progresses more rapidly when compared with adults [3, 4]. Therefore, to avoid the need for corneal transplantation, it is imperative to stop the progression of the disease in childhood.

Corneal collagen cross-linking (CXL) can halt the progression of keratoconus by increasing the biomechanical rigidity of the corneal stroma via an interaction of riboflavin and ultraviolet radiation (UV) [5, 6]. Many publications have reported on the safety and efficacy of CXL in the treatment of pediatric keratoconus patients [7–10], but treatment by accelerated transepithelial corneal collagen cross-linking (ATE-CXL) [11, 12], which maintains the integrity of the corneal epithelium layer in pediatric keratoconus patients with a higher irradiation intensity of UV

* Correspondence: doctzhouxingtao@163.com
Department of Ophthalmology, Eye and ENT Hospital of Fudan University, Myopia Key Laboratory of the Health Ministry, No.19 Baoqing Road, Shanghai 200031, People's Republic of China

light and a reduced duration of irradiation, has not reported. The present study aimed to assess the safety and efficacy of ATE-CXL in children with progressive keratoconus.

Methods

Subjects

All subjects in the present study were recruited from patients who underwent ATE-CXL at Eye and ENT Hospital of Fudan University in Shanghai, China. Criteria for inclusion were age = 10–17 years, progressive keratoconus (≥1.00 D increase in maximal keratometry in the last year, or ≥1.00 D increase in astigmatic degree in the last year), minimal corneal thickness ≥ 400 μm. Exclusion criteria were a history of ocular disease (except keratoconus), previous ocular surgeries, and a history of systemic diseases. Finally, 18 eyes of 17 patients (male:female = 15:2) with a mean age of 14.44 ± 1.98 years were enrolled in this study. The mean spherical error of all the subjects was -4.17 ± 3.88 D. The mean cylindrical error was -3.35 ± 2.44 D, and the mean spherical equivalent refraction was -5.84 ± 4.13 D. Every patient underwent a 1-year follow-up after the operation.

This study adhered to the tenets of the Declaration of Helsinki and was approved by the Ethics Committee of the Eye and ENT Hospital of Fudan University in Shanghai, China. Written informed consent was obtained from at least one parent or legal guardian of each subject after a detailed explanation of the procedure, and all the procedures were carried out with the subjects' consent.

Ophthalmologic examinations

All patients underwent slit-lamp biomicroscope examination, best corrected visual acuity (BCVA) and manifest refraction assessment, preoperatively and at 1, 6, and 12 months postoperatively. Steepest meridian keratometry (K1), flattest meridian keratometry (K2), maximum keratometry (Kmax), and thinnest corneal thickness (TCT) were measured by the Pentacam imaging system (Oculus GmbH, Wetzlar, Germany) before the treatment and at each follow-up time point.

Posterior elevation data for the cornea were also obtained by the Pentacam software. The reference best-fit sphere (BFS) was defined in the central 8-mm region of the cornea, which was set to be the same across the images from each patient. Posterior central elevation (PCE) and posterior mean elevation (PME) were measured in the central 4-mm area above the BFS. The change in the posterior elevation (ΔPCE and ΔPME) was found by subtracting preoperative data from postoperative data for each patient.

Surgical procedures

All surgeries were performed by the same surgeon. Before the surgery, topical anesthetic eye drops were applied. After a lid speculum was used, a trephine (Model 52503B; 66 vision Tech Co, Ltd., Suzhou, China) was placed in the center of the cornea. ParaCel Solution (0.25% riboflavin-5-phosphate, hydroxylpropyl methylcellulose, NaCl, ethylenediaminetetraaceticacid, Tris, and benzalkonium chloride; Medio-Haus-Medizinprodukte GmbH, Kiel, Germany) was dripped into the trephine to cover the corneal epithelium for 4 min. The cornea was then continually infiltrated with Vibex-Xtra Solution (riboflavin phosphate 2.80 mg/mL and NaCl, Avedro, Inc.) for 6 min. After the cornea was rinsed with balanced salt solution (BBS), UV treatment was administered using Avedro's KXL System (Avedro, Inc) for 5 min and 20 s with 365-nm UV-A light and 45 mW/cm2 irradiation in the pulsed mode (one second on, next second off). BBS was used to keep the ocular surface moist during irradiation. A bandage contact lens was applied after the procedure. Postoperative medications included levofloxacin (4 times daily for 1 week), 0.1% fluorometholone (7 times daily initially, then gradually reduced for 3 weeks), and artificial tears (4 times daily for 4 weeks).

Statistical analysis

Statistical analysis was performed using the Statistical Package for the Social Sciences (SPSS, Inc., Armonk, NY). Continuous parameters were described as mean ± standard deviation. Repeated measures analysis of variance (ANOVA) with Bonferroni-adjusted post hoc comparisons and Friedman rank test were performed to evaluate the significance of differences between preoperative and postoperative data. A P value less than 0.05 was considered statistically significant.

Results

All procedures were completed successfully, and no intraoperative or postoperative complications were observed. All corneas maintained integrity, but had mild to moderate edema on the first postoperative day. There were no cases of corneal haze or infection.

Refractive parameters at 1, 6, and 12 months of follow-up showed the results displayed in Table 1. At 12-month postoperatively, improvement in the BCVA was noted in 7 (38.89%) eyes, stabilization in 8 (44.44%) eyes, and worsening in 3 (16.67%) eyes. There were no statistically significant differences in SD, CD, SE and BCVA before and after ATE-CXL over the 12-month follow-up ($P > 0.05$).

Changes in topographic parameters after ATE-CXL are shown in Table 2. At 12 months postoperatively, the Kmax value decreased in 11 (61.11%) eyes, stabilized in 1

Table 1 Changes in refractive parameters after ATE-CXL($n = 18$)

	Preoperative	Post 1mo	Post 6mo	Post 12mo
SD	−4.17 ± 3.88	−4.19 ± 3.50	−4.29 ± 3.71	−4.71 ± 4.14
CD	−3.35 ± 2.44	−3.35 ± 2.71	−3.42 ± 2.56	−2.99 ± 2.49
SE	−5.84 ± 4.13	−5.87 ± 3.98	−6.00 ± 4.10	−6.20 ± 4.41
BCVA	0.64 ± 0.32	0.69 ± 0.30	0.64 ± 0.29	0.69 ± 0.32

SD spherical degree, *CD* cylindrical degree, *SE* spherical equivalent, *BCVA* best corrected visual acuity

(5.56%) eye, and increased in 6 (33.33%) eyes. There were no statistically significant differences in K1, K2, Kmax, or TCT before and after ATE-CXL over the 12-month follow-up ($P > 0.05$).

Changes in PCE and PME (ΔPCE and ΔPME; Δ values were defined by subtracting preoperative data from postoperative data) after ATE-CXL are shown in Figs. 1 and 2. There were no statistically significant differences between ΔPCE and ΔPME over the 12-month follow-up ($P > 0.05$). The topographic map changes in the typical case are shown in Fig. 3.

Discussion

Although keratoconus is frequently diagnosed during or after adolescence, the ectatic process begins at a much younger age. When it manifests at a pediatric age, progression is more rapid, leading to severe visual impairment with a possible need for corneal transplantation [4, 13]. Corneal CXL is a relatively new and promising treatment that halts the progression of the disease at the corneal ectasia stage. Several studies [7–10] have provided evidence that CXL is safe and effective in slowing or halting the progression of keratoconus, but most of these studies examined conventional CXL (C-CXL). To our knowledge, this study is the first to report the safety and efficacy of ATE-CXL in pediatric keratoconus patients.

All subjects in the present study had progressive keratoconus with an increase in Kmax of 1.00 D or more, or an increase in astigmatism degree greater than 1.00 D. This study showed that the value of BCVA increased from 0.64 ± 0.32 preoperatively to 0.69 ± 0.32 postoperatively, and Kmax decreased from 56.67 ± 9.60 preoperatively to 55.94 ± 8.46 postoperatively at the 1-year follow-up, suggesting

Table 2 Changes in topographic parameters after ATE-CXL ($n = 18$)

	Preoperative	Post 1mo	Post 6mo	Post 12mo
K1	45.70 ± 3.96	45.79 ± 4.14	45.47 ± 3.65	45.76 ± 3.61
K2	49.22 ± 5.83	49.46 ± 5.81	49.08 ± 5.39	49.14 ± 5.64
Kmax	56.67 ± 9.60	56.19 ± 8.55	56.08 ± 8.85	55.94 ± 8.46
TCT	473.50 ± 36.19	473.33 ± 40.14	473.61 ± 39.28	472.72 ± 34.77

K1 teepest meridian keratometry, *K2* flattest meridian keratometry, *Kmax* Maximum keratometry, *TCT* thinnest corneal thickness

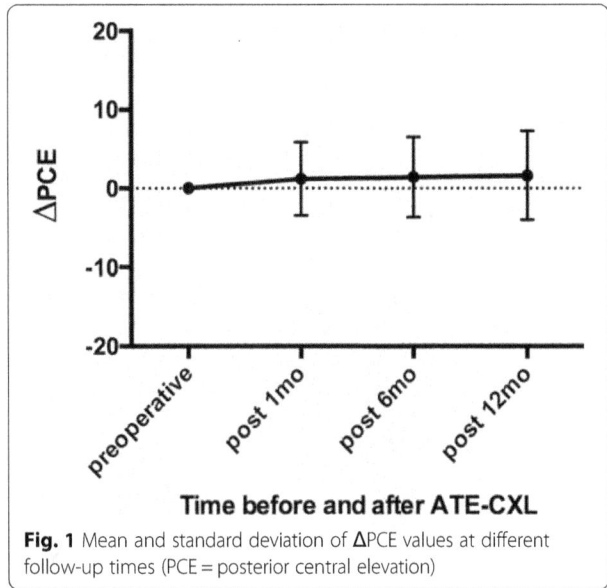

Fig. 1 Mean and standard deviation of ΔPCE values at different follow-up times (PCE = posterior central elevation)

that ATE-CXL is an effective procedure that can halt the progression of keratoconus in pediatric patients. In previous studies of C-CXL for the pediatric keratoconus throughout the 1-year follow-up, Stephanie et al. [9] found that BCVA in 39 eyes changed from 0.34 ± 0.27 to 0.34 ± 0.23, and Kmax decreased from 48.49 ± 5.44 D to 48.24 ± 4.47 D, while Ömür et al. [14] found that Kmax in 40 eyes decreased from 58.4 ± 5.5 D to 57.6 ± 6.0 D, which are similar to our results. Previous studies on ATE-CXL for progressive keratoconus have been conducted in adults, and this study is the first to report the effectiveness of ATE-CXL for pediatric keratoconus.

In this study, the values of K1, K2, Kmax and TCT tended to be stable over 1 year of follow-up, suggesting

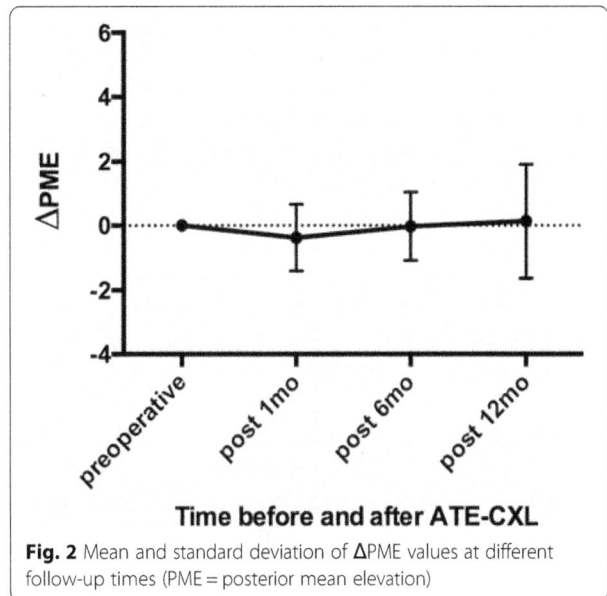

Fig. 2 Mean and standard deviation of ΔPME values at different follow-up times (PME = posterior mean elevation)

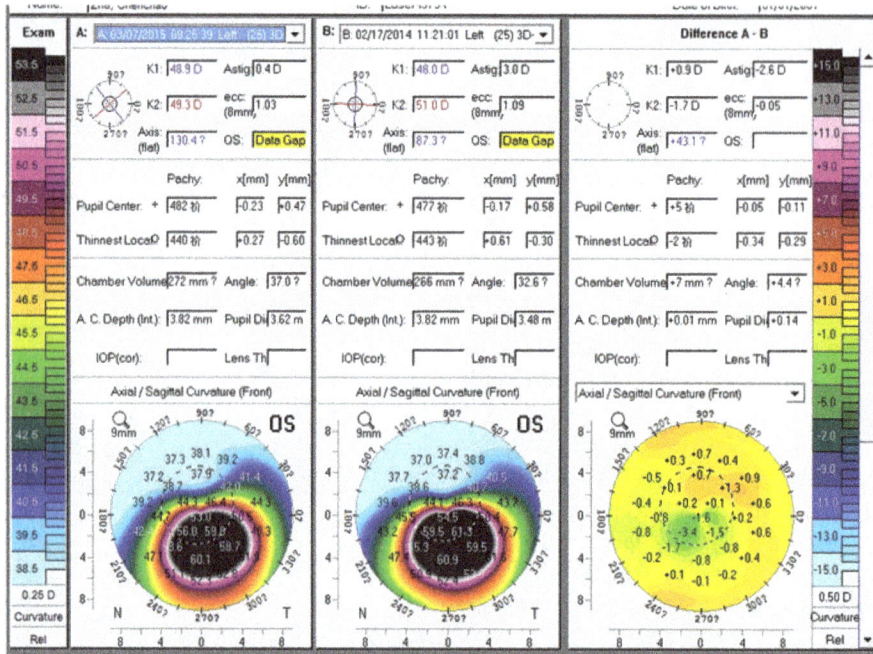

Fig. 3 One-year topographic map changes in a typical case. (Comparison of topographic maps preoperatively and at 1 year postoperatively, showing an increase in K1 of 0.9 D, and a decrease in K2 of 1.7 D)

that ATE-CXL showed good stability in the treatment of progressive keratoconus in pediatric patients. Previous studies have reported that after C-CXL, the corneal thickness of patients was significantly decreased compared to the preoperative values, [7, 15] while in our study, we found that ATE-CXL could keep the corneal thickness stable at each follow-up time point because of its retention of the corneal epithelium. The previous studies typically evaluated the stability of CXL for keratoconus in terms of visual acuity, corneal thickness and keratometry value, and the corneal posterior elevation could also be used as a reliable way of evaluating the stability of the corneal structure. A positive change of the posterior corneal surface indicated an ectatic change of the cornea. This study showed that 1 year postoperatively, the PCE and PME values had no statistically significant differences from the preoperative values, which indicates that ATE-CXL could stabilize the structure of the cornea by preventing corneal expansion. To our knowledge, this is the first prospective clinical study in which corneal posterior elevation had been observed in keratoconus after ATE-CXL.

The current study reported no intraoperative and postoperative complications in pediatric patients, indicating the safety of ATE-CXL. Corneal epithelial defects and corneal haze have been reported for C-CXL treatment of keratoconus [16, 17], but these were not observed for the ATE-CXL treatment. C-CXL treatment with low UV radiation energy (3 mW/cm2) and long

exposure time (30 min) required a long recovery time for the patients, because of removal of the epithelium and the resulting risk of haze. However, ATE-CXL in our study not only maintained the integrity of the corneal epithelium, but also shortened the time of infiltration (10 min) and irradiation (5 min and 20 s). Therefore, ATE-CXL produced mild corneal irritation symptoms and light postoperative reactions, so that patients felt more comfortable in the treatment process, which is more suitable for patients with thin corneas and pediatric patients.

This study demonstrated that ATE-CXL is a safe and effective treatment for progressive keratoconus in pediatric patients. The principle limitation of this study was that the sample size was small, and a longer follow-up of ATE-CXL for pediatric patients is needed to validate the findings.

Conclusions

ATE-CXL is a safe and effective treatment for pediatric progressive keratoconus patients. The long-term effects of ATE-CXL in pediatric patients need further observation.

Abbreviations

ATE-CXL: Accelerated transepithelial corneal collagen cross-linking; BCVA: Best corrected visual acuity; C-CXL: Conventional corneal collagen cross-linking; CD: Cylindrical degree; K1: Steepest meridian keratometry; K2: Flattest meridian keratometry; Kmax: Maximum keratometry; PCE: Posterior central elevation; PME: Posterior mean elevation; SD: Spherical degree; SE: Spherical equivalent; TCT: Thinnest corneal thickness

Acknowledgements
Not applicable.

Funding
This work was supported by a grant from the National Natural Science Foundation of China: Grant No. 81570879 (Xingtao Zhou) and Project of Shanghai Science and Technology: Grant No. 17140902900 (Xingtao Zhou).

Authors' contributions
Concept and design (MT and XTZ); analysis the data (MT and WJ); writing the article (MT and XTZ); critical revision of the article (MT, WJ and XTZ); data collection (MT, YS, LS and XYZ); provision of materials, patients or resources (XTZ); and administrative, technical or logistic support (LS, YS and XYZ). All authors have reviewed the manuscript. All authors read and approved the final manuscript.

Competing interests
The authors declare that they have no competing interests.

References
1. Krachmer JH, Feder RS, Belin MW. Keratoconus and related noninflammatory corneal thinning disorders[J]. Surv Ophthalmol. 1984;28(4):293–322.
2. Tuft SJ, Moodaley LC, Gregory WM, et al. Prognostic factors for the progression of keratoconus[J]. Ophthalmology. 1994;101(3):439–47.
3. Reeves SW, Stinnett S, Adelman RA, et al. Risk factors for progression to penetrating keratoplasty in patients with keratoconus[J]. Am J Ophthalmol. 2005;140(4):607–11.
4. Chatzis N, Hafezi F. Progression of keratoconus and efficacy of pediatric [corrected] corneal collagen cross-linking in children and adolescents[J]. J Refract Surg. 2012;28(11):753–8.
5. Spoerl E, Huhle M, Seiler T. Induction of cross-links in corneal tissue[J]. Exp Eye Res. 1998;66(1):97–103.
6. Wollensak G, Spoerl E, Seiler T. Stress-strain measurements of human and porcine corneas after riboflavin-ultraviolet-A-induced cross-linking[J]. J Cataract Refract Surg. 2003;29(9):1780–5.
7. Kumar KS, Arsiwala AZ, Ramamurthy D. One-year clinical study on efficacy of corneal cross-linking in Indian children with progressive keratoconus[J]. Cornea. 2014;33(9):919–22.
8. Viswanathan D, Kumar NL, Males JJ. Outcome of corneal collagen crosslinking for progressive keratoconus in paediatric patients[J]. Biomed Res Int. 2014;2014:140461.
9. Wise S, Diaz C, Termote K, et al. Corneal cross-linking in pediatric patients with progressive keratoconus[J]. Cornea. 2016;35(11):1441–3.
10. Schuerch K, Tappeiner C, Frueh BE. Analysis of pseudoprogression after corneal cross-linking in children with progressive keratoconus[J]. Acta Ophthalmol. 2016;94(7):e592–9.
11. Shen Y, Jian W, Sun L, et al. One-year follow-up of changes in corneal densitometry after accelerated (45 mW/cm2) transepithelial corneal collagen cross-linking for keratoconus: a retrospective study[J]. Cornea. 2016;35(11):1434–40.
12. Zhang X, Sun L, Chen Y, et al. One-year outcomes of Pachymetry and epithelium thicknesses after accelerated (45 mW/cm(2)) transepithelial corneal collagen cross-linking for keratoconus patients[J]. Sci Rep. 2016;6:32692.
13. El-Khoury S, Abdelmassih Y, Hamade A, et al. Pediatric keratoconus in a tertiary referral center: incidence, presentation, risk factors, and treatment[J]. J Refract Surg. 2016;32(8):534–41.
14. Ucakhan OO, Bayraktutar BN, Saglik A. Pediatric corneal collagen cross-linking: long-term follow-up of visual, refractive, and topographic outcomes[J]. Cornea. 2016;35(2):162–8.
15. Vinciguerra P, Albe E, Frueh BE, et al. Two-year corneal cross-linking results in patients younger than 18 years with documented progressive keratoconus[J]. Am J Ophthalmol. 2012;154(3):520–6.
16. Chow VW, Chan TC, Yu M, et al. One-year outcomes of conventional and accelerated collagen crosslinking in progressive keratoconus[J]. Sci Rep. 2015;5:14425.
17. Nawaz S, Gupta S, Gogia V, et al. Trans-epithelial versus conventional corneal collagen crosslinking: a randomized trial in keratoconus[J]. Oman J Ophthalmol. 2015;8(1):9–13.

15

A meta-analysis of the effect of a dexamethasone intravitreal implant versus intravitreal anti-vascular endothelial growth factor treatment for diabetic macular edema

Ye He[1], Xin-jun Ren[1†], Bo-jie Hu[1†], Wai-Ching Lam[2] and Xiao-rong Li[1*]

Abstract

Background: This meta-analysis evaluated the effectiveness and safety of dexamethasone (DEX) implant and intravitreal anti-vascular endothelial growth factor (VEGF) treatment for diabetic macular edema (DME).

Methods: The PubMed, Embase, clinicaltrials.gov website and Cochrane Library databases were comprehensively searched for studies comparing DEX implant with anti-VEGF in patients with DME. Best-corrected visual acuity (BCVA), central subfield thickness (CST) and adverse events were extracted from the final eligible studies. Review Manager (RevMan) 5.3 for Mac was used to analyze the data and GRADE profiler were used to access the quality of outcomes.

Results: Based on four randomized clinical trials assessing a total of 521 eyes, the DEX implant can achieve visual acuity improvement for DME at rates similar to those achieved via anti-VEGF treatment (mean difference [MD] = − 0.43, $P = 0.35$), with superior anatomic outcomes at 6 months (MD = − 86.71 μm, $P = 0.02$), while requiring fewer injections, in comparison to anti-VEGF treatment. Although the mean reduction in CST did not showed significant difference at 12 months (MD = − 33.77 μm, $P = 0.21$), the significant in BCVA from baseline to 12 months supported the anti-VEGF treatment (MD = − 3.26, $P < 0.00001$). No statistically significant differences in terms of the serious adverse events. However, use of the DEX implant has higher risk of intraocular pressure elevation and cataract than anti-VEGF treatment.

Conclusions: Compared with anti-VEGF, DEX implant improved anatomical outcomes significantly. However, this did not translate to improved visual acuity, which may be due to the progression of cataract. Therefore, the DEX implant may be recommended as a first chioce for select cases, such as for pseudophakic eyes, anti-VEGF-resistant eyes, or patients reluctant to receive intravitreal injections frequently.

Keywords: Diabetic macular edema, Ozurdex, Dexamethasone implant, Anti-VEGF, Meta-analysis

Background

Macular edema (ME) is not an independent disease, but a common phenomenon in various retinal diseases in which fluid and protein accumulate in the extracellular space within the retina [1, 2]. Diabetic macular edema (DME) is macular thickening secondary to diabetic retinopathy (DR) that may be present in any of the stages of this disease, although it manifests more commonly in the non-proliferative diabetic retinopathy stage. In patients with DR, aged 20 to 79 years, the global prevalence for DME is 6.8% [3]. The prevalence of DME is reported to be related to the duration of the diabetes [4, 5]. DME is the foremost cause of central vision loss, and even blindness, and has a great influence on life quality of patients. Thus, reduction of ME may be associated with improved vision.

However, the treatment of DME remains controversial among vitreoretinal specialists. In addition to glycemic

* Correspondence: xiaorli@163.com
†Equal contributors
[1]Department of Retina, Tianjin Medical University Eye Hospital, 251 Fukang Road, Tianjin 300384, China
Full list of author information is available at the end of the article

control, a variety of treatment alternatives exist for patients presenting with DME, including focal or grid photocoagulation, which has been the standard therapy since the 1970s, and more recently, intravitreal injection (anti-VEGF or corticosteroids) has been applied to DME, and vitrectomy in patients with DME with vitreomacular traction. As understanding of the pathophysiology of DME has improved, focal or grid photocoagulation is no longer the first choice for the treatment of DME. Treatment now targets the causal factor specifically, VEGF. To date, anti-VEGF drugs, including aflibercept, ranibizumab, and bevacizumab, have been proven in many clinical trials with efficacy for DME. The RESOLVE [6], RISE/RIDE [7, 8], and READ-2 [9] studies have all shown that ranibizumab is a good choice for the treatment of DME. The BOLT [10] randomized trial showed that bevacizumab is superior to laser monotherapy for persistent center-involving clinically significant macular edema.

Anti-VEGF drugs is still the first-line for treating DME, but also may impose a significant burden for patients who either do not have good respond to anti-VEGF or have recurrent ME, require frequent anti-VEGF injections [11]. Indeed, a study by the Diabetic Retinopathy Clinical Research Network (DRCR. Net), Protocol I revealed that more than 40% of ranibizumab-treated eyes still had CST ≥ 250 μm at 2 years post-treatment. The limited visual gains or resolution of DME in those naive patients are believed to be related to the pathophysiology of DME. Although the contribution of VEGF to the development of DME is indisputable, the role of other non-VEGF pathways has also been considered. Many studies have demonstrated that the inflammation is involved in the DR progression. With the increased recognition of the role of inflammation in the development of DME, sustained-release implants of steroids have shown good anatomical benefit and have also, to some extent, reduced the number of intravitreal injections that is needed in most cases.

Dexamethasone, it has the highest relative clinical efficacy of any corticosteroid applied to ophthalmological practice, and exerts its multiple-effects via its influence on multiple signal transduction pathways. The 0.7 mg intravitreal DEX implant is a biodegradable solid polymer drug-delivery system (Ozurdex®, Allergan, Inc.), which uses the following characteristic mode of drug release by diffusion, in a biphasic fashion: an initial high-concentration phase and a second low-concentration phase, which facilitates continued efficacy of the treatment for up to 6 months [12]. The U.S. Food & Drug Administration (FDA) first approved the Ozurdex for retinal vein occlusion-induced ME treatment in 2009. It was then approved for non-infectious uveitis treatment. In 2014, the FDA and most European countries approved Ozurdex for the treatment of DME, based on results of the MEAD study [13]. Studies of treatment of DME have demonstrated that Ozurdex may be an alternative treatment for patients who do not have good respond to serial anti-VEGF injections or in recalcitrant cases [14–19]. In addition, Ozurdex may be considered as primary treatment for DME [20].

To date, no systematic review has discussed the therapeutic effect and safety of intravitreal anti-VEGF versus DEX implant in DME. We performed a systematic review and meta-analysis to quantify the effect of these two treatments on BCVA and CST in DME. Additionally, we report the adverse events described with these therapies.

Methods
Search strategy
The study was conducted in accordance with Cochrane Handbook for Systematic Reviews and Meta-Analysis (PRISMA) guidelines (Additional file 1) [21]. The following databases were screened: including PubMed, Embase, clinicaltrials.gov, and the Cochrane Library, up to August 2017 (Additional file 2, Table 1). Keywords, including macular edema, dexamethasone intravitreal implant, dexamethasone, anti-VEGF, and Ozurdex were used to maxmise the search accuracy. The literature selections are shown in the PRISMA flow diagram in Fig. 1.

Inclusion and exclusion criteria
Studies were regarded eligible if they accord with the following criterias: (1) the study population included patients with DME; (2) the DEX implant (Ozurdex) was included as an intervention; (3) there was a comparison between the DEX implant (Ozurdex®) and anti-VEGF. Through our analysis of the studies, we determined the following primary outcomes. First, the mean BCVA and mean improvement from baseline in BCVA [time points: baseline, 6 months, and 12 months]. BCVA was obtained using the Early Treatment Diabetic Retinopathy Study (ETDRS). Second, the mean CST and mean change from baseline in CST or foveal thickness, and central macular thickness (CMT) was demonstrated on optical coherence tomography (OCT) [time points: baseline, 6 months, and 12 months]. Additional outcomes collected included the following: 1) total number of serious adverse events (SAEs) at the end of each study; 2) elevation of intraocular pressure (IOP>21 mmHg, required glaucoma agents for IOP control, or IOP elevation by at least 5 mmHg from baseline at any follow-up visit; 3) the number of cataracts; 4) the mean number of intravitreal injections; and 5) the study design should be randomized controlled trials (RCTs).

We designed the study to have no limitations on dose. Patients taking bevacizumab and ranibizumab were placed in the anti-VEGF group. The two authors, Ye He and Bojie Hu assessed all eligible studies independently. A consensus was reached if there were any cases of disagreement. The exclusion criteria included studies with insufficient data, non-RCTs, case reports, review articles.

Table 1 Summary of the characteristics of the included studies

Study	Place	Conditions	Participants numbers	Interventions details	Total number of treatments	Age (years)	Female sex, no. (%)	BCVA at baseline	CST/CMT (μm) at baseline	Follow-up duration (months)
Gillies et al. 2014 <The BEVORDEX Study> [23]	Australia	DR	DEX: 46 IVB: 42	DEX: 0.7 mg every 16 weeks + PRN IVB: 0.5 mg every 4 weeks + PRN	DEX: 2.7 IVB: 8.6	DEX: 61.4 ± 9.0 IVB: 62.2 ± 10.5 ($P = 0.71$)	DEX: 16 (35%) IVB: 16 (38%) ($P = 0.83$)	DEX: 55.5 ± 12.5 IVB: 56.3 ± 11.9 ($P = 0.75$)	DEX: 474.3 ± 95.9 IVB: 503 ± 140.9 ($P = 0.38$)	12
Allergan 2015 [27]	Multiple countries: Belgium, Denmark, France, Germany, Israel, Italy, Netherlands, Portugal, South Africa, Spain, United Kingdom, United States	DR	DEX: 181 IVR: 182	DEX: 0.7 mg on Day 1, Month 5, and Month 10 IVR: 0.5 mg into the study eye on Day 1. Patients may receive additional injections on a monthly basis, as needed, for disease progression	NA	NA	DEX: 69 (38%) IVR: 66 (36%)	DEX: 60.2 ± 9.74 IVR: 60.4 ± 9.34	DEX: 465.1 ± 136.09 IVR: 471.2 ± 139.51	12
Shah et al. 2016 [24]	Indiana, United States	DR	DEX: 27 IVB: 23	DEX: 0.7 mg given every 3 months over 6 month period with a maximum of 3 injections IVB: 1.25 mg given monthly during a 6 month period	DEX: 2.7 ± 0.5 IVB: 7.0 ± 0.2 ($P < 0.001$)	DEX: 65 ± 11 IVB: 61 ± 9 ($P = 0.209$)	DEX: 15 (56%) IVB: 10 (44%) ($P = 0.571$)	DEX: 59 ± 12 IVB: 59 ± 13 ($P = 0.770$)	DEX: 458 ± 100 IVB: 485 ± 122 ($P = 0.508$)	7
Gallemore et al. 2017 [26]	California, United States	DR	DEX: 10 IVB: 10	DEX: Ozurdex, 0.7 mg given at initial visit and at month 4 (visit 5) IVB: 1.25 mg given at initial visit and Q1 month for a total of 5 treatments	NA	DEX: 63.9 ± 1.8 IVB: 61.2 ± 2.9	DEX: 5 (50%) IVB: 3 (30%)	DEX: 67.8 ± 3.8 IVB: 71.9 ± 2.9	DEX: 385.9 ± 43.0 IVB: 341.5 ± 11.3	6

NA not available, *PRN* pro re nata

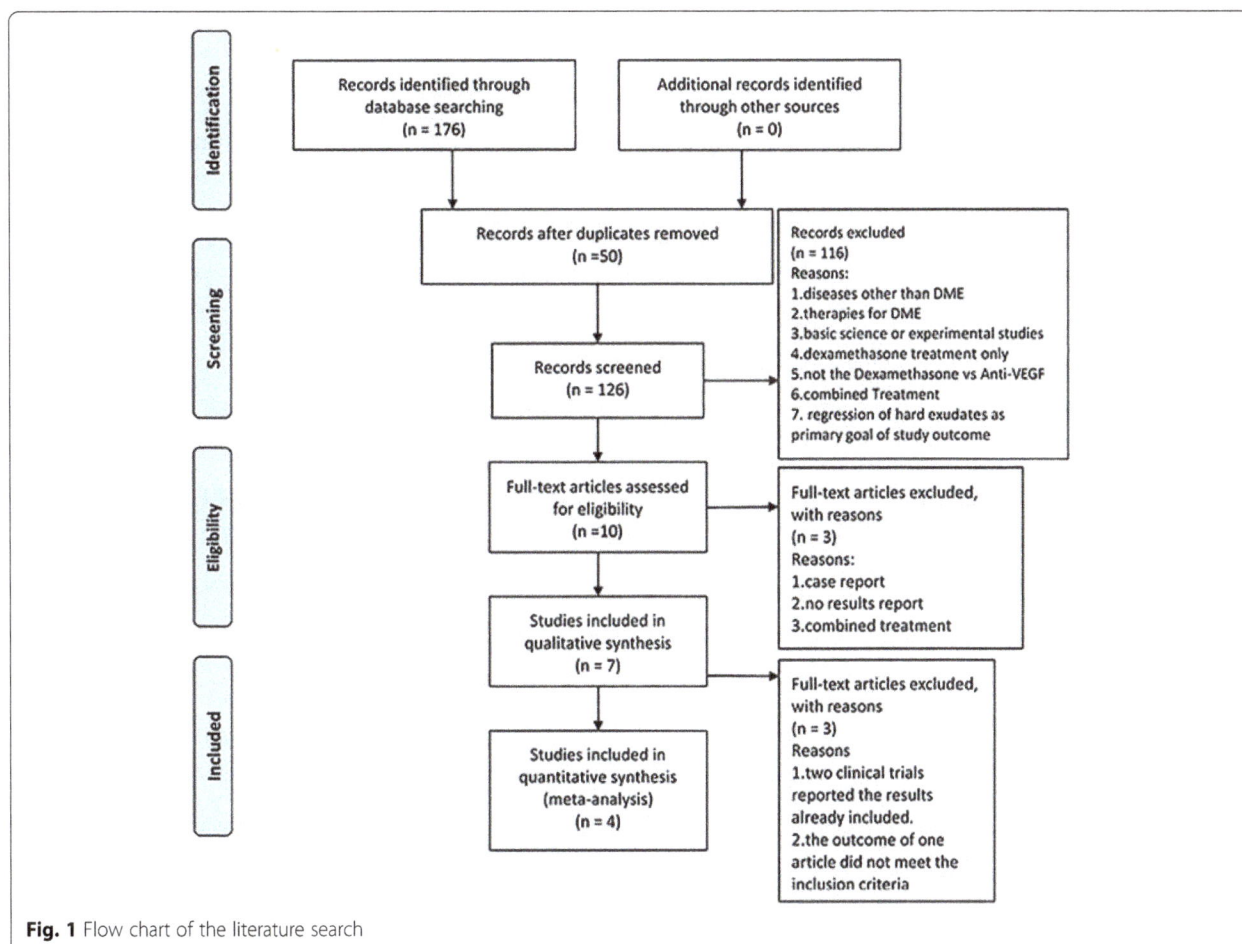

Fig. 1 Flow chart of the literature search

Data extraction and risk of bias assessment

The relevant data from the articles were extracted by two reviewers (Ye He and Bo-jie Hu) independently, using a standard data extraction form. The extracted data included the first author(s) or the information provider, publishing date, study design, sample size, geographical location of the research, interventions details, age, sex, outcomes and follow-up periods. We emailed the corresponding authors of the studies for which we had unanswered questions to ensure completeness of our study, and to acquire incomplete and missing data. Data are showed in the format: mean ± standard deviation (SD). We used the formula that $SD = SE*\sqrt{N}$) to calculate SD if the data was reported as standard error (SE). Afterwards, we used Get Data software to estimate the mean and the SD from the reported graph. The Cochrane Collaboration's tool was applied to assess the risk of bias in each study based on the Cochrane Handbook.

Statistical analysis

RevMan 5.3 was applied to integration collected data statistics and analysis. The mean difference (MD) and risk ratio (RR) were used to assess continuous variable outcomes and dichotomous outcomes with a 95% confidence interval

[CI], respectively. The heterogeneity of studies was accessed using the chi-square test based on the values of P and I^2. The random-effects model was applied for the meta-analysis. I^2 results between 50 and 100% represented substantial heterogeneity. P values < 0.05 were considered statistically significant.

Quality of the evidence

The evidence quality of all included outcomes was evaluated based on the GRADE system [22]. Initially, RCTs were regarded as high-quality evidence for the estimation of study effects. Factors such as risk of bias, imprecision and inconsistency of results etc., all of which can result in rating down the quality of evidence for specific outcomes, reduced the level of confidence in estimating the study effects. The GRADE evidence was divided into the four categories (High, Moderate, Low and Very low-quality evidence).

Results

Search results

A total of 176 potential records up to August 2017 were identified with the electronic-based search (PubMed = 83, Embase = 52, clinicaltrials.gov=38, and the Cochrane

Library = 3). After eliminating 50 duplicates, a total of 126 potentially eligible studies were retrieved. After reading the title and abstract, 116 of these studies were excluded. We further excluded three studies after reading the full text due to ineligible for criteria. Among the 7 studies included in the qualitative synthesis, two clinical trials (ClinicalTrials.gov identifier: NCT01298076; NCT02036424) were duplicates, because the data had already been published. Among these published articles [23–25], the outcome of one article did not meet the inclusion criteria [25]. After looking through all eligible studies, four studies comprising 521 study eyes were used in our meta-analysis (Fig. 1) [23, 24, 26, 27].

All of included studies were RCTs and the characteristics of these studies are summarized in Table 1. The sample size of the four studies ranged from 20 to 363. Two studies were published in 2014 and 2016. Two studies reported their

results online and verified the results in January 2015 and April 2017, respectively. In all included studies, the dose of the DEX implant was the same. However, in the study by Shah et al., dexamethasone (0.7 mg) was given every 3 months instead of every 4 months as in the other included studies. Among them, Gillies et al., Shah et al., and Gallemore et al. performed intravitreal bevacizumab (IVB) injection, while Allergan study used intravitreal ranibizumab (IVR) injection. The risk of bias assessment and the results of the GRADE evidence are presented in Fig. 2 and Additional file 2: Table S2, respectively.

Meta-analysis results
Mean BCVA at 6 months
Data from three studies assessing 157 eyes (82 eyes with DEX treatment, 75 eyes with anti-VEGF treatment) reported the BCVA at 6 months. No difference in the treatment effect

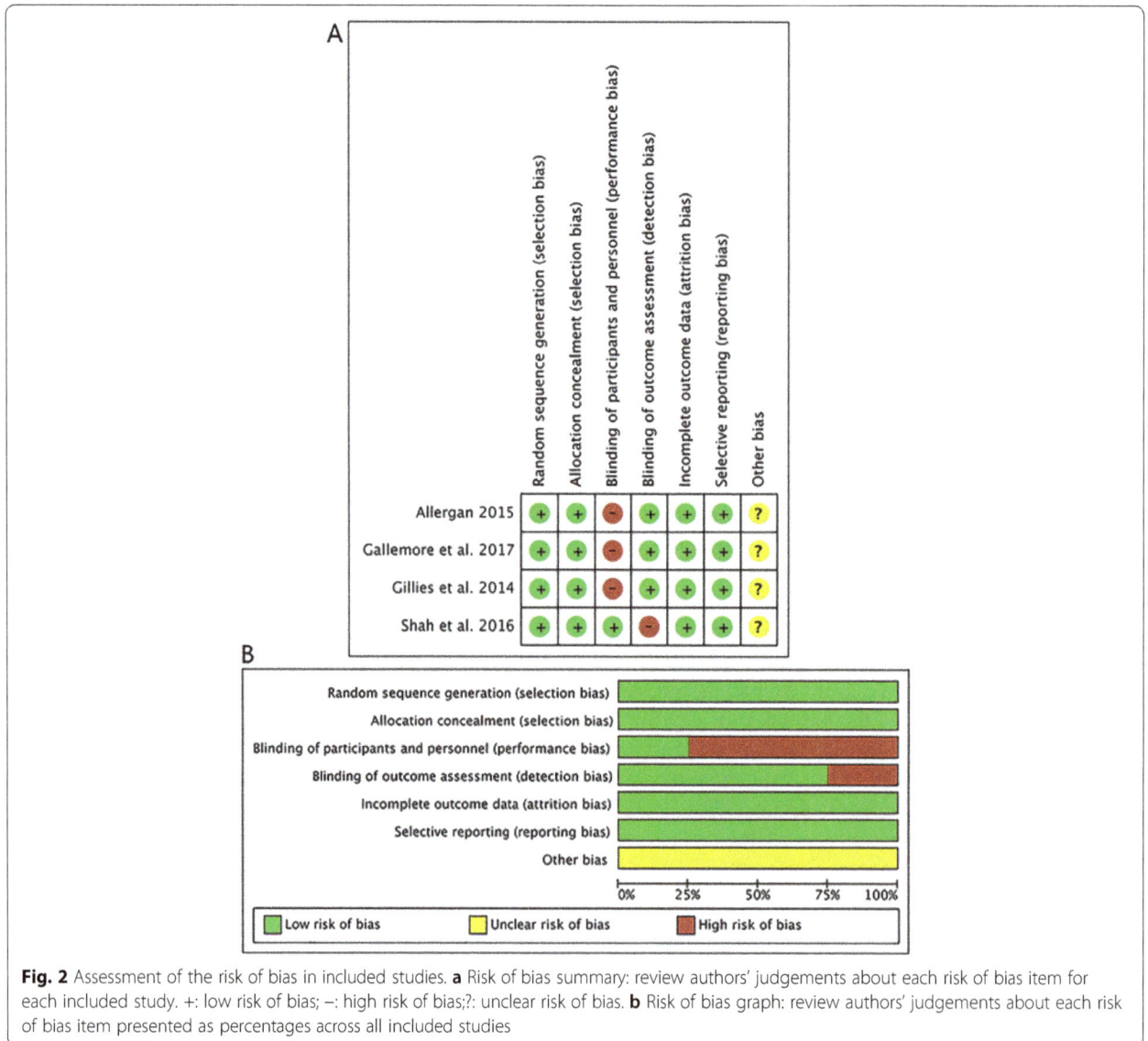

Fig. 2 Assessment of the risk of bias in included studies. a Risk of bias summary: review authors' judgements about each risk of bias item for each included study. +: low risk of bias; –: high risk of bias;?: unclear risk of bias. b Risk of bias graph: review authors' judgements about each risk of bias item presented as percentages across all included studies

on BCVA at 6 months between the two treatment arms; the MD in visual acuity of the three trials was − 0.43 (95% CI: -1.32 to 0.47, $P = 0.35$, Fig. 3). No statistical heterogeneity was found (chi^2 = 0.26, $P = 0.88$, I^2 = 0%).

Mean change in BCVA at 6 months and 12 months

At 6 months, data from three studies assessing 157 eyes reported the an improvement in BCVA from baseline. Because the clinical effect in 6 months was similar to that in 7 months, we used the data from month 7 to represent month 6 in the study by Shah et al. [24]. The DEX group reported a similar mean change in BCVA from baseline compared with the anti-VEGF group (MD = 0.32; 95% CI, − 2.54 to 3.17; $P = 0.83$; Fig. 4), and no heterogeneity was found ($P = 0.99$, I^2 = 0%). A meta-analysis at 12 months was conducted using two studies of 451 eyes to assess the improvement in BCVA from baseline. Statistically significant differences were discovered between the DEX implant and anti-VEGF treatment groups, in favor of the anti-VEGF group (MD = − 3.26, 95% CI: -4.66 to − 1.86, $P < 0.00001$; Fig. 4) and no heterogeneity was found ($P = 0.99$, I^2 = 0%).

Mean CST at 6 months

Three studies of 157 eyes included data on CST at 6 months after the initial treatment. Meta-analysis demonstrated that all studies except that by Gallemore et al. [26] showed a marked reduction in CST from baseline in the DEX group. The MD for all studies at 6 months was statistically significant (MD = − 86.71 μm, 95% CI: − 161.61 to − 11.82, $P = 0.02$) in favor of DEX treatment over anti-VEGF treatment, and showed high heterogeneity ($P < 0.00001$, I^2 = 95%; Fig. 5).

Mean change in CST at 6 months and 12 months

Data from three studies assessing 157 eyes reported the mean change from baseline to 6 months in terms of the reduction of CST was significantly greater in the DEX groups (MD = − 88.74, 95% CI: -122.85 to − 54.63, $P < 0.00001$, Fig. 6). However, this superiority was no longer observed at 12 months. Data from two studies assessing 417 eyes at 12 months, with a combined mean difference in CST of − 33.77 μm, did not show statistically significant differences (95% CI: -86.72 to − 19.18, $P = 0.21$), and showed a large amount of heterogeneity between the two studies ($P = 0.08$, I^2 = 68%, Fig. 6).

Total serious adverse events

All four studies reported complications during the follow-up period, such as increased IOP, cataract, and vitreous hemorrhage. In these studies, the study by Gallemore et al. reported no serious adverse events during the follow-up period. The total SAEs reported by the three studies are presented in the forest plot (Fig. 7). Analysis of the available data demonstrated a lower incidence of serious adverse events in the DEX arm (RR = 0.89), with no heterogeneity ($P = 0.44$, I^2 = 0%), however the differences were not statistically significant (95% CI: 0.63 to 1.26; $P = 0.51$).

Elevation of IOP

All cases demonstrated increased IOP after injection of DEX/anti-VEGF; this was mostly controllable by medication or surgery. Low heterogeneity was detected between studies (I^2 = 43%, $P = 0.15$, Fig. 8). Analysis using a random-effects model demonstrated a statistically significant difference between DEX and anti-VEGF treatment (RR = 4.14; 95% CI: 1.89 to 8.65; $P = 0.0002$).

Adverse events: cataract

Three studies involving 501 eyes reported post-operative cataract. Statistically significant difference was founded between the DEX and anti-VEGF groups (RR =2.68, 95% CI: 1.54 to 4.68, $P = 0.0005$), without heterogeneity ($P = 0.44$, I^2 = 0%, Fig. 9).

Mean number of intravitreal injections

In the study by Shah et al. [24], more injections were required in the IVB group (7.0 ± 0.2) compared to the DEX group ($P = 0.001$) over a follow-up period. Similarly, no statistically significant difference in BCVA according to Gillies et al., but a lower treatment frequency was required for the DEX implant (mean number: 2.7), which was an obvious advantage over IVB treatment (mean number: 8.6) [23].

Discussion

In our study, we evaluated four RCTs to evaluate the efficacies of DEX implants and anti-VEGF in the treatment of DME. We found that both DEX implant and anti-VEGF could achieve significant functional and anatomical improvement during early treatment. We did not find statistically significant differences in terms of BCVA and with no statistical

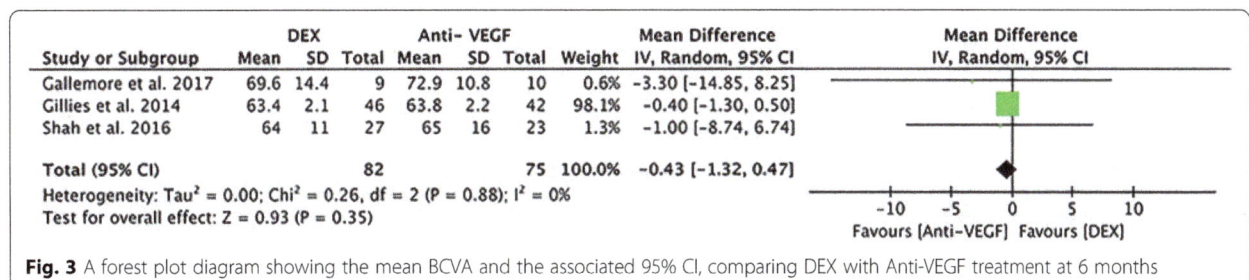

Study or Subgroup	DEX Mean	DEX SD	DEX Total	Anti−VEGF Mean	Anti−VEGF SD	Anti−VEGF Total	Weight	Mean Difference IV, Random, 95% CI
Gallemore et al. 2017	69.6	14.4	9	72.9	10.8	10	0.6%	−3.30 [−14.85, 8.25]
Gillies et al. 2014	63.4	2.1	46	63.8	2.2	42	98.1%	−0.40 [−1.30, 0.50]
Shah et al. 2016	64	11	27	65	16	23	1.3%	−1.00 [−8.74, 6.74]
Total (95% CI)			82			75	100.0%	−0.43 [−1.32, 0.47]

Heterogeneity: Tau^2 = 0.00; Chi^2 = 0.26, df = 2 (P = 0.88); I^2 = 0%
Test for overall effect: Z = 0.93 (P = 0.35)

Fig. 3 A forest plot diagram showing the mean BCVA and the associated 95% CI, comparing DEX with Anti-VEGF treatment at 6 months

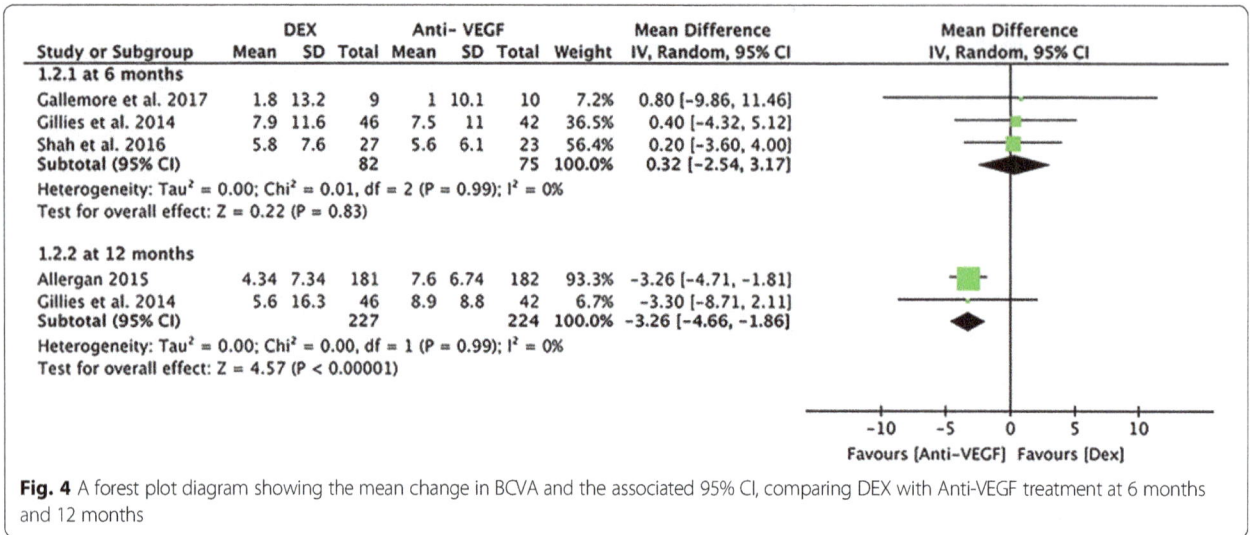

Fig. 4 A forest plot diagram showing the mean change in BCVA and the associated 95% CI, comparing DEX with Anti-VEGF treatment at 6 months and 12 months

heterogeneity between these two treatment arms at 6 months. However, the anti-VEGF group revealed significant improvement in BCVA at 12 months, compared to the DEX implant group, and without statistical heterogeneity. These findings are in line with the Protocol I in DRCR.net, whereby the ranibizumab group had better visual acuity than the triamcinolone group.

Even with good treatment effects, repeated injections carry increased risks, such as infectious endophthalmitis, intraocular inflammation, and even stroke or myocardial infarction [28]. Therefore, anti-VEGF treatment may not be a good therapy for all patients. DME has been shown to be a complex multifactorial disease; in addition to VEGF, inflammation may be another pathophysiological feature of these treatment-naive patients. Diabetics are found to have high concentrations of pro-inflammatory cytokines, such as interleukin 6 (IL-6), IL-1β, tumor necrosis factor α (TNFα), and intracellular adhesion molecule (ICAM)-1. All of these cytokines induce retina with persistent chronic inflammation, which leads to leukostasis, increased vascular permeability and dysfunction of the blood-retinal barrier (BRB) [29, 30]. Additionally, according to an investigation by Jonas et al. [31], DME was shown to be related to elevated cytokines in the aqueous humor or vitreous, such as ICAM-1, IL-6, transforming growth factor beta (TGF-β) and monocyte chemotactic protein 1 (MCP-1). Among the cytokines,

ICAM-1 is closely related with diabetes characteristics. Thus, treatment principally aims to block the effect of these two pathogenic pathways. Corticosteroids have anti-inflammatory, anti-permeability, and angiostatic effects when treating DME [32]. Thus, DEX implant could be a better alternative for DME.

Our analysis demonstrated that DEX implant treatment could significantly reduce CST at 6 months, compared to anti-VEGF treatment. Unfortunately, this effect can not last until 12 months. This can be explained by the characteristics of the DEX implant. There are two phases in the DEX implant treatment. Higher concentrations of DEX are found in the initial phase, followed by lower concentrations in the final phase. The drug reaches its peak efficacy less than two months after administration. Afterwards, the drug continues to provide treatment, but, at lower levels in months 2–6 [12]. Regarding heterogeneity, we could not perform a subgroup analysis to interpret the potential source of heterogeneity, due to the limited studies. We suspect that, at 6 months, the heterogeneity mainly derives from the small sample size of the study by Gallemore et al. Moreover, the results of CST may be affected by other factors, including initial retinal thickness, the dosage of bevacizumab, and previous treatment (laser or anti-VEGF). The mean change in CST at 12 months showed heterogeneity mainly caused by the

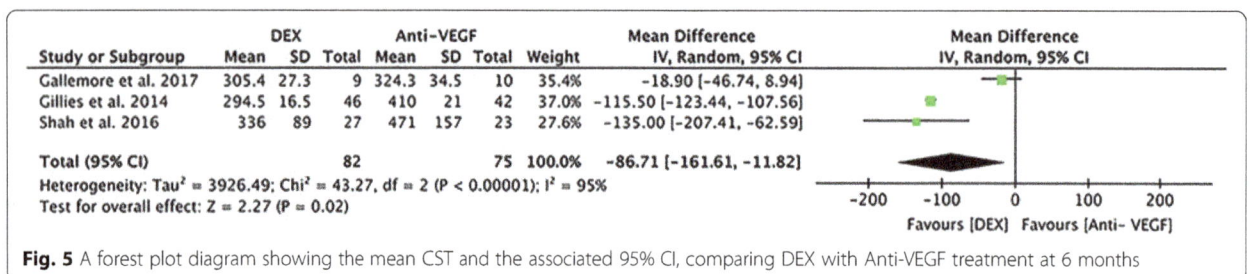

Fig. 5 A forest plot diagram showing the mean CST and the associated 95% CI, comparing DEX with Anti-VEGF treatment at 6 months

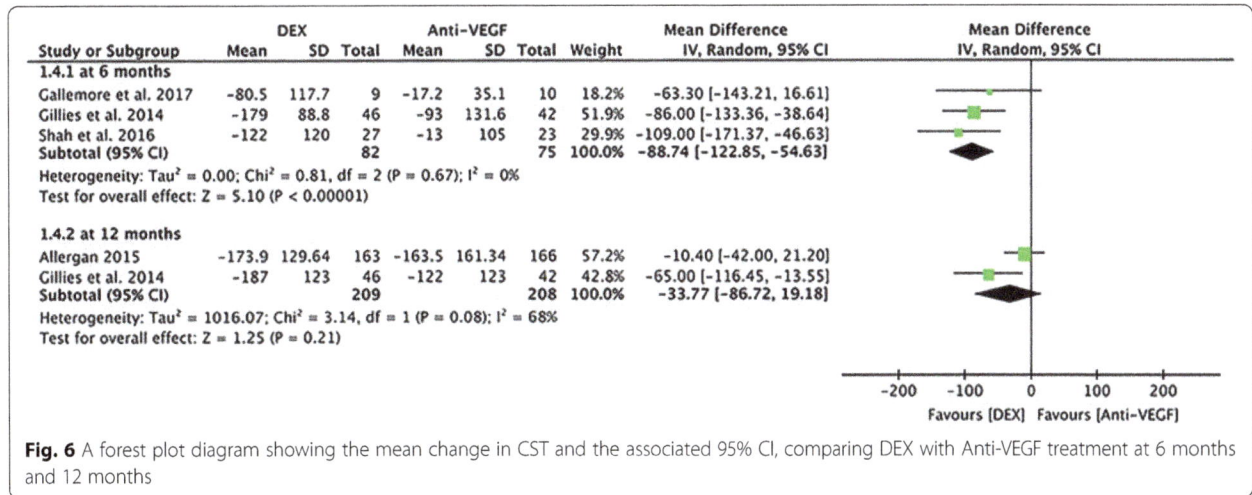

Fig. 6 A forest plot diagram showing the mean change in CST and the associated 95% CI, comparing DEX with Anti-VEGF treatment at 6 months and 12 months

type of anti-VEGF drugs used. In the Allergan 2015 study [27], patients received 0.5 mg ranibizumab. However, in the BEVORDEX study [23], 0.5 mg bevacizumab was given to the patients. It has been reported that ranibizumab and bevacizumab do not differ in terms of functional outcomes, but that ranibizumab was more effective in terms of CST reduction [33]. Factors such as race, dosage, age, and baseline states may have attributed to heterogeneity. To some extent, these factors were unavoidable. In terms of CST, at 6 months, Ozurdex showed superior reduction in CST, which indicates that patients with DME can achieve superior anatomical outcomes with fewer injections. Similar to our results, the results from the MEAD study evaluating the DEX implant showed that a mean number of 4.1 DEX treatments were administered after 3 years of follow-up. Compared to the sham group, the DEX group acquired a CST reduction of 112 μm, nearly three times than the sham group (42 μm).

Notably, the improved anatomical outcomes in our data did not translate to improved visual acuity outcomes. Results from other clinical trials were consistent with the four studies included here. In the CHROME study [34], significant reduction in retinal thickness were occurred in the Ozurdex group: 190.9 ± 23.5 μm for DME (*P* < 0.0001). The greatest mean improvements in

BCVA in terms of number of lines of vision observed in the eyes with DME (0.7 ± 0.5; *P* > 0.05). Similarly, compared to monthly IVB monotherapy (– 30 μm), the combination therapy with DEX and bevacizumab led to a significantly greater change of CST (– 45 μm) in the study by Maturi et al.; nevertheless, visual acuity improvement was not statistically significant [35]. The limited visual gains in these patients may have been related to the duration of macular edema, neural damage, retinal pigment epithelium changes, and subretinal fibrosis caused by chronic macular edema prior to treatment, as well as the result of structural damage from repeated macular laser therapy, and the natural course of DR [7].

Additionally, we suspect that it may be due to DEX-induced progression of cataract, based on previous studies. In the DRCR Protocol I, when controlling for cataract formation, in pseudophakic eyes, the group that received triamcinolone observed similar BCVA results to the ranibizumab group. Similar to this study, the CHROME study also showed that the pseudophakic eyes with DME acquired a average gain of 1.4 ± 0.5 lines, but a average loss of 0.6 ± 0.6 lines was shown in phakic eyes [34]. These results are also in agreement with those of the BEVORDEX study, which found exhibited no significant effect for pseudophakic eyes. Compared to 10.4

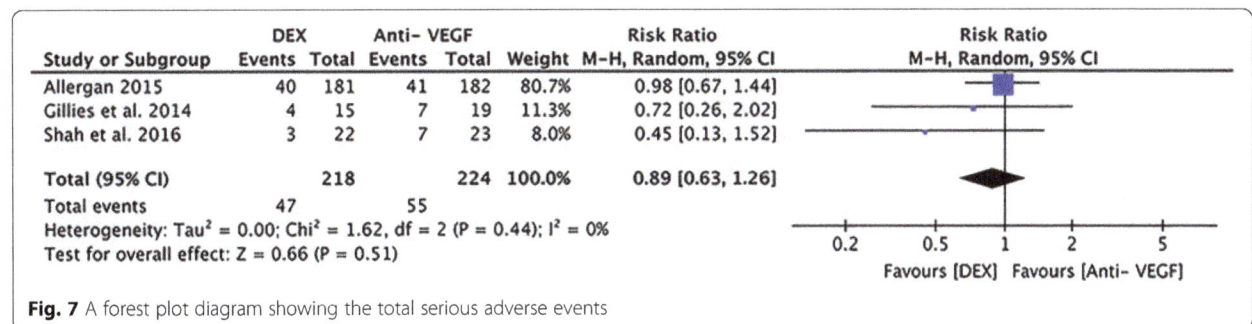

Fig. 7 A forest plot diagram showing the total serious adverse events

Study or Subgroup	DEX Events	Total	Anti-VEGF Events	Total	Weight	Risk Ratio M–H, Random, 95% CI
Allergan 2015	65	181	12	182	46.9%	5.45 [3.05, 9.73]
Gallemore et al. 2017	1	10	0	10	5.2%	3.00 [0.14, 65.90]
Gillies et al. 2014	21	46	8	42	41.5%	2.40 [1.19, 4.82]
Shah et al. 2016	14	27	0	23	6.4%	24.86 [1.56, 395.09]
Total (95% CI)		264		257	100.0%	4.14 [1.98, 8.65]
Total events	101		20			

Heterogeneity: Tau^2 = 0.21; Chi^2 = 5.27, df = 3 (P = 0.15); I^2 = 43%
Test for overall effect: Z = 3.78 (P = 0.0002)

Fig. 8 A forest plot diagram showing the elevation of IOP

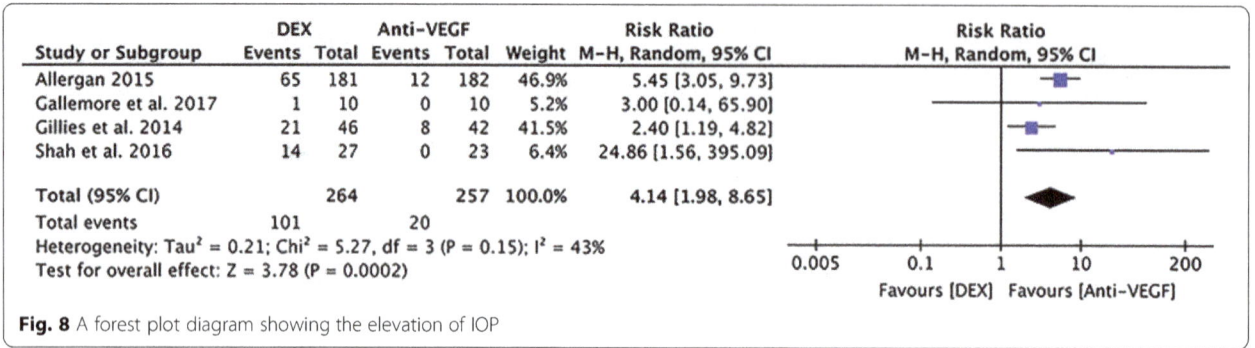

letters in the dexamethasone group, the mean change in BCVA for the bevacizumab group was 7.7 letters ($P = 0.47$). Moreover, visual acuity may be affected by postoperative complications, such as Irvine–Gass syndrome or cataract secondary to pars plana vitrectomy prior to DEX or anti-VEGF treatment.

In addition to having different efficacies for treating DME, DEX implants and anti-VEGF injection are associated with varying degrees of increased risk of systemic and/or local complications over the period of treatment. The systemic adverse event rate has been reported to be higher with anti-VEGF treatment in some clinical trials [36]. In the study by Avery et al., the increased potentially cerebrovascular accidents may be link to anti-VEGF treatment, especially after two years therapy [37]. Similar to previous studies, our data demonstrated that a lower incidence of SAEs in the DEX implant group, but this was not statistically significantly different between the DEX and anti-VEGF group. These results suggest that we should be cautious in using anti-VEGF in patients with myocardial infarction and stroke [38]. The deterioration of hypertension was the most frequent systemic adverse event encountered in the BEVORDEX study. Other adverse events, such as cardiac disorders, also occurred in the studies included in this meta-analysis, except in the study by Gallemore et al. High IOP and secondary cataract are the most common ocular adverse events of DEX implants. Our meta-analysis agrees with these findings, which demonstrated a statistically significant difference between the two groups in

terms of increased IOP and cataract. The groups receiving DEX had a higher risk of a rise in IOP and cataract progression than the anti-VEGF groups for DME. This suggests that the ophthalmologist should take care when using DEX implants in patients with high IOP or in young patients with a clear lens.

The relative benefits and costs should also be considered when applying therapies. In terms of cost-effectiveness, intravitreal corticosteroid injections are relatively cheaper than anti-VEGF therapies, although this is not true for ranibizumab. One study calculated the amount of money (USD) saved per line of visual acuity improvement for each of the various therapies as follows: DEX implant—$5666, bevacizumab—$1329–$2246, and ranibizumab—$11,372–$11,609. In addition, the dollars per quality-adjusted life year for these therapies were as follows: DEX implant—$9446, bevacizumab—$2013–$4260, and ranibizumab—$19,251–$23,119 [39].

Currently, dexamethasone delivery systems and anti-VEGF therapies have a positive effect on the course of DME. However, these two different types of drugs have different pharmacological properties and side-effect characteristics. Given the results of clinical trials and the pathophysiology of DME, Ozurdex is considered to be the preferred treatment for patients who have chronic DME and are anti-VEGF-resistant, as an alternative to switching between anti-VEGF drugs [40, 41]. Ozurdex may be recommended as a first choice for the following cases: 1. pseudophakic eyes, or patients who are under consideration for cataract surgery in the near future; 2.

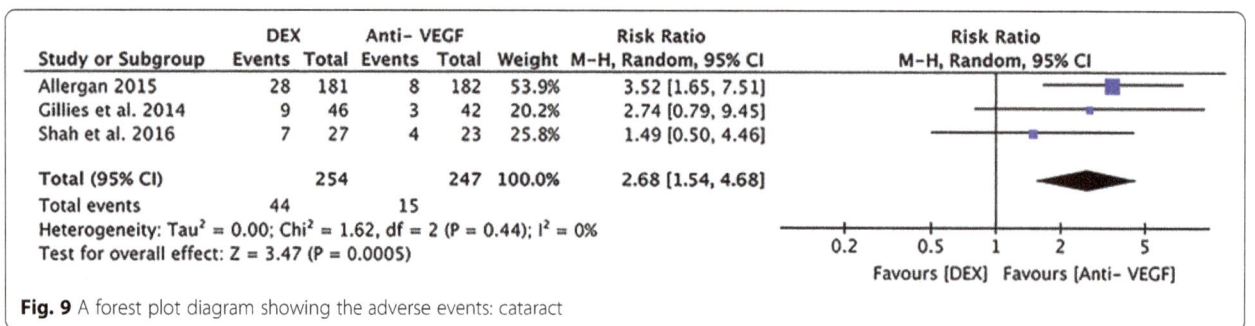

Study or Subgroup	DEX Events	Total	Anti-VEGF Events	Total	Weight	Risk Ratio M–H, Random, 95% CI
Allergan 2015	28	181	8	182	53.9%	3.52 [1.65, 7.51]
Gillies et al. 2014	9	46	3	42	20.2%	2.74 [0.79, 9.45]
Shah et al. 2016	7	27	4	23	25.8%	1.49 [0.50, 4.46]
Total (95% CI)		254		247	100.0%	2.68 [1.54, 4.68]
Total events	44		15			

Heterogeneity: Tau^2 = 0.00; Chi^2 = 1.62, df = 2 (P = 0.44); I^2 = 0%
Test for overall effect: Z = 3.47 (P = 0.0005)

Fig. 9 A forest plot diagram showing the adverse events: cataract

patients who are anti-VEGF-resistant [42]; 3. patients who have a history of cardiovascular and cerebrovascular diseases [42]; 4. post-vitrectomy patients [18]; 5. patients without a high IOP risk at baseline; 6. patients who are reluctant to receive frequent injections. In all cases, the IOP should to be monitored frequently. Reinjection of Ozurdex can be considered after approximately 3–6 months if remains evidence of impaired vision and residual ME.

Our study was limited by the following factors: (1) We only included four studies assessing a total of 521 eyes. (2) The clinical trails duration was quite short in some of the that were included, and thus we may have underestimated the drug-induced adverse events. (3) Heterogeneity was inevitable due to the different regimens of anti-VEGF therapies used. Previous studies indicated that the efficacy of aflibercept, ranibizumab or bevacizumab for DME was different but the relative efficacy depended on baseline BCVA. At the 1-year follow-up, aflibercept exhibited some advantage over bevacizumab and ranibizumab, especially among patients with an initial baseline BCVA letter score of less than 69. However, ranibizumab and bevacizumab did not show significant differences [28, 33]. A previous meta-analysis study also confirmed that bevacizumab and ranibizumab did not differ in terms of BCVA, but ranibizumab was more effective in terms of CST reduction with a low-certainty of evidence [43]. To reinforce the validity of our meta-analysis, clinical trials comparing the 3 anti-VEGF agents with the DEX implant as well as extended follow-up trials should be conducted in the future.

Conclusions

In summary, this meta-analysis of data from four randomized clinical trials revealed that despite some ocular adverse events, DEX-treated eyes had relatively superior anatomic outcomes compared with anti-VEGF, and showed similar rates of vision improvement, while requiring fewer injections, especially in pseudophakic patients. However, considering for the restrictions of indications, the DEX implant may not be recommended as a first-line therapy for DME. In the future, randomization of these treatments would allow a definite conclusion about whether switching to a DEX implant is more beneficial rather than anti-VEGF treatment. Additionally, new treatments (monotherapy or combined therapy) should be investigated to optimize clinical efficacy and reduce side-effects.

Abbreviations
BCVA: Best corrected visual acuity; CI: Confidence interval; CMT: Central macular thickness; CST: Central subfield thickness; DEX implant: Dexamethasone intravitreal implant; DRCR. Net: Diabetic Retinopathy Clinical Research Network; ETDRS: Early Treatment Diabetic Retinopathy Study; FDA: Food & Drug Administration; IVB: Intravitreal bevacizumab; IVR: Intravitreal ranibizumab; MD: Mean difference; ME: Macular edema; NA: Not available; OCT: Optical coherence tomography; PRN: Pro re nata; RCTs: Randomized controlled trials; RevMan: Review Manager; RR: Risk ratio; SAEs: Serious adverse events; SD: Standard deviation; SE: Standard error; VEGF: Vascular endothelial growth factor

Acknowledgements
The authors thank Ming-jie Kuang for helping with the statistical analysis.

Authors' contributions
YH designed this study. BJH and YH collected and analyzed the data and generated the figures. WCL reviewed and revised the manuscript. XRL, XJR and BJH involved with the manuscript development, proofreading and approved the final version of the manuscript. All authors read and approved the final manuscript.

Competing interests
The authors declare that they have no competing interests.

Author details
[1]Department of Retina, Tianjin Medical University Eye Hospital, 251 Fukang Road, Tianjin 300384, China. [2]Department of Ophthalmology, The University of Hong Kong, Hong Kong, China.

References
1. Ferris FL 3rd, Patz A. Macular edema. A complication of diabetic retinopathy. Surv Ophthalmol. 1984;28 Suppl:452–61.
2. Patz A, Schatz H, Berkow JW, Gittelsohn AM, Ticho U. Macular edema–an overlooked complication of diabetic retinopathy. Trans Am Acad Ophthalmol Otolaryngol. 1973;77:Op34–42.
3. Yau JW, Rogers SL, Kawasaki R, Lamoureux EL, Kowalski JW, Bek T, Chen SJ, Dekker JM, Fletcher A, Grauslund J, et al. Global prevalence and major risk factors of diabetic retinopathy. Diabetes Care. 2012;35:556–64.
4. Klein R, Klein BE, Moss SE, Davis MD, DeMets DL. The Wisconsin epidemiologic study of diabetic retinopathy. IV. Diabetic macular edema. Ophthalmology. 1984;91:1464–74.
5. Williams R, Airey M, Baxter H, Forrester J, Kennedy-Martin T, Girach A. Epidemiology of diabetic retinopathy and macular oedema: a systematic review. Eye (Lond). 2004;18:963–83.
6. Massin P, Bandello F, Garweg JG, Hansen LL, Harding SP, Larsen M, Mitchell P, Sharp D, Wolf-Schnurrbusch UE, Gekkieva M, et al. Safety and efficacy of ranibizumab in diabetic macular edema (RESOLVE study): a 12-month, randomized, controlled, double-masked, multicenter phase II study. Diabetes Care. 2010;33:2399–405.
7. Brown DM, Nguyen QD, Marcus DM, Boyer DS, Patel S, Feiner L, Schlottmann PG, Rundle AC, Zhang J, Rubio RG, et al. Long-term outcomes of ranibizumab therapy for diabetic macular edema: the 36-month results from two phase III trials: RISE and RIDE. Ophthalmology. 2013;120:2013–22.
8. Nguyen QD, Brown DM, Marcus DM, Boyer DS, Patel S, Feiner L, Gibson A, Sy J, Rundle AC, Hopkins JJ, et al. Ranibizumab for diabetic macular edema: results from 2 phase III randomized trials: RISE and RIDE. Ophthalmology. 2012;119:789–801.
9. Nguyen QD, Shah SM, Khwaja AA, Channa R, Hatef E, Do DV, Boyer D, Heier JS, Abraham P, Thach AB, et al. Two-year outcomes of the ranibizumab for edema of the mAcula in diabetes (READ-2) study. Ophthalmology. 2010;117: 2146–51.
10. Rajendram R, Fraser-Bell S, Kaines A, Michaelides M, Hamilton RD, Esposti SD, Peto T, Egan C, Bunce C, Leslie RD, Hykin PG. A 2-year prospective randomized controlled trial of intravitreal bevacizumab or laser therapy (BOLT) in the management of diabetic macular edema: 24-month data: report 3. Arch Ophthalmol. 2012;130:972–9.
11. Sim DA, Keane PA, Tufail A, Egan CA, Aiello LP, Silva PS. Automated retinal image analysis for diabetic retinopathy in telemedicine. Curr Diab Rep. 2015;15:14.
12. Chang-Lin JE, Attar M, Acheampong AA, Robinson MR, Whitcup SM, Kuppermann BD, Welty D. Pharmacokinetics and pharmacodynamics of a sustained-release dexamethasone intravitreal implant. Invest Ophthalmol Vis Sci. 2011;52:80–6.

13. Boyer DS, Yoon YH, Belfort R Jr, Bandello F, Maturi RK, Augustin AJ, Li XY, Cui H, Hashad Y, Whitcup SM, Ozurdex MSG. Three-year, randomized, sham-controlled trial of dexamethasone intravitreal implant in patients with diabetic macular edema. Ophthalmology. 2014;121:1904–14.

14. Sharma A, Madhusudhan RJ, Nadahalli V, Damgude SA, Sundaramoorthy SK. Change in macular thickness in a case of refractory diabetic macular edema with dexamethasone intravitreal implant in comparison to intravitreal bevacizumab: a case report. Indian J Ophthalmol. 2012;60:234–5.

15. Garweg JG, Zandi S. Longterm treatment of diabetic macular edema with dexamethasone Im plant after unsatisfactory response to anti- VEGF therapy. Investig Ophthalmol Vis Sci. 2015;56:217.

16. Giralt J, Alforja S, Keller J, Latasiewicz M, Fontecilla C, Civera AA. Intravitreal dexamethasone implant in eyes with chronic refractory diabetic macular oedema. Investig Ophthalmol Vis Sci. 2014;55:1782.

17. Sun HJ, Lee SJ. Reduced efficacy of intravitreal dexamethasone implant in diabetic macular edema with subfoveal cystoid spaces. Investig Ophthalmol Vis Sci. 2016;57:3249.

18. Boyer DS, Faber D, Gupta S, Patel SS, Tabandeh H, Li XY, Liu CC, Lou J, Whitcup SM, Ozurdex CSG. Dexamethasone intravitreal implant for treatment of diabetic macular edema in vitrectomized patients. Retina. 2011;31:915–23.

19. Augustin AJ, Kuppermann BD, Lanzetta P, Loewenstein A, Li X-Y, Cui H, Hashad Y, Whitcup SM. Dexamethasone intravitreal implant in previously treated patients with diabetic macular edema: subgroup analysis of the MEAD study. BMC Ophthalmol. 2015;15. PMID: 26519345. https://doi.org/10.1186/s12886-015-0148-2.

20. Cui QN, Stewart JM. Intravitreal dexamethasone implant (Ozurdex) as primary treatment for diabetic macular edema. Investig Ophthalmol Vis Sci. 2014;55:1780.

21. Moher D, Liberati A, Tetzlaff J, Altman DG, The PG. Preferred reporting items for systematic reviews and meta-analyses: the PRISMA statement. PLoS Med. 2009;6:e1000097.

22. Atkins D, Best D, Briss PA, Eccles M, Falck-Ytter Y, Flottorp S, Guyatt GH, Harbour RT, Haugh MC, Henry D, et al. Grading quality of evidence and strength of recommendations. BMJ. 2004;328:1490.

23. Gillies MC, Lim LL, Campain A, Quin GJ, Salem W, Li J, Goodwin S, Aroney C, McAllister IL, Fraser-Bell S. A randomized clinical trial of intravitreal bevacizumab versus intravitreal dexamethasone for diabetic macular edema: the BEVORDEX study. Ophthalmology. 2014;121:2473–81.

24. Shah SU, Harless A, Bleau L, Maturi RK. Prospective randomized subject-masked study of intravitreal bevacizumab monotherapy versus dexamethasone implant monotherapy in the treatment of persistent diabetic macular edema. Retina. 2016;36:1986–96.

25. Aroney C, Fraser-Bell S, Lamoureux EL, Gillies MC, Lim LL, Fenwick EK. Vision-related quality of life outcomes in the BEVORDEX study: a clinical trial comparing Ozurdex sustained release dexamethasone intravitreal implant and bevacizumab treatment for diabetic macular edema. Invest Ophthalmol Vis Sci. 2016;57:5541–6.

26. Gallemore RP. Ozurdex for treatment of recalcitrant diabetic macular edema. 2017. May 31, 2017 edition: ClinicalTrials.gov.

27. Allergan: Safety and efficacy study of dexamethasone versus ranibizumab in patients with diabetic macular edema. 2015. January 29, 2015 edition: ClinicalTrials.gov.

28. Wells JA, Glassman AR, Ayala AR, Jampol LM, Bressler NM, Bressler SB, Brucker AJ, Ferris FL, Hampton GR, Jhaveri C, et al. Aflibercept, bevacizumab, or ranibizumab for diabetic macular edema: two-year results from a comparative effectiveness randomized clinical trial. Ophthalmology. 2016;123:1351–9.

29. Tang J, Kern TS. Inflammation in diabetic retinopathy. Prog Retin Eye Res. 2011;30:343–58.

30. Adamis AP, Berman AJ. Immunological mechanisms in the pathogenesis of diabetic retinopathy. Semin Immunopathol. 2008;30:65–84.

31. Jonas JB, Jonas RA, Neumaier M, Findeisen P. Cytokine concentration in aqueous humor of eyes with diabetic macular edema. Retina. 2012;32:2150–7.

32. Ciulla TA, Walker JD, Fong DS, Criswell MH. Corticosteroids in posterior segment disease: an update on new delivery systems and new indications. Curr Opin Ophthalmol. 2004;15:211–20.

33. Wells JA, Glassman AR, Ayala AR, Jampol LM, Aiello LP, Antoszyk AN, Arnold-Bush B, Baker CW, Bressler NM, Browning DJ, et al. Aflibercept, bevacizumab, or ranibizumab for diabetic macular edema. N Engl J Med. 2015;372:1193–203.

34. Lam WC, Albiani DA, Yoganathan P, Chen JC, Kherani A, Maberley DA, Oliver A, Rabinovitch T, Sheidow TG, Tourville E, et al. Real-world assessment of intravitreal dexamethasone implant (0.7 mg) in patients with macular edema: the CHROME study. Clin Ophthalmol. 2015;9:1255–68.

35. Maturi RK, Bleau L, Saunders J, Mubasher M, Stewart MW. A 12-month, single-masked, randomized controlled study of eyes with persistent diabetic macular edema after multiple anti-vegf injections to assess the efficacy of the dexamethasone-delayed delivery system as an adjunct to bevacizumab compared with continued bevacizumab monotherapy. Retina. 2015;35:1604–14.

36. Virgili G, Parravano M, Menchini F, Evans JR. Anti-vascular endothelial growth factor for diabetic macular oedema. Cochrane Database Syst Rev 2014:Cd007419. PMID:25342124. https://doi.org/10.1002/14651858.CD007419.pub4.

37. Avery RL, Gordon GM. Systemic safety of prolonged monthly anti-vascular endothelial growth factor therapy for diabetic macular edema: a systematic review and meta-analysis. JAMA Ophthalmol. 2016;134:21–9.

38. Csaky K, Do DV. Safety implications of vascular endothelial growth factor blockade for subjects receiving intravitreal anti-vascular endothelial growth factor therapies. Am J Ophthalmol. 2009;148:647–56.

39. Smiddy WE. Economic considerations of macular edema therapies. Ophthalmology. 2011;118:1827–33.

40. Thomas BJ, Yonekawa Y, Wolfe JD, Hassan TS. Contralateral eye-to-eye comparison of intravitreal ranibizumab and a sustained-release dexamethasone intravitreal implant in recalcitrant diabetic macular edema. Clin Ophthalmol. 2016;10:1679–84.

41. Lazic R, Lukic M, Boras I, Draca N, Vlasic M, Gabric N, Tomic Z. Treatment of anti-vascular endothelial growth factor-resistant diabetic macular edema with dexamethasone intravitreal implant. Retina. 2014;34:719–24.

42. Schmidt-Erfurth U, Garcia-Arumi J, Bandello F, Berg K, Chakravarthy U, Gerendas BS, Jonas J, Larsen M, Tadayoni R, Loewenstein A. Guidelines for the Management of Diabetic Macular Edema by the European Society of Retina Specialists (EURETINA). Ophthalmologica. 2017;237:185–222.

43. Virgili G, Parravano M, Evans JR, Gordon I, Lucenteforte E. Anti-vascular endothelial growth factor for diabetic macular oedema: a network meta-analysis. Cochrane Database Syst Rev. 2017;6:CD007419.

16

The Chinese Catquest-9SF: validation and application in community screenings

Zequan Xu[1†], Song Wu[2†], Wenzhe Li[3], Yan Dou[4] and Qiang Wu[1*]

Abstract

Background: The purpose of this study was to validate the Chinese Catquest-9SF questionnaire in community screenings and explore the correlation between Catquest-9SF scores and Lens Opacities Classification System (LOCS) III cataract grading.

Methods: This was a prospective questionnaire validation study. The Catquest-9SF questionnaire was translated into Chinese and was completed by 104 Chinese cataract patients who were diagnosed in community screening. Rasch analysis was used to assess its psychometric properties, and Spearman correlation coefficient was employed to determine the correlation between Catquest-9SF scores and LOCS III cataract grading.

Results: The Catquest-9SF questionnaire demonstrated ordered response categories and unidimensionality (item fit statistics range: 0.70–1.35); the PSI and PR of the category probability curves were 2.00 and 0.80, respectively. There was a fair but statistically significant correlation between Catquest-9SF (Q6, Q7, and Q8) and LOCS III scores and a moderate correlation between Q4 in Catquest-9SF and subcapsular components for the better eye ($r = -0.546$, $p < 0.001$).

Conclusion: The Chinese version of Catquest-9SF is a valid and reliable questionnaire in community screenings. Thus, this questionnaire may be expected to be an auxiliary tool for preliminary cataract screening use.

Keywords: Catquest-9SF, Questionnaires, Patient-reported outcomes, Validation, Rasch analysis

Background

Patient-reported outcomes (PROs), together with Clinician-reported outcomes (CROs) and laboratory tests (or device measurements) are three types of endpoints of diseases. The major representative of formal PROs is reliable and validated multi-item questionnaires [1]. There are many vision-related functional questionnaires [2–4], such as Visual Functioning 14 (VF-14) [5], NEI-visual functioning questionnaire 25 (NEI-VFQ 25) [6] and Catquest nine-item short-form (Catquest-9SF) [7, 8]. Catquest-9SF has been adopted by the International Consortium for Health Outcomes Measurement (ICHOM) to specifically measure the risk factors for and outcomes of cataracts, which are the main global cause of blindness and vision impairment [9].

Originally, Catquest-9SF contained 19 questions, was available in Swedish and was used by the National Swedish Cataract Register to evaluate the visual disability of cataract patients [10]. However, its nine-item short-form Rasch-scaled version (Catquest-9SF) was shown to be more reliable and valid in measuring the visual disability outcomes of cataract surgery [7].

Currently, Catquest-9SF has been translated and culturally adapted, as well as validated, in Australia [11], Germany and Austria [12], Italy [13], and the Netherlands [14], among other countries. Recently, this questionnaire has been assessed by using Rasch analysis in Chinese populations [15, 16].

However, unsolved problems issues arise on the Chinese Catquest-9SF. On the one hand, the results of Chinese Catquest-9SF is still controversial, one study claimed that all nine questions of Chinese Catquest-9SF are valid and reliable [15], while the other study suggested that it is better remove item 7, for item 7 is misfitting [16].

* Correspondence: qiang.Wu@shsmu.edu.cn
†Equal contributors
[1]Department of Ophthalmology, Shanghai Jiao Tong University Affiliated Sixth People's Hospital, No. 600, Yishan Road, Xuhui District, Shanghai 200233, People's Republic of China
Full list of author information is available at the end of the article

On the other hand, the aim of the study was also to find the direct evidence that the Catquest-9SF would be used as a routine clinical tool in community screening. Previous studies have mainly focused on the validation of cataract surgery candidates in a hospital setting, but a questionnaire valid in a hospital setting serves only as an indirect evidence it is also valid community screening. There is a usually overlooked difference between the two groups: for patients who were diagnosed as cataract in a community screening could have no awareness of their disease while cataract patients who go to a hospital to ask for clinical help usually are fully aware of the troubles which cataract bring to them. And to prove that Catquest-9SF could be used as a routine clinical tool in community screening, the direct evidence on the validity of Catquest-9SF in a community based population are needed. And the function of Catquest-9SF would be extended if it could be used in community screening.

Furthermore, as an indicator of CROs, Lens Opacities Classification System (LOCS) III cataract grading has been widely used to assess lens opacities [5]. Thus, by determining the correlation between Catquest-9SF scores and LOCS III cataract grading, we can further discover whether Catquest-9SF could reflex the opacity of lens.

Methods

Catquest-9SF questionnaire

The Catquest-9SF questionnaire was translated from English into Chinese. Five individuals were included on the translation team: one professor of medical English at a medical university; two independent, bilingual native Chinese ophthalmologists; one senior consultant; and one bilingual translation coordinator. The translation procedures were completed via the following steps: 1 The professor of medical English helped to define the conceptual meaning behind each item; 2 The two

bilingual native Chinese ophthalmologists translated the Catquest-9SF questionnaire from English into Chinese independently; 3 The senior consultant reconciled the Chinese translations, which were then back translated into English by a third translator; 4 By comparing the original version and the back-translated version, discrepancies between the two versions were identified; 5 The questionnaire was revised and was tested on five other ophthalmologists and five cataract patients to ensure that the items on the questionnaire could be adequately understood; and 6 After thorough discussion of minor revisions, the questionnaire was finalized. In our final version (presented in Table 1), we tried to be more specific in each item to make the questionnaire more understandable to Chinese people, and we also switched the order of Item 7 and Item 8.

The Catquest-9SF questionnaire contains 9 questions. Seven of the questions cover the perceived difficulties in performing daily-life activities, and one of two global questions is about general difficulties in everyday life. The response options are as follows: 1 = very great difficulty; 2 = great difficulty; 3 = some difficulty; 4 = no difficulty; and 5 = cannot decide. There is also one global question about general satisfaction. The response options are as follows: 1 = very dissatisfied; 2 = rather dissatisfied; 3 = fairly satisfied; 4 = very satisfied; and 5 = cannot decide. The response category "cannot decide" is treated as missing data in the analysis [14].

Data collection

The subject data were collected in the Gumei community (Xuhui District, Shanghai) in community screenings that aimed to identify cataract patients between June 2016 and July 2016. We included patients who were diagnosed as age-related cataracts and willing to participate in this study. All of them received an ophthalmic examination included best-corrected visual acuity, slit-

Table 1 Final version of the Chinese Catquest-9SF and English version of Catquest-9SF

Item	Chinese Catquest-9SF	English Catquest-9SF
Q1	Vision difficulty in everyday life	Vision difficulty in everyday life
Q2	Vision satisfaction in general	Vision satisfaction in general
Q3	Reading text in the newspaper	Reading text in the daily paper
Q4	Recognizing the faces of people around you	Recognizing the faces of people you come across
Q5	Seeing prices of goods when shopping, or descriptions on medicine bottles or bank receipts, electricity bill, water account, etc.	Seeing prices when shopping
Q6	Seeing to walk on uneven ground	Seeing to walk on uneven ground
Q7	Reading text on TV or in movie or on advertising board	Seeing to do handiwork, woodworking, etc.
Q8	Seeing to do delicate work (needlework, handiwork, carpentry, etc.)	Reading text on TV
Q9	Seeing to carry on an activity/hobby you are interested in, such as photography, calligraphy, Mah-jongg playing	Seeing to carry on an activity/hobby you are interested in

lamp (and LOCS III cataract grading) intraocular pressure and funduscopy. And all of the involved patients completed Catquest-9SF with the help of an ophthalmologist (the coordinator of the translation team). Patients who had difficulty with the Chinese language (Mandarin) and patients who were with diseases that may potentially affect eye sight (have a history of ocular pathology, corneal or intraocular trauma ocular surgery, or with severe subjective dry eye symptoms etc.) and/or a disease that influences daily-life activities (other than cataracts) were excluded. Written informed consent, was obtained from all subjects. And this study was approved by the Office of Research Ethical Committee of Shanghai Jiao Tong University Affiliated Sixth People's Hospital, The Declaration of Helsinki was strictly followed in all procedures.

Statistical analysis

Rasch analysis

Rasch analysis is a psychometric model widely used in the assessment of questionnaires that measures both person ability and item difficulty on the same scale. In the current study, Rasch analysis was used to determine how well the items (questions) (1), fit the vision function; (2), separated the patients; (3), targeted the patients' ability. The data from Catquest-9SF were assessed in the Rasch analysis using WINSTEPS software (version 3.72.3, Chicago, IL) with Andrich's rating scale model. To validate the Chinese version of Catquest-9SF, five key indicators were used, which included the following: (1) Information-weighted (infit) and outlier-sensitive (outfit) mean-square (MnSq) statistics. MnSq values between 0.7 and 1.3 were considered acceptable for unidimensionality [15]. A value > 1.3 implies too much variance, while < 0.7 implies too little variance [14]. (2) Principal component analysis (PCA). PCA of the residuals was performed, which is also an indicator of unidimensionality. Two criteria were used. The first was that the variance explained by the first component should be adequate (> 50%). The second was that the unexplained variance in the first contrast of the residuals should be less than 3.0 eigenvalue units [15]. (3) Category threshold order. The category threshold order, which is reflected by the category probability curves, is an important parameter for demonstrating the usage of response categories, and it is essential for the calculation of person and item calibrations. Disorder thresholds occur when patients have difficulty discriminating between ordered response options. (4) Person separation index (PSI) and person reliability (PR). The PSI and PR are indicators of measurement precision, aiming to reflect the ability to separate people. For a questionnaire with 3 strata, a PSI of 2.0 represents an acceptable level of separation, while 3.00 represents an excellent level, and a PR > 0.8 represents good

reliability, while > 0.9 represents excellent reliability (PR range from 0 to 1) [15]. (5) Person-item map. In the present study, a person-item map shows person measures ranked by their ability level and item difficulties ranked by difficulty. It provides a way to visualize how well the items target the ability of the patients.. The person-item map was expressed in logit values,the logit (or log-odds units) is the natural logarithm of the odds of a participant being successful at a specific task or an item being successfully carried out. A more positive value means more visual disability of cataract patients or more difficulties of items. Ideally, the difference between patients and item measure should be approximately 0 logits, which means the visual disability of cataract patients are targeted to difficulties of items. Most research defined that a difference between the mean person and item measure of more than 1.0 logits generally indicates significant mistargeting [13, 15, 16], while less than 1.0 logits generally indicates slight mistargeting. (6) Cronbach's α. Cronbach's α is an indicator of reliability that represents how much confidence can be placed in the consistency of the measurement. A Cronbach's $\alpha > 0.8$ represents a good consistency, while > 0.9 represents excellent consistency (ranging from 0 to 1).

Other statistics

An assessment of Catquest-9SF was also performed by determining the correlation between LOCS III cataract grading and Catquest-9SF scores. Spearman correlation analysis was performed using SPSS (Version 21.0, IBM Corp., Armonk, NY) and was used to determine the relationship. LOCS III is a subjective grading system that has good reproducibility in cataract grading [17]. The correlation was classified as follows [13]: strong, > 0.8, moderate, 0.5–0.8; fair, 0.3–0.5; and poor, < 0.3.

Sample size

There is no consistent guidance on the issue of sample size of pre-test of a questionnaire. For an instrument item (question), different studies suggest different participants, including 5-8, [18] 5-15(Health Outcomes Group (2004). Available from: http://www.Healthoutcomesgroup.com/Tables/ translation.html.), 7-10 (Merkus MP, Dekker FW. Kidney Disease Quality of Life-Short-Form: Translation Document. Amsterdam, The Netherlands. 1997.), 8-15 (Evidence Clinical and Pharmaceutical Research (2004). Available from: http://www.evidence-cpr. com/ieo/qlf.html), 10-15, [19] 10-30 (Fayers, P. M., & Machin, D. (2000). Quality of life. Assessment, analysis and interpretation. New York: Wiley.) According to these previous studies, "10 question for an item" was mostly recommended, thus the recommended sample size was 90 (for 9 questions). Besides, the sample size of a previous validation study on Chinese Catquest-9SF

Table 2 LOCS III cataract grading of all 104 participants

LOCS III cataract grading of 104 participants	Better eye (mean ± SD)	Worse eye (mean ± SD)
Cortical	1.87 ± 1.11	2.05 ± 1.21
Posterior subcapsular	1.08 ± 0.58	1.13 ± 0.71
Nuclear colour	2.94 ± 0.84	3.00 ± 0.86
Nuclear opalescence	2.88 ± 0.78	2.99 ± 0.78

was 102 [15]. Considering all mentioned above, we set the sample size as 90-100.

Results
Characteristics of the patients
A total of 104 people participated in the study. There were slightly more females (59%), and the median age was 67 (60-87) years. The basic LOCS III scores of the patients are presented in Table 2. The scores of the Chinese Catquest-9SF questionnaire are presented in Table 3.

Unidimensionality
Unidimensionality is an important assumption of Rasch analysis. As mentioned above, MNSQ and PCA are both indicators of unidimensionality.

For the MNSQ, both the "infit" and the "outfit" MNSQ values (presented in Table 3) for each item were acceptable (0.7- 1.3). For PCA, the residuals explained 51.3% (> 50%) of the raw variance, while the unexplained variance in the 1st contrast was 2.0 (< 3.0) eigenvalue units. Both of these outcomes suggested that there was no evidence of multidimensionality.

Threshold order
No evidence of disordered thresholds was found in the category probability curves, as the category calibration increased in an orderly way (presented in Fig. 1). Four response categories were found for all items, suggesting three thresholds for each item.

Separation
Acceptable PSI (2.00) and good PR (0.80) values were respectively found in the analysis, suggesting adequate separation ability for Catquest-9SF.

Person-item map
By comparing item difficulty with person ability, the person-item map was used to determine and visualize whether the item difficulties targeted the person abilities in the sample. The person-item map is shown in Fig. 2. On the left dashed line, the less disabled participants (represented by '#' or '.'; each '#' and each '.' represents two participants and one participant, respectively) are located at the bottom of the diagram; on the right dashed line, items with lower difficulties are located at the bottom of the diagram. In the present study, item difficulty had a spread from − 1.27 to 1.01 logits (mean value = 0 logits), while patient ability had a spread of − 2.05 to 5.66 logits (mean value = 1.39 logits). Thus, the difference between the item and the person means was 1.39 logits (> 1 logit indicates mistargeting). The mistargeting between patient ability and item difficulty suggested that the specified tasks were relatively easy to perform.

Reliability: Cronbach's α
Cronbach's α was 0.854, and removing any of the items decreased the Cronbach's α value (presented in Table 3).

Correlation between LOCS III cataract grading and Catquest-9SF scores
Spearman rank correlation coefficients were used to assess the correlation, and the results are presented in Table 4. A statistically significant ($p < 0.05$ or $p < 0.01$) correlation was found between each question and the LOCS III cataract grading (cortical, posterior subcapsular, nuclear colour and nuclear opalescence). Meanwhile, a moderate correlation was observed between "Recognizing the faces of people around you (Q4)" and posterior subcapsular grading for both the better eye ($r = 0.532$, $p < 0.0001$) and

Table 3 Rasch validation of the Chinese Catquest-9SF

Item	Score (mean ± SD)	Response category "cannot decide" rate	Item difficulty (logit)	Infit MNSQ	Outfit MNSQ	Cronbach's α after removing the item
Q1	2.89 ± 0.78	0.96%	0.53	0.70	0.74	0.832
Q2	2.77 ± 0.85	1.92%	0.89	0.78	0.79	0.839
Q3	2.86 ± 0.97	0	0.56	1.14	1.09	0.839
Q4	3.36 ± 0.81	0	−0.82	1.25	1.11	0.843
Q5	2.78 ± 0.99	0	0.78	1.07	0.72	0.826
Q6	3.52 ± 0.68	0.96%	−1.27	0.93	0.90	0.834
Q7	3.25 ± 0.82	0	−0.43	0.91	0.82	0.832
Q8	2.84 ± 1.10	6.73%	1.01	0.82	0.68	0.851
Q9	3.80 ± 0.83	18.27%	−1.26	1.10	1.01	0.847

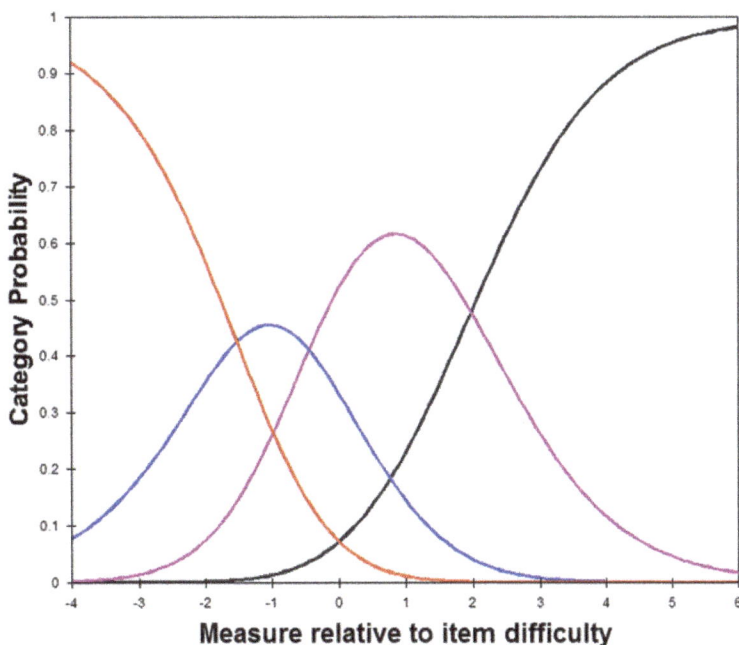

Fig. 1 Category probability curves. Category probability curves for the global "difficulties in your daily life" item, which illustrates ordered threshold. The four curves from left to right represent 4 response categories (1 = very great difficulty; 2 = great difficulty; 3 = some difficulty; 4 = no difficulty)

the worse eye ($r = 0.546$, $p < 0.0001$). In addition, fair correlations were observed between Q6, Q7 and Q8 with and cortical grading ($r > 0.3$, $p < 0.01$) for the better eye. Fair correlations were observed between Q1 and nuclear colour and nuclear opalescence grading ($r > 0.3$, $p < 0.01$) for the better eye.

Discussion

The subjects of previous studies on Catquest-9SF validation were mostly hospitalized patients expecting cataract

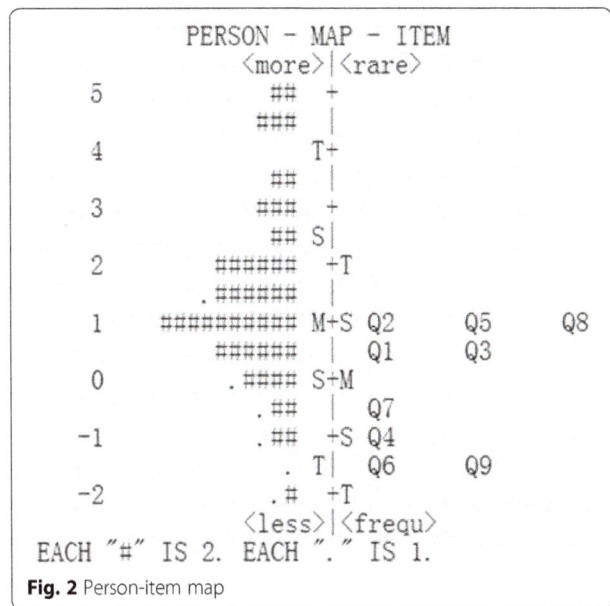

Fig. 2 Person-item map

surgery (patients awaiting cataract operation [7, 12–16]) because they were not satisfied with their present vision and had visual disability. The results of our study showed that the Chinese Catquest-9SF was also valid and reliable for assessing cataract patients in community screening and that Catquest-9SF scores have a statistically significant correlation with LOCS III cataract grading. Both of these outcomes suggest that the Chinese Catquest-9SF partly reflects the severity of cataracts in Chinese population-based community screening.

Based on the MNSQ values and PCA, the Chinese Catquest-9SF has demonstrated good unidimensionality. Similar results were found in a study by Lin et al..... [15] and for versions in other languages [7, 11–14]. However, in a study by Wang et al, the question about "Seeing to do delicate work (Q8)" was removed from the questionnaire because it was deemed "ambiguous" and failed to demonstrate a good fit (outfit value > 1.3) [16]. Wang et al attributed the misfit to the ambiguity of the word "delicate". In our study, we elaborated on "delicate work" as "needlework, handiwork, carpentry, etc." to ensure that patients thoroughly and accurately understood the meaning.

Our study demonstrated an ordered threshold in the category probability curves, which means that patients who responded that they had more visual disability for a certain item indeed had more visual disability for that item than people who claimed that they had less disability. The combination of a good PSI and good PR suggested that the measurement precision of Catquest-9SF

Table 4 Correlation between LOCS III cataract grading and Catquest-9SF

Item	Cortical	Posterior subcapsular	Nuclear colour	Nuclear opalescence
Q1				
Better eye	−0.183	−0.285**	−0.310**	− 0.340**
Worse eye	−0.172	−0.336**	− 0.232*	−0.288**
Q2				
Better eye	−0.085	−0.226*	− 0.084	−0.150
Worse eye	−0.159	−0.287**	− 0.062	−0.101
Q3				
Better eye	−0.179	−0.167	− 0.231*	−0.242*
Worse eye	−0.253**	−0.128	− 0.228*	−0.299**
Q4				
Better eye	−0.202*	−0.532**	− 0.113	−0.029
Worse eye	−0.171	−0.546**	− 0.071	−0.083
Q5				
Better eye	−0.150	−0.472**	− 0.119	−0.097
Worse eye	−0.149	−0.450**	− 0.155	−0.130
Q6				
Better eye	−0.304**	−0.324**	− 0.089	−0.178
Worse eye	−0.233*	−0.297*	− 0.182	−0.259**
Q7				
Better eye	−0.348**	−0.401**	− 0.143	−0.208*
Worse eye	−0.304**	−0.353**	− 0.098	−0.150
Q8				
Better eye	−0.319**	−0.275**	− 0.152	−0.098
Worse eye	−0.269**	−0.173	− 0.118	−0.090
Q9				
Better eye	−0.183	−0.027*	− 0.258**	−0.281**
Worse eye	−0.167	−0.149	− 0.275**	−0.242*
General score				
Better eye	−0.301**	−0.490**	− 0.221*	−0.247*
Worse eye	−0.313**	−0.441**	− 0.203*	−0.236*

**: $p < 0.01$ (two-sided test), significant correlation
*: $p < 0.05$ (two-sided test), significant correlation

was good, which means that the instrument could accurately distinguish between low and high performers. In the case of Catquest-9SF, this finding specifically means that the measure could accurately distinguish between people with and without cataract-related visual disturbances. Our results were consistent with previous studies, regardless of the Catquest-9SF version used [7, 11–16].

The person-item map showed significant mistargeting (1.39-logit difference in means) of persons and items, suggesting that the specified tasks were relatively easy for the cataract patients, even with decreased visual abilities. Better targeting was found in the study by Wang et al... [16]. This discrepancy may be partially due to the fact that we assessed cataract patients within a

community-based population, who tend to have more satisfaction with their present vision and less visual disability in general than hospitalized patients expecting cataract surgery. Meanwhile, mistargeting (1.61 logits) was also found in the study by Lin et al [15] and in studies of a Swedish version (1.95-logit difference in means) [20], Italian version (2.04-logit difference in means) [13], and Dutch version (1.64-logit difference in means) [14]. Thus, the inclusion of additional items that could facilitate better targeting of items for visual abilities should be considered in future studies.

Significant correlation was found between some questions on Catquest-9SF and LOCS III grading, while a moderate correlation was observed for Q4 and posterior subcapsular grading. In addition, fair correlations were observed between "Seeing to walk on uneven ground (Q6)", "Reading text on TV, in movie or on advertising board (Q7)" and "Seeing to do delicate work (needle-work, handiwork, carpentry, etc.) (Q8)" and cortical grading for the better eye. Fair correlations were observed between "Vision difficulty in everyday life (Q1)" and nuclear colour and nuclear opalescence grading for the better eye. In a previous study by Skiadaresi et al....., no correlation was found between the general score on the Italian Catquest-9SF and LOCS III grading [13]. However, in another previous study by Pan et al, a significant and moderate correlation was found between the general score on another vision-related functional questionnaire (VF-14) and LOCS III grading (especially nuclear opalescence grading) [5]. Instead of calculating the general score for all questions, we specifically calculated the score for each question. In addition, the sample size of the study by Skiadaresi et al was too small (only 24 patients with nuclear cataracts, 3 with cortical cataracts, and 25 with posterior subcapsular cataracts) to obtain significant results. Thus, Catquest-9SF can reflect lens opacities to some extent.

This study has a few limitations. First, all patients were recruited only from a single community, so larger and more representative samples are needed in future studies. Second, we only investigated the relationship between LOCS III grading and Catquest-9SF, other objective methods, such as lens density and objective scatter index measurement, could be used in future studies. Third, to determine whether Catquest-9SF could be useful as a screening tool, future studies between patients with and without cataract-related visual disturbances might be still needed.

Conclusion

In conclusion, the Chinese Catquest-9SF is a concise, valid and reliable questionnaire that is easy to understand and quick to complete for Chinese-speaking patients in Chinese community. Moreover, Catquest-9SF scores had a certain correlation with LOCS III grading. Thus, the Chinese Catquest-9SF is expected to be an auxiliary tool for preliminary cataract screening use.

Acknowledgements

This research was presented in part as an oral presentation at the 30th Asia-Pacific Association of cataract and Refractive Surgeons (APACRS) Annual Meeting.

Funding

This research was supported by the Health Bureau of Shanghai City (201440029).

Authors' contributions

Conceived and designed the experiments: ZX, QW. Performed the experiments: ZX, WL. Analysed the data: SW, ZX. Contributed reagents/materials/analysis tools: ZX, YD. Wrote the paper: ZX. Critically revised the manuscript: YD. All authors have read and approved the manuscript, and ensure that this is the case.

Competing interests

The authors declare that they have no competing interests.

Author details

¹Department of Ophthalmology, Shanghai Jiao Tong University Affiliated Sixth People's Hospital, No. 600, Yishan Road, Xuhui District, Shanghai 200233, People's Republic of China. ²School of Integrated Traditional and Western Medicine, Anhui University of Traditional Chinese Medicine, No. 103, Meishan Road, Hefei, Anhui 230038, People's Republic of China. ³Clinical Medical College, Tianjin Medical University, No. 176 Xueyuan Road, Dagang District, Tianjin 100270, People's Republic of China. ⁴Department of Foreign Languages, Hainan Medical University, No. 3, College Road, Longhua District, Haikou City, Hainan Province 571100, People's Republic of China.

References

1. Willke RJ, Burke LB, Erickson P. Measuring treatment impact: a review of patient-reported outcomes and other efficacy endpoints in approved product labels. Control Clin Trials. 2004;25(6):535–52.
2. Khadka J, Mcalinden C, Gothwal VK, Lamoureux EL, Pesudovs K. The importance of rating scale design in the measurement of patient-reported outcomes using questionnaires or item banks. Invest Ophthalmol Vis Sci. 2012;53(7):4042–54.
3. Khadka J, Mcalinden C, Pesudovs K. Quality assessment of ophthalmic questionnaires: review and recommendations. Optom Visi Sci. 2013;90(8):720–44.
4. Mahmud I, Kelley T, Stowell C, Haripriya A, Boman A, Kossler I, Morlet N, Pershing S, Pesudovs K, Goh PP. A proposed minimum standard set of outcome measures for cataract surgery. JAMA Ophthalmol. 2015;133(11):1247–52.
5. Pan AP, Wang QM, Huang F, Huang JH, Bao FJ, Yu AY. Correlation among Lens opacities classification system III grading, visual function Index-14, Pentacam nucleus staging, and objective scatter index for cataract assessment. Am J Ophthalmol. 2015;159(2):241–7.
6. Petrillo J, Cano SJ, McLeod LD, Coon CD. Using classical test theory, item response theory, and Rasch measurement theory to evaluate patient-reported outcome measures: a comparison of worked examples. Value Health. 2015;18(1):25–34.
7. Lundstrom M, Pesudovs K. Catquest-9SF patient outcomes questionnaire: nine-item short-form Rasch-scaled revision of the Catquest questionnaire. J Cataract Refract Surg. 2009;35(3):504–13.
8. Lundstrom M, Roos P, Jensen S, Fregell G. Catquest questionnaire for use in cataract surgery care: description, validity, and reliability. J Cataract Refract Surg. 1997;23(8):1226–36.
9. Pascolini D, Mariotti SP. Global estimates of visual impairment: 2010. Br J Ophthalmol. 2011;96(5):614–8.
10. Behndig A, Montan P, Stenevi U, Kugelberg M, Lundstrom M. One million cataract surgeries: Swedish National Cataract Register 1992-2009. J Cataract Refract Surg. 2011;37(8):1539–45.
11. Gothwal VK, Wright TA, Lamoureux EL, Lundstrom M, Pesudovs K. Catquest questionnaire: re-validation in an Australian cataract population. Clin Exp Ophthalmol. 2009;37(8):785–94.
12. Harrer A, Gerstmeyer K, Hirnschall N, Pesudovs K, Lundstrom M, Findl O. Impact of bilateral cataract surgery on vision-related activity limitations. J Cataract Refract Surg. 2013;39(5):680–5.
13. Skiadaresi E, Ravalico G, Polizzi S, Lundstrom M, Gonzalez-Andrades M, McAlinden C. The Italian Catquest-9SF cataract questionnaire: translation, validation and application. Eye Vis (London, England). 2016;3:12.
14. Visser MS, Dieleman M, Klijn S, Timman R, Lundström M, Busschbach JJ, Reus NJ. Validation, test-retest reliability and norm scores for the Dutch Catquest-9SF. Acta ophthalmologica. 2017;95(3):312.
15. Lin X, Li M, Wang M, Zuo Y, Zhu S, Zheng Y, Lin X, Yu M, Lamoureux EL. Validation of Catquest-9SF questionnaire in a Chinese cataract population. PLoS One. 2014;9(8):e103860.

16.   Khadka J, Huang J, Chen H, Chen C, Gao R, Bao F, Zhang S, Wang Q, Pesudovs K. Assessment of cataract surgery outcome using the modified Catquest short-form instrument in China. PLoS One. 2016;11(10):e0164182.
17.   Jr CL, Wolfe JK, Singer DM, Leske MC, Bullimore MA, Bailey IL, Friend J, Mccarthy D, Wu SY. The Lens Opacities Classification System III. The Longitudinal Study of Cataract Study Group. Arch Ophthalmol. 1993;111(6):831–36.
18.   Wild D, Grove A, Martin M, Eremenco S, McElroy S, Verjee-Lorenz A, Erikson P. Principles of good practice for the translation and cultural adaptation process for patient-reported outcomes (PRO) measures: report of the ISPOR task force for translation and cultural adaptation. Value Health. 2005;8(2):94–104.
19.   Sprangers MA, Cull A, Groenvold M, Bjordal K, Blazeby J, Aaronson NK. The European Organization for Research and Treatment of Cancer approach to developing questionnaire modules: an update and overview. EORTC Quality of Life Study Group. Qual Life Res. 1998;7(4):291.
20.   Lundstrom M, Behndig A, Kugelberg M, Montan P, Stenevi U, Pesudovs K. The outcome of cataract surgery measured with the Catquest-9SF. Acta Ophthalmol. 2011;89(8):718–23.

17

Comparative study of inverted internal limiting membrane (ILM) flap and ILM peeling technique in large macular holes: a randomized-control trial

Naresh Babu Kannan[*], Piyush Kohli, Haemoglobin Parida, O. O. Adenuga and Kim Ramasamy

Abstract

Background: The anatomical success rate of macular hole surgery ranges around 93–98%. However, the prognosis of large macular holes is generally poor. The study was conducted to compare the anatomical and visual outcomes of Internal Limiting Membrane (ILM) peeling vis-a-vis inverted ILM flap for the treatment of idiopathic large Full-Thickness Macular Holes (FTMH).

Methods: This was a prospective randomized control trial. The study included patients with idiopathic FTMH, with a minimum diameter ranging from 600 to 1500 μm. The patients were randomized into Group A (ILM peeling) and Group B (inverted ILM flap). The main outcome measures were anatomical and visual outcome at the end of 6 months. Anatomical success was defined as flattening of macular hole with resolution of the subretinal cuff of fluid and neurosensory retina completely covering the fovea.

Results: There were 30 patients in each group. The mean minimum diameters in Group A and B were 759.97 ± 85.01 μm and 803.33 ± 120.65 μm respectively ($p = 0.113$). The mean base diameter in group A and B was 1304.50 ± 191.59 μm and 1395.17 ± 240.56 μm respectively ($p = 0.112$). The anatomical success rates achieved in Group A and B were 70.0 and 90.0% respectively ($p = 0.125$). The mean best-corrected visual acuity (BCVA) after 6 months was logMAR 0.65 ± 0.25 (Snellen equivalent, 20/89) in Group A and logMAR 0.53 ± 0.20 (Snellen equivalent, 20/68) in Group B ($p = 0.060$). The mean improvement in BCVA was 1.4 lines and 2.1 lines in groups A and B respectively ($p = 0.353$). BCVA$\geq$20/60 was achieved by 13.3 and 20.0% in group A and B respectively ($p = 0.766$).

Conclusion: The anatomical and functional outcome of Inverted ILM flap technique in large FTMH is statistically similar to that seen in conventional ILM peeling.

Keywords: 600 μm, Inverted ILM flap, Large macular hole, Muller cells, Type 1 closure

Background

Vitrectomy is the gold standard for the treatment of macular holes. The anatomical success rate of macular hole surgery is 93–98% [1–4]. However, the anatomical success rate of large macular holes is as low as 40 to 80% [5–10]. Poor prognosis demoralizes most surgeons from operating upon such patients [11–13].

Michalewska et al., first described a novel technique of inverted internal limiting membrane (ILM) flap for the treatment of large macular holes [14]. They found that their technique achieved better anatomical and visual outcomes compared to conventional ILM peeling (ILMP). In last couple of years, a number of studies have suggested that inverted ILM flap technique (IFT) may be better for the treatment of large macular holes [14–24]. A systemic review and single-arm meta-analysis showed that the anatomical closure and visual improvement rates after IFT for FTMH with minimum diameter (MD)

---

* Correspondence: cauveryeye@gmail.com
Department of Vitreo-retinal services, Aravind Eye Hospital and Post graduate Institute of Ophthalmology, Madurai, Tamil Nadu, India

> 400 μm were 95 and 75% respectively [19]. But most of these studies were either retrospective in nature or lacked a control arm and included macular hole with MD < 600 μm.

We performed a randomized control trial to compare the anatomical and visual outcome of inverted ILM flap technique (IFT) vis-à-vis conventional ILM peeling (ILMP) in idiopathic large macular holes with MD > 600 μm.

Methods

This was a prospective randomized control study done at Aravind Eye Hospital, Madurai, India, after obtaining approval from Institutional Review Board (IRB) of Aravind Medical Research Foundation (Registration No. ECR/182/Inst/TN/2013 dated 20.04.2013). This study adheres to the tenets of Declaration of Helsinki. The nature and aim of the study was explained to the patients, and a written consent for participation was taken from each patient before the surgery. Patients with idiopathic full thickness macular hole (FTMH) with a MD > 600 μm were included. Patients with MD > 1500 μm, traumatic macular holes, myopic macular holes, presence of co-existing ocular pathologies affecting vision and patients refusing randomization were excluded from the study.

The presenting best-corrected visual acuity (BCVA) and intraocular pressure (IOP) were recorded. The Snellen visual acuity was converted into a logarithm of the minimum angle of resolution i.e. logMAR for statistical analysis. FTMH parameters and indices were gauged with Heidelberg Spectralis Spectral-Domain Optical Coherence Tomography (SD-OCT) (Heidelberg Engineering, Inc., Heidelberg, Germany) using high definition 5-line raster scans and 3-dimensional 512×128 macular cube scans passing through the fovea, before and after the surgery [6, 7, 9]. All the surgeries in both the groups were performed by a single surgeon (Dr NB) with more than 15 years of post-fellowship experience of performing high volume vitreoretinal surgeries. All the patients were randomized into two groups. System-generated random number were used to recruit the patients into two groups. The patients in group A underwent 25G Pars Plana Vitrectomy (PPV) with ILMP while the patients in group B underwent 25G PPV with IFT.

Surgical technique

In both groups, phacoemulsification with implantation of intraocular lens was followed by core vitrectomy and induction of posterior vitreous detachment. ILM was then stained with 0.05% solution of Heavy Brilliant Blue G dye (HBBG), prepared by mixing Brilliant Blue G dye (Ocublue plus, Aurolab, India) with 10% dextrose in 1:2 proportions. HBBG was injected slowly under balance salt solution (BSS) [25]. The stained ILM was pinched with a 25G end gripping forceps (Grieshaber Asymmetrical Forceps, DSP, Alcon, Fort Worth, Texas, USA) and peeled off in a circular fashion for approximately 2-disc diameters around the hole.

In the ILM peeling group, the ILM was discarded. In the inverted ILM flap group, the margins of the ILM were left attached to the edges of the hole. The margins were later trimmed with the vitrectomy cutter. Only adequate amount of ILM required to tuck into the hole was retained. Fluid-air exchange (FAE) was done and the ILM flap was tucked into hole with Tano diamond-dusted membrane scraper (DDMS; Synergetics, Inc., O'Fallon, MO, USA).

In both groups, FAE was done multiple times to ensure complete fluid removal. The superonasal and superotemporal cannulae were then removed and the conjunctiva was repositioned to cover the sclerotomy sites. Two mL pure SF_6 was injected with a 30-gauge needle, while the air-infusion line was used for venting. After the syringe was flushed, the infusion line was clamped and the digital tension of the globe was assessed. The infusion cannula was then removed and the inferotemporal sclerotomy sealed [26]. Post-operative prone positioning was recommended for first 48 h.

Post-operative evaluation

Post-operative visits were scheduled at day1, 2 weeks, 1 month and 6 months. Frequent follow-ups were scheduled, in case of any complication. At each follow-up visit BCVA, IOP and SD-OCT were recorded. The main outcome measures were anatomical and visual outcome at the end of 6 months. Anatomical closure was defined as the flattening of the hole with resolution of subretinal cuff of fluid. Anatomical success was defined as Type 1 anatomical closure i.e. flattening of macular hole with resolution of subretinal cuff of fluid and neurosensory retina (NSR) completely covering the fovea [27]. Type 2 anatomical closure, i.e. when the whole rim of the NSR around the macular hole was attached to the underlying retinal pigment epithelium (RPE) but NSR was absent above the fovea, was also considered anatomical failure.

Statistical analysis

Statistical analysis was performed by using statistical software STATA 14.1, (Texas, USA). Continuous variables were expressed as mean (±standard deviation) or median (range) and categorical variables were expressed as percentages. Chi-square test/ Fisher's exact test was used to assess the association of categorical variables. Student's t-test/ Mann-Whitney U test was used to find out the significant difference of continuous variables between the two study groups. Wilcoxon sign rank test was used to find out the difference between pre- and post-operative visual acuity. *P*-value less than 0.05 considered as statistically significant.

Sample size calculation

The type 1 closure rate obtained by Michalewska et al., i.e. 69% in ILMP group and 96% in IFT group, was used as reference [14]. By keeping the power of the study as 80% and the confidence interval as 95%, a sample of 60 subjects (30 in each arm) was calculated. The following formula was used:

$$H_o : P_1 = P_2; \quad H_a : P_1 \neq P_2$$

$$n = \frac{\left\{ Z_{1-\frac{\alpha}{2}} \sqrt{2\overline{P}\left(1-\overline{P}\right)} + Z_{1-\beta} \sqrt{P_1\left(1-P_1\right) + P_2\left(1-P_2\right)} \right\}^2}{\left(P_1 - P_2\right)^2}$$

Where,

$$\overline{P} = \frac{P_1 + P_2}{2}$$

P_1 : Proportion in the first group
P_2 : Proportion in the second group
α : Significance level
$1-\beta$: Power

Results

The study included 30 patients in each of the two groups. The mean MD in group A (ILMP) and group B (IFT) was 759.97 ± 85.01 μm and 803.33 ± 120.65 μm respectively ($p = 0.113$). The mean base diameter in group A and B was 1304.50 ± 191.59 μm and 1395.17 ± 240.56 μm respectively ($p = 0.112$). The mean BCVA in group A and B was logMAR 0.79 ± 0.24 (Snellen equivalent 20/123) and logMAR 0.75 ± 0.22 (Snellen equivalent 20/112) respectively ($p = 0.471$) (Table 1).

Anatomical closure was achieved in 76.7% ($n = 23/30$) and 90% ($n = 27/30$) eyes in Group A and B respectively ($p = 0.166$). Type 1 closure was achieved in 70.0% ($n = 21/30$) and 90% (n = 27/30) eyes in Group A and B respectively (Fig. 1). A two-line improvement was seen in 43.3% ($n = 13/30$) and 40.0% ($n = 12/30$) eyes in Group A and B respectively ($p = 0.793$). Mean BCVA at post-operative 1-month in Group A and Group B was logMAR 0.68 ± 0.25 (Snellen equivalent 20/96) and logMAR 0.54 ± 0.19 (Snellen equivalent 20/69) ($p = 0.016$) respectively. Mean BCVA at post-operative 6-month in Group A and B was logMAR 0.65 ± 0.25 (Snellen equivalent 20/89) and logMAR 0.53 ± 0.20 (Snellen equivalent 20/68) respectively ($p = 0.060$). The mean improvement in BCVA was 1.4 and 2.1 lines in groups A and B respectively ($p = 0.353$) (Table 2).

The three holes that did not close in the IFT group had a MD of 906 μm, 986 μm and 1007 μm. All the holes in IFT group with MD ≤ 900 μm achieved a Type 1 closure. On the contrary, four out of the seven failed surgery in ILMP group had MD < 700 μm. Anatomical closure rate 66.7% ($n = 6/9$) and 50% ($n = 3/6$) was achieved in FTMH with MD > 850 μm in IFT and ILMP group respectively. The data is available as Additional files 1 and 2.

Discussion

Internal limiting membrane peeling relieves the tractional forces responsible for causing the hole by removing the template upon which glial tissue proliferates as well as triggers reparative gliosis by injuring the muller cells, which constitute the framework of ILM [28–32]. However, large neural defects are difficult to bridge by the glial tissue. Hence, large macular holes have a propensity to remain open or close in a Type 2 manner [6, 10, 13, 33]. Chhablani et al... concluded that probability of Type1 closure with ILM peeling was 100% only if the MD of the hole was less than 300 μm [10].

Table 1 The baseline characteristics of the two groups

	Group A ILM Peeling	Group B ILM inverted flap	p value
Number	30	30	–
Male: Female	17:13	11:19	0.121[a]
Mean Age	61.17 ± 7.42 years (46.00–71.00 years)	59.37 ± 6.71 years (41.00–70.00 years)	0.328[d]
Mean Minimum Diameter	759.97 ± 85.01 μm (638.00–947.00 μm) 95% CI (728.22–791.71 μm)	803.33 ± 120.65 μm (603.00–1007.00 μm) 95% CI (758.28–848.38 μm)	0.113[d]
Mean Base Diameter	1304.50 ± 191.59 μm (873.00–1712.00 μm) 95% CI (1232.96–1376.04 μm)	1395.17 μm ± 240.56 (1005.00–1968.00 μm) 95%CI (1305.34–1484.99 μm)	0.112[d]
Mean Baseline visual acuity	logMAR 0.79 ± 0.24 (Snellen equivalent, 20/123) 95% CI (logMAR 0.70-logMAR 0.89)	logMAR 0.75 ± 0.22 (Snellen equivalent, 20/112) 95%CI (logMAR 0.66-logMAR 0.83)	0.471[c]

ILM Internal limiting membrane, [a]Chi-square test, [c]Mann-Whitney U test, [d]independent t-test

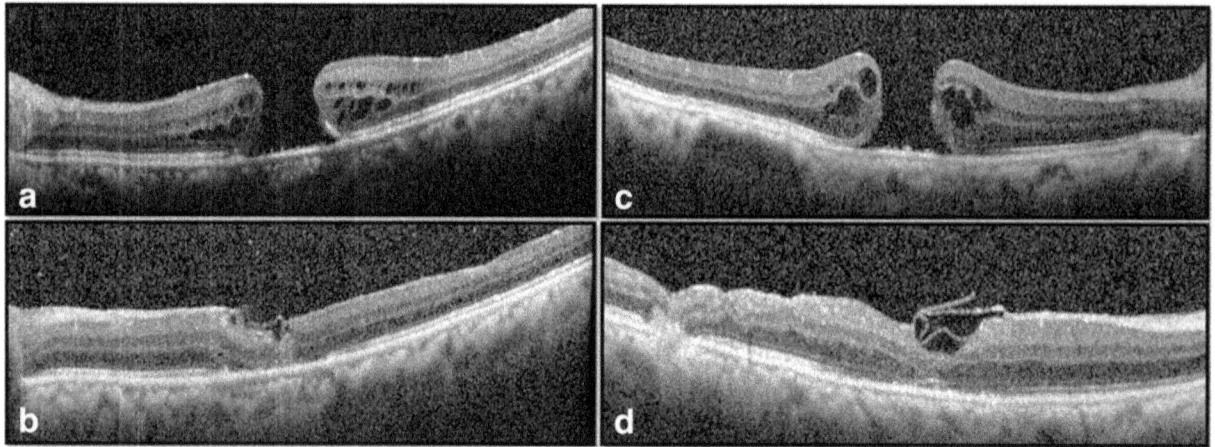

Fig. 1 Pre-operative (**a**, **c**) and 6 months post-operative (**b**, **d**) images of two patients who underwent surgery with inverted Internal limiting membrane flap technique and achieved anatomical success

In our study, a trend towards a higher anatomical success rate and a better functional outcome was noticed with inverted ILM flap technique. However, this difference did not reach statistical significance. The trend can be explained by the fact that the IFT provides a smooth and gap-free natural scaffold for the migration of glial cells and photoreceptors towards the fovea [14, 34]. Shiode et al experimentally proved that the neurotrophic and growth factors retained on the surface of the ILM flap enhanced the proliferation and migration of the muller cells. The migrating muller cells secrete neurotrophic factors and growth factors that may promote the survival of retinal neurons and photoreceptor cells. Some markers of cell proliferation like Ki-67 were also found in contact with the inverted ILM flap [35]. The technique has even been found to be superior in

achieving anatomical success in case of retinal detachment associated with FTMH [36].

There have been few studies comparing the anatomical and functional outcome of IFT with conventional ILMP in case of large macular hole. However, there is no conclusive evidence suggesting the superiority of the novel technique. There are few studies which suggest that IFT is better than conventional ILMP. Michalewska et al.. performed a prospective trial including 50 eyes in each group. They found that anatomical closure rate was 98% in IFT group (mean MD-759 μm) and 88% in ILMP group (mean MD-698 μm) [14]. Type 1 anatomical closure rates in the IFT and ILMP groups were 96 and 69% respectively. The post-operative BCVA was significantly higher in the IFT group. Similarly, Manasa et al. did a prospective trial including 50 eyes in each group (mean

Table 2 Anatomical and functional outcome in both the groups

	Group A ILM Peeling	Group B ILM inverted flap	p value
Anatomical closure	76.7% (n = 23/30)	90.0% (n = 27/30)	0.166[a]
Anatomical success i.e. Type 1 closure	70.0% (n = 21/30)	90.0% (n = 27/30)	0.125[b]
Type 2 closure	6.7% (n = 2/30)	0	
No closure	23.3% (n = 7/30)	10.0% (n = 3/30)	
1-line improvement	46.7% (n = 14/30)	53.3% (n = 16/30)	0.606[a]
2-line improvement	43.3% (n = 13/30)	40.0% (n = 12/30)	0.793[a]
Mean BCVA at 1 month	logMAR 0.68 ± 0.25 (Snellen equivalent, 20/96).	logMAR 0.54 ± 0.19 (Snellen equivalent, 20/69)	*0.016[c]*
Mean BCVA at 6 months	logMAR 0.65 ± 0.25 (Snellen equivalent, 20/89)	logMAR 0.53 ± 0.20 (Snellen equivalent, 20/68)	*0.060[c]*
Mean improvement in BCVA	1.4 lines	2.1 lines	0.353[d]
BCVA≥20/60	26.7% (n = 8/30)	23.3% (n = 7/30)	0.766[a]

ILM Internal limiting membrane, *BCVA* Best-corrected visual acuity, [a]Chi-square test, [b]Fisher's exact test, [c]Mann-Whitney U test, [d]independent t-test, in italics - statistically significant value

MD around 650 μm in each group) [20]. They found that Type 1 closure rate was significantly better in the IFT group (62.8%) than ILMP (33.3%). Also, the functional outcome was significantly better in the IFT group. Rizzo et al. (mean MD not mentioned) in their retrospective analysis of 620 eyes, showed that both the anatomical and the functional outcome was statistically better in the IFT group (95.6%) than the ILMP group (78.6%) [21].

Other studies have found no significant difference between the two techniques. Yamashita et al. retrospectively analyzed the outcome in 165 eyes with large FTMH [22]. They found that the anatomical closure rate in the ILMP group was 95.2, 86 and 69.2% in holes with MD ≤550 μm, > 550 μm and > 700 μm respectively. On the contrary, the anatomical closure rate in the IFT group was 100% irrespective of the macular hole size. However, there was no statistically significant difference in either the anatomical or the functional outcome between the two groups. Similarly, Narayanan et al.. in their retrospective analysis of 36 eyes (mean MD around 550 μm in each group), found no statistically significant difference in either the anatomical or the functional outcome between the two groups [23]. Their results showed 88.9% closure rate in IFT group and 77.8% in ILM peeling group. Velez-Montoya et al performed a prospective trial with 12 patients in each group (mean MD around 600 μm in each group) [24]. They found that there was no statistically significant difference in the anatomical success rates between the two groups (91.7% in both groups). However, the functional outcome was significantly better in the IFT group.

The anatomical success rates in our study were similar to that reported in the literature. Our study showed that IFT showed a trend towards better anatomical and visual outcome in case of large macular holes. However, this difference did not reach statistically significance. In spite of not reaching clinical significance, our results show that holes with MD > 850 μm have a higher probability of closing with inverted ILM flap.

Conclusions

The main limitation of our study was the small sample size. However, as large macular hole is an uncommon condition, it is difficult to take a large sample size operated by a single surgeon in a limited time period. Although the new technique has shown significantly better results for MH > 400 μm, it seems to be only marginally better for very large holes, especially in case of functional outcome. Larger comparative studies need to be performed to conclusively demonstrate any significant benefit of the inverted ILM flap technique.

Abbreviations

BCVA: Best-corrected visual acuity; DDMS: Diamond-dusted membrane scraper; FAE: Fluid-air exchanged; FTMH: Full-Thickness macular holes; HBBG: Heavy Brilliant Blue G dye; ILM: Internal limiting membrane; IOP: Intraocular pressure; IRB: Institutional review board; MD: Minimum diameter; NSR: Neurosensory retina; RPE: Retinal pigment epithelium; SD-OCT: Spectralis Spectral-Domain Optical Coherence Tomography; SF_6: Sulphur hexafluoride

Authors' contributions

NBK - Research Design, Data Interpretation, Manuscript Preparation. PK - Data Interpretation, Manuscript Preparation. HP - Research Design, Data Acquisition, Data Interpretation, Manuscript Preparation. OOA - Data Interpretation, Manuscript Preparation. KR - Research Design, Data Interpretation. All authors read and approved the final manuscript.

Competing interests

The authors declare that they have no competing interests.

References

1. Rahimy E, MCCannel CA. Impact of internal limiting membrane peeling on macular hole reopening. A systematic review and meta-analysis. Retina. 2016;36:679–87. https://doi.org/10.1097/IAE.0000000000000782.
2. Lai MM, Williams GA. Anatomical and visual outcomes of idiopathic macular hole surgery with internal limiting membrane removal using low-concentration indocyanine green. Retina. 2007;27:477–82. https://doi.org/10.1097/01.iae.0000247166.11120.21.
3. Park DW, Sipperley JO, Sneed SR, Dugel PU, Jacobsen J. Macular hole surgery with internal-limiting membrane peeling and intravitreous air. Ophthalmology. 1999;106:1392–8. https://doi.org/10.1016/S0161-6420(99)00730-7.
4. Wolf S, Reichel MB, Wiedemann P, Schnurrbusch UE. Clinical findings in macular hole surgery with indocyanine greenassisted peeling of the internal limiting membrane. Graefes Arch Clin Exp Ophthalmol. 2003;241:589–92. https://doi.org/10.1007/s00417-003-0673-1.
5. Ip MS, Baker BJ, Duker JS, Reichel E, Baumal CR, Gangnon R, et al. Anatomical outcomes of surgery for idiopathic macular hole as determined by optical coherence tomography. Arch Ophthalmol. 2002;120:29–35.
6. Ullrich S, Haritoglou C, Gass C, Schaumberger M, Ulbig MW, Kampik A. Macular hole size as a prognostic factor in macular hole surgery. Br J Ophthalmol. 2002;86:390–3.
7. Kusuhara S, Teraoka MF, Fujii S, Nakanishi Y, Tamura Y, Nagai A, et al. Prediction of postoperative visual outcome based on hole configuration by optical coherence tomography in eyes with idiopathic macular holes. Am J Ophthalmol. 2004;138:709–16. https://doi.org/10.1016/j.ajo.2004.04.063.
8. Haritoglou C, Neubauer AS, Reiniger IW, Priglinger SG, Gass CA, Kampik A. Long-term functional outcome of macular hole surgery correlated to optical coherence tomography measurements. Clin Exp Ophthalmol. 2007;35:208–13. https://doi.org/10.1111/j.1442-9071.2006.01445.x.
9. Ruiz-Moreno JM, Staicu C, Piñero DP, Montero J, Lugo F, Amat P. Optical coherence tomography predictive factors for macular hole surgery outcome. Br J Ophthalmol. 2008;92:640–4. https://doi.org/10.1136/bjo.2007.136176.
10. Chhablani J, Khodani M, Hussein A, Bondalapati S, Rao HB, Narayanan R. Role of macular hole angle in macular hole closure. Br J Ophthalmol. 2015; 99:1634–8. https://doi.org/10.1136/bjophthalmol-2015-307014.
11. Scott RA, Ezra E, West JF, Gregor ZJ. Visual and anatomical results of surgery for long standing macular holes. Br J Ophthalmol. 2000;84:150–3.
12. Stec LA, Ross RD, Williams GA, Gregor ZJ. Vitrectomy for chronic macular holes. Retina. 2004;24:341–7.
13. Shukla SY, Afshar AR, Kiernan DF, Hariprasad SM. Outcomes of chronic macular hole surgical repair. Indian J Ophthalmol. 2014;62:795–8. https://doi.org/10.4103/0301-4738.138302.
14. Michalewska Z, Michalewski J, Adelman RA, Nawrocki J. Inverted internal limiting membrane flap technique for large macular holes. Ophthalmology. 2010;117:2018–25. https://doi.org/10.1016/j.ophtha.2010.02.011.
15. Mahalingam P, Sambhav K. Surgical outcomes of inverted internal limiting membrane flap technique for large macular hole. Indian J Ophthalmol. 2013;61:601 3. https://doi.org/10.4103/0301-4738.121090

16. Shanmugam MP, Ramanjulu R, Kumar M, Rodrigues G, Reddy S, Mishra D. Inverted ILM peeling for idiopathic and other etiology macular holes. Indian J Ophthalmol. 2014;62:898–9. https://doi.org/10.4103/0301-4738.141077.

17. Khodani M, Bansal P, Narayanan R, Chhablani J. Inverted internal limiting membrane flap technique for very large macular hole. Int J Ophthalmol. 2016;9:1230–2. https://doi.org/10.18240/ijo.2016.08.22.

18. Chen Z, Zhao C, Ye JJ, Sui RF. Inverted internal limiting membrane flap technique for repair of large macular holes: a short-term follow-up of anatomical and functional outcomes. Chin Med J. 2016;129:511–7. https://doi.org/10.4103/0366-6999.176988.

19. Gu C, Qiu Q. Inverted internal limiting membrane flap technique for large macular holes: a systematic review and single-arm meta-analysis. Graefes Arch Clin Exp Ophthalmol 2018 [Ahead of print]. doi: https://doi.org/10.1007/s00417-018-3956-2.

20. Manasa S, Kakkar P, Kumar A, Chandra P, Kumar V, Ravani R. Comparative evaluation of standard ILM peel with inverted ILM flap technique in large macular holes: a prospective, randomized study. Ophthalmic Surg Lasers Imaging Retina. 2018;49:236–40. https://doi.org/10.3928/23258160-20180329-04.

21. Rizzo S, Tartaro R, Barca F, Caporossi T, Bacherini D, Giansanti F. Internal limiting membrane peeling versus inverted flap technique for treatment of full-thickness macular holes: a comparative study in a large series of patients. Retina 2017 Dec 8 [Ahead of print]. doi:https://doi.org/10.1097/IAE.0000000000001985.

22. Yamashita T, Sakamoto T, Terasaki H, Iwasaki M, Ogushi Y, Okamoto F, et al. Best surgical technique and outcomes for large macular holes: retrospective multicentre study in Japan. Acta Ophthalmol 2018 Apr 19 [Ahead of print]. doi: https://doi.org/10.1111/aos.13795.

23. Narayanan R, Singh SR, Taylor S, Berrocal MH, Chhablani J, Tyagi M, et al. Surgical outcomes after inverted internal limiting membrane flap versus conventional peeling for very large macular holes. Retina 2018 Apr 23 [Ahead of print]. doi:https://doi.org/10.1097/IAE.0000000000002186.

24. Velez-Montoya R, Ramirez-Estudillo JA, Sjoholm-Gomez de Liano C, Bejar-Cornejo F, Sanchez-Ramos J, Guerrero-Naranjo JL, et al. Inverted ILM flap, free ILM flap and conventional ILM peeling for large macular holes. Int J Retina Vitreous. 2018;4:8. https://doi.org/10.1186/s40942-018-0111-5.

25. Shukla D, Kalliath J, Patwardhan A, Kannan NB, Thayyil SB. A preliminary study of heavy brilliant blue G for internal limiting membrane staining in macular hole surgery. Indian J Ophthalmol. 2012;60:531–4. https://doi.org/10.4103/0301-4738.103786.

26. Kannan NB, Adenuga OO, Kumar K, Ramasamy K. Outcome of 2 cc pure sulfur hexafluoride gas tamponade for macular hole surgery. BMC Ophthalmol. 2016;16:73. https://doi.org/10.1186/s12886-016-0254-9.

27. Landolfi M, Zarbin MA, Bhagat N. Macular holes. Ophthalmol Clin N Am. 2002;15:565–72.

28. Smiddy WE, Feuer W, Cordahi G. Internal limiting membrane peeling in macular hole surgery. Ophthalmology. 2001;108:1471–6.

29. Gupta D. Face-down posturing after macular hole surgery. A Review. Retina. 2009;29:430–43. https://doi.org/10.1097/IAE.0b013e3181a0bd01.

30. Funata M, Wendel RT, de la Cruz Z, Green WR. Clinicopathologic study of bilateral macular holes treated with pars plana vitrectomy and gas tamponade. Retina. 1992;12:289–98.

31. Madreperla SA, Geiger GL, Funata M, de la Cruz Z, Green WR. Clinicopathologic correlation of a macular hole treated by cortical vitreous peeling and gas tamponade. Ophthalmology. 1994;101:682–6.

32. Rosa RH Jr, Glaser BM, de la Cruz Z, Green WR. Clinicopathologic correlation of an untreated macular hole and a macular hole treated by vitrectomy, transforming growth factor-b2, and gas tamponade. Am J Ophthalmol. 1996;122:853–63.

33. Kang SW, Ahn K, Ham DI. Types of macular hole closure and their clinical implications. Br J Ophthalmol. 2003;87:1015–9.

34. Michalewska Z, Michalewski J, Dulczewska-Cichecka K, Adelman RA, Nawrocki J. Temporal inverted internal limiting membrane flap technique versus classic inverted internal limiting membrane flap technique: a comparative study. Retina. 2015;35:1844–50. https://doi.org/10.1097/IAE.0000000000000555.

35. Shiode Y, Morizane Y, Matoba R, Hirano M, Doi S, Toshima S, et al. The role of inverted internal limiting membrane flap in macular hole closure. Invest Ophthalmol Vis Sci. 2017;58:4847–55. https://doi.org/10.1167/iovs.17-21756.

36. Yuan J, Zhang LL, Lu YJ, Han MY, Yu AH, Cai XJ. Vitrectomy with internal limiting membrane peeling versus inverted internal limiting membrane flap technique for macular hole-induced retinal detachment: a systematic review of literature and meta-analysis. BMC Ophthalmol. 2017;17:219. https://doi.org/10.1186/s12886-017-0619-8.

A rodent model of anterior ischemic optic neuropathy (AION) based on laser photoactivation of verteporfin

Jing-yu Min[1,2,3], Yanan Lv[1,2,3], Lei Mao[1,2,3], Yuan-yuan Gong[1,2,3]* ⓘ, Qing Gu[1,2,3] and Fang Wei[1,2,3]

Abstract

Background: A rodent model of photodynamic AION resulting from intravenous verteporfin is presented. The analysis of the morphological function, the pathological changes and the potential mechanism of action were further investigated.

Methods: Photodynamic treatment was conducted on the optic nerve head (ONH) following administration of the photosensitizer. The fellow eye was considered as sham control. Fundus Fluorescein angiography (FFA), spectral domain optical coherence tomography (SD-OCT) and Flash-visual evoked potential (F-VEP) recordings were conducted at different time points. Immunohistochemistry was used to observe apoptotic cell death (TUNEL) and macrophage infiltration (ED-1/Iba-1). Retrograde labeling of retinal ganglion cells (RGCs) was used to evaluate the loss of RGCs.

Results: After laser treatment, SD-OCT indicated optic nerve edema, while FFA indicated late leakage of the ONH. F-VEPs were distinctly reduced compared to control eyes. The number of apoptotic RGCs peaked on day 14 (5.71 ± 0.76, $p < 0.01$). The infiltration of ED-1 and Iba-1 increased on the 3rd day following PDT, while it peaked on day 14 (67.5 ± 9.57 and 77.5 ± 12.58 respectively, $p < 0.01$). Following 3 weeks of AION, the densities of RGCs in the central retinas of the normal and AION eyes were 3075 ± 298/mm^2 and 2078 ± 141/mm^2 ($p < 0.01$), respectively.

Conclusions: Verteporfin photodynamic treatment on rodents ONH can lead to functional, histological, and pathological changes. This type of animal model of AION is easy to establish and stable. It can be used for studying the mechanism and neuroprotective medicine of AION injury.

Keywords: Anterior ischemic optic neuropathy, Verteporfin, Laser photoactivation, RGCs

Introduction

Anterior ischemic optic neuropathy (AION) is the leading cause of sudden optic nerve-related (ON-related) vision loss in elderly people. Approximately 11.7% of these cases experience central vision abnormalities [1]. In addition, AION was notably noted in one eye, according to a previous study conducted in China, with an incidence rate of 0.03+/– 0.03% (mean +/– standard error) per 5 years (1:16,000 subjects annually) [2].

Based on clinical studies, AION is considered a secondary symptom to ischemia, which is predominantly caused by the posterior ciliary arteries [3], although the exact pathophysiology that leads to axonal degeneration remains undiscovered. In addition, there are a lot of risks, scuh as diabetes mellitus, hypertension, hypercholesterolemia, and crowded structure of the optic disc with small cup to disc ratio. To date no effective method has been reported to prevent vision loss following the development of AION. Thus, it is necessary to establish an animal model of AION that can be used to assess the potential benefits of neuroprotective strategies.

Bernstein et al. conducted the first study that used a photodynamic model of AION in rats by photoactivating rose Bengal with a 532 nm laser [4]. Since then, this

* Correspondence: gyydr@alumni.sjtu.edu.cn
[1]Department of Ophthalmology, Shanghai General Hospital, Shanghai Jiao Tong University School of Medicine, NO.100, Haining Road, Hongkou District, Shanghai 200080, China
[2]Shanghai Key Laboratory of Ocular Fundus Diseases, NO.100, Haining Road, Hongkou District, Shanghai 200080, China
Full list of author information is available at the end of the article

model had been further investigated by several neuro-protective agents [5–8]. Differences had been noted among the severity of this disease in rodents due to a variety of factors, such as the differences of operation and individuals worked, and the very short half-life of rose Bengal, which required a rapid operation of photo-activation following administration. Furthermore, the photosensitizing agent mesoporphyrin IX dihydrochloride was used in establishing the model of AION via intraperi-toneal injection [9], although this type of model had not been widely used due to its short time of discovery.

Verteporfin is a benzoporphyrin derivative and is pro-posed for treating several eye diseases, such as choroidal neovascularization (CNV), pathological myopia, and/or polypoidal choroidal vasculopathy (PCV). Photodynamic treatment following intravenous injection of verteporfin in rodents can lead to edema of the normal choroid and retina [10]. Hence this type of photosensitizer was used in the development of the AION model. Furthermore, verteporfin exhibits a longer half-life than rose Bengal, whereas the photosensitizing agents that were used in the present study were recycled by the discarded parts used for the clinical procedures required for AION examination. Consequently, verteporfin was selected to construct the AION model in the current study.

In the present study, we describe an alternative ap-proach to induce AION inrodents. Furthermore, we studied the morphology, function, and the mechanism of action of this model.

Method
Animals
All animal experiments adhered to the ARVO statement for the Use of Animals in Ophthalmic and Vision Re-search. Adult male Sprague Dawley (S-D) rats weighing 180–200 g were purchased from the Shanghai Labora-tory Animal Center of the Chinese Academy of Sciences and were used for all the experiments. All animals were housed in cages at constant temperature, fed with a standard diet ad libitum and maintained under a 12-h light/12-h dark photoperiod. All types of surgery and ma-nipulation were conducted in the Shanghai Key Laboratory of Fundus Disease. All procedures were carried out under sedation. Sedation was achieved by intraperitoneal injection of 10% (w/v) chloral hydrate(3.5 ml/kg). The pupils of anesthetized rats were dilated with one drop of 5% tropica-mide, and the corneal was anesthetized with one drop of 0.4% oxybuprocaine hydrochloride. The number of animals used for the morphological and functional analyses of each group was $N = 6$.

Induction of AION
A total of 6 mg/m^2 of verteporfin (Novartis Ophthalmics Europe Ltd., Basel, Switzerland) was injected intravenously through the tail vein in order to induce optic nerve head ischemia. Following administration of the photosensitizer for 1 to 10 min duration, the laser was applied on the ONH of the left eye of each animal. The optic nerve head was subjected to a laser beam at a wavelength of 689 nm across a 500-µm diameter spot size for 158 consecutive secs. The laser energy used was 600 mW/cm^2. The laser beam was used for the fellow eye at the ONH with no laser emission and the same operation parameters as stated above.

Fluorescein angiography and optical coherence tomography
Fundus fluorescein angiography (FFA), and spectral do-main optical coherence tomography (SD-OCT) were conducted on days 0, 1, 3 and 7 following treatment to observe the progress of the optic nerve head edema and the related retinal response. A solution of 10% Fluores-cein sodium (Alcon Laboratories Inc. Switzerland) was injected intraperitoneally. The angiographs were recorded following the change in coloration of the conjunctiva that appeared yellow in color (Heidelberg Engineering, Heidelberg,Germany). Retinal structure and retinal thickness were measured using SD-OCT (Heidelberg Engineering). Retinal scans were centered on the optic disc in both control and injured eyes.

Flash-visual evoked potentials (F-VEPs)
The F-VEP was conducted on days 1, 7, 14 and 21 following treatment with a Ganzfeld system (RetiPort, Roland Consult, Brandenburg, Germany). All animals had their pupils dilated and were anesthetized. Upon examination of one of the two eyes of each animal, the contralateral eye was covered. The settings of F-VEPs were based on previous reports [6, 11], including no background illumination, a flash intensity of Ganzfeld 0 dB, a single flash with a flash rate of 1.9 Hz and a flash intensity of 3 cd.s/m^2. The average test was conducted at 80 sweeps, whereas the threshold for rejecting artifacts was set at 50 mV and a sample rate of 2,000 Hz was used. The amplitudes of P1 for each F-VEP wave within the initial 100-ms interval were determined and used for the amplitude analysis (amplitude of P_1 = amplitude of P_1- amplitude of N_2) [6, 12].

Immunohistochemistry
Animals were euthanized on days 1, 4, 7, 14 and 21 fol-lowing laser application. The eyes were enucleated, fixed in 4% paraformaldehyde (PFA) in PBS for 24 h and the anterior segment was removed. Subsequently, certain eyes were dehydrated in 30% sucrose overnight and em-bedded in Tissue-Tek O.C.T compound (Sakura, Tor-rance, CA) Cross sections of 10-µm in diameter were performed. The sections were incubated with mouse

anti-CD68 monoclonal antibody(Serotec Ltd., Oxford, UK) at a 1:100 dilution and/or rabbit anti-Iba-1 monoclonal antibody (Abcam Inc. Cambridge, MA) at a 1:100 dilution, at 4 °C overnight in order to identify macrophages and microglia. FITC conjugated goat anti-mouse IgG and/or FITC conjugated goat anti-rabbit IgG (Jackson Immunoresearch, West Point, PA) were incubated with the sections for 1 h. Finally, sections were counterstained with 4′,6-diamidino-2-phenylindole (DAPI) nuclear stain.

The remaining eyes that were not examined were dehydrated with a posterior eyecup and embedded in paraffin. Retinal cross sections (5 mm thick) were then cut and stained with hematoxylin and eosin (Sigma, MO,USA). The sections were photographed and measured at approximately 2 to 3 disc diameters from the optic nerve using a microscope (Olympus BX53; Olympus, Tokyo, Japan). The thickness of the retinal tissues was determined by cell counts over a distance scale of 200 mm. The retinal thickness and cell number were calculated as the mean values of at least 3 measurements in adjacent sections [13].

TdT-mediated dUTP Nick-end labeling (TUNEL) assay

On days 1, 4, 7 and/or 14 following laser application, paraffin-embedded retinal tissue sections were deparaffinized, rehydrated, fixed with 4% PFA for 15 min at 4 °C and then subjected to enzymatic digestion with 20 mg/ml proteinase K for 8 to 10 min at room temperature. Induction of apoptosis was examined by TUNEL assay using a DeadEnd™ Fluorometric TUNEL System, according to the manufacturer's instructions. 4′,6-diamidino-2-phenylindole (DAPI) was used to stain the nuclear regions of the tissues. TUNEL-positive cells were examined using a laser scanning confocal microscope (Zeiss LSM 510, Carl Zeiss,Germany) in vitro in 6 random fields (at least 100 DAPI-positive cells per field) for each experimental group. The level of apoptosis was expressed as the ratio of the number of TUNEL-positive cells to that of DAPI-positive cells [13].

Retrograde labeling of RGCs with FluoroGold and morphometry of the RGCs

Following deep anesthesia, the rat heads were fixed in a stereotactic apparatus (Stoelting Kiel, Germany) and the skin covering the skull of the rats was incised. Fluoro-Gold (FG;Biotium, Hayward, CA, USA) was injected (2 μl of 4% FG in distilled H_2O) into the superior colliculus (SC) on each side using a microsyringe, and was retained for 10 min. The animals were maintained for 1 week post-labeling and subsequently the eyes were enucleated and fixed with 4% PFA for 1 h. The retinas were examined with an Olympus BX53 fluorescence microscope (Olympus, Tokyo, Japan) with UV excitation (excitation filter, 350–400 nm; barrier filter, 515 nm) and a digital imaging system. The RGCs were examined by division into 4 quadrants (superior, inferior, nasal,and

temporal), which were further divided into central (0.8–1.2 mm from the optic disc), middle (1.8–2.2 mm from the optic disc), and peripheral regions (0.8–1.2 mm from the retinal border). A total of 2 standard square areas (200 × 200 μm²) were measured in each region. The density of RGCs in each group of rats was expressed as the number of labeled RGCs/mm² compared with the counted retinal area [14].

Statistical analysis

The quantitative data were presented as mean ± SD. Statistical analyses were conducted using SPSS version 20 (SPSS, IL, USA). An unpaired Student's t-test for two-group data and one-way analysis of variance followed by a post hoc Bonferroni's multiple comparison test for three groups or more. A p value of lower than 0.05 ($p < 0.05$) was considered statistically significant. Each experiment was conducted three times.

Results
Morphology of ONH following AION induction

The control eye had no abnormal changes (Fig. 1a, d). In the photodynamically treated eyes, FFA indicated fluorescein leakage from the ONH vasculature on day 1, (Fig. 1b, c) which was consistent with the swelling of the retina tissue as demonstrated by the SD-OCT images. On day 3, the optic nerve edema was more pronounced (Fig. 1e). However, a resolution of the edema was noted on day 7.

Flash-visual evoked potentials (F-VEPs)

F-VEPs were recorded at the first, second and third week, following AION induction in order to evaluate the function of ON (Fig. 2). The F-VEPs of the treated eyes were compared with the fellow eyes of each animal in order to eliminate the variations in the F-VEP amplitude within the animal groups [15]. F-VEP amplitudes in the treated eyes ($N = 6$) were estimated to 87.3 ± 11%, 67.6 ± 11.5% and 35.9 ± 13.6% of the fellow control eyes at the first, second and third week, respectively ($P < 0.05$). F-VEP latencies in the two data sets exhibited no statistical significance, as demonstrated in previous experiments [15].

Induction of apoptosis and death in the RGC layer

The induction of apoptosis was evident by the presence of TUNEL-positive cells in the outer nuclear layer (ONL), inner nuclear layer (INL) and RGC layers of the control eyes. The present study analyzed solely the induction of apoptosis in the RGC layer in treated and sham eyes. On the 1st and the 3rd day following AION induction, negligible induction of apoptosis was noted by the presence of TUNEL- positive cells in GCL, which were not demonstrated in the corresponding figure. On

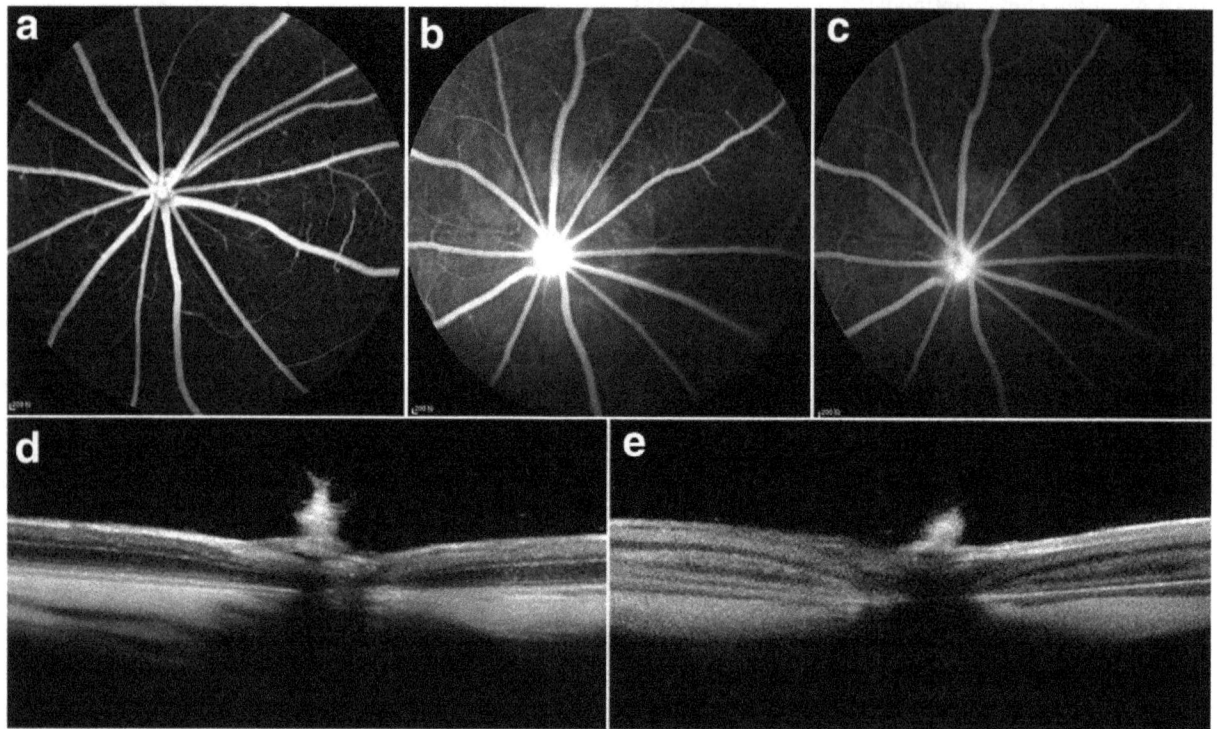

Fig. 1 Fundus fluorescein angiography (FFA) and spectral domain optical coherence tomography (SD-OCT). **a, d** The control fellow eye had no abnormal changes. **b** In the mid-phase, hyperfluorescence can be dectected at the ONH in PDT eye at 1 day post-AION. **c** In the late-phase, subdued fluorescence at ONH in the same PDT eye. **e** SD-OCT showed the swelling of the retina tissue of treated eyes at 3 days post-AION

day 7, the number of TUNEL-positive cells significantly increased, and reached a peak (5.71 ± 0.76, $p < 0.01$) by day 14, (Fig. 3b, d) then reduced. At 3 weeks post-AION, the densities of RGCs in the central retinas were $3,075 \pm 298$ /mm^2 and $2,078 \pm 141$ /mm^2 in the normal and AION eyes, respectively, while in the mid-peripheral retinas the corresponding densities were $2,615 \pm 138$ /mm^2 and $1,691 \pm 142$ /mm^2, respectively (Fig. 3a, c). The densities of RGCs exhibited significant variation in the treated group compared with the sham group ($N = 6$ in each group, all $p < 0.01$).

The inflammatory response in retina and ON

In control ONs, occasional ED-1(+) cells were noted in the peripapillary choroid and in the anterior ON surrounding a blood vessel. By contrast, distributed Iba-1(+) cells were noted in the ON, in the peripapillary choroid, and around the blood vessels (Fig. 4). Following 3 days of treatment, scattered ED-1(+) cells exhibited a moderate increase notably in the choroid and in close proximity to the blood vessels compared with the normal eyes, while Iba-1(+) cells exhibited a significant localization on the anterior ON. On day 14, ED(+) and Iba-1(+) cells were widely distributed on ON, and both reached their maximum number (67.5 ± 9.57 and 77.5 ± 12.58 respectively, $p < 0.01$) during the whole process of the study. Subsequently, ED-1

cells tended to disappear, whereas Iba-1(+) cells exhibited a considerable decrease to a certain number of cells.

Discussion

In the present study, we aimed to establish an alternative experimental model of laser photoactivation that can be applied for the development of neuroprotective agents against AION. Bernstein et al. were the first to develop a photodynamic model of AION in rats by photoactivating rose Bengal with a 532 nm laser [4]. Since then, this model had been further utilized by various research groups [15–18]. However, the biological half-life of rose Bengal in rats is solely 2 min [19], which indicates that the delay of operation post-injection may weaken the effect of photodynamic treatment on the ON. In the present study, the immediate operation with laser on ON was conducted following injection that can be technically challenging and can lead to variable injured levels of ON. Depending on our clinical experience and previous studies [20, 21], we selected an alternative treatment to induce AION using a dye with easier acquisition and longer half-life.

Preliminary experiments were conducted in order to simplify the experimental operation. Verteporfin was injected via intraperitoneal rather than intravenous injection, but it proved unsuccessful despite the high dose

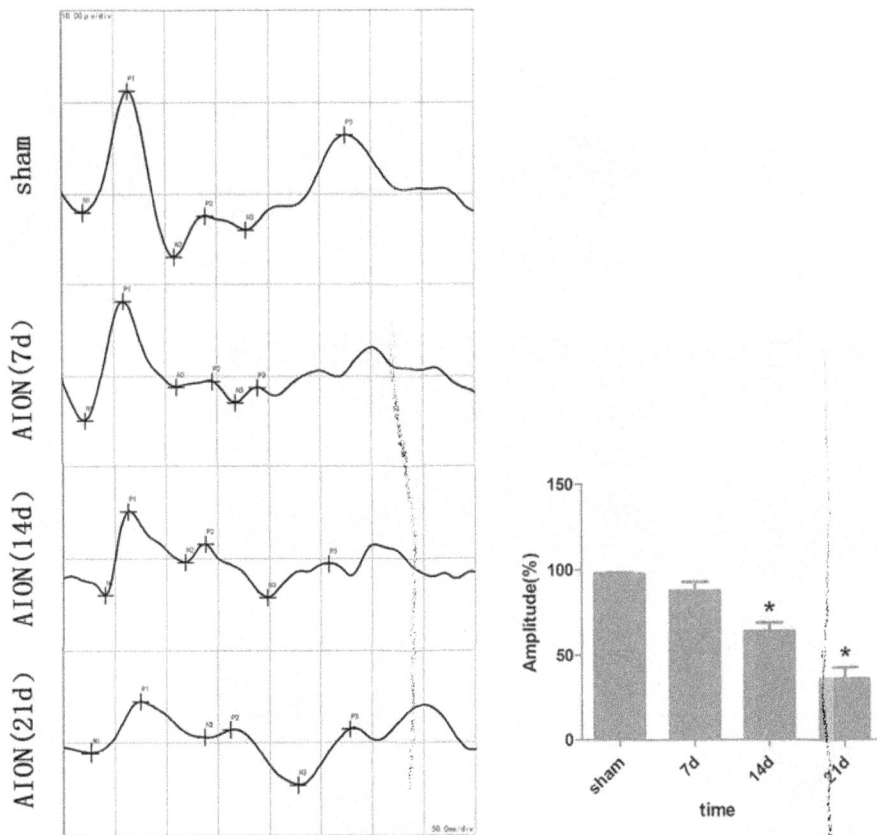

Fig. 2 Flash-Visual Evoked Potentials (F-VEPs) in AION. F-VEP amplitudes of P1 in treated eyes measured $87.3 \pm 11\%$ of the fellow control eyes at 1 week, $67.6 \pm 11.5\%$ at 2 week, and $35.9 \pm 13.6\%$ at 3 week. We did not compare F-VEP latencies in the two data sets because of the indistinctive statistics. (*$P < 0.05$ in the 14d and 21d groups compared with the sham group, $N = 6$ in each group)

of the photosensitizer and the high energy emission of the laser beam. Considering the fact that the intraperitoneal injection with verteporfin has not been previously reported in rodents [20–22], the present study indicates that the slow accumulation of verteporfin in the retinal circulation may have resulted by the slow peritoneal absorption. Furthermore, the intraperitoneal injection of verteporfin is impractical due to the inability to test the peak plasma concentration and the difficulty of mastering the illumination time. Consequently, the mode of delivery was changed from intraperitoneal injection to intravenous injection. Angiography was carried out with verteporfin at a dose of 6 mg/m^2 as demonstrated by a previous study [10], in order to test the time duration of the flow of this compound through the choroidal and retinal circulation. Verteporfin was readily detected and was immediately visible in the vascular circulation following the intravenous injection. Following 5 min of injection, verteporfin was visible in both the choroidal and retinal circulation, and after that time period verteporfin appeared to wash out of the vascular circulation. The detection of verteporfin was not possible in the vascular circulation following

10 min of injection. Hence, the operating time was estimated to 10 min post-injection. This time period was sufficient to complete the laser operation and construct an ideal model for AION.

SD-OCT and FFA images of the treated group indicated significant optic nerve edema compared with the sham group on day 1 following the induction of injury. The development of the edema peaked on day 3 and began to decline from day 7. Based on the SD-OCT images, it was noted that certain treated rats had subretinal fluid on day 1. A similar finding has been demonstrated previously in human AION cases [9, 23] and in experimental AION models [24]. The presence of subretinal fluid may promote the death of retinal cells, indicating that the detection of TUNEL-positive cells was possible outside the ganglion cell layer [9]. A wide, non-perfused choroidal vasculature was noted in a certain rat. This unexpected injury may have resulted from individual differences and/or inadvertent operation, and this rat was removed from the study.

TUNEL staining was used to evaluate the apoptotic cell death. Certain parts of TUNEL-positive cells were detected in the outer nuclear layer (ONL) and inner

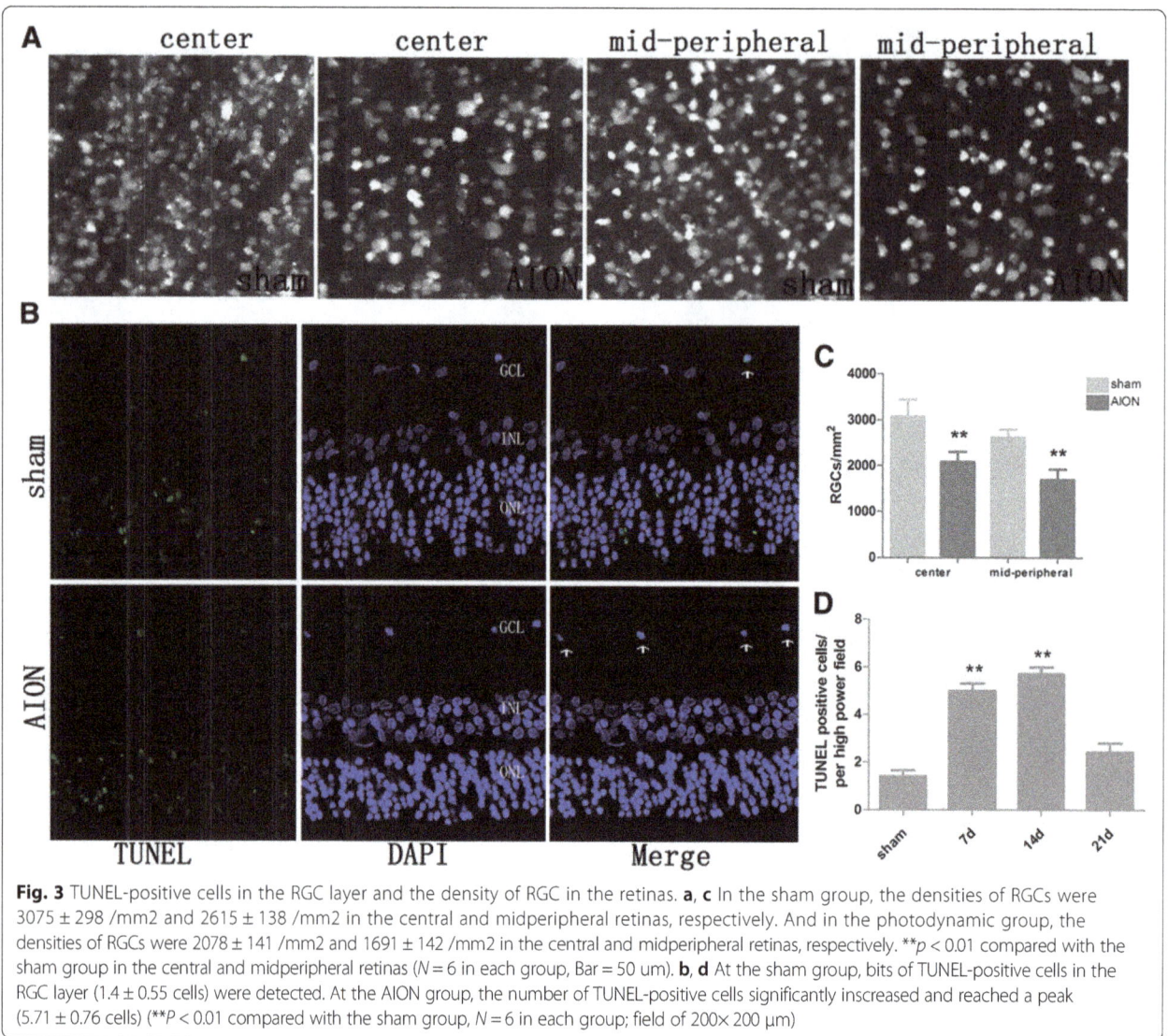

Fig. 3 TUNEL-positive cells in the RGC layer and the density of RGC in the retinas. **a, c** In the sham group, the densities of RGCs were 3075 ± 298 /mm2 and 2615 ± 138 /mm2 in the central and midperipheral retinas, respectively. And in the photodynamic group, the densities of RGCs were 2078 ± 141 /mm2 and 1691 ± 142 /mm2 in the central and midperipheral retinas, respectively. **p < 0.01 compared with the sham group in the central and midperipheral retinas (N = 6 in each group, Bar = 50 um). **b, d** At the sham group, bits of TUNEL-positive cells in the RGC layer (1.4 ± 0.55 cells) were detected. At the AION group, the number of TUNEL-positive cells significantly inscreased and reached a peak (5.71 ± 0.76 cells) (**P < 0.01 compared with the sham group, N = 6 in each group; field of 200× 200 µm)

nuclear layer (INL) both in the treated and control eyes, although there was no statistically significant difference (P = 0.3) between the two groups. In the treated group, TUNEL-positive cells were demonstrated in the ganglion cell layer by day 7. The percentage of positive cells peaked by day 14 post-ischemia and subsequently declined, which suggested delayed apoptosis following the ON infarct compared to the previous studies [25, 26]. This diversity may have resulted from individual variation and different modeling methods. In the current model, at 3 weeks post-infarct, we could still detect approximately 60% of all RGCs through retrograde labeling of RGCs with Fluoro-Gold. This time period coincided with the seventh day following the peak of apoptosis. Slater et al. [27] demonstrated that at 2–3 weeks post-ischemia, approximately 50% of RGCs were still present. As a result, we speculated that the number of RGCs may be reduced considerably after the

3rd week of treatment until the RGC densities were approximately 30% [8]. The aforementioned findings demonstrated that a prolonged "treatment window" is potentially present in the current model, while the induction of treatment within 7 days post- ischemia may preserve the RGC number. Similarly, such a treatment window may exist in the human AION.

Following injury, extrinsic macrophages were recruited, and resident microglia were activated, at the core of the ischemic ON [8, 28]. This suggests the breakdown of the blood–ON barrier. Activated macrophages exert a dual fuction: They can enhance remyelination and regeneration [29], while they may produce harmful substances –such as pro-inflammatory mediators which can aggravate the neruronal injury. Due to the individual variation and different modeling methods, the current model exhibited a delay of inflammatory response compared to

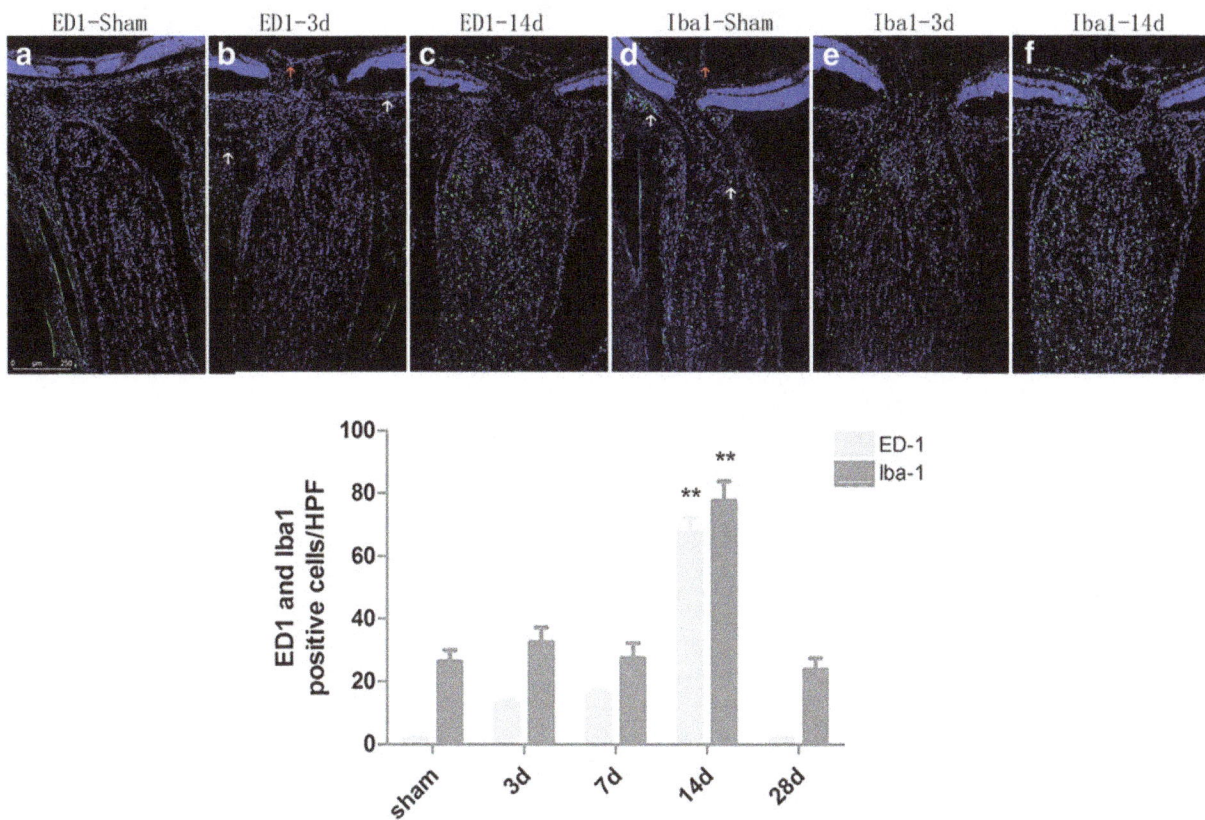

Fig. 4 Infiltration of ED-1(+) cells and Iba-1(+) cells both were detected in the ONs post-AION. **a, d** At sham group, occasional ED-1(+) cells and distributed Iba-1(+) cells were found in the peripapillary choroid(white arrows) as well as in the anterior ON surrounding a blood vessel(red arrows); **b, e** At 3 days post-AION, scattered ED-1(+) cells had a moderate increase especially in the choroid and next to the blood vessels; Iba-1(+) cells had a significat gatheration on the anterior ON; **c, f** At 14 days post-AION, ED-1(+) as well as Iba-1(+) cells widely distributed on ON, and both reached the peak (67.5 ± 9.57 cells/HPF and 77.5 ± 12.58 cells/HPF, respectively), **$P < 0.01$ compared with the sham group ($N = 6$ in each group)

previous studies [5, 28, 30]. Both numbers of ED(+) and Iba-1(+) cells peaked on the 14th day post-infarct and they were subsequently decreased. This suggests additional time for the modulation of the inflammatory process at an early stage.

The functional deficits were demonstrated by gradually decreasing the amplitude of P1 on F-VEP. According to our histological and pathological findings, the decline of vision resulted from the activation of macrophages and the loss of RGCs. We detected subnormal P1 amplitudes on the 7th day. These observations were more profound on the 14th day post-treatment and suggested that cellular degeneration proceeded following the resolution of the ON edema. The visual function was affected by the progressive damage, which is consistent with the findings reported in previous studies [9, 31, 32].

Conclusion

An AION model was successfully produced as demonstrated by FFA, SD-OCT and F-VEP images. The model can provide the estimation of inflammation by immunofluorescent staining and the estimation of the number of RGCs. The current study provided a steady, technically simple and controlled model, which can be used to examine the potential neuroprotective effects of certain agents and explore the pathological mechanism of AION.

Abbreviations

AION: Anterior ischemic optic neuropathy; CNV: Choroidal neovascularization; DAPI: 4',6-diamidino-2-phenylindole; FFA: Fundus Fluorescein angiography; F-VEP: Flash-visual evoked potential; ON: Optic nerve; ONH: Ptic nerve head; PCV: Polypoidal choroidal vasculopathy; RGCs: Retinal ganglion cells; SD-OCT: Spectral domain optical coherence tomography

Funding
This study was supported by National Natural Science Foundation of China (no. 81300774), the opening project of Shanghai key laboratory of Fundus Diseases (no.07Z22911).

Authors' contributions

MJY and GYY were primarily responsible for experimental concept and design, and was major contributors in writing the manuscript. LYN raised all the experimental rats and helped to operated on them. ML performed the histological examination of the retina and optic nerve. GQ and WF performed data acquisition and analysis. All authors reviewed and approved the final manuscript.

Competing interests

The authors declare that they have no competing interests.

Author details
[1]Department of Ophthalmology, Shanghai General Hospital, Shanghai Jiao Tong University School of Medicine, NO.100, Haining Road, Hongkou District, Shanghai 200080, China. [2]Shanghai Key Laboratory of Ocular Fundus Diseases, NO.100, Haining Road, Hongkou District, Shanghai 200080, China. [3]Shanghai Engineering Center for Visual Science and Photomedicine, NO.100, Haining Road, Hongkou District, Shanghai 200080, China.

References

1. Biousse V, Newman NJ. Ischemic optic neuropathies. N Engl J Med. 2015; 372:2428–36. https://doi.org/10.1056/NEJMra1413352.
2. Xu L, Wang Y, Jonas JB. Incidence of nonarteritic anterior ischemic optic neuropathy in adult Chinese: the Beijing eye study. Eur J Ophthalmol. 2007; 17:459–60.
3. Hayreh SS. Management of ischemic optic neuropathies. Indian J Ophthalmol. 2011;59:123–36. https://doi.org/10.4103/0301-4738.77024.
4. Bernstein SL, Guo Y, Kelman SE, Flower RW, Johnson MA. Functional and cellular responses in a novel rodent model of anterior ischemic optic neuropathy. Invest Ophthalmol Vis Sci. 2003;44:4153–62.
5. Wen YT, Huang TL, Huang SP, Chang CH, Tsai RK. Early applications of granulocyte colony-stimulating factor (G-CSF) can stabilize the blood-optic-nerve barrier and ameliorate inflammation in a rat model of anterior ischemic optic neuropathy (rAION). Dis Model Mech. 2016;9:1193–202. https://doi.org/10.1242/dmm.025999.
6. Huang TL, Wen YT, Chang CH, Chang CW, Lin KH, Tsai RK. Efficacy of intravitreal injections of triamcinolone Acetonide in a rodent model of Nonarteritic anterior ischemic optic neuropathy. Invest Ophthalmol Vis Sci. 2016;57:1878–84. https://doi.org/10.1167/iovs.15-19023.
7. Mathews MK, Guo Y, Langenberg P, Bernstein SL. Ciliary neurotrophic factor (CNTF)-mediated ganglion cell survival in a rodent model of non-arteritic anterior ischaemic optic neuropathy (NAION). Br J Ophthalmol. 2015;99:133–7. https://doi.org/10.1136/bjophthalmol-2014-305969.
8. Huang TL, Huang SP, Chang CH, Lin KH, Chang SW, Tsai RK. Protective effects of systemic treatment with methylprednisolone in a rodent model of non-arteritic anterior ischemic optic neuropathy (rAION). Exp Eye Res. 2015;131:69–76. https://doi.org/10.1016/j.exer.2014.12.014.
9. Mantopoulos D, Bouzika P, Tsakris A, Pawlyk BS, Sandberg MA, Miller JW, Rizzo Iii JF, Vavvas DG, Cestari DM. (TUNEL!!!) an experimental animal model of photodynamic optic nerve head injury (PONHI). Curr Eye Res. 2016:1–9. https://doi.org/10.3109/02713683.2015.1135960.
10. Zacks DN, Ezra E, Terada Y, Michaud N, Connolly E, Gragoudas ES, Miller JW. Verteporfin photodynamic therapy in the rat model of choroidal neovascularization: angiographic and histologic characterization. Invest Ophthalmol Vis Sci. 2002;43:2384–91.
11. Denny CA, Alroy J, Pawlyk BS, Sandberg MA, d'Azzo A, Seyfried TN. Neurochemical, morphological, and neurophysiological abnormalities in retinas of Sandhoff and GM1 gangliosidosis mice. J Neurochem. 2007;101: 1294–302. https://doi.org/10.1111/j.1471-4159.2007.04525.x.
12. Jiang B, Zhang P, Zhou D, Zhang J, Xu X, Tang L. Intravitreal transplantation of human umbilical cord blood stem cells protects rats from traumatic optic neuropathy. PLoS One. 2013;8:e69938. https://doi.org/10.1371/journal.pone.0069938.
13. Xiong S, Xu Y, Ma M, Wang H, Wei F, Gu Q, Xu X. Neuroprotective effects of a novel peptide, FK18, under oxygen-glucose deprivation in SH-SY5Y cells and retinal ischemia in rats via the Akt pathway. Neurochem Int. 2017. https://doi.org/10.1016/j.neuint.2017.02.015.
14. Chen YJ, Huang YS, Chen JT, Chen YH, Tai MC, Chen CL, Liang CM. Protective effects of glucosamine on oxidative-stress and ischemia/reperfusion-induced retinal injury. Invest Ophthalmol Vis Sci. 2015;56:1506–16. https://doi.org/10.1167/iovs.14-15726.
15. Touitou V, Johnson MA, Guo Y, Miller NR, Bernstein SL. Sustained neuroprotection from a single intravitreal injection of PGJ2 in a rodent model of anterior ischemic optic neuropathy. Invest Ophthalmol Vis Sci. 2013;54:7402–9. https://doi.org/10.1167/iovs.13-12055.
16. Huang SP, Tsai RK. Efficacy of granulocyte-colony stimulating factor treatment in a rat model of anterior ischemic optic neuropathy. Neural Regen Res. 2014;9:1502–5. https://doi.org/10.4103/1673-5374.139472.
17. Fard MA, Ebrahimi KB, Miller NR. RhoA activity and post-ischemic inflammation in an experimental model of adult rodent anterior ischemic optic neuropathy. Brain Res. 2013;1534:76–86. https://doi.org/10.1016/j.brainres.2013.07.053.
18. Bernstein SL, Guo Y. Changes in cholinergic amacrine cells after rodent anterior ischemic optic neuropathy (rAION). Invest Ophthalmol Vis Sci. 2011; 52:904–10. https://doi.org/10.1167/iovs.10-5247.
19. Klaassen CD. Pharmacokinetics of rose bengal in the rat, rabbit, dog and Guinea pig. Toxicol Appl Pharmacol. 1976;38:85–100.
20. She H, Nakazawa T, Matsubara A, Connolly E, Hisatomi T, Noda K, Kim I, Gragoudas ES, Miller JW. Photoreceptor protection after photodynamic therapy using dexamethasone in a rat model of choroidal neovascularization. Invest Ophthalmol Vis Sci. 2008;49:5008–14. https://doi.org/10.1167/iovs.07-1154.
21. Renno RZ, Terada Y, Haddadin MJ, Michaud NA, Gragoudas ES, Miller JW. Selective photodynamic therapy by targeted verteporfin delivery to experimental choroidal neovascularization mediated by a homing peptide to vascular endothelial growth factor receptor-2. Arch Ophthalmol. 2004; 122:1002–11. https://doi.org/10.1001/archopht.122.7.1002.
22. Matsubara A, Nakazawa T, Noda K, She H, Connolly E, Young TA, Ogura Y, Gragoudas ES, Miller JW. Photodynamic therapy induces caspase-dependent apoptosis in rat CNV model. Invest Ophthalmol Vis Sci. 2007;48:4741–7. https://doi.org/10.1167/iovs.06-1534.
23. Hedges TR 3rd, Vuong LN, Gonzalez-Garcia AO, Mendoza-Santiesteban CE, Amaro-Quierza ML. Subretinal fluid from anterior ischemic optic neuropathy demonstrated by optical coherence tomography. Arch Ophthalmol. 2008; 126:812–5. https://doi.org/10.1001/archopht.126.6.812.
24. Yu C, Ho JK, Liao YJ. Subretinal fluid is common in experimental non-arteritic anterior ischemic optic neuropathy. Eye (Lond). 2014;28:1494–501. https://doi.org/10.1038/eye.2014.220.
25. Zhang C, Guo Y, Slater BJ, Miller NR, Bernstein SL. Axonal degeneration, regeneration and ganglion cell death in a rodent model of anterior ischemic optic neuropathy (rAION). Exp Eye Res. 2010;91:286–92. https://doi.org/10.1016/j.exer.2010.05.021.
26. Slater BJ, Mehrabian Z, Guo Y, Hunter A, Bernstein SL. Rodent anterior ischemic optic neuropathy (rAION) induces regional retinal ganglion cell apoptosis with a unique temporal pattern. Invest Ophthalmol Vis Sci. 2008; 49:3671–6. https://doi.org/10.1167/iovs.07-0504.
27. Tsai RK, Chang CH, Wang HZ. Neuroprotective effects of recombinant human granulocyte colony-stimulating factor (G-CSF) in neurodegeneration after optic nerve crush in rats. Exp Eye Res. 2008;87:242–50. https://doi.org/10.1016/j.exer.2008.06.004.
28. Salgado C, Vilson F, Miller NR, Bernstein SL. Cellular inflammation in nonarteritic anterior ischemic optic neuropathy and its primate model. Arch Ophthalmol. 2011;129:1583–91. https://doi.org/10.1001/archophthalmol.2011.351.
29. Yin Y, Henzl MT, Lorber B, Nakazawa T, Thomas TT, Jiang F, Langer R, Benowitz LI. Oncomodulin is a macrophage-derived signal for axon regeneration in retinal ganglion cells. Nat Neurosci. 2006;9:843–52. https://doi.org/10.1038/nn1701.
30. Zhang C, Guo Y, Miller NR, Bernstein SL. Optic nerve infarction and post-ischemic inflammation in the rodent model of anterior ischemic optic neuropathy (rAION). Brain Res. 2009;1264:67–75. https://doi.org/10.1016/j.brainres.2008.12.075.
31. Bernstein SL, Johnson MA, Miller NR. Nonarteritic anterior ischemic optic neuropathy (NAION) and its experimental models. Prog Retin Eye Res. 2011; 30:167–87. https://doi.org/10.1016/j.preteyeres.2011.02.003.
32. Slater BJ, Vilson FL, Guo Y, Weinreich D, Hwang S, Bernstein SL. Optic nerve inflammation and demyelination in a rodent model of nonarteritic anterior ischemic optic neuropathy. Invest Ophthalmol Vis Sci. 2013;54:7952–61. https://doi.org/10.1167/iovs.13-12064.

19

Evidence for alterations in fixational eye movements in glaucoma

Giovanni Montesano[1,2]* (iD), David P. Crabb[2], Pete R. Jones[2], Paolo Fogagnolo[1], Maurizio Digiuni[1] and Luca M. Rossetti[1]

Abstract

Background: Fixation changes in glaucoma are generally overlooked, as they are not strikingly evident as in macular diseases. Fundus perimetry might give additional insights into this aspect, along with traditional perimetric measures. In this work we propose a novel method to quantify glaucomatous changes in fixation features as detected by fundus perimetry and relate them to the extent of glaucomatous damage.

Methods: We retrospectively analysed fixation data from 320 people (200 normal subjects and 120 with glaucoma) from the Preferred Retinal Locus (PRL) detection of a Compass perimeter. Fixation stability was measured as Bivariate Contour Ellipse Area (BCEA), and using two novel metrics: (1) Mean Euclidean Distance (MED) from the Preferred Retinal Locus, and (2) Sequential Euclidean Distance (SED) of sequential fixation locations. These measures were designed to capture the spread of fixation points, and the frequency of position changes during fixation, respectively.

Results: In the age corrected analysis, SED was significantly greater in glaucomatous subjects than controls ($P = 0.002$), but there was no difference in BCEA ($P = 0.15$) or MED ($P = 0.054$). Similarly, SED showed a significant association with Mean Deviation ($P < 0.001$), but neither BCEA nor MED were significantly correlated ($P > 0.14$ for both).

Conclusion: Changes in the scanning pattern detected by SED are better than traditional measures of fixation spread (BCEA) for describing the changes in fixation stability observed in glaucoma.

Keywords: Fundus perimetry, Fixation, Glaucoma, Eye movements, Visual field

Background

Primary Open Angle Glaucoma (POAG) is a progressive optic neuropathy usually associated with increased intra-ocular pressure (IOP), progressive damage to the visual field and characteristic changes in the optic nerve and the inner retina [1]. Both structural and functional measurements are employed in the diagnosis of POAG, most notably Optical Coherence Tomography (OCT) for the structural assessment, and Visual Field testing (VF) for the functional assessment [2].

VF testing (static white-on-white perimetry), measures the differential light sensitivity (DLS) by presenting light points of variable intensity, in order to assess patient's detection threshold at various retinal locations. VF testing is one of the most useful means of diagnosing and staging glaucoma and assessing progression [3]. However, classical VF testing requires the patient to be able to fixate a central target throughout the test. To assess the accuracy of the exam, the Humphrey Field Analyzer (HFA) is able to report fixation performances on the final printout both as a descriptive plot from a simple eye tracker and as an estimate of fixation loss with the classical Heijl-Krakau technique [4].

Fundus Automated Perimetry (FAP), also known as microperimetry, has been introduced to allow reliable testing in patients with central vision impairment, such as in macular degenerations, who are usually not able to maintain a stable central fixation. FAP uses continuous infrared Scanning Laser Ophthalmoscope (SLO) imaging to track the retina and compensates for eye movements during the presentation of the stimuli [5]. Despite this, very unsteady fixation is still likely to be a confounding factor [6], due to limited temporal resolution or poor image quality during tracking.

* Correspondence: giovmontesano@gmail.com
[1]ASST Santi Paolo e Carlo, University of Milan, 20142 Milan, Italy
[2]City, University of London, Optometry and Visual Sciences, Northampton Square, EC1V 0HB, London, UK

Furthermore, even with a perfect control of fixation shifts in perimetry, fixation data might contain useful information that can be exploited [7]. Recent works have analysed fixational movements during central static fixation with microperimetry [8, 9], reporting partially contrasting results. At the same time there has been an interest in eye movement behaviour in people with glaucoma and how it differs from visually healthy peers when undergoing different visual tasks [10–13]. A better understanding of fixation alterations in glaucomatous patients might be useful to improve visual field testing accuracy by gathering additional functional information on individual VF loss [14].

Some attempts have been made to produce a quantitative evaluation of the gaze tracking data [15]. The Bivariate Contour Ellipse Area (BCEA) [16] is commonly used to quantify the spatial extent of fixations collected over a period of time. The BCEA has limitations since it assumes that fixations are normally distributed in space. Moreover, the BCEA disregards the temporal sequence of fixation movements [17].

In short, fixation analysis has the potential to be an additional tool in characterizing functional changes in glaucoma, but current tools might be not adequate to characterize fixation features to their full extent.

In the present study, we aim to analyse fixation in patients with different severity of VF loss and people without VF loss (normal subjects) using data obtained during the Preferred Retinal Locus (PRL) registration performed prior to automated perimetry assessment in fundus perimetry. For this, we used a Compass perimeter (CenterVue, Padova, Italy), a recently introduced fundus perimeter for glaucoma testing [18, 19]. We aim to capture fixation information and relate it to measures of VF damage. We also propose two new measures of fixation instability that may better characterize the changes in fixation in glaucomatous patients (Fig. 1):

- The *Mean Euclidean Distance* (MED), which is a measure of central dispersion of fixation positions around the barycentre.
- The *Sequential Euclidean Distance* (SED), which is a measure of how frequently the subject is changing fixation location independently of the spatial spread of the points and is designed to encode the temporal instability of subjects' fixation.

Methods
Data overview
The present study retrospectively analyses data from the validation study of the Compass perimeter [18]. The dataset contains 320 eyes of 320 people (200 normal subjects and 120 with a clinical diagnosis of glaucoma). All subjects underwent a standard ophthalmological evaluation and performed a visual field test using the Compass perimeter. This was carried out monocularly (random eye), using a 24–2 grid and a 4–2 staircase strategy.

Inclusion/exclusion criteria
Details of inclusion and exclusion criteria for the study are reported in Rossetti et al. [18] Inclusion criteria for all subjects were: age between 20 and 80 years; best-corrected decimal visual acuity > 0.8 (for subjects < 50 years old) or > 0.6 (over 50) in both eyes; spherical refraction within ±5D; astigmatism within ±2D. For normal subjects: normal visual field in both eyes from Humphrey Field Analyzer (HFA) testing; normal appearance of the optic disc in both eyes; and an IOP ≤ 21 mmHg in both eyes. Glaucoma subjects were selected based on clinical diagnosis and structural damage to the optic nerve head (evident from fundus examination or OCT), independently of the visual field (i.e. preperimetric glaucoma subjects were included). Subjects with general or ocular conditions other than glaucoma that could affect visual field test results were not recruited. The study adhered to the tenets of the Declaration of Helsinki and all participants gave written informed consent. The local ethical committee ("San Paolo Hospital Ethics Committee", n. 734 of July 30th, 2013—Studio GSD 2013) approved the original study and subsequent use of data in anonymized form for research purposes.

PRL assessment and data extraction
Eye-tracking data were extracted from the Preferred Retinal Locus (PRL) assessment phase of the Compass perimeter. PRL assessment consists of a 10 s period prior to testing, during which time no stimuli are projected and the subject is asked to fixate the central target while retinal displacements are measured using an eye tracker. Eye tracking is performed using an infrared SLO picture of the subject's retina with a temporal resolution of 25 times/sec. The theoretical spatial resolution is 0.03 degrees (derived from the 32 degrees/pixel resolution in the SLO picture) but may vary depending on the image quality. These data are used by the instrument to calculate the PRL for fixation, later set as the centre of the visual field testing grid.

The whole track of the PRL assessment consists of a list of horizontal and vertical displacements in degrees sampled every 40 ms (250 samples) along with a quality score of the tracking values provided by the instrument, based on the correlation coefficient between the fundus image at each time point and the reference image.

Data analysis
All data were analysed in anonymized form. For each PRL assessment we selected only values with reliable tracking quality (Quality Score > 700). We excluded from

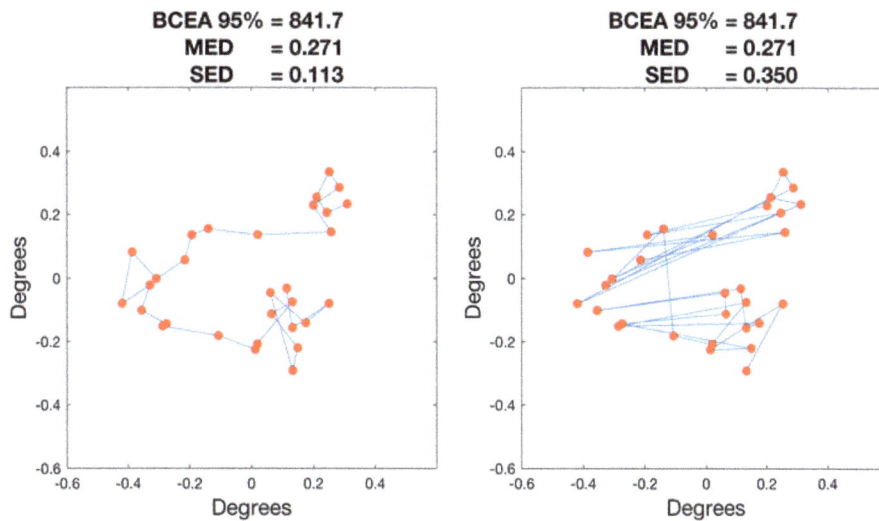

Fig. 1 Schematic representation of the differences between the two proposed MED and SED indices. The left and right tracks represent two fictional fixation patterns ($n = 30$ points). The red dots represent the individual displacements of fixation and the blue lines join subsequent locations in the sequence. Both fixation patterns have the same point coordinates (the red dots) but the sequence is different. In the pattern on the left each displacement tends to be very close to the previous location in the sequence. In the pattern on the right, fixation shifts randomly from one point to another. As a result, indices that only account for fixation point locations (the BCEA and the MED) do not change. On the contrary, the SED index, calculated as the average of distances between successive points in the sequence, is greatly increased in the pattern on the right, capturing the continuous movement from one position to the other

our analysis subjects that had less than 150 reliable samples (< 60%). This resulted in 28 (8.75%) of the subjects being excluded (11 normal subjects and 17 glaucoma subjects).

For the remaining 292 participants, each participant's data were processed independently to compute three metrics of fixation stability:

1. *Bivariate Contour Ellipse Area (BCEA):* BCEA is considered the current 'Gold Standard' measure of fixation stability [16] and is defined as an ellipse which encompasses fixation points for a given proportion of eye positions during one fixation trial. It assumes the distribution of the data to follow a Normal distribution along the two axes of the ellipse. Moreover, it only accounts for spatial alterations in the fixation pattern [17], ignoring the temporal sequence of the fixation displacements or simply the order of their occurrence.

2. The *Mean Euclidean Distance* (MED): MED is a measure of central dispersion of fixation positions around the mean position of the cloud of points (barycentre, see Fig. 1). It is computed by averaging the Euclidean distances of each tracked position from the location of the PRL. Differently from BCEA, it does not assume an elliptically shaped distribution of the points.

3. The *Sequential Euclidean Distance* (SED): SED is a measure of how frequently the subject is changing fixation location independently of the spatial spread

of the points. It is computed by averaging the Euclidean distances of each tracked position from the subsequent location in the temporal sequence of displacements (see Fig. 1). Since some samples were excluded due to low tracking quality, gaps could appear in the temporal sequence. This issue was accounted for in the computation by measuring the distances only between temporally subsequent points both classified as reliable with the quality check.

The conceptual difference between the MED and SED is shown in the diagram in Fig. 1. BCEA 95% was calculated as reported in Crossland et al. [17].

As explained below (section on statistical analysis), log-transformed values of these indices were used for the analysis. They are denoted as log-BCEA, log-MED and log-SED respectively.

MATLAB (The MathWorks, Inc., Natick, Massachusetts, US) was used to extract the raw data and compute the various metrics.

Visual (VF) field testing

Mean Deviation (MD) and Pattern Standard Deviation (PSD) were calculated from visual field data. We also divided the visual field into sectors following a map described by Garway-Heath et al. [20] and calculated sector-wise MD values. Values from the temporal visual field sector were discarded and the remaining clusters were grouped in 3 categories (peripheral, mid-peripheral and central, see Fig. 2) to assess the local glaucoma visual field loss at increasing eccentricities.

Statistical analysis

Although all calculations were performed in degrees (deg) for the MED and SED and in minutes of arc for the BCEA, we will report the indices as adimensional. The BCEA, MED and SED measures are strictly positive and exhibited a strong positive skew. To compensate for such skewness, their values were log-transformed prior to statistical analysis. The log-transformed measures are denoted as log-BCEA, log-MED andlog-SED respectively. The skewness of the residuals using log-transformed values was computed and evaluated. A skewness value outside the range – 0.5 and 0.5 was considered indicative of a non-symmetric distribution of the residuals [21].

We used linear models both to compare the control and glaucomatous groups and to analyse associations between fixation stability indices and the MD. All models included age as predictor to account for any possible changes in fixation with aging. To assess whether the age could have a non-linear effect on fixation metrics, we also fit the models using cubic basis splines, which are a common standard method to assess the presence of non-linear relationships [22]. Improvement in the goodness-of-fit with basis splines was evaluated using the Akaike Information Criterion (AIC) [22].

In order to assess which part of the visual field was affecting fixation the most when damaged, the correlation of fixation indices with the local MD values was analysed. In this analysis, we estimated a single model for each fixation index and used interactions to model different slopes for each visual field region (peripheral, mid-peripheral and central, see Fig. 2) and used the central region as the reference level. This was designed to investigate if damages to more peripheral parts of

the visual fields would have an additional significant effect on the fixation indices. This could be considered to be a repeated measure design (with three regional MD values for each subject). Yet, the independent variable in this analysis was the same fixation index value (log-transformed BCEA, MED or SED) repeated three times, once for each regional MD value, yielding a perfect within subject correlation on the response variable. Therefore, since the variation of the response variable in each subject was equal to zero, this is the same as fitting a simple linear model, and no correction for repeated measures was used.

Model estimates are denoted as *ME*, Standard Errors as *SE* and Standard Deviations as *SD*.

All statistical analyses were carried out in R (https://www.r-project.org/).

Results

Demographics for the study participants are reported in Table 1. Data from 292 subjects (189 normal subjects and 103 glaucoma subjects) were analysed (see Methods).

Differences between the normal and glaucoma group are shown in Table 1. As expected we found a significant difference in the MD values ($P < 0.001$). Glaucoma patients were older on average (see Table 1) than the normal subjects; hence all analyses on the fixation indices included age as a covariate.

As shown in Table 2 (row 6), mean log-MED values appeared lower in glaucoma patients (-1.47 ± 0.7) than controls (-1.24 ± 0.86), and the non age corrected comparison yielded a statistically significant difference ($P = 0.02$). However, we did not observe a statistically significant difference in log-MED index once age was corrected for via multivariate analysis (estimated difference 0.16 ± 0.12, $ME \pm SE$, $P = 0.16$, Table 2).

We performed an equivalent analysis on the log-BCEA, with similar results. Log-BCEA values for the glaucoma

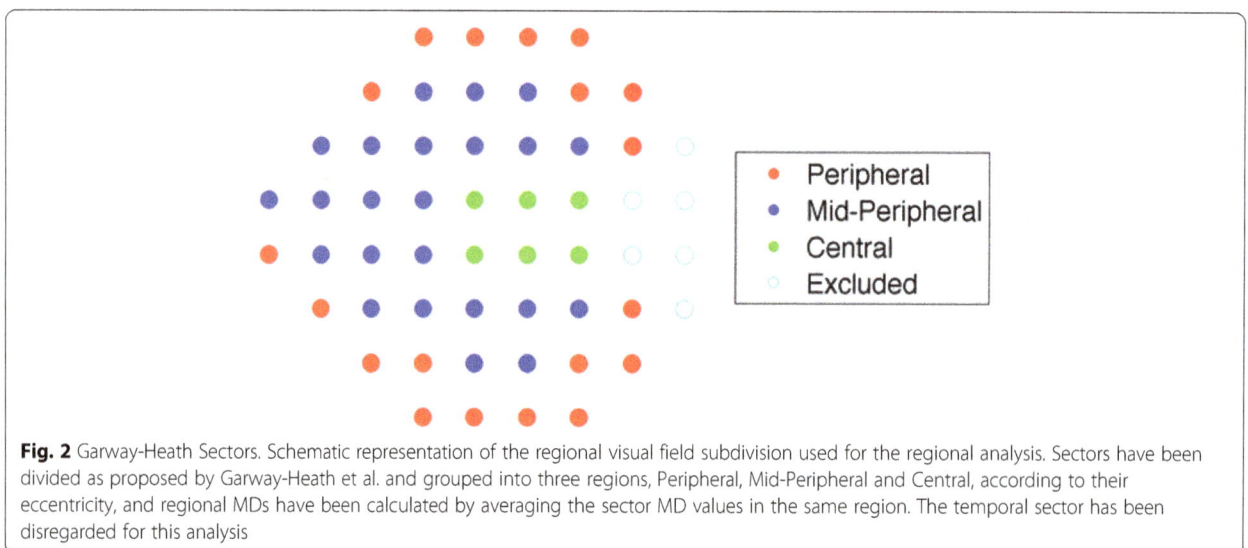

Fig. 2 Garway-Heath Sectors. Schematic representation of the regional visual field subdivision used for the regional analysis. Sectors have been divided as proposed by Garway-Heath et al. and grouped into three regions, Peripheral, Mid-Peripheral and Central, according to their eccentricity, and regional MDs have been calculated by averaging the sector MD values in the same region. The temporal sector has been disregarded for this analysis

Table 1 Demographics of the final sample (n = 292). MD = Mean Deviation; PSD = Pattern Standard Deviation

	Normal	Glaucoma	p
Age	49.9 ± 15.21	71.14 ± 9.07	< 0.0001
MD	0.1 ± 1.38	−6.24 ± 6.93	< 0.0001
PSD	2.14 ± 0.56	6.1 ± 3.68	< 0.0001

group were higher and significantly different in the non age corrected comparison ($P = 0.006$), but we could not find a statistically significant effect in the age corrected multivariate analysis (estimated difference 0.28 ± 0.15, $ME \pm SE$, $P = 0.054$, Table 2).

Then, sequential instability was measured with the log-SED index. Statistical analysis showed a significant difference in the non age corrected comparison ($P < 0.0001$), but, in contrast with the previous indices, a statistically significant effect could be identified even in the age corrected comparison ($P = 0.002$), glaucoma patients having a higher log-SED value (-2.48 ± 0.55, Mean $\pm SD$) compared to normal subjects (-2.84 ± 0.57, Mean $\pm SD$), yielding a 14.5% difference on the log-scale.

To analyse the relationship between fixation changes and the individual visual field loss, we also correlated the two indices with the MD, in a multivariate model with age as a covariate. The results are reported in Table 3. Both the log-BCEA and the log-MED were not significantly correlated with the MD values (all $P > 0.14$). In contrast the log-SED index had a highly significant association with the MD values ($P = 0.00002$). The results are depicted in the scatter plot in Fig. 3. We did not observe an improvement in the goodness-of-fit (i.e. reduction in the AIC) in any of the aforementioned models when evaluating non-linear effects of age on fixation metrics.

When analysing the correlation between the fixation indices and the local MD values for different regions of the visual field (peripheral, mid-peripheral and central, see Fig. 2), we found a significant correlation only for the log-SED and, as expected, the MD of the central region was the only significant predictor in the multivariate

analysis ($P = 0.005$), with minimal non-significant contribution from the peripheral and mid-peripheral regions. The results are reported in Table 4. With marginal effect we refer to the effect that the change in the MD value of a non-central region has on the fixation indices when the MD of the central region is equal to 0. With additional effect we refer to the effect that the change in the MD value of a non central region has on the fixation indices when the MD of the central region is also affected. In this latter analysis, the goodness-of-fit was mildly increased for the log-SED and log-BCEA models when non linear effect of age was explored. However, this did not change the significance of the log-SED correlation and caused a very limited change in the estimate of its effect (-0.016 ± 0.007, Mean $\pm$ SE, $p = 0.03$).

The skewness of the residuals was within the critical range (-0.5, 0.5) for all the aforementioned models.

Discussion

This study retrospectively analysed eye-movement data obtained from the Compass perimeter in a large number of people with and without glaucoma. Fixation stability in glaucomatous subjects was shown to differ from normals when it was described by a measure of how frequently the subject is changing fixation location independently of the spatial spread of the points (log-SED). However, measures of stability based on traditional notions of dispersion (like BCEA and log-MED) did not show any significant differences. Furthermore, the log-SED better correlated with worsening visual field loss (measured with the MD) and better reflected the loss of the central visual field in the regional analysis. Taken as a whole, these findings indicate that glaucoma can affect some aspects of fixation, especially when the central visual field is involved, although not greatly altering the dispersion of fixation locations.

To our knowledge, only two previous papers have analysed fixation data measured with fundus perimetry in glaucoma patients, with mixed results [8, 9].

Longhin et al. analysed the differences between what they defined 'static' (during a pure fixation task) and 'dynamic' (during the microperimetric test) fixation, in four different

Table 2 Results of the group analysis of the fixation indices

	Normal	Glaucoma	P	Age corrected P
N° of Samples	229.8 ± 20.8	224.5 ± 24.73	0.053	0.18
BCEA	732.47 ± 778.97	1050.86 ± 950.22	0.002	
MED	0.31 ± 0.28	0.42 ± 0.4	0.005	
SED	0.07 ± 0.05	0.1 ± 0.06	< 0.0001	
log-BCEA	6.2 ± 0.88	6.52 ± 1.05	0.006	0.054
log-MED	− 1.47 ± 0.7	− 1.24 ± 0.86	0.02	0.16
log-SED	−2.84 ± 0.57	−2.48 ± 0.55	< 0.0001	0.002

BCEA Bivariate Contour Ellipse Area (at 95% in our study), MED Mean Euclidean Distance from the PRL, SED Sequential Euclidean Distance, log-BCEA log-transformed BCEA, log-MED log-transformed MED, log-SED log-transformed SED

Table 3 Multivariate regression coefficients for global MDs

log-BCEA			log-MED			log-SED		
MD (SE)	Age (SE)	Intercept (SE)	MD (SE)	Age (SE)	Intercept (SE)	MD (SE)	Age (SE)	Intercept (SE)
− 0.006	0.006	6.295***	− 0.008	0.007*	6.268***	− 0.019***	0.005	6.227***
(0.012)	(0.004)	(0.061)	(0.009)	(0.004)	(0.395)	(0.007)	(0.004)	(0.093)

*$p < 0.1$; **$p < 0.05$; ***$p < 0.01$
SE Standard Error, *MD* Mean Deviation, *log-BCEA* log-transformed BCEA, *log-MED* log-transformed MED, *log-SED* log-transformed SED

diseases compared to normals, including POAG. In all groups they observed an increase in the BCEA values in the dynamic fixation compared to static fixation [9]. In our work we analysed data from the first 10 s of the examination, when no stimuli are projected and the subject is asked to fixate the central target for PRL detection. Therefore, our analysis is comparable to what they defined as 'static' fixation, i.e. during a pure fixation task. Longhin et al. reported stable fixation in 100% of the POAG subjects (based on the BCEA classification) in the 'static' fixation and did not perform formal testing to compare BCEA values in POAG to normal subjects. They did not report numerical values of the BCEA, but it can be deduced from the graphical depictions that BCEA values in POAG patients were not very different from those in normal subjects. This is in agreement with our results. Indeed we found only mild differences in the indices of pure fixation spreading (log-BCEA and log-MED) that were not statistically significant in the multivariate analysis corrected by age (see Table 2 and the Results section).

Shi et al. performed a more detailed analysis comparing glaucoma patients at different stages with normal subjects, analysing fixation data recorded during the microperimetric test; this procedure was analogous to the 'dynamic' fixation according to Longhin et al. They found a statistically significant effect when comparing the POAG patients with normal subjects in terms of number fixation points falling within the central 2 degrees (one degree around the foveal point) but not when comparing the number of points within the central 4 degrees [8]. They also reported a significant correlation with the sensitivity of the inferior temporal and superior temporal sectors [8]. These results might be explained by the fact that the central 2 degrees and the temporal sectors were the ones with the highest difference in sensitivity between normal subjects and glaucoma patients in their dataset [8]. In turn, this might simply be explained by glaucoma subjects in their specific sample not fixating with the more damaged parts of their visual fields. Moreover, since this analysis was performed on data acquired during the perimetric test, results might

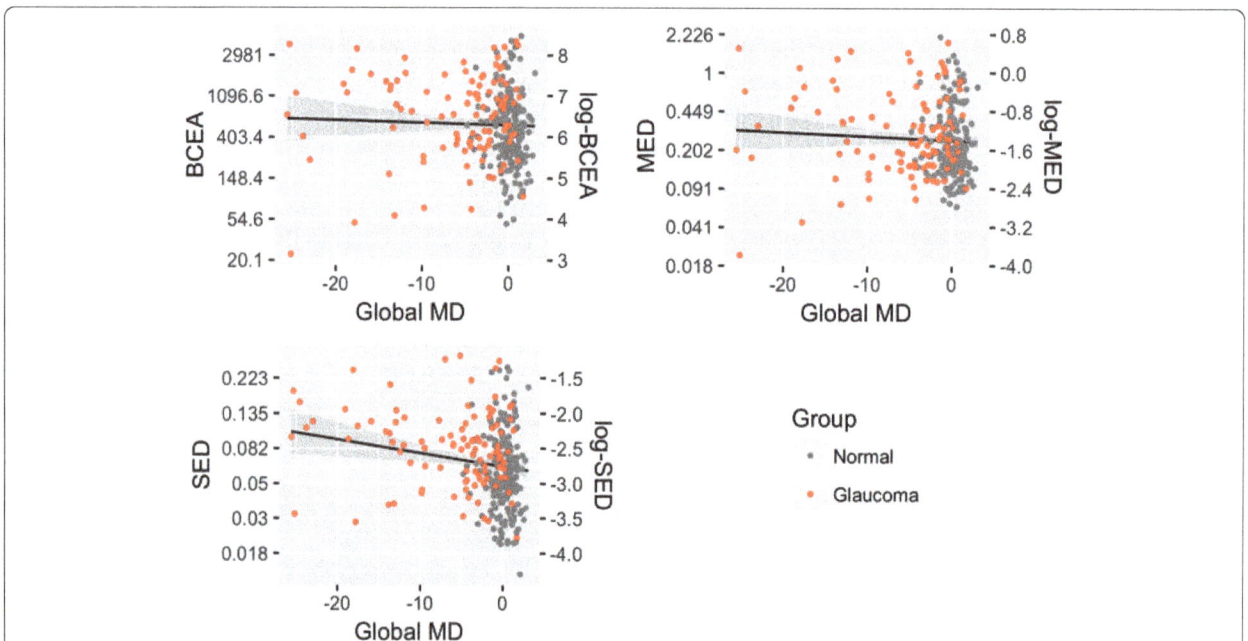

Fig. 3 Fixation indices and MDs. Scatter plots and regression lines for the three fixation indices (log-BCEA, log-MED and log-SED) showing the relationship with the global MD value. Normal subjects are in green while glaucoma subjects are in red. The shaded region represents the 95% confidence interval of the estimate. The regression estimate was obtained from a multivariate model accounting for the age of the subject and the depicted line has been calculated at the mean age of the sample (57.4 years). The scale on the right vertical axis represents the values of the log transformed measures, while the left vertical axis reports the corresponding values in the linear scale

Table 4 Multivariate regression coefficients for regional MDs

	log-BCEA	log-MED	log-SED
Age (SE)	0.006***	0.005***	0.006***
	(0.002)	(0.002)	(0.001)
Central MD (SE)	− 0.002	− 0.003	− 0.020***
	(0.012)	(0.01)	(0.007)
Marginal effect of the mid-peripheral region (SE)	−0.016	−0.018	− 0.011
	(0.084)	(0.068)	(0.049)
Marginal effect of the peripheral region (SE)	−0.003	−0.006	− 0.005
	(0.084)	(0.068)	(0.049)
Additional effect of the mid-peripheral region (SE)	−0.006	−0.007	0.002
	(0.016)	(0.013)	(0.009)
Additional effect of the peripheral region (SE)	−0.001	− 0.002	0.004
	(0.016)	(0.013)	(0.009)
Intercept (SE)	6.305***	−1.392***	−2.748***
	(0.059)	(0.047)	(0.035)

*p < 0.1; **p < 0.05; ***p < 0.01

SE Standard Error, MD Mean Deviation, log-BCEA log-transformed BCEA, log-MED log-transformed MED, log-SED log-transformed SED

also be influenced by the gaze attraction towards more sensitive regions during the projection of the stimuli. In this perspective, although clearly showing that glaucoma can influence fixation, their results are more likely to reflect characteristics of the specific sample analysed, rather than general features of fixation in glaucoma patients.

In our analysis we found that, both in uncorrected and age corrected analysis, the log-SED index, which was designed to better capture the temporal fixation instability even in relatively restricted fixation areas, was significantly different in glaucoma patients compared to normal patients (see Table 2). This index of fixation instability was significantly correlated to the global MD (Table 3). When we analysed the correlation of the log-SED with the regional MD values, we found that the correlation with the global MD was mostly due to central impairment, with minimal non significant contributions from more peripheral regions of the visual field (Table 4).

These findings might be explained by patients with glaucoma typically not having a visual field loss starting in the foveal region and expanding peripherally. In contrast to macular degeneration, patients with glaucoma usually experience a progressive restriction of their central visual field, which is independent across the median raphe [23]. Therefore, an extremely widespread and displaced area of fixation points, as with retinal diseases, is not expected. This view is coherent with our data and data from the literature [8, 9] regarding the distribution of the fixation points, where POAG patients did not show strong differences from normal subjects when corrected by age.

Our working hypothesis is that patients with glaucoma might change the temporal features of their fixation, rather

then exhibiting important fixation spread. This is reflected in the much stronger differences we have found when analysing the log-SED index. We speculate that these observations are coherent with the processing of visual information performed by the ganglion cells, which is more targeted to highlight variations rather than steady states [24]. Indeed, fixational eye movements have been involved in contrast sensitivity and stimulus detection, since they might prevent stimulus fading due to perceptual adaptation [24]. Moreover, in experimental setup on animal models, greater ganglion cell responses have been detected with wobbling stimuli compared to stationary stimuli [24]. Our results might reflect the idea of glaucoma patients trying to enhance the perception of the fixation target by frequent shifting between different positions. This idea would have to be tested further and this could be the subject of future work.

One limitation in the original database was that glaucomatous and normal subjects were not age matched. This feature was inherited from the study design and we accounted for that by using a multivariate analysis with age as a covariate. Such a mismatch might explain why we had different results when analyses were not age corrected. Non corrected analyses showed significantly increased values for all fixation metrics, including BCEA and log-MED, in glaucoma patients. This might be related to an age dependent effect on fixation features and highlights the importance of performing age corrected comparisons. From our analysis, the age effect on fixation indices appeared to be fairly linear, although some mild increase in the goodness-of-fit was noted when using basis spline in two of the models used to explore the effect of the local MD values. However, our analysis was not designed to test and analyse this aspect in particular, and modelling a non linear relationship with age only had minor effects on the estimates of the parameters of interest.

Future works could couple imaging data from the Compass perimeter with the structural information from OCT scans. In this way it might be possible to assess how local changes in the retinal nerve fibre layer and in the retinal ganglion cell complex might shape and modify the temporal and spatial pattern of fixation in glaucomatous patients, both during a pure fixation task and during the perimetric test. Indeed, Mallery et al. [25] recently showed that local ganglion cell loss is able to shape the fixation pattern in patients with optic neuropathies. Furthermore, other fixation stability parameters could be better derived from other statistical approaches such as Kernel Density Estimators [17, 25] and Brownian motion [26] modelling. In turn these might provide more information on the fine spatial and temporal modification of fixation in glaucoma damage.

Conclusions

In conclusion, we provide evidence that in glaucoma subjects subtle changes in fixation are present, but are better described by features of the temporal sequence of displacements rather than by usual metrics of dispersion, like BCEA. Further investigations will be needed to understand the implications of this finding in visual tasks and perimetric testing.

Abbreviations

BCEA: Bivariate Contour Ellipse Area; DLS: Differential light sensitivity; FAP: Fundus Automated Perimetry; HFA: Humphrey Field Analyzer; IOP: Intraocular pressure; MD: Mean Deviation; ME: Model estimates; MED: Mean Euclidean Distance; OCT: Optical Coherence Tomography; POAG: Primary Open Angle Glaucoma; PRL: Preferred Retinal Locus; SD: Standard Deviation; SE: Standard Error; SED: Sequential Euclidean Distance; SLO: Scanning Laser Ophthalmoscopy; VF: Visual field

Funding

No funding was received for the analysis presented in this work, however the original data collection was funded by CenterVue, Padua, Italy.

Authors' contributions

DC, PF, LR and GM conceptualized the research. GM drafted the manuscript and analysed the data. DC, PF, LR, PJ and MD contributed to the interpretation of the results, critical revision and writing of the manuscript. All authors read and approved the final manuscript.

Competing interests

David P. Crabb, Paolo Fogagnolo and Luca Rossetti are consultants for CenterVue, Padua, Italy.

References

1. Quigley HA. Glaucoma. Lancet. 2011;377(9774):1367–77.
2. Malik R, Swanson WH, Garway-Heath DF. Structure-function relationship' in glaucoma: past thinking and current concepts. Clin Exp Ophthalmol. 2012; 40(4):369–80.
3. Zhu H, Russell RA, Saunders LJ, Ceccon S, Garway-Heath DF, Crabb DP. Detecting changes in retinal function: analysis with non-stationary Weibull error regression and spatial enhancement (ANSWERS). PLoS One. 2014;9(1): e85654.
4. Heijl A, Krakau CE. An automatic static perimeter, design and pilot study. Acta Ophthalmol. 1975;53(3):293–310.
5. Hanout M, Horan N, Do DV. Introduction to microperimetry and its use in analysis of geographic atrophy in age-related macular degeneration. Curr Opin Ophthalmol. 2015;26(3):149–56.
6. Jones PR, Yasoubi N, Nardini M, Rubin GS. Feasibility of macular integrity assessment (MAIA) Microperimetry in children: sensitivity, reliability, and fixation stability in healthy observers. Invest Ophthalmol Vis Sci. 2016;57(14): 6349–59.
7. Crabb DP, Smith ND, Zhu H. What's on TV? Detecting age-related neurodegenerative eye disease using eye movement scanpaths. Frontiers in aging neuroscience. 2014;6:312.
8. Shi Y, Liu M, Wang X, Zhang C, Huang P. Fixation behavior in primary open angle glaucoma at early and moderate stage assessed by the MicroPerimeter MP-1. J Glaucoma. 2013;22(2):169–73.
9. Longhin E, Convento E, Pilotto E, Bonin G, Vujosevic S, Kotsafti O, Midena E. Static and dynamic retinal fixation stability in microperimetry. Canadian journal of ophthalmology Journal canadien d'ophtalmologie. 2013;48(5): 375–80.
10. Glen FC, Smith ND, Crabb DP. Saccadic eye movements and face recognition performance in patients with central glaucomatous visual field defects. Vis Res. 2013;82:42–51.
11. Burton R, Smith ND, Crabb DP. Eye movements and reading in glaucoma: observations on patients with advanced visual field loss. Graefes Arch Clin Exp Ophthalmol. 2014;252(10):1621–30.
12. Crabb DP, Smith ND, Rauscher FG, Chisholm CM, Barbur JL, Edgar DF, Garway-Heath DF. Exploring eye movements in patients with glaucoma when viewing a driving scene. PLoS One. 2010;5(3):e9710.
13. Smith ND, Glen FC, Crabb DP. Eye movements during visual search in patients with glaucoma. BMC Ophthalmol. 2012;12:45.
14. Wyatt HJ. Automated perimetry: using gaze-direction data to improve the estimate of scotoma edges. Invest Ophthalmol Vis Sci. 2011;52(8):5818–23.
15. Ishiyama Y, Murata H, Mayama C, Asaoka R. An objective evaluation of gaze tracking in Humphrey perimetry and the relation with the reproducibility of visual fields: a pilot study in glaucoma. Invest Ophthalmol Vis Sci. 2014; 55(12):8149–52.
16. Crossland MD, Dunbar HM, Rubin GS. Fixation stability measurement using the MP1 microperimeter. Retina. 2009;29(5):651–6.
17. Crossland MD, Sims M, Galbraith RF, Rubin GS. Evaluation of a new quantitative technique to assess the number and extent of preferred retinal loci in macular disease. Vis Res. 2004;44(13):1537–46.
18. Rossetti L, Digiuni M, Rosso A, Riva R, Barbaro G, Smolek MK, Orzalesi N, De Cilla S, Autelitano A, Fogagnolo P. Compass: clinical evaluation of a new instrument for the diagnosis of glaucoma. PLoS One. 2015;10(3):e0122157.
19. Fogagnolo P, Modarelli A, Oddone F, Digiuni M, Montesano G, Orzalesi N, Rossetti L. Comparison of compass and Humphrey perimeters in detecting glaucomatous defects. Eur J Ophthalmol. 2016;26(6):598–606.
20. Garway-Heath DF, Poinoosawmy D, Fitzke FW, Hitchings RA. Mapping the visual field to the optic disc in normal tension glaucoma eyes. Ophthalmology. 2000;107(10):1809–15.
21. Bulmer MG. Principles of statistics. New York: Dover Publications; 1979.
22. Faraway JJ. Extending the linear model with R : generalized linear, mixed effects and nonparametric regression models. Chapman & Hall/CRC: Boca Raton; 2006.
23. Schiefer U, Papageorgiou E, Sample PA, Pascual JP, Selig B, Krapp E, Paetzold J. Spatial pattern of glaucomatous visual field loss obtained with regionally condensed stimulus arrangements. Invest Ophthalmol Vis Sci. 2010;51(11):5685–9.
24. Martinez-Conde S, Macknik SL, Hubel DH. The role of fixational eye movements in visual perception. Nat Rev Neurosci. 2004;5(3):229–40.
25. Mallery RM, Poolman P, Thurtell MJ, Wang JK, Garvin MK, Ledolter J, Kardon RH. The pattern of visual fixation eccentricity and instability in optic neuropathy and its spatial relationship to retinal ganglion cell layer thickness. Invest Ophthalmol Vis Sci. 2016;57(9):429–37.
26. Rolfs M. Microsaccades: small steps on a long way. Vis Res. 2009;49(20): 2415–41.

20

A qualitative study on gender barriers to eye care access in Cambodia

Camille Neyhouser[1,2]* (iD), Ingrid Quinn[3], Tessa Hillgrove[1], Renee Chan[1], Chhorvann Chhea[4], Seang Peou[5] and Pol Sambath[5]

Abstract

Background: The Fred Hollows Foundation (FHF) Cambodia recently partnered with the Ministry of Women's Affairs (MoWA) and National Program for Eye Health (NPEH, part of the Ministry of Health) to establish the *Gender Equality in Eye Health Project*. As part of this project, a qualitative study was carried out to identify barriers affecting women's access to eye health in Cambodia.

Methods: A cross-sectional qualitative study was conducted in four provinces in both urban and rural locations between May and June 2015. Purposive sampling was used to identify respondents from a range of age groups, geographical locations, and experiences to explore different perceptions regarding access barriers to eye health care. Thirteen women experiencing eye problems (age range 45–84 years; mean age 63 years) and 25 eye health professionals took part in in-depth interviews. Eleven focus groups discussions were held with 69 participants (50 women, 19 married men) to capture the views and experiences of both younger and older women, as well as household decision makers' perspectives.

Results: Gender-based differences in decision-making, access and control over resources and women's social status all contributed to impeding women's access to eye health services. Women relied predominantly on informal sources of information about health, and these channels might be utilised to address barriers to information and access. Disparities in perceived costs of eye health treatment were evident between eye healthcare providers and users: costs were not perceived as a barrier by service providers due to health financing support for poor patients, however, many users were not aware of the availability of the scheme.

Conclusion: Demand-side and supply-side elements interact to reduce women's ability to seek eye treatment.

Keywords: Barriers, Cambodia, Eye care, Gender role

Background

Women make up approximately 60% of the estimated 223.4 million people who live with avoidable blindness or visual impairment [1]. A major cause of blindness is cataract, which can be successfully treated by surgery [1]. Globally, although women bear the greater burden of cataract, they are less likely to receive surgery [2]. Cambodia is no exception. A rapid assessment of avoidable blindness (RAAB) conducted in 2007 estimated the prevalence of blindness to be higher among women over 50 years at 3.4%, compared to 2% of the male population of the same age [3]. Only 31% of women requiring surgery were receiving it, compared to 40% of men [3].

Previous studies conducted in Cambodia on eye health promotion and service provision have suggested potential barriers to uptake for women. These have included: cost [3, 4]; fear of surgery and poor outcomes [3–5]; fear of hospitals [5]; poor awareness of eye health issues and treatment [3–5]; and a lack of social support [3, 4, 6]. The majority of these studies focussed on individual determinants of eye health behaviours. However, factors promoting health-seeking behaviours are not rooted solely within the individual. Women are vulnerable as a result of broader social constructs and in Cambodia, it is not well understood how these constructs influence

* Correspondence: camille.neyhouser@gmail.com
[1]The Fred Hollows Foundation, Level 2, 61 Dunning Avenue, Rosebery, Sydney, NSW 2018, Australia
[2]School of Public Health and Community Medicine, Faculty of Medicine, University of New South Wales, Kensington, NSW 2052, Australia
Full list of author information is available at the end of the article

access to eye health care. In addition, these previous studies did not explore provider-side barriers to understand aspects inherent to the health system that hinder service uptake, nor the perspectives of men on women's eye health.

The purpose of this study was to inform projects aiming to increase women's access to eye health services for The Fred Hollows Foundation (FHF), which is a secular non-profit non-government organisation (NGO) with a vision for a world where no one is needlessly blind [7]. FHF currently has programs running in more than 25 countries and has been operating in Cambodia since 1998 [7]. Therefore this study aimed to broaden our understanding of the socio-ecological determinants for women accessing eye health care in Cambodia with a view to design an evidence-based intervention to ensure delivery of gender equitable eye services in Cambodia in collaboration with the Cambodian Ministry of Women's Affairs.

The research objectives were:

1. To identify demand-side (consumer) barriers for women accessing eye health care
2. To identify supply-side (provider) barriers for women accessing eye health care
3. To identify barriers to accessing eye health care for a vulnerable sub-group of women

This paper aims to identify barriers affecting women's access to eye health in Cambodia in order to inform the development of an evidence-based intervention addressing these barriers. Specifically, this paper describes demand-side barriers, supply-side barriers and intersecting barriers affecting a vulnerable sub-group of women.

Methods
Study area
The study was conducted in urban and rural locations in four provinces of Cambodia: Siem Reap, Kampot, Pursat and Tbong Khmum. Provinces were pre-selected based on purposive criteria including poverty levels and availability of eye health programs/services. Exact study locations were selected by the Cambodian researcher (CC) in consultation with FHF Cambodia. The local eye health researcher has an in-depth knowledge of the Cambodia context since he belongs to the National Institute for Public Health (NIPH). Siem Reap was also selected, as it is a hub for FHF Cambodia, which has many partnerships in the area. The selection was not intended to be representative for the whole country, but rather to provide insights into the barriers to eye health care access for women in a diverse range of settings in Cambodia. A map of Cambodia showing the study areas is depicted in Fig. 1.

Study design and sampling
This qualitative study engaged a gender equity approach which is concerned with the role of gender relations in the production of vulnerability to ill-health or disadvantage within health care systems [8]. This study utilised focus-group discussions (FGDs), in-depth interviews (IDIs), and key informant interviews (KIIs) to collect information on perceptions and experiences regarding access barriers to eye health care amongst different subgroups of women, men and service providers in Cambodia.

The FGDs were conducted at the community level. A non-probability purposive sampling approach was used, with participants selected according to their demographic and social characteristics, including gender, level of education, socio-economic status (as measured by income) and geographic location (urban/rural) in each study location. Groups identified for inclusion are shown in Table 1.

IDIs were conducted to collect information on perceptions and experiences of individual women experiencing eye health problems. Participants were selected through a combination of convenience and purposive sampling. IDIs were conducted with patients seeking eye treatment on a selected day at each of the four provincial referral hospitals, identified by Eye Unit personnel. Participants with an existing eye problem but who had not sought eye treatment were identified by Village Health Volunteers (VHVs), who were familiar with the health needs of local community members. A list of IDI participants' demographic characteristics is shown in Table 2.

KIIs were conducted to gain an understanding of health sector service provider perceptions regarding barriers to accessing eye health care for women. Key informants were selected for interviews through purposive sampling at the provincial and district levels based on their knowledge of eye health care management/operations and of eye health service delivery. A list of key informants' positions and gender is shown in Table 3.

Data collection
Data collection took place over 3 weeks between May 2015 and June 2015. The international researcher (IQ) conducted the FGDs, IDIs and KIIs with the assistance of a national research assistant/translator (BC). All were conducted using simultaneous Khmer-English translation with the exception of the KIIs with the eye health service provider in Siem Reap, FHF Cambodia Country Manager and National Program for Eye Health (NPEH) Coordinator, all conducted in English. Three semi-structured interview guides were developed in English, reviewed by the local eye health consultant, translated, pilot tested and used to conduct the FGDs, IDIs and KIIs. IDIs were conducted in provincial eye hospitals, in eye units of district referral hospitals or in district health centres. KIIs took

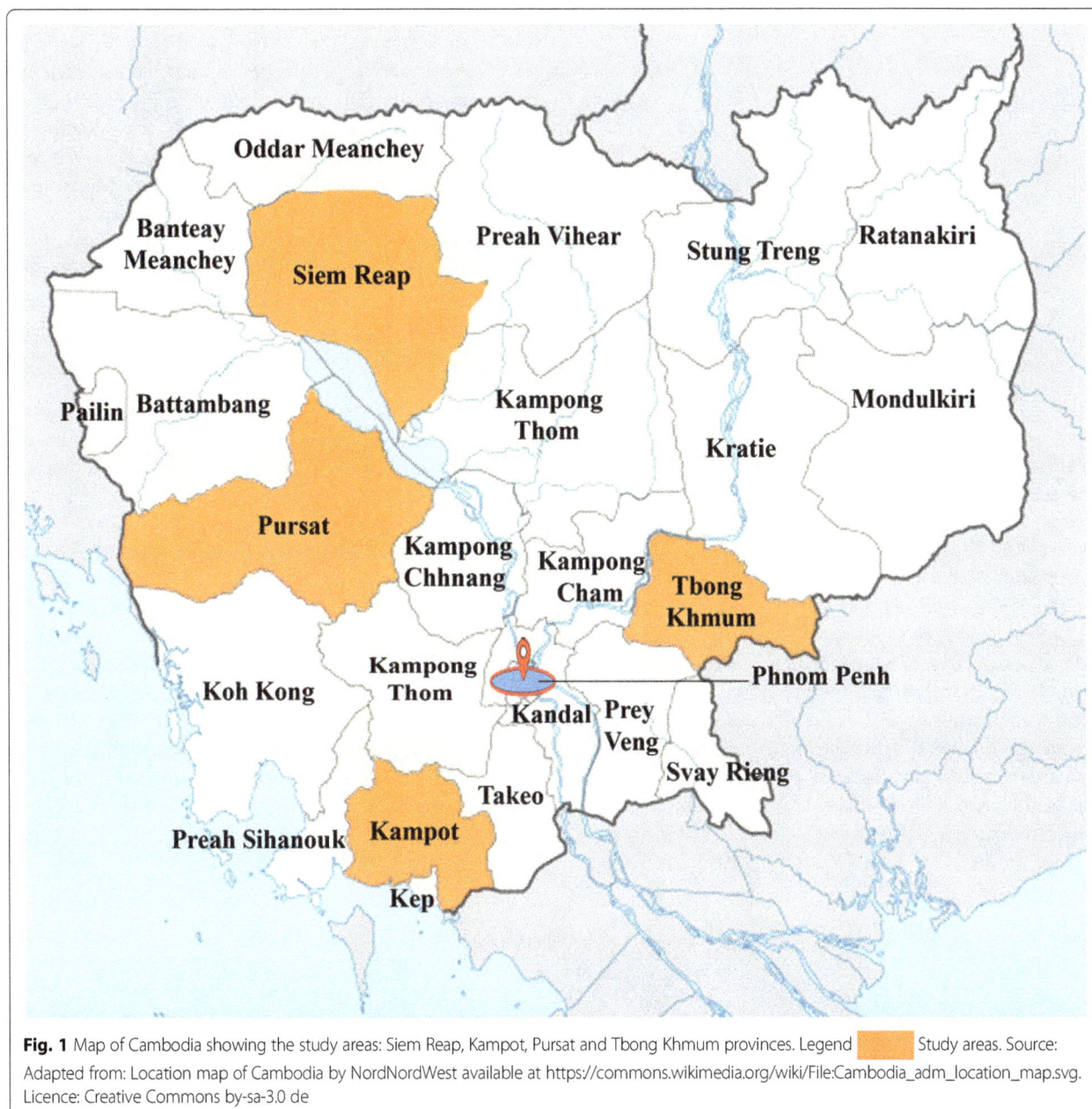

Fig. 1 Map of Cambodia showing the study areas: Siem Reap, Kampot, Pursat and Tbong Khmum provinces. Legend � Study areas. Source: Adapted from: Location map of Cambodia by NordNordWest available at https://commons.wikimedia.org/wiki/File:Cambodia_adm_location_map.svg. Licence: Creative Commons by-sa-3.0 de

place at the workplace location of each interviewed participant. FGDs were conducted at district health centres in each province with the meeting area enclosed for privacy wherever possible. Each FGD was approximately 2 h long while IDIs and KIIs lasted approximately 1 h.

Data analysis

Field audio recordings in Khmer were transcribed to English by BC, while audio recordings from interviews in English were transcribed verbatim by IQ. IQ was responsible for undertaking data analysis with support from BC. The data were analysed by using a systematic manual text-analysis procedure. First, a preliminary

review of the raw data was conducted to reduce and generate specific thematic categories and codes. The codes included key words that represented topics conveyed in the transcripts. More specific descriptive sub-codes were assigned to data grouped under these broad categories. Searches were then conducted for each sub-code to bring together text from all FGDs and individual interviews related to each theme. As part of this step, tables were created to list main themes, subthemes, and all quotes related to each subtheme, to determine patterns in the data according to source and summarize perceptions on barriers to access to eye health service use.

Table 1 Demographic characteristics of focus-group discussion (FGD) participants

	Marital status	Age group	No. of participants
1.	Urban women	<50 years	7
2.	Urban women	>50 years	12
3.	Rural women	<50 years	11
4.	Rural women	>50 years	20
	Sub-total women in FGDs		50
5.	Urban married men	<50 years	9
6.	Rural married men	<50 years	5
7.	Rural married men	>50 years	5
	Sub-total men in FGDs		19
	Total FGD participants		69

Results

Characteristics of the study population

A total of 108 participants (72 women, 36 men) were interviewed. Eleven FGDs were held with a total of 69 participants (50 women,19 married men). The women for the FGDs were selected to provide a perspective of female eye health consumers. Men were selected to provide a perspective of married men as heads of household. In addition, 13 face-to-face IDIs were conducted with women whose ages ranged between 45 and 84 years (mean age 63 years) experiencing eye problems to provide more insight into barriers for women in accessing eye health care. Out of these 13 women, six were currently receiving eye treatment at one of the provincial referral hospitals in Siem Reap, Tbong Khmum, Kampot or Pursat. Five were from rural areas and one woman was from an urban area. Seven women who were all from a rural area had eye problems but did not seek eye treatment. Most IDI participants were illiterate or had low education levels. Furthermore, KIIs were conducted with 25 participants (9 women, 16 men) who were representatives of relevant line ministries and government departments, professional eye health care providers and health facilitators at commune level. The purpose of the KIIs was to explore barriers to eye health care access for women from a supply side perspective.

Demand-side barriers to accessing eye health care for women

In IDIs and FGDs, study participants were asked about the barriers they encountered in accessing eye health care services. Four main themes emerged: socio-cultural factors, access and control over resources, organisational/institutional factors, and economic factors.

Socio-cultural factors are related to socio-cultural realities in Cambodia. They are the result of larger power differentials embedded within the community leading to patriarchal attitudes and deep-rooted gender stereotypes. Men's health is prioritised due to the societal perception that the potential benefits to both the household and the community is higher for men than women. Because women have less agency over their own health than men and are traditionally the primary caretakers, they reported often having to negotiate with their husbands and/or family to organise their childcare and household duties in order to access health care:

Table 2 Demographic characteristics of in-depth interview (IDI) participants

No.	Age	Education	Place Interviewed
Women with eye problems who sought eye treatment			
1	60	Illiterate	Siem Reap Provincial Hospital, Eye Hospital
2	69	Illiterate	Siem Reap Provincial Hospital, Eye Hospital
3	63	Informal education	Kampot Referral Hospital, Eye Unit
4	66	Grade 4	Tbong Khmum Referral Hospital, Eye Unit
5	84	Illiterate	Pursat Referral Hospital, Eye Unit
6	50	Illiterate	Pursat Referral Hospital, Eye Unit
Women with eye problems who did not seek eye treatment			
7	68	Grade 2	Popel Health Centre
8	60	Illiterate	Popel Health Centre
9	58	Grade 6	Tany Health Centre
10	45	Grade 6	Tany Health Centre
11	80	Illiterate	Tbong Khmum Referral Hospital
12	58	Illiterate	Chi Peang Health Centre
13	59	Grade 1	Chi Peang Health Centre
	Total IDI participants: 13		

Table 3 List of key informant interview (KII) participants per function and gender

Key informant interview (KII) participant's role	Male	Female
Coordinator, National Program for Eye Health (NPEH)	1	0
Country Director, Fred Hollows Foundation Cambodia	1	0
Director or Deputy Directors of Provincial Health Department	4	0
Referral Hospital Eye Health Providers	3	0
Health Centre Facility Managers	4	0
Commune Committee for Women and Children (CCWC) Representatives	0	4
Village Health Volunteers	3	5
Total KII participants per gender	16	9

If I had eye surgery, I would stay in bed and who will look after me? And who will look after my grandchildren? I decided not to go. (Female participant, 60 years old, rural area)

Many female participants also displayed a number of beliefs about eye health. Most deemed eye problems, including visual impairment, as being 'not serious' enough to seek treatment, unless experiencing pain. Further, many female respondents believed vision impairment to be an inevitable but natural consequence of aging and that eye treatment interventions require surgery and a prolonged recovery period. A fear of surgery further served as a deterrent to seeking eye treatment.

Access and control over resources relates to household resources and access to accurate health-related information. Because of women's lack of access over household resources, attitudes of male heads of household were important in either supporting or discouraging women from seeking eye health care, including financially:

I would not go if my husband does not give me the money. (Female participant, 55 years old, urban area)

For elderly women undergoing eye treatment, the cost of treatment is often shared between adult children and decision-making is a collective process requiring consensus. Adult children are therefore an important source of information, as well as financial and psychological support for women:

I was encouraged by my sons and daughters to go to the hospital for treatment. (Female participant, 60 years old, urban area)

In spite of the availability of a wide range of information sources in the community, it was found that the status of women prevented them from accessing accurate information and effective communications:

Men have more opportunities [to access information] than women. For example, men can go out to the coffee shop, or join the meeting or public discussion... but for women, few go out, they just stay at home. (Director, Referral Hospital, male)

Participant perceptions of eye health care were largely determined by informal sources of information such as word of mouth and treatment outcomes observed in their direct environment, rather than by information from health services. Unsurprisingly, women who decided to seek treatment were often motivated to do so by their family circle or social networks:

I was encouraged by my sons and daughters to go to the hospital for treatment. (Female participant, 60 years old, urban area)

However, these informal sources were often shown to be inaccurate resulting in misconceptions regarding eye treatment:

Some people say I have to spend hundreds of dollars for the treatment, particularly surgery. (Female participant, 68 years old, rural area)

In terms of *institutional/organisational factors*, neither female nor male participants sought eye health care at the health centre (HC), as participants perceived that eye health services at HCs were at best limited.

I don't come because I don't think the health centre has the medicine that I need for eye health problems. (Female participant, 57 years old, rural area)

However, women were less likely to be able to access eye health units of provincial referral hospitals due to costs incurred by long travel distances and cultural norms dictating that they should not travel alone. In addition, their lack of experience and familiarity with health systems and structures was seen as a significant barrier, particularly for elderly and poorly educated women. For instance, a lack of support/assistance with hospital administrative processes was reported by several participants.

Economic constraints posed a considerable barrier to accessing eye health care for women, both in terms of perceived direct costs (user fees/treatment costs) as well as indirect costs (transportation, opportunity costs e.g. lost income):

I have never had any [eye] treatment, this is my first time... the problem I have is not serious and the cost of the treatment... I think I have to pay a lot of money and the transportation is also costly, so I just ignore it. (Female participant, 68 years old, rural area)

In addition, although in Cambodia poor patients are entitled to receive free or discounted care at public facilities through equity cards, in practice they reported this was rarely the case. It was evident that participants were often unable to effectively utilize these financial support schemes due to a lack of awareness of health financing support and/or a lack of understanding of how to navigate the system to obtain financial support.

Supply-side barriers to accessing eye health care for women

KIIs with service providers explored barriers to eye health care access for women from a supply side perspective across four dimensions: accessibility, availability, affordability and acceptability.

In this study, *accessibility of services* refers to location of services, transportation and opportunity costs including travel time. Limited availability of eye services at the HCs and long distance to the referral hospitals emerged as significant challenges for women seeking eye treatment. Eye specialists are primarily located in urban areas, which contributes to the up-front transportation costs for rural patients, particularly for women who have less access to resources and limited decision-making power regarding health care expenditure. In addition, cultural norms dictate that women should not travel alone, particularly long distances and that patients are accompanied for the duration of hospital treatment. The challenge of finding an accompanying person, particularly for elderly and visually impaired women, was reported as a barrier to access.

The success of eye outreach programmes and eye camps organised by NGOs, in collaboration with the government shows that, in the absence of such initiatives, accessibility issues disproportionately impact women. This is reflected in the increase in female patients attending provincial hospital eye units for treatment following referral, as observed at one referral hospital:

More and more patients come here for eye treatment and the number of female patients who come to the eye hospital is higher than men. (Eye Health Professional, Referral Hospital, male)

Limited *availability* of eye health human resources was acknowledged by service providers as contributing to extending patient waiting times. For women in urban higher income groups, waiting times were reported as an important factor in decision-making. Similarly, FGDs showed that waiting times were a barrier for rural women seeking eye health care, tied to opportunity costs including travel time and lost income. In addition, supply-side respondents recognised that amongst female eye health consumers, availability of information required to make informed decisions regarding eye health was limited. At community level, VHVs recognized that whilst women in rural areas often relied on health messages delivered by VHVs, reaching vulnerable sub-groups, especially elderly women was a continued challenge:

Currently, people trust VHV's information. [However] If we call people for meeting, very few people come... Elderly women who stay at home are unable to access health information. (VHV, female)

A number of providers recognized that for patients unfamiliar with the health system, particularly visually impaired patients from remote areas, the modern hospital environment may be perceived as complex and intimidating. This may act as a deterrent to eye health utilization, particularly amongst poor rural women.

In terms of *affordability*, patient treatment costs were not perceived as a barrier to access by the majority of service providers due to the range of health financing support mechanisms in place for poor patients (e.g. user fee exemptions for equity card holders). In reality, however, these mechanisms have not resulted in the removal of cost barriers for eye health consumers, as described in the paragraph on economic constraints of the Demand-side section. One provider recognized the broad financial implications of accessing eye care services for patients, including indirect costs:

Yes, of course it is a burden for the [poor] patients...When they come and stay at the hospital, they have to pay... for treatment fees and their living expenses... they may need their relatives such as sons or daughters to come along and look after them. So those relatives cannot work or earn any money for the family. That really makes the situation worse. (Deputy Director, Provincial Health Department, male)

Strong traditional beliefs as well as fear of surgery and negative treatment outcomes were cited by service providers as *acceptability barriers* for women:

> *They are afraid of the result of the operation. Some believe that their eyes may get worse after the surgery... that surgery might be painful, and... that the result may be unsatisfactory... This may deter women from seeking treatment.* (Commune Committee for Women and Children Representative, female)

They also recognised that the effectiveness of the referral system is limited and its shortcomings disproportionately impacted women.

> *We need to strengthen referral system and make consumers/patients aware of services at the health centre.* (Eye Health Professional, Referral Hospital, male)

Health providers acknowledged that women's multiple roles and responsibilities acted as barriers and that the interaction of gender-specific barriers had an important influence on their ability to seek eye health services, particularly elderly women.

> *I think the problems is not having caretakers; there is no one to replace them, to take over their responsibilities... grandparents that have to look after the household and prepare food for children. If they have eye surgery, they have to take a rest and somebody else has to do the work...* (Eye Health Professional, Referral Hospital, male)

A table summarising the study results in terms of demand- and provider-side barriers is presented in Table 4.

Most vulnerable subgroups

Elderly women from lower socio-economic backgrounds living in remote rural areas were the most vulnerable group to demand-side barriers to accessing eye health. They were more likely to have lower levels of education and be less mobile. Therefore, they were more likely to experience a vision impairment compared to their urban and younger peers or married men. Multiple barriers intersect for them.

Socio-cultural factors were found to have more impact amongst those sub-groups of the population with the strongest traditional beliefs:

> *Some older people...said that it is due to aging and it [eyesight] may get better... when your children are grown.* (Female participant, 46 years old, rural area)

Widowed and elderly female heads of households were even less likely to have access to information, be aware of treatment options or to seek treatment. As a result of visual impairment, their social networks were more likely weaker than other subgroups (e.g. urban married women). Due to their eye health condition, they were at a higher risk of being dependent on others at the same time as socially isolated:

> *I could not do anything, even pressing the phone buttons. I cannot do anything besides staying at home and cleaning the house.* (Female participant, 60 years old, urban area)

Discussion

This qualitative study demonstrated how women encounter barriers at various steps of their journey towards better eye health – from their individual beliefs and attitudes towards eye health to socio-cultural barriers in the household and the wider community to economic constraints and institutional barriers. Overall, a lack of access to information, fear of surgery and negative outcomes, costs of accessing eye health services and their limited availability are the most significant barriers to women's access to eye health care services. The socio-cultural status of women means they are often not in a position to prioritise their own health. These findings are consistent with what is known about gender barriers to accessing health care services from previous research [4, 5, 7, 8].

This research shows that the demand and supply side elements interact to influence women's ability to seek eye treatment. However, while female consumers were not aware of user fee exemptions for poor patients, and identified significant direct and indirect costs of accessing services, the vast majority of service providers did not think that costs were a barrier to access for women, citing the existence of financial support mechanisms for the most vulnerable. This is an important issue which should be addressed by policy makers and service providers. The equity card scheme currently in place is not used by those who are entitled to it, which represents a threat in terms of health financing. If poor women fail to access eye care services at the early stage of an eye health condition because of financial concerns, they might end up using the service when their eye condition has become significantly worse (e.g. when experiencing pain as reported by several women), risking a higher cost for the health financing system. Another risk is that patients may become irreversibly blind as a result of not accessing the services, compounding the disadvantage for their family, their community and the broader society.

Addressing socio-cultural barriers is an important step towards better eye health for women. Across all age groups and locations, women seek advice and approval

Table 4 Summary of barriers to accessing eye health care for women in Cambodia from a demand- and provider-side perspective

Demand-side barriers to accessing eye health care for women in Cambodia				Provider-side barriers to accessing eye health care for women in Cambodia			
Socio-cultural factors	Access to and control over resources	Institutional & organisational factors	Economic factors	Accessibility	Availability	Affordability	Acceptability
Status of women in Cambodian society Women as primary caretakers Beliefs about eye health Women's limited agency in healthcare decision-making	Lack of control over household resources Limited access to accurate eye health information	Poor perceived quality of eye health care from service user perspective Limited eye health services at health centre level Lack of experience and familiarity with health systems and structures esp. referral Long travel distances to eye health services	Direct costs (user fees/treatment costs) Indirect costs (transportation, opportunity costs e.g. lost income) Unable to use financial schemes available for poor patients	Limited availability of eye services at the HCs Long distances to the referral hospitals Cultural norms dictate that women should not travel alone Difficult to find an accompanying person	Limited availability of eye health human resources Long waiting times for patients Limited availability of information required to make informed decisions on eye health Complexity of modern hospital environment	Patient treatment costs not perceived as a barrier to access by the majority of service providers	Strong traditional beliefs Fear of surgery and negative treatment outcomes Shortcomings in the referral system Women's multiple roles and responsibilities

from their social networks in weighing the advantages and disadvantages of seeking treatment and different treatment options. Women are more vulnerable to poor, inaccurate or distorted information because their main source of information is word of mouth. If social networks are strong and well informed, women may be more likely to seek eye health care. Eye health services should therefore seek to influence informal information channels, especially adult children who are an important part of the decision-making process. The socio-cultural barriers were largely mitigated by the intervention of outreach programmes for those women who were able to obtain eye treatment. This shows that if other key barriers such as cost and transport are addressed, social-cultural barriers can also be overcome.

Strengths and limitations

The current study adds to the existing evidence because it comprehensively articulates the different barriers and identifies the most vulnerable subgroups by comparing barriers for men and women as well as for urban and rural women. In addition, it compares and contrasts the barriers identified by respondents from the demand side and supply side.

This study had some limitations. This paper documents a qualitative study. Qualitative research provides access to rich information that allows us to explore and understand complex social phenomena, and is therefore meant to yield results that are explorative rather than definitive. Although consumer-side participants were selected according to pre-defined criteria, local authorities were responsible for inviting demand-side participants to take part in the research. This may have introduced selection bias towards those familiar with the health care system. In some locations, FGDs were organised with participants other than those requested by the research team (i.e. different demographic groups). Furthermore, although every effort was made to ensure a gender-balanced representation of provider-side stakeholders, there are more men than women in healthcare management positions in Cambodia. Therefore, gender equality among KII participants could not be reached. Finally, the primary researcher does not speak Khmer. It is possible subtleties of meaning were lost in the translation process. The focus of the translation process was therefore on meaning rather than terminology.

Conclusions

This study has identified a range of barriers to accessing eye health services for women in Cambodia and provides some insights into strategies to overcome them. Fear of surgery and gender-based differences in decision-making, access, control over resources and social status disempower Cambodian women. These demand-side barriers interact with supply-side barriers to further impede women's ability to seek eye health services. Vulnerable women such as older rural women are more likely to rely on informal sources of information, including social networks and adult children. These channels are key in influencing women's eye health-seeking behaviour and might be utilised to address barriers to information and access. Providing these informal sources with accurate information is an important component to improve women's access to eye health services.

In addition, there is a disparity or inconsistency between perceptions of eye care costs between health providers and users: costs were not perceived as a barrier by service providers due to health financing support for poor patients, however, many users were not aware of the availability of the scheme. Further research is necessary to investigate the reasons for high failure rates amongst users applying for healthcare fee exemptions, as well as to inform the establishment and implementation of policies resulting in adequately reduced direct costs for vulnerable eye health consumers in Cambodia.

Findings from this research will inform the joint development through a partnership between FHF and the Cambodian Ministry of Women's Affairs of an evidence-based intervention that will address some of the barriers identified to ensure delivery of gender equitable eye services in Cambodia.

Abbreviations
FGD: Focus-group discussion; FHF: The Fred Hollows Foundation; HC: Health Centre; IDI: In-depth interview; KII: Key informant interview; MoH: Ministry of Health; MoWA: Ministry of Women's Affairs; NECHR: National Ethics Committee for Health Research; NGO: Non-government organisation; NIPH: National Institute for Public Health; NPEH: National Program for Eye Health; RAAB: Rapid assessment of avoidable blindness; VHV: Village Health Volunteer

Acknowledgements
We wish to thank the Cambodian Ministry of Women's Affairs for supporting this study. We also would like to thank all the study participants who gave us their time and trust.

Funding
This research was funded by The Fred Hollows Foundation. The authors declare that they have no competing interests related to this submission.

Authors' contributions
CN, RC and TH conceived the study; CC, CN, IQ and TH designed the study protocol; CC and IQ carried out the data collection with support from PS and SP; CC, IQ, CN, TH and RC analysed and interpreted these data; CN and IQ drafted the manuscript; PS, RC, SP and TH critically revised the manuscript for intellectual content. All authors read and approved the final manuscript. CN is the guarantor of the paper.

Competing interests

The authors declare that they have no competing interests.

This submission has not been published anywhere previously and it is not simultaneously being considered for any other publication. This paper was reviewed and rejected by the International Health Journal. The reason stated by the journal editor was that the findings outlined in the paper are likely to be of more interest to a regional audience than to an international one. We have not changed the manuscript as a result, as we think that the barriers identified by this study are actually valid in other contexts based on other research projects on barriers to eye care for women conducted (but not yet published) in Kenya and Bangladesh by The Fred Hollows Foundation.

Author details

[1]The Fred Hollows Foundation, Level 2, 61 Dunning Avenue, Rosebery, Sydney, NSW 2018, Australia. [2]School of Public Health and Community Medicine, Faculty of Medicine, University of New South Wales, Kensington, NSW 2052, Australia. [3]Siem Reap, Cambodia. [4]Phnom Penh, Cambodia. [5]The Fred Hollows Foundation Cambodia, Phnom Penh 12301, Cambodia.

References

1. Abou-Gareeb I, Lewallen S, Bassett K, Courtright P. Gender and blindness: a meta-analysis of population-based prevalence surveys. Ophthalmic Epidemiol. 2001;8:39–56.
2. Lewallen S, Courtright P. Gender and use of cataract surgical services in developing countries. Bull World Health Organ. 2002;80(4):300–3.
3. Seiha D, Limburg H. Summary Report of the Rapid Assessment of Avoidable Blindness in Cambodia, 2007. Phnom Penh: National Program for Eye Health, Ministry of Health; 2013.
4. Langdon T, Mörchen M, Nimeth E, Bonn TS, Tomic N, Keeffe J. Rapid assessment for avoidable blindness (RAAB) in Takeo Province, Cambodia 2012. Phnom Penh: AusAID; 2012.
5. Cains S, Sophal S. Creating demand for cataract services: a Cambodian case study. Commun Eye Health. 2006;19(60):65–6.
6. Ormsby G, Arnold AL, Busija L, Morchen M, Bonn TS, Keefe J. The impact of knowledge and attitudes on access to eye-care services in Cambodia. Asia Pac J Ophthalmol. 2012;1(6):331–5.
7. The Fred Hollows Foundation. Annual Report 2015. In: The Fred Hollows Foundation website; 2015. http://www.hollows.org/getattachment/au/Annual-Report-2015/2015-Annual-Report.pdf.aspx. Accessed 13 Oct 2016.
8. Gender GJ. Globalization and health in a Latin American context. Basingstoke: Palgrave Macmillan; 2014.

21

Conventional immunosuppressive therapy in severe Behcet's Uveitis: the switch rate to the biological agents

Hande Celiker[1][*], Haluk Kazokoglu[1] and Haner Direskeneli[2]

Abstract

Background: To report the switch rate of conventional immunosuppressive (CIS) therapies to the biological agents (BA) in patients with refractory Behcet's uveitis (BU).

Methods: In this retrospective study, clinical records were reviewed of 76 patients' 116 eyes presenting with BU who had been treated with immunosuppressive drug therapy. Mann Whitney U test was used for the intergroup comparisons of parameters without normal distribution as well as calculation of descriptive statistical methods (mean, standard deviation, median, frequency and rate). Wilcoxon Signed Ranks test was used for the intragroup comparisons of parameters without normal distribution. Pearson's Chi-Square test and Fisher-Freeman-Halton test were used for the comparisons of qualitative data.

Results: Except for one, all patients were first treated with CIS regimens for BU. Thirty-one patients (41.3%) who were unresponsive to CIS regimens were switched to IFNα2a therapy. After that, eight of these cases were switched to the anti-TNF-α treatments. The presence of initial ocular complications were found to be statistically higher in BA treated patients than the CIS treated cases ($p < 0.001$). Both in CIS treated and in BA treated cases, an increase in visual acuity (VA) was observed during the last examination compared to the initial examination and was significant ($p < 0.001$ and $p = 0.018$, respectively).

Conclusions: CIS treatment was found to be effective and safe, as suggested in the management guidelines for severe BU. Biological therapy was also found effective for the improvement of the VA. We observed that 58.7% of cases could be treated with strong immunosuppressive therapies, however, nearly half of the patients could have lost their VA if BAs were not existent. During the treatment course of severe cases with BU, classical therapy stage must still be protected as the first-line therapy due to the their reasonable activity and safety.

Keywords: Anti-TNF-α therapy, Behçet's uveitis, Immunosuppressive therapy, Interferon therapy, Uveitis

Background

Behcet's disease (BD) is a systemic vasculitis of unknown etiology manifesting mainly with oral/genital ulcers, skin lesions and uveitis. BD was first described as a distinct clinical entity by Hulusi Behcet [1]. This ubiquitous disorder is endemically higher in Turkey, Iraq, Iran, Korea, and Japan, the population derived historically from the ancient Silk Road, from the Mediterranean to the Far East and Middle Eastern countries [2]. Ocular manifestations of BD mostly include bilateral panuveitis, and retinal vasculitis with a chronic repetitive relapsing-remitting course. Systemic corticosteroids are still widely used in the therapy of ocular BD with or without conventional immunosuppressive (CIS) therapies [3]. Visual impairment has been prevented in recent years with the increasing use of immunosuppressive therapies such as azathioprine (2–3 mg/kg per day), cyclosporine-A (3–5 mg/kg per day), methotrexate (7.5–20 mg per week) or mycophenolat mofetil (500 mg- 2 g/per day) [4]. Recently, interferons and other biological agents have been suggested as a second choice to CIS therapy in

* Correspondence: drhandeceliker@yahoo.com
[1]Department of Ophthalmology, Marmara University School of Medicine, Fevzi Çakmak Mah. Muhsin Yazıcıoğlu Cad. No:10 Pendik, Istanbul, Turkey
Full list of author information is available at the end of the article

patients with refractory Behçet uveitis (BU) [5, 6]. Although they are shown to be superior compared to CIS therapies, biological agents are relatively new drugs and their efficacy and safety are still being investigated [7]. Use of biological agents in uveitis remains mostly limited to cases refractory to conventional treatment regimens due to their costs and our limited understanding of their long-term results [8]. Lately, in the literature, regarding BU or other uveitis treatments, most of the studies investigate the efficacy and safety profile of biological agents. Nonetheless, some of the patients with severe BU could still be treated with CIS agents. However, the reports of studies on the proportion of patients who have been changed to biological agents for the treatment of BU from CIS drugs is lacking. Thus, in this study we aimed to investigate the switch ratio from the conventional treatments to the biological therapy in patients with refractory BU in our Clinic.

Methods

The study protocol was approved by the local Institutional Ethics Board and conducted according to the tenets of the Declaration of Helsinki. Informed consent was obtained for all procedures. In our tertiary interdisciplinary uveitis clinic, clinical records were reviewed of 76 patients' 116 eyes presenting with severe uveitis due to BD who had been treated with immunosuppressive drug therapies from January 2008 to December 2016. Thirty-two of these cases who were treated with a biological agent (IFNα2a) were further evaluated. The patients were diagnosed on the basis of the International Study Group Criteria for BD [9]. Patients were systematically followed in both the Ophthalmology Clinic and the combined Behçet's Clinics in our institution. Uveitis terminology was described by the Standardization of Uveitis Nomenclature (SUN) Working Group [10]. Inactive anterior uveitis was defined as 0.5 cells or less. Severe uveitis was defined as a decrease of visual acuity (VA) < 20/100, vitritis > 2+, panuveitis, or failing to respond to 1 or more conventional immunosuppressive drugs and/or requiring intermediate doses of oral corticosteroids (> 10 mg per day). Inflammation of the posterior segment was defined by the presence of retinal vasculitis, retinitis, cystoid macular edema, and papillitis. Control of intraocular inflammation reported as quiescence was documented as inactivity of anterior chamber and absence of posterior segment intraocular inflammatory signs. Remission was defined as an inactive disease for at least 3 months after discontinuation of all immunosuppressive therapy [10]. Uveitis was defined as refractory when patients were receiving the highest anti-inflammatory or immunosuppressant regimen in their lives and it was insufficient to maintain the disease under control, defined as having a history of at least 1 relapse of the disease in a year before admission that needed an escalation of the dose of oral corticosteroid or other immunosuppressive agents, including azathioprine, methotrexate, cyclosporine A, IFNα2a, infliximab, or adalimumab to control the relapse [11]. The switch criteria was defined as any patient with the diagnosis of refractory BU; using an ineffective therapy, consisting of at least 1 additional immunosuppressant drug besides corticosteroids that was not able to maintain the patient without relapses and that needed an elevation of the oral corticosteroid or other immunosuppressant dosage to control the inflammation in a year, frequency of attacks (at least one severe relapse), presence of severe uveitis complications, CIS treatment resistant leakage on fundus fluorescein angiography, level of VA (decrease of VA < 20/100 or visual loss of 2 acuity lines). We use IFNα2a as a second-line treatment in refractory BU cases. Then, we switch to anti-TNF-α therapy according to the interferon-response status or the side-effects developed.

Complete ophthalmologic examination included best corrected VA testing, biomicroscopic evaluation, tonometry, fundus examination, and optical coherence tomography (OCT) performed during the all visits. Digital color fundus photographs and fluorescein angiography (FA) were performed in all patients at least once and whenever necessary during the course.

All of the 76 patients were treated initially with corticosteroids or a CIS therapy. Thirty-two of these patients, who suffered from sight-threatening uveitis and refractory to CIS agents, were given IFNα2a therapy (Roferon-A®; Roche Pharmaceuticals, Whitehouse Station, New Jersey, US). All patients underwent evaluation by a rheumatologist at the begining of treatments. Hematologic, tyroid, and hepatic functions were analysed by rheumatologists before final inclusion into the treatment group. For treatment of patients with BU, a standardized clinical algorithm was used. In case of anterior uveitis, topical prednisolone acetate 1% every hour and topical cyclopentolate hydrochloride 1% twice per day were prescribed. If it was necessary, pulse corticosteroid therapy was used (1 g/day, for 3–5 days) for severe uveitic attacks. Systemic therapy was started generally with using corticosteroids (CS, methylprednisolone, 1 mg/kg/day) in combination with azathioprine (AZA, 2–3 mg/kg per day), methotrexate (MTX, 7.5–20 mg per week) or cyclosporine A (CsA, 3–5 mg/kg per day). If the dual combinations did not work, as a third-line treatment, a triple combination of CS, AZA, and CsA was initiated to the cases with refractory BU. When all these drugs were not efficacious or serious side effects were observed, treatments were switched to the biological agents. All other immunosuppressant therapies were discontinued the day before the initial IFNα2a treatment, except colchicine and topical and/or systemic CS. IFNα2a therapy was started subcutaneously at a dosage of 3.0 million IU (MIU) per day for 2 weeks as the remission induction phase. All patients received paracetamol and pheniramine maleate before and after injections to avoid flu-like symptoms At the end of the remission induction period, maintenance dose of IFNα2a was continued with 3.0 million MIU 3 times per week. Doses of steroids were tapered based on clinical improvement of uveitis and according to the severity of the systemic symptoms of BD after induction of IFNα2a therapy. In case of limitation of clinical improvement, or if steroids could not be tapered, the dosage of IFNα2a was escalated in sequences of 4.5, 6.0, and 9.0 MIU 3 times per week for each severe inflammatory attacks [12]. When IFNα2a was ineffective or untolerable adverse events were observed, anti-TNF-α (infliximab 5 mg/kg i.v.or adalimumab 40 mg sc every other week) or the other therapies were introduced.

VA was assessed in European decimals (with Snellen chart), then converted to the logarithm of the minimum angle of resolution (logMAR) for computing. NCSS (Number Cruncher Statistical System) 2007 Statistical Software (Utah, USA) program was used for the statistical analysis. During the evaluation of the study data, Mann Whitney U test was used for the intergroup comparisons of parameters without normal distribution as well as calculation of descriptive statistical methods (mean, standard deviation, median, frequency and rate) and Wilcoxon Signed Ranks test was used for the intragroup comparisons of parameters without normal distribution. Pearson's Chi-Square test and Fisher-Freeman-Halton test were used for the comparisons of qualitative data.

Results
Patient characteristics
Seventy-six Behcet's patients were included the study. Except for one patient, all of them were treated first with a CIS treatment regimen for BU. One patient (1.3%) was treated with IFNα2a directly due to severe systemic BD symptoms. Thirty-one patients (41.3%) who were unresponsive to CIS regimens were switched to IFNα2a therapy. The relapse features of CIS treated patients before the IFNα2a treatment were one relapse 14 (43.7%), two relapses 14 (43.7%), three relapses 2 (6.3%), and four relapses 2 (6.3%). After this step, during the therapy or after the discontinuation, non-responder eight of these cases were switched to the anti-TNF-α treatment. Forty-four cases (58.7%) continued to the CIS treatments. Treatment stepwise and distribution of the treated patients shown in Fig. 1. The mean age was 31.46 ± 8.75 years

(range, 18 to 58 years). Fifty-one patients (67.1%) were men and 25 (32.9%) were women. The mean duration of follow-up was 38.70 ± 25.62 months (range, 6 to 96 months). Of BU patients, 40 (52.6%) had bilateral disease and 36 (47.4%) had unilateral ocular involvement (20 right and 16 left eyes). The most frequent type of uveitis was panuveitis ($n = 48$, 63.2%), followed by recurrent severe anterior uveitis ($n = 16$, 21.1%) and posterior uveitis ($n = 12$, 15.7%). Patients' general characteristics and extraocular symptoms of cases are summarized in Table 1. Of 88 eyes in 116 eyes, 132 severe ocular complications were detected at the first examination. Initial ocular clinical manifestations of all patients are presented in Table 2.

Descriptive characteristics of patients
Between the CIS treated patients and biological agent-treated cases, there were no statistically significant differences in terms of mean age, duration of BD, gender, pathergy positivity, presence of HLA-B51, and first attack treatment approach ($p > 0.05$). Follow-up periods of the biological agent-treated patients were significantly longer than the conventional treatment patients ($p < 0.001$). In the biological agent-treated group, the percentage of panuveitis was found to be statistically higher than the conventional drug treated patients ($p < 0.001$). Presence of initial ocular clinical complications were also significantly higher in biological agent-treated patients compared to conventional drug treated cases ($p < 0.001$). The bilaterality ratio of the biological agent-treated patients were significantly higher than the conventional drug treated patients ($p < 0,05$).

Visual acuity
Both groups (CIS and BA patients) had significant improvement in VA at last visit when compared to baseline ($p = 0.003$, $p = 0.030$, respectively), although VA scores were higher in the CIS group for both time points ($p < 0.001$). In biological agent-treated cases, the increase in VA observed during last examination compared to initial examination was also determined to be statistically significant ($p = 0.018$). Distribution of LogMAR VA of two treatment groups is shown in Fig. 2. After the discontinuation of IFNα2a treated 3 cases who was started anti-TNF-α agents during this period, significantly loss of vision (logMAR ≥ 2.0) occured in 3 eyes due to the severe former relapses of disease and in one eye rhegmatogenous retinal detachment also happened. These cases had experienced severe uveitis attacks during the all treatment period, before anti-TNF-α agents was started.

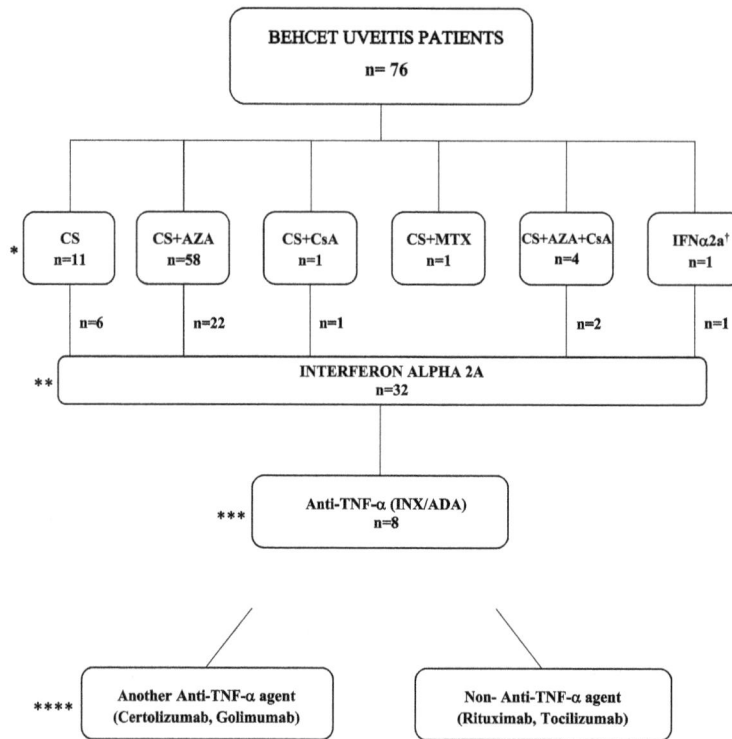

Figure 1. Our stepwise therapeutic approach for the patients with Behcet's uveitis and distribution of the cases

*First Line Therapy: AZA: azathioprine, CS: corticosteroid, CsA: cyclosporine A, IFNα2a: interferon alpha2a, MTX: methotrexate

† *except one case*

**Second Line Therapy: Interferon alpha2a

***Third Line Therapy: ADA: adalimumab, Anti-TNF-α: Anti tumor necrosis factor alpha, INX: infliximab

****Fourth Line Therapy: this line is used if necessary

Fig. 1 Our stepwise therapeutic approach for the patients with Behcet's uveitis and distribution of the cases. *First Line Therapy: AZA: azathioprine, CS: corticosteroid, CsA: cyclosporine A, IFNα2a: interferon alpha2a, MTX: methotrexate. † *except one case*. **Second Line Therapy: Interferon alpha2a. ***Third Line Therapy: ADA: adalimumab, Anti-TNF-α: Anti tumor necrosis factor alpha, INX: infliximab. ****Fourth Line Therapy: this line is used if necessary

Adverse effects

We did not observe severe side effects related to CIS therapy. Adverse effects related to IFNα2a therapy occurred in the following frequencies: flu-like syndrome associated with myalgia and fever (at the initiation phase of the treatment) (100%, $n = 32$), fatigue (12.5%, $n = 4$), loss of weight (6.25%, $n = 2$), mild leukopenia ($> 2.000/\mu l$) (6.25%, $n = 2$), elevation of serum liver enzymes (alanine transaminase (ALT, range 0–55 U/L), aspartate transaminase (AST, range 5–34 U/L)) (6.25%, $n = 2$), severe diarrhea (3.1%, $n = 1$), dissemine and intractable fibromyalgia (3.1%, $n = 1$), loss of appetite (3.1%, $n = 1$), hair loss (3.1%, $n = 1$), dryness of the mouth (3.1%, $n = 1$). Flu-like syndrome associated with myalgia and fever was well controlled with premedication using paracetamol and pheniramine maleate in all patients. Depression and aggressiveness were no observed. IFN-α2a therapy was discontinued due to adverse events in two patients (severe diarrhea and excessive weight loss). Nevertheless, these patients were non-responder to IFNα2a therapy at the same time (despite escalating of IFNα2a treatment dosages). As a consequence, their treatment was changed to anti-TNF-α agents. During the anti-TNF-α agent treatment (adalimumab), one patient have suffered for tuberculosis infection. The drug was discontinued, the patient is still being followed by us and infectious disease specialists.

Discussion

BD is a multiorgan disease characterized by an immune-mediated occlusive vasculitis [4]. Although BD represents a multisystemic disease, ocular involvement may reduce quality of life more than other complications of the disorder for many Behcet's patients. The use of advanced immunosuppressive drugs have virtually prevented the loss of vision in many patients with BU. Nonetheless, due to uncontrolled progression of the disease, a substantial proportion of patients with BU cannot be treated sufficiently with these

Table 1 Patient's descriptive characteristics and extraocular symptoms

(n = 76)		Mean ± sd (Min-Max)
Age (year)		31.46 ± 8.75 (18–58)
Follow-up time (month)		38.70 ± 25.62 (6–96)
		n (%)
Gender	Male	51 (67.1)
	Female	25 (32.9)
Uveitis type	Anterior	16 (21.1)
	Posterior	12 (15.7)
	Panuveitis	48 (63.2)
Laterality	Unilateral (right/left)	36 (20/16) (47.4, 26.3/21.1)
	Bilateral	40 (52.6)
HLAB51	Positive	8 (10.5)
	Negative	5 (6.6)
	Not performed	63 (82.9)
Pathergy	Positive	9 (11.8)
	Negative	18 (23.7)
	Not performed	49 (64.5)
First line therapy	CS	11 (14.5)
	CS + AZA	58 (76.3)
	CS + CsA	1 (1.3)
	CS + MTX	1 (1.3)
	CS + AZA + CsA	4 (5.3)
	IFNα2a	1 (1.3)
Extraocular symptoms	Recurrent oral ulcers	76 (100)
	Genital ulceration	52 (68.4)
	Folliculitis	47 (61.8)
	Arthritis	41 (53.9)
	Erythema Nodosum	19 (25.0)
	CNS involvement	9 (11.8)
	Thrombophlebitis	4 (5.2)

AZA azathioprine, *CS* corticosteroid, *CsA* cyclosporine, *IFNα2a* interferon alpha2a

Table 2 Distribution of ocular manifestations at initial examination

	n (%)
Ocular Complications	
None	28 (24.1)
Vasculitis	60 (51.7)
Macular edema	23 (19.8)
Retinitis	18 (15.5)
Papillitis	18 (15.5)
Opaque media	4 (3.4)
Vitreoretinal Adhesions	2 (1.7)
Lamellar Macular Hole	2 (1.7)
Epiretinal membrane	2 (1.7)
Keratitis	1 (0.9)
Optic atrophy	1 (0.9)
Recurrent hypopion	1 (0.9)

Multiple complications were seen in one eye

in review). Our main purpose in the present study was to report our renunciation from the conventional agents therapy in patients with BU and also the switch ratio of powerful immunosuppressants to the biological agents in our clinic. We did not aim to make direct comparisons between two patient groups, as a selection bias was present for the biological treatment group. Due to this selection, the percentage of panuveitis and presence of initial ocular clinical complications were found to be statistically higher in biological agent-treated patients than with CIS group. As known, these parameters are predictors of probable advance treatment requirements in the future.

CIS agent's activity and safety profile have been known for many years, therefore studies on these drugs are no longer published. Recently, most of the studies have been evaluating the efficacy and safety of IFNα2a and anti-TNF-α agents in BU. We believe that the studies which are related to CIS agents are still valuable, since we still are able to treat many patients with BU with these conventional drugs. In the present study, we could treat more than half of our cases of severe BU with these agents.

In the present study, we obtained accomplished VA results from the patients who were treated with conventional agents. In the biological agent-treated cases, the increase in VA during last examination was also acquired. As a result of assessment of VA in the whole cases, at the initial and the last examination, the VA of patients who were treated with immunosuppressant agents was determined to be statistically significantly higher than the patients treated only with biological agents. Due to the existence of more severe ocular inflammation in biological agent-treated patients than the others, this was an expected result. Therefore,

conventional agents. In 1986, Tsambos introduced for the first time the successful interferon treatment of three patients with BD, as herpes simplex virus type 1 was regarded to be involved in the etiopathogenesis in BD [13]. TNF-α inhibitors have also been shown to be effective and safe for the treatment of various diseases like rheumatoid arthritis, ankylosing spondylitis, juvenile idiopathic arthritis, Crohn's Disease, sarcoidosis and also uveitis. We intended to report our 8-year experience with the treatment of patients with BU. We previously evaluated risk factors of the patients who needed to the biological agents. Being young was detected as a poor prognostic factor in the multivariable analyses (unpublished data, Celiker et al., manuscript

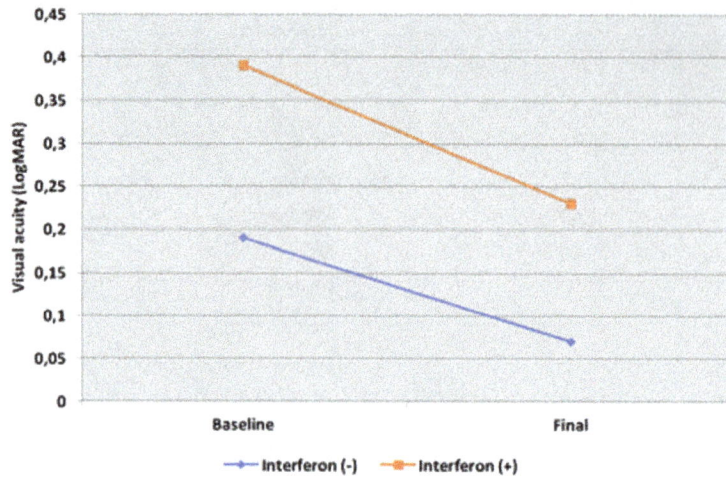

Fig. 2 Distribution of LogMAR visual acuity of conventional agent treated patients and Interferon alpha 2a treated cases

both treatment modalities demonstrated powerful efficacy in the treatment of patients with BU.

For our country, we calculated the costs for treatment regimens for a patient with BU of 60 kg of body weight. For anti-TNF-α treatment (adalimumab), the cost will be US $15,600 (induction and maintenance dose regimen: 40 mg/0.8 ml two times per month) per year. For IFNα2a (Roferon-A®; Roche Pharmaceuticals), the cost will be US $1485/year (induction and maintenance dose regimen: 3.0 MIU 3 times per week). For the same patient, AZA (Imuran® Glaxo Smithkline Pharmaceuticals Ltd., 150 mg per day) + CsA (Sandimmun Neoral® Novartis Pharmaceuticals Ltd., 200 mg per day) combination treatment cost will be US $882 per year. In comparison, there is a significant difference in terms of costs of the drugs. Of course, drug choice should always be considered in favor of the patient, however, the cost-effectivity should also be taken into consideration when selecting the eligible agent. Kötter et al. emphasized that there is a need for studies with IFNα2a using standardized outcome measures and pre-and post-treatment observation periods in this era of evidence-based medicine [7]. Besides the efficacy of a drug, cost-effectiveness should be compared with standard immunosuppressants to determine its hierarchy in the treatment of BD [7]. In our opinion, in the fashion of the present study, the reports about comparing the cost-effectiveness of both treatment regimens may be important for the establish of the BU therapy algorithm.

In some uveitis clinics, due to their well documented intense effects to control BU, anti-TNF-α agents' are being used as a second line therapy after single or combination CIS treatment. However, according to our stepwise therapeutic approach, anti-TNF-α agents are used as a third line therapy for BU patients who fail or do not tolerate second line IFNα2a treatment. Furthermore, it is also important that each clinic's treatment algorithms should be determined according to the healthcare system of their own country.

Conclusions

CIS treatment was effective and safe as has been known for a long time in the management of BU. Biological therapies were also found to be effective for the improvement of the VA. Comparative studies of the two treatment modalities may lead to bias due to the fact that patients in the biological-agent group do not respond to the conventional treatment. However, in our opinion, despite the new biological agents, it is still important to know how often we can treat our patients with classical immunosuppressive drugs. In the present study we observed that while 58.7% of cases could be treated with strong immunosuppressive therapies, nevertheless, 41.3% of patients had to be treated with biological agents. Namely, according to the outcomes of the present study, nearly half of the our patients could have lost their VA if biological agents have not been existent. The cost-effectiveness of the biological agents compared with the standard immunosuppressive drugs also should be considered during the selection of appropriate treatments, particularly as a first-line agent. In our opinion, during the treatment course of severe cases with BU, in the treatment algorithm, the classical therapy stage must be protected as a first-line therapy due to the strong activity and safety. Nonetheless, as known by all BD specialists, BU can lead to irreversible visual loss, especially in younger individuals, thus, the choice of the appropriate prompt treatment is essential for these patients. Therefore, in our opinion, there is a need for more controlled, randomized studies with conventional strong immunosuppresive drugs and biological agents using standardized outcome measures, and their efficacy and cost-effectiveness should be compared to determine their hierarchy in the treatment of BU.

Abbreviations

ADA: Adalimumab; ALT: Alanine transaminase; Anti-TNF-α: Anti tumor necrosis factor alpha; AST: Aspartate transaminase; AZA: Azathioprine; BA : Biological agents; BD: Behcet's disease; BU: Behcet's uveitis; CIS: Conventional immunosuppressive; CS: Corticosteroid; CsA: Cyclosporine A; FA: Fluorescein angiography; IFNα2a: Interferon alpha2a; INX: Infliximab; MTX: Methotrexate; OCT: Optical coherence tomography; SUN: Standardization of Uveitis Nomenclature; VA: Visual acuity

Authors' contributions

The authors alone are responsible for the content and writing of the paper. HC: substantial contribution to conception and design, acquisition of data, analysis and interpretation of data, writing of manuscript. HK: critical revision of the manuscript for important intellectual content, analysis and interpretation of data, administrative, technical, ot material support supervision. HD: critical revision of the manuscript for important intellectual content, statistical anaysis, substantial contribution to conception and design, writing of manuscript. All authors have read and approved the manuscript.

Competing interests

The authors declare that they have no competing interests.

Author details

[1]Department of Ophthalmology, Marmara University School of Medicine, Fevzi Çakmak Mah. Muhsin Yazıcıoğlu Cad. No:10 Pendik, Istanbul, Turkey. [2]Division of Rheumatology, Marmara University School of Medicine Fevzi Çakmak Mah, Muhsin Yazıcıoğlu Cad. No:10 Pendik, Istanbul, Turkey.

References

1. Behçet H. Über rezidivierende aphthöse durch ein virus verursachte Geschwüre am Mund, am Auge, und an den Genitalien. Dermatol Wochenschr. 1937;105:1152–7.
2. Michelson JB, Chisari FV. Behçet's disease. Surv Ophthalmol. 1982;26:190–203.
3. Kaçmaz RO, Kempen JH, Newcomb J, Gangaputra S, Daniel E, Levy-Clarke GA, et al. Ocular inflammation in Behçet disease: incidence of ocular complications and of loss of visual acuity. Am J Ophthalmol. 2008;146:828–36.
4. Deuter CM, Kotter I, Wallace GR, Murray PI, Stübiger N, Zierhut M. Behcet's disease: ocular effects and treatment. Prog Retin Eye Res. 2008;27:111–36.
5. Gueudry J, Wechsler B, Terrada C, Gendron G, Cassoux N, Fardeau C, et al. Long-term efficacy and safety of low-dose interferon alpha2a therapy in severe uveitis associated with Behcet disease. Am J Ophthalmol. 2008;146:837–44.
6. Sobaci G, Erdem U, Durukan AH, Erdurman C, Bayer A, Köksal S, et al. Safety and effectiveness of interferon alpha-2a in treatment of patients with Behcet's uveitis refractory to conventional treatments. Ophthalmology. 2010;117:1430–5.
7. Kotter I, Gunaydin I, Zierhut M, Stübiger N. The use of interferon alpha in Behçet disease: review of the literature. Semin Arthritis Rheum. 2004; 33:320–35.
8. Imrie FR, Dick AD. Biologics in the treatment of uveitis. Curr Opin Ophthalmol. 2007;18:481–6.
9. Criteria for diagnosis of Behçet's disease. International study Group for Behçet's disease. Lanset. 1990;335(8697):1078–80.
10. Jabs DA, Nussenblatt RB, Rosenbaum JT. Standardization of uveitis nomenclature (SUN) working group. Standardization of uveitis nomenclature for reporting clinical data: results of the first international workshop. Am J Ophthalmol. 2005;140:509–16.
11. Díaz-Llopis M, Salom D, Garcia-de-Vicuña C, Cordero-Coma M, Ortega G, Ortego N, Suarez-de-Figueroa M, et al. Treatment of refractory uveitis with adalimumab: a prospective multicenter study of 131 patients. Ophthalmology. 2012;119:1575–81.
12. Onal S, Kazokoglu H, Koc A, Akman M, Bavbek T, Direskeneli H, et al. Long-term efficacy and safety of low-dose interferon alfa-2a therapy in refractory Behcet uveitis. Arch Ophthalmol. 2011;129:288–94.
13. Tsambaos D, Eichelberg D, Goos M. Behcet's syndrome: treatment with recombinant leukocyte alphainterferon. Arch Dermatol Res. 1986;278:335–6.

22

Optical coherence tomography patterns and outcomes of contusion maculopathy caused by impact of sporting equipment

Danjie Li[1,2]*, Hideo Akiyama[1] and Shoji Kishi[3]

Abstract

Background: To describe the patterns and outcomes of contusion maculopathy after ocular contusions resulting from accidental impact with sporting equipment.

Methods: We conducted a retrospective study of interventional case series. Patient Population: Twenty-one eyes of 21 patients who sustained blunt ocular trauma while playing a sport. Intervention/Observation Procedure(s): Surgery or observation by optical coherence tomography (OCT). Main Outcome Measure(s): The morphologic changes within the macula in the early stages after injury and changes in visual function in the early and recovery stages after injury.

Results: In the early stage, OCT visualized four injury patterns: type I, commotio retinae (14.3%, 3 eyes) with increased reflectivity of the ellipsoid zone and retinal pigment epithelium; type II, incomplete macular hole(38.1%, 8 eyes) with three structural changes, i.e., a partial V-shaped macular hole, a jar-shaped macular hole with retinal tissue at the bottom, and a connective bridge attached to retinal tissues; type III, full-thickness macular hole (33.3%, 7 eyes); and type IV, foveal hemorrhage (14.3%, 3 eyes). During recovery, OCT images of types I and II showed almost normal macular morphology with better visual acuity (mean ± SD,0.02 ± 0.1 and 0.14 ± 0.21logMAR.). In types III and IV, the visual prognosis was poor (0.52 ± 0.34 and 0.22 ± 0.16), OCT images showed retinal atrophy at the fovea despite vitrectomy and sulfur hexafluoride (SF6) gas tamponade.

Conclusion: Early OCT images identified four patterns of contusion maculopathy with different treatment outcomes. In types I and II, the visual function and retinal morphology remained intact. With types III and IV, respectively, the treatments of vitrectomy and SF6 gas tamponade for patients were effective.

Keywords: Optical coherence tomography (OCT), Contusion maculopathy, Commotio retinae, Incomplete macular hole, Full-thickness macular hole, Foveal hemorrhage

Background

About half (54%) of all ocular injuries are minor superficial ocular or periocular injuries. Ocular contusions account for 23%; followed by chemicals and burns (13%), fractures (5%), lid wounds (3%), open globe injuries (2%) and optic nerve injuries (1%) [1]. inadvertent contact with sporting equipment, and tools used during work are the main causes of ocular contusions. Among young people in Japan, sports that include use of a ball; including but not limited to baseball, football, and basketball, are very popular. In these types of sports, blunt traumatic maculopathy resulting from being struck by the balls is the most common mechanism of injury in clinical ophthalmology. However, traumatic macular holes are disproportionly more common in the pediatric and adolescent populations [2]. Treatment success is multifactorial and depends on both ophthalmic factors, e.g., identified diagnostics, treatment methods, timing of surgery, and patient factors, e.g., patient requirements and social barriers.

Optical coherence tomography (OCT) is a relatively new medical diagnostic imaging modality that is being used extensively to observe Retinopathy. By using echo

* Correspondence: 2015lidanjie@sina.com
[1]Department of Ophthalmology, Gunma University School of Medicine, 3-39-15 Showa-machi, Maebashi, Gunma 371-8511, Japan
[2]Aier eye hospital (Cheng Du), 115 Xiyiduan, Yihuanlu,, Chengdu 610041, China
Full list of author information is available at the end of the article

time delay and intensity of backscattered light; OCT can view internal microstructures in biologic tissue with incredible resolution [3, 4]. Coupled with the ability to view multiple cross-sectional images; OCT is a great tool to view macular lesions secondary to macular trauma.

Previous studies [4, 5] using OCT have observed retinal changes in eyes with contusion maculopathy of commotion retinae and traumatic macular hole. Commotio retinae has been known to have good prognosis without interventional therapy. However, there are mixed opinions regarding the benefits of surgical intervention in the treatment of macular holes. In this study, we examine the retinal characteristics of patients diagnosed with contusion maculopathy secondary to sport related ocular trauma using OCT. The question regarding whether surgical or minimally invasive therapy is beneficial will be explored and hopefully better elucidated.

Methods

In this retrospective study we reviewed the medical records files of twenty-one patients with contusion maculopathy between January 2008 and April 2017 at the Gunma University Hospital. Inclusion criteria included blunt injury and nonpenetrating trauma only. All penetrating trauma were excluded from the study.

All patients underwent a routine ophthalmic examination that included measurement of the best-corrected visual acuity (BCVA), color fundus photography, and OCT examination at multiple time points. We defined 1 week after the ocular injury as the early-period stage. The final examination was defined as that performed after at least 1 month or when the patient refused to undergo examination and treatment. The VA was measured using a decimal chart and converted to the logarithm of the minimum angle of resolution for statistical analysis. When the VA was finger counting, 0.001 was considered the equivalent decimal VA. The data of VA on initial visit were statistically compared with those in final visit with the paired t test $P < .05$ was statistically significant.

In our study, the type of OCT system includes SD-OCT (Topcon, Tokyo, Japan), Cirrus high-definition OCT (Carl Zeiss Meditec, Inc., Dublin, CA), and SS-OCT (DRI OCT-1 Atlantis; Topcon, Tokyo, Japan). For OCT examinations, we selected a transverse or vertical display, after generating a macular cube scan (6 × 6 mm area centered on the fovea) and observed changes in the retinal layers of the macula. We evaluated the morphologic changes of retina within the macula during an early stage after injury (within a week after injury) and described the patterns of maculopathy after ocular contusion. The contusion maculopathy was defined as four types: type i: macular commotio retinae, type ii: incomplete macular hole; type iii: macular hole, and type iv: macular hemorrhage. During follow-up, all patients

with an ocular contusion received general treatment and/or surgical treatments for macular disorders, which included vitrectomy and sulfur hexafluoride (SF6) gas tamponade.

The study was conducted according to the Declaration of Helsinki. The institutional review board of Gunma University approved the study.

Results

Twenty-one eyes (11 right eyes, 10 left eyes) of 21 patients (20 males, 1 female) with a macular disorder from blunt ocular trauma were included (Table 1). The ocular contusions resulted from direct injury to the eyeball after being hit by a ball or shuttlecock while playing a sport. Fourteen patients were hit by baseballs, four by footballs, two by shuttlecocks, and one by a tennis ball. The mean patient age at the initial visit was 18.3 years (range, 9–53 years). The mean duration of follow-up was 10.7 months (range, 1–60 months).

At the initial visit, the decimal BCVA ranged from 20 cm/n.d to 1.2 (mean: 1.08 logMAR). The final BCVA were increased ($P < .001$), these ranged from 0.15 to 1.2 (mean: 0.26 logMAR) (Fig. 1). In addition to contusion maculopathy, other findings included dilated pupils (cases 6 and 12), traumatic iris (cases 2, 3, 6,10,14 and 18), hyphema (cases4, 5, 12,15,18, and 21), angle recession (cases 2, 3, 5, and 15), lens subluxation (case 3), traumatic cataract (case 15), and varying degrees of retinal edema or/and hemorrhage outside the macular region (all cases).

Oct images

OCT was performed at the initial visit -within one week after injury. The Table 1 summarizes all OCT retinal features in all cases. According to the changes in the macular retinal morphology seen on the initial OCT images, the contusion maculopathy was divided into four types: macular commotio retinae, incomplete macular hole; macular hole, and macular hemorrhage.

Type I

Commotio retinae was seen on the second day after injury. In cases 1,2, and 3 (14.3%, 3 eyes), the fundus examination showed commotio retinae in the retinal posterior pole. The OCT images showed a merging area of increased reflectivity in the ellipsoidal zone (EZ) and retinal pigment epithelium (RPE) (Fig. 2); a funduscopic photograph showed an opaque white spot on the fovea. After 1 month, a normal retinal structure was seen (Fig. 2). Other OCT changes (Fig. 2) of commotion retinae included a vertical band of high reflectivity with the outer nuclear layer (ONL) on the fovea in addition to the high reflectivity of the EZ and RPE lines. In case 3, during follow up; the OCT showed partial EZ irregularity on the fovea.

Table 1 Characteristics of the Subject Population

No	Age[a]	R/L	Equipment	initial VA	Follow period (M)	Final VA	Initial OCT imaging on the fovea	Type	Treatment	Final OCT imaging on the fovea
1	B	L	Tennis	1.2	1	1.2	Outer retinal layer shows thickened and high reflection	I	No	Normal
2	C	R	Baseball	0.8	1	1.2	Vertical high reflective lesion on the fovea	I	No	Normal
3	F	R	Badminton	0.3	11	0.8	EZ irregularity and high reflective lesion on the fovea	I	Lens removal surgery	Normal
4	B	L	Baseball	0.5	3.5	1.2	Macular hole of inner-retinal (V-shaped)	II	No	Normal
5	D	L	Baseball	0.06	1	0.6	Macular hole of inner-retinal (V-shaped)	II	No	EZ disorder
6	C	L	Baseball	0.2	2	0.8	Remaining some retinal tissues on the macular hole-like (V-shaped)	II	No	EZ disorder
7	B	R	Football	0.2	10	1.0	Remaining some retinal tissues on the bottom of hole-like (jar-shaped)	II	No	EZ disorder
8	A	R	Football	0.01	24	0.5	In the center there was a bridge-like retinal tissue	II	No	Retinal atrophy on fovea
9	B	L	Baseball	0.3	8	1.2	In the center there was a bridge-like retinal tissue	II	No	Normal
10	B	R	Baseball	0.1	2.5	0.3	In the center there was a bridge-like retinal tissue	II	No	EZ defect; Retinal atrophy
11	B	L	Baseball	0.6	1	0.7	In the center there was a bridge-like retinal tissue	II	No	Vertical high reflective lesion on the fovea
12	B	R	Baseball	0.001	29	0.8	Full-thickness macular hole and gradually expanded	III	SF6 gas tamponade, vitreous surgery	EZ defect
13	B	R	Baseball	0.2	12	0.9	Full-thickness macular hole and gradually expanded	III	Vitreous surgery	EZ defect
14	B	R	Baseball	0.2	4	0.3	Full-thickness macular hole and gradually expanded	III	No	Full-thickness macular hole
15	C	L	Badminton	0.03	14	0.3	Full-thickness macular hole	III	SF6 gas tamponade vitreous surgery, IOL	Retinal atrophy
16	C	R	Football	0.01	8	0.15	Full-thickness macular hole	III	SF6 gas tamponade, vitreous surgery	[a]Full-thickness macular hole
17	B	R	Football	0.1	20	0.15	Full-thickness macular hole	III	No	Retinal atrophy
18	B	R	Baseball	0.04	6	0.15	Full-thickness macular hole	III	No	EZ defect; retinal atrophy
19	C	L	Baseball	0.01	7	0.7	Submacular hemorrhage, Macular hole?	IV	SF6 gas tamponade	EZ defect; Retinal atrophy
20	B	L	Baseball	0.08	1.5	0.4	Submacular hemorrhage	IV	SF6 gas tamponade	EZ defect
21	D	L	Baseball	0.01	60	0.8	Submacular hemorrhage	IV	Vitrectomy in the fourth year	Full-thickness macular hole

R = right; L = left; VA = visual acuity; M = months; OCT = optical coherence tomography; IOL = intraocular lens; SF$_6$ = sulfur hexafluoride; EZ = ellipsoidal zone
Age[a]: providing ages as age-range, A: 1–9, B: 10–19; C: 20–29; D: 30–39; D: 40–49; E: 50–59

In type I, the mean BCVA improved without treatment from the initial level of 0.18 ± 0.31 logMAR (mean ± SD) to a final level of-0.02 ± 0.1 (mean ± SD) logMAR (Fig. 1). In case 3 with traumatic subluxation, lens replacement surgery was performed and the BCVA improved to 0.8 after 11 months. The morphologic structures of the retina on OCT returned to the baseline level in the three cases, after 1 month (case 1 and 2), and 11 months (case 11).

Type II
OCT showed an incomplete macular hole in cases 4 to 11 (38.1%, 8 eyes) at the initial visit (Fig. 3) that we defined as type II contusion maculopathy. The OCT images of cases 4,5, and 6 (Fig. 3) appear as separation of the inner retinal layer at the fovea with a complete EZ. As seen in case 4; a V-shaped macular hole in an 11-year-old boy, had an initial BCVA of 0.5 in the left

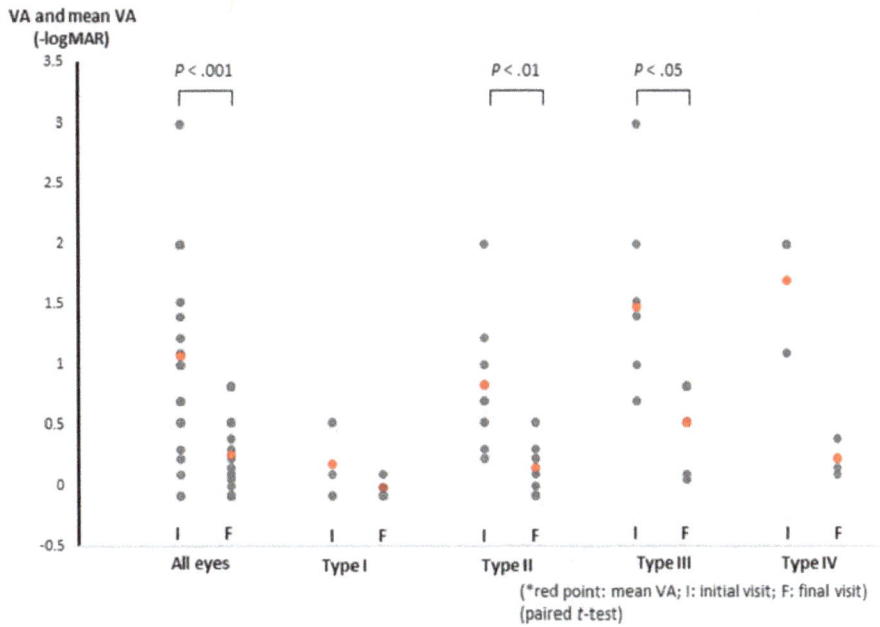

Fig. 1 The mean visual acuity (VA) associated with each type of injury during the early and final stages of recovery after contusion maculopathy. logMAR = logarithm of the minimum angle of resolution

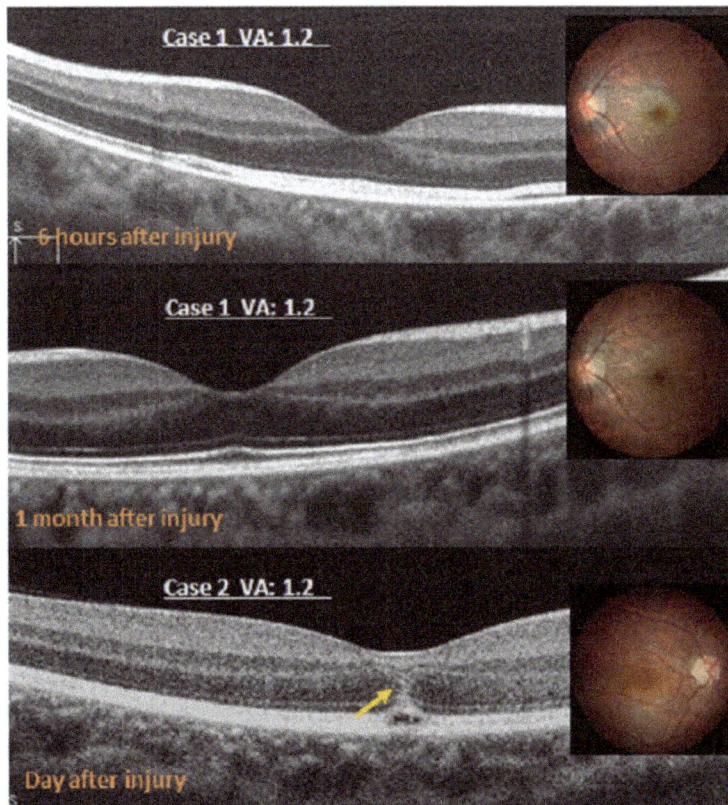

Fig. 2 The optical coherence tomography images of a type 1 injury with color photography. Top, Case 1 has abnormal increased reflectivity of the ellipsoid zone (EZ) and retinal pigment epithelium (RPE). Middle, In case 1, the retina is normal after 1 week. Bottom, In case 2, vertical bands of high reflectivity (arrow) on the fovea are seen in addition to the high reflectivity of the EZ and RPE line on the fovea. VA = visual acuity

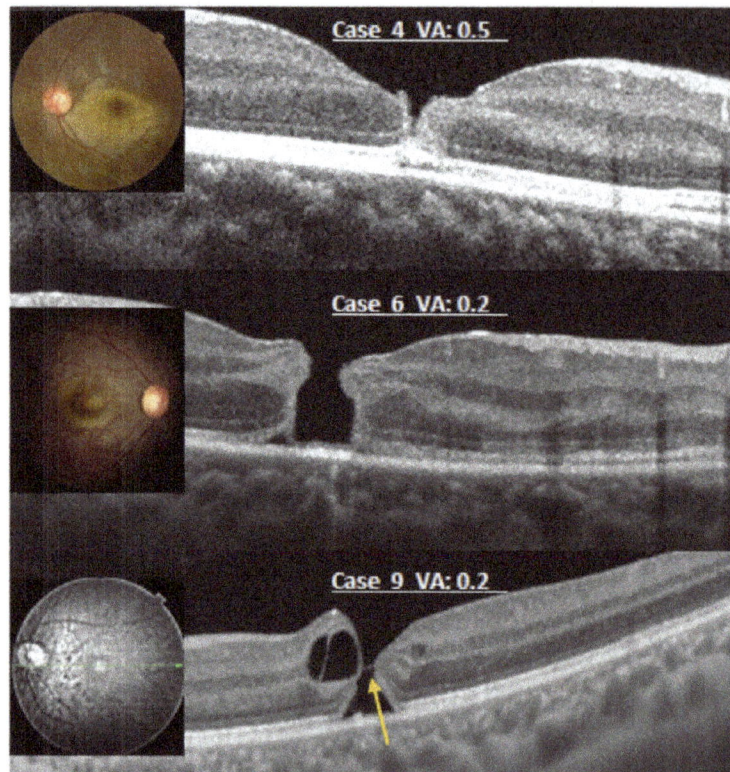

Fig. 3 Theoptical coherence tomography images of a type 2 injury with color photography. Top, The image shows a V-shaped separation of the inner retinal layer at the fovea. The bottom of the hole-like has a complete ellipsoidal zone (EZ). Middle, The image shows an incomplete jar-shaped macular hole with a complete EZ. Bottom, A bridge (arrow) is seen connected to the retinal tissues in the middle of a macular hole-like structure. VA = visual acuity.

eye immediately after he sustained the ocular trauma. 3.5 months later, the BCVA recovered to 1.2 without treatment. OCT images of the fovea showed a normal retina. In cases 5 and 6, after 2 weeks and 2 months, respectively, without surgical treatment, OCT showed normal macular concavity with a disrupted EZ. The BCVAs recovered from the initial levels of 0.06 and 0.2 respectively, to the final levels of 0.2 and 0.8.

Case 7 appeared to be a macular hole (Fig. 3); however, in the inferior fovea, an irregular layer of outer retinal tissue with EZ contributed to a skewed contour, which we described as "jar-like". After 10 months without surgical treatment, OCT showed the retina had a slight EZ defect. The BCVA increased from the initial level of 0.2 to1.0.

The OCT feature in cases 8 to 11 demonstrated a bridge connected to the retinal tissue in the middle of the macular holes (Fig. 3). The bridge appeared at different levels in the macular holes. Without surgical treatment, the OCT images in case 9 were normal, and the other eyes experienced some recovery. However, each case showed varying degrees of EZ defect and macular dystrophy.

During follow-up, in these eyes with type II, no retinal detachments occurred around the macular holes, and these hole-like defects tended to close; thus, we did not perform surgery. The mean BCVA (Fig. 1) increased from the initial level of 0.83 ± 0.57logMAR (mean $\pm$ SD) to 0.14 ± 0.21 logMAR ($P < .01$). The final OCT images of the fovea of patient 8 and 10 showed retinal dystrophy with a final BCVA of 0.5 and 0.3, the other eyes showed a normal retina or EZ defect with better final vision.

Type III
OCT showed full-thickness macular holes in cases 12 to 18 (33.3%, 7 eyes) during the early stage after injury (Fig. 4). The mean BCVA in type III increased from the initial level of 1.47 logMAR to 0.52logMAR ($P < .05$) (Fig. 1). Figure 4a shows a full-thickness macular hole that was not surrounded by a localized retinal detachment on the day after the injury (case 12). During follow-up, the hole expanded gradually, and a retinal detachment developed gradually around the hole. On the third week, 0.3 ml of pure SF6 was injected into the vitreous cavity; however, the macular hole did not close postoperatively. Two weeks later, we repaired the macular hole during vitrectomy. The final OCT image showed a localized EZ on the fovea, and the BCVA recovered to 0.8. The macular holes in cases 13 and 14 also enlarged gradually similarly to case 12. The final BCVA in case 13

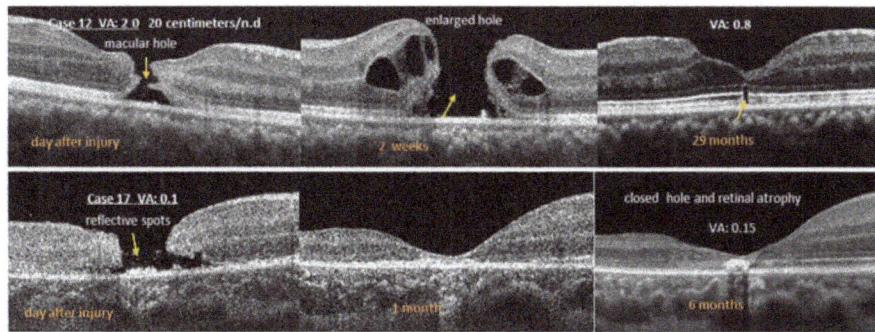

Fig. 4 Top, An optical coherence tomography (OCT) image of case 12 shows a full-thickness macular hole on the left. After 2 weeks, the hole expanded gradually with a retinal detachment around the hole (middle). The final OCT image shows that the hole closed with a defect of the ellipsoidal zone (EZ) defect at the fovea (right). Middle, The left OCT image in case 17 shows a full-thickness macular hole 2 days after the injury and some reflective spots in the middle of the hole (arrow). The middle OCT image shows that the hole closed 1 month after the injury. After 6 months, the hole is closed and an atrophic scar is seen on the fovea (right)

reached 0.9 after vitrectomy. In case 14, the patient refused surgery and 3 months after the injury, the macular hole remained open and the final BCVA was only 0.3.

In cases 15 and 16, same as case 12, after pure SF6 was injected into the vitreous cavity, the holes remained open, but they closed after vitrectomy. The final OCT image showed macular retinal dystrophy in cases 15. Case 16 had recurrence of macular hole, and he terminated his treatment. The final BCVAs were 0.3 and 0.15, respectively.

In cases 17 and 18, some spots of reflectivity of varying sizes were seen within the macular holes on OCT (Fig. 4). The holes were gradually reduced during follow-up visits. Although no surgery was performed, the macular holes closed after1 month. The final OCT images showed an extremely thin retina at the fovea and macular dystrophy, and the BCVAs were poor at 0.15.

Type IV

Macular hemorrhages developed during the early stage after injury in cases 19, 20, and 21 (14.3%, 3 eyes). The OCT images showed elevation of the retina (Fig. 5), as well as a completed RPE line and Bruch's membrane.

Some blood was visible between the separated foveal pit, on the retinal surface, and in the vitreous cavity. Cases 19 and 20 were treated with pure SF6 on the thirteenth and seventeenth day respectively after injury. One month later, OCT images showed a deeper fovea with EZ defect and a thinning retina in case 19. Comparatively; case 20 only had an EZ defect. The blunt traumatic maculopathy observed in case 21 was not treated surgically; it was characterized by an emerging macular pseudo-hole 1 year after the injury. Four years after the injury, a full-thickness macular hole was seen, and vitrectomy was performed. In all three cases, their mean BCVA from initial 1.7 logMAR (0.01, 0.08, 0.01, respectively) increased to 0.22 logMAR (0.7, 0.4, 0.8, respectively).

Discussion

In the current retrospective study, we evaluated the OCT images of contusion maculopathy in 21 patients. Blunt sports-related trauma resulting from balls and shuttlecocks hitting the eyes were the main mechanisms of injuries. Based on the OCT images obtained during the early stage of ocular injury (within 1 week), we divided the

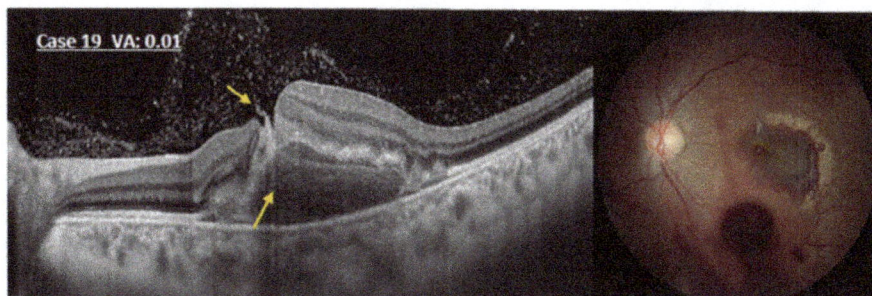

Fig. 5 An optical coherence tomography image of the eye in case 19 shows that the retina is elevated. Some blood (arrows) is seen between the separated fovea, on the retinal surface, and the subretinal hemorrhage

contusion maculopathy into four types: I, commotio retinae (14.3%); II, incomplete macular holes (38.1%); III, macular holes (33.3%); and IV, macular hemorrhage (14.3%). The proportion of macular holes with incomplete (type III) and full-thickness (type IV) contusion maculopathy are larger, about 71% (38.3% + 33.3%). Our results reveal differing treatment approaches which alter prognosis in the two types of contusion maculopathy. Based on these results, it is important to distinguish these two forms of contusion maculopathy by OCT features.

The term commotio retinae describes the damage to the outer retinal layers caused by shock waves that traverse the eye from the site of impact after blunt trauma. Using OCT, Itakura and Kishi [5] reported acute abnormalities of the EZ in commotio retina and restoration of the photoreceptor architecture accompanied by improvement in BCVA. In the three patients with a type I injury, the OCTs on the initial visit showed not only thickened and increased reflectivity of the EZ and RPE but also injury in the outer nuclear layer (ONL) (Fig. 2). Although this has been attributed to extreme paretic vasodilatation, it is more likely caused by a change in the transparency of the intracellular proteins of the retina. Change in transparency of retina likely results as a direct response to either contusion or brief ischemia secondary to injury of choroidal or retinal blood vessels. During the early stages in a type I injury, we did not find EZ defects. However, during the retinal recovery stage, we noticed an evanescent EZ defect phase. This phase might be considered as retinal edema in the early stages, eventually leading to small amounts of photoreceptor cell damage. Depending on the degree of damage, the times to complete recovery varied from 1 month to 11 months. In the end their BCVA recovered to normal 1.0.

In routine fundus examination, the eyes suspected of macular holes were diagnosed as incomplete macular holes after detailed OCT analysis. Based on the OCT images, 38.1% of all cases were classified with incomplete macular holes (type II injury). Their images included the following three retinal changes: 1) AV-shaped macular hole, 2) Jar shaped macular hole, and 3) Bridge shaped macular hole. The AV-shaped appearance was characterized by a separation between the retinal surface and the ONL; the outer retinal tissues of the external limiting membrane and EZ layers remained at the bottom of the hole (Fig. 3). The jar-shaped appearance was characterized by the EZ on the wide bottom of the macular hole (Fig. 3). The bridge-shaped appearance was characterized by a bridge connected to retinal tissue in the middle of the full-thickness macular hole (Fig. 3). As a result, residual macular retinal atrophy was observed. The eyes with type II injury had better BCVA (mean ± SD, 0.14 ± 0.21 logMAR) compared to type III (mean ± SD, 0.52 ± 0.34 logMAR), and had natural closing of the macular

hole. It can be inferred OCT examination of eyes with contusion maculopathy can directly assess the prognosis of the patients.

In this study, we found that the cases with three retinal changes in type II injury were significantly correlated with visual and retinal morphologic improvements. In addition, no cases with a type II injury progressed to full-thickness macular holes (type III), despite appearance of residual retinal EZ defect and atrophy at the fovea. These changes are similarly observed in idiopathic lamellar macular holes. Some researchers have reported that lamellar macular holes usually remain stable over time, with few eyes evolving into full-thickness macular holes, and some cases resolve spontaneously [6–8].

We observed that the early OCT images of traumatic macular holes (type III) did not show localized retinal detachments around the macular holes, but the holes expanded gradually. This differed from idiopathic macular holes [9, 10], which are thought to result from focal shrinkage of the vitreous cortex in the foveal area. In contrast, traumatic macular holes result from traumatic shock. The results in the current cases indicated that SF6 gas tamponade was ineffective, while vitrectomy was the more effective treatment method as with idiopathic macular holes [11–14]. The current results indicated that although surgery can be successful, once the macular holes have formed, it is easy for macular atrophy to occur, and recovery of visual function is not good. The final mean BCVA is less than 0.3 (mean ± SD, 0.52 ± 0.34 logMAR), while in eye with type II injury is more than 0.5 (mean ± SD, 0.14 ± 0.21 logMAR). Even if our number of cases is relatively small, we still think that if there are punctate high reflective tissues in the macular hole, or the hole has no tendency to expand, it may eventually close naturally (case 17 and 18), otherwise surgical intervention is recommended.

A high spontaneous closure rate was observed, with a trend toward smaller OCT dimensions. Surgical intervention was less successful at hole closure when elected after 3 months [2]. In our study cases, all eyes of Type II injury had successful spontaneous hole closure as compared to type III where vitrectomy was required. Therefore, it is very important to distinguish incomplete and full-thickness macular hole by OCT features at the early stage of trauma.

Bruch's membrane is an elastin- and collagen-rich extracellular matrix that acts as a molecular sieve. Blunt trauma of the eye can cause Bruch's membrane tear and choroidal rupture, resulting in vitreous and subretinal bleeding. In our type IV cases, Bruch's membranes were complete on OCT. This suggests subfoveal and vitreous hemorrhages may originate from retinal vessels excluding ruptures. In the early phase of injury, due to retinal or vitreous hemorrhage in the fovea/macula; it was difficult to

Optical coherence tomography patterns and outcomes of contusion maculopathy caused...

159

determine if macular holes were present. Type IV contusion maculopathy was defined once a definite macular hole was established. One treatment with SF6 gas tamponade for eyes with type IV can promote absorption of bleeding and early retinal anatomic recovery. In cases 19 and 20, the result of our treatment was effective. Ocular trauma in younger patients demonstrate proliferation of vitreous cortex after absorption of macular hemorrhage. This may be in part facilitated by the presence of a macular hole [12, 14–16]. Case 21 is an example of this. Long-term clinical follow-up of traumatic maculopathy after ocular contusion is important. OCT becomes an important imaging modality in differentiating types of contusion maculopathy. As seen in the cases presented in our study, treatment outcomes and prognosis are directly related to type of OCT imaging seen during follow-up.

Conclusion

The current retrospective study indicated that the changes associated with contusion maculopathy in the early stage (within 1 week) after blunt injury can be divided to four patterns with different outcomes: type 1, macular commotio retinae; type II, incomplete macular hole; type III, macular hole; and type IV macular hemorrhage. Eyes with types I and II can achieve better visual outcomes without surgery (mean ± SD, logMAR. 0.02 ± 0.1 and 0.14 ± 0.21). With types III and IV, a more invasive approach involving vitrectomy and SF6 gas tamponade was required for adequate response in results. OCT imaging is effective in differentiating Type I/II from Type III/IV contusion maculopathy, ultimately altering treatment decision and overall prognosis for patients.

Abbreviations
BCVA: Best-corrected visual acuity; EZ: Ellipsoidal zone; OCT: Optical coherence tomography; ONL: The outer nuclear layer; RPE: Retinal pigment epithelium

Authors' contributions
DL designed the study, and collected data and wrote the manuscript; HA and SK performed the data analysis and revised the manuscript. All authors made substantial contribution to this manuscript meeting authorship criteria, agreed to be accountable for all aspects of the work and have read and approved the final version.

Competing interests
The authors declare that they have no competing interests.

Author details
[1]Department of Ophthalmology, Gunma University School of Medicine, 3-39-15 Showa-machi, Maebashi, Gunma 371-8511, Japan. [2]Aier eye hospital (Cheng Du), 115 Xiyiduan, Yihuanlu,, Chengdu 610041, China. [3]Maebashi Central Eye Clinic, Maebashi, Gunma, Japan.

References
1. Sahraravand A, Haavisto AK, Holopainen JM, Leivo T. Ocular traumas in working age adults in Finland - Helsinki ocular trauma study. Acta Ophthalmol. 2017;95(3):288–94.
2. Miller JB, Yonekawa Y, Eliott D, et al. Long-term follow-up and outcomes in traumatic macular holes. Am J Ophthalmol. 2015;160(6):1255–8.
3. R S, Kusaka S, Ohji M, Gomi F, Ikuno Y, Tano Y. Optical coherence tomographic evaluation of a surgically treated traumatic macular hole secondary to Nd: YAG laser injury. Am J Ophthalmol. 2003;135(4):537–9.
4. WC W, Drenser KA, Trese MT, Williams GA, Capone A. Pediatric traumatic macular hole: results of autologous plasmin enzyme-assisted vitrectomy. Am J Ophthalmol. 2007;144(5):668–72.
5. Itakura H, Kishi S. Restored photoreceptor outer segment in commotio retinae. Ophthalmic Surg Lasers Imaging. 2011;42(3):e29–31. https://doi.org/10.3928/15428877-20110224-03.
6. Schumann RG, Compera D, Schaumberger MM, et al. Epiretinal membrane characteristics correlate with photoreceptor layer defects in lamellar macular holes and macular pseudoholes. Retina. 2015;35(4):727–35.
7. Itoh Y, Levison AL, Kaiser PK. Prevalence and characteristics of hyporeflective preretinal tissue in vitreomacular interface disorders. Br J Ophthalmol. 2016;100(3):399–404.
8. Govetto A, Dacquay Y, Farajzadeh M, et al. Lamellar macular hole: two distinct clinical entities? Am J Ophthalmol. 2016;164:99–109.
9. Hee MR, Puliafito CA, Wong C, et al. Optical coherence tomography of macular holes. Ophthalmology. 1995;102(12):748–56.
10. Takahashi H, Kishi S. Optical coherence tomography images of spontaneous macular hole closure. Am J Ophthalmol. 1999;128(4):519–20.
11. Gass J. Reappraisal of biomicroscopic classification of stages of development of a macular hole. Am J Ophthalmol. 1995;119(6):752–9.
12. Gonvers M, Machemer R. A new approach to treating retinal detachment with macular hole. Am J Ophthalmol. 1982;94(4):468–72.
13. JS R, Glaser BM, Thompson JT, Sjaarda RN, Pappas SS, Murphy RP. Vitrectomy, fluid-gas exchange and transforming growth factor-beta-2 for the treatment of traumatic macular holes. Ophthalmology. 1995;102(12):1840–5.
14. JT T, Glaser BM, Sjaarda RN, Murphy RP. Progression of nuclear sclerosis and long-term visual results of vitrectomy with transforming growth factor beta-2 for macular holes. Am J Ophthalmol. 1995;119(1):48–54.
15. Schepens CL. Fundus changes caused by alterations of the vitreous body. Am J Ophthalmol. 1955;39(5):631-3.
16. Haruhiko Y, Akemi S, Eri Y, Tetsuya N, Miyo M. Spontaneous closure of traumatic macular hole. Am J Ophthalmol. 2002;134(3):340–5.

23

Shielding effect of the smoke plume by the ablation of excimer lasers

Csaba Szekrényesi[1*] (iD), Huba Kiss[2], Tamás Filkorn[2] and Zoltán Zsolt Nagy[1,2]

Abstract

Background: Shielding and scattering effect of the smoke plume column ejected from the laser ablated material is a well-known phenomenon. Debris evacuation system of the excimer laser equipment removes these particles, but insufficient air flow can result in undesired refractive outcomes of the treatment. The aim of this study was to reveal the effect of the air flow speed on the actual ablation depth.

Methods: SCWIND AMARIS 500E flying spot excimer laser was tested in this study. A 150 μm phototherapeutic keratectomy (PTK) profile with 8 mm diameter was applied to the surface of polymethyl methacrylate (PMMA) plates. The velocity of the air flow was changed with adjustable air aspiration system. Ablation depth was measured with highly-precise contact micrometer.

Results: The prediction model was statistically significant, $F(1,8) = 552.85$, $p < 0.001$, and accounted for approximately 98.7% of variance of ablation ($R^2 = 0.987$, $R^2_{adj} = 0.986$). Lower air flow speed resulted in a weaker ablation capability of the excimer laser.

Conclusion: Air flow generated by the aspiration equipment is a key factor for the predictable outcomes of refractive treatment. Therefore, manufacturer inbuilt debris removal system should be regularly checked and maintained to ensure proper clinical and predictable refractive results.

Keywords: Excimer lasers, PMMA, Laser ablation, Refractive surgery

Background

Excimer laser devices are used worldwide for reshaping of the cornea and to change the refractive power of the corneal surface to achieve emmetropia. The high-precision, 193 nm laser pulses created by the excimer laser absorbed by the surface of the cornea and ablated a part of the corneal tissue with a 1 μm precision. The effects of the environmental factors regarding the fluence and efficacy of the excimer laser pulses are an investigated and deeply-researched area, and both of them is important and might have a long-term effect on the results of the excimer laser procedure [1–4]. Other general factors as temperature and humidity in the operation theater have to be kept in a given range. They might have an influence on the stable function and pre-set parameters of the optical system of the excimer laser and on the energy settings as well. The smoke plume generated during by the excimer laser pulses is a well-known phenomenon [5–7]. Beer-Lambert Law shows a non-linear relationship between the laser fluence (F) and depth of the ablation (d).

$$d = 1/\alpha * \ln(F/F_{th})$$

Where F_{th} is the ablation threshold and α is the ablation coefficient. These last two parameters depend on the material to be ablated [8]. The laser energy is absorbed by the material, surface molecules are photoablated and particles are ejaculated from the surface. The generated smoke plume shields and scatters the next laser pulses, decreases the energy load and the achieved ablated depth as well. Therefore to reach the planned ablation depth and profile, by the design of the excimer lasers the smoke plume evacuation system or debris module is an essential part of the device.

To the precise performance of the excimer lasers, PMMA (polymethyl methacrylate) plates are used for the calibration procedure and for regular maintenance

* Correspondence: szekrenyesics@se-etk.hu
[1]Faculty of Health Sciences, Semmelweis University, Vas u. 17, Budapest 1088, Hungary
Full list of author information is available at the end of the article

[9]. Test treatments are applied to the surface of the PMMA plates. The ablated area is measured with contact or non-contact methods [10–15].

The study presented by Dorronsoro et al. [16] shows that the shielding and scattering effect produced by the smoke plume column has a significant influence to the ablation depth by shielding the laser fluence. In this experimental setting the ablation depth on PMMA plates were measured with 4 different air flow settings. Significant relationship was found by the speed of the air flow. From these three air speed settings a mathematical model was created, which suggests that the air flow speed should depends on the repetition rate.

In the present study the ablation depth was investigated during precise experimental conditions and by 10 different air flow speed settings and a statistical relationship was found between the air flow speed caused by the smoke plume evacuation system. Compared to the results of Dorronsoro in this article authors evaluated more technical settings of the smoke plume evacuation unit in order to reveal more accurate statistical relationship and clinical significance to achieve precise ablation depth and the best postoperative refraction.

Methods

Last-generation SCHWIND AMARIS 500E flying spot excimer platform (SCHWIND eye-tech solutions Gmbh, Kleinostheim, Germany) was used in this study. This laser platform is able to perform myopic, hyperopic, astigmatic and higher order customized treatments as well. Relevant parameters are: 193 nm wavelength, 0.54 mm Super-Gaussian laser-spot profile, 500 Hz repetition rate, flying-spot ablation strategy.

The air flow speed was measured with TESTO 405-V1 anemometer (accuracy: ± (0.3 m/s ± 5% of mv)).

The SCHWIND AMARIS 500E used to these study works with a manufacturer-modified plume evacuator system, which based on the suction only. The fix speed, external plume evacuator offered by the manufacturer was exchanged in this study to adjustable external smoke evacuation equipment (Smoke Evacuator) (Edge Systems Corporations, Redondo Beach, CA, USA). Only the evacuator equipment was exchanged. The patient-side mechanics, the debris suction module, the debris nozzle, the air-pipelines and the main tube which leads to the external evacuator were identical with the manufacturer-offered plume evacuation system in all cases during the study. The experimental layout can be seen on the Fig. 1.

The voltage and current of the rotor of the evacuation system were adjusted manually with a button on the control panel of the equipment continuously from 1 to 9 scaled linearly. The evacuator system is able to work standalone, without the control of the laser device as well. The laser starts and stops the external evacuator, but it is possible to start and stop manually. Every suction speed measurement was conducted with the anemometer at the mouth of the debris suction nozzle in the same position.

Airflow speed was measured after the evacuator was set to a certain step. 150 μm PTK treatments were performed in 8 mm diameter on three PMMA plates without changing the setting of the evacuator. After finishing three treatments on the same level of suction speed, the airflow was measured again to find out, if the airflow speed was changed during the treatments. This

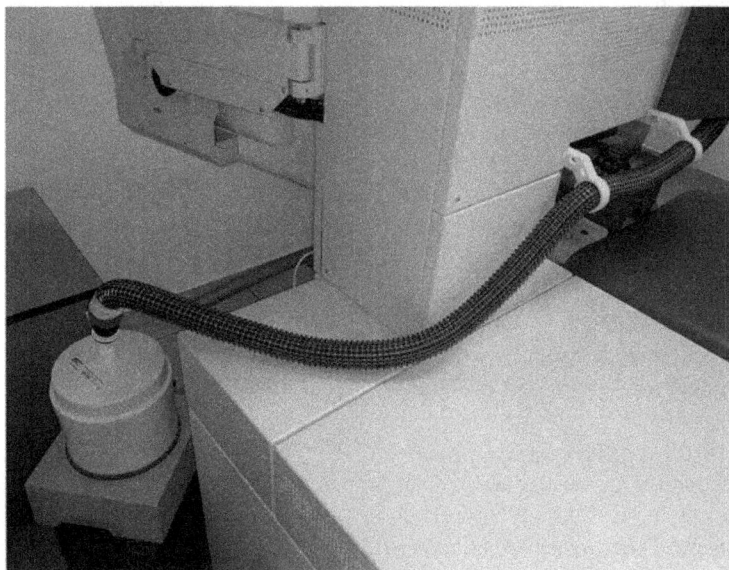

Fig. 1 Photo about the experimental layout of the study

procedure was repeated on 9 different settings of the evacuator from the lowest possible airflow to the maximum suction level, the air speed values were in the range of 4.6 to 7.4 m/s.

According to our experiences the suction speed was unchanged before and after the measurement of a certain setting of the evacuator. This indicates a steady, constant relation between the setting of the evacuator and the suction power. Since the suction characteristic of the evacuation system was unknown, the measured air velocity values were used for the statistical calculations. Once the evacuator was adjusted to a certain airflow setting, three ablations on three different PMMA plates were performed without any adjustment of the evacuator. Therefore the error of the evacuator was taken in the statistical calculation as a constant value, regarding to our airflow speed measurements before and after the ablation. Therefore the study did not calculate with the error propagation.

This external evacuation system is equipped with HEPA (high-efficiency particulate arrestance) pre- and main filter combination.

Round shaped flat PMMA plates (28 mm diameter, 4 mm height) were used for the measurement of the ablation depth of the test treatment. This plate is equal to the PMMA plate used by daily calibration procedure of the Wavelight Allegretto 400 (Alcon Wavelight, Erlangen, Germany) provided by the company. Energy calibration was performed and flatness of each PMMA plate was checked before the ablation with zeroing of the micrometer. Manufacturer-offered mechanical adapter holding a spirit level was applied to ensure the central position and the tilting of the surface of the samples to ensure the exactly perpendicular position of the optical axis of the instrument. Tilting of the adapter was corrected with thin metal sheets. The height and the horizontal adjustment were maintained during the whole measurement procedure. The PMMA plates are transparent, an artificial pupil was used by the backside surface of the PMMA made from a paper sheet with a round-shaped 4 mm diameter hole, to direct the position of the test treatment within the center of the round-shaped surface.

Humidity was during the measurement 35% ± 5%, temperature was 22.5 °C ± 0.5 °C in the operation theatre.

The achieved central ablation depth was measured with a calibrated contact micrometer, Inductive Dial Comparator 2000 (Mahr, Göttingen, Germany) with 901 R type standard contact point (accuracy: ±0.2 μm). The contact point of the micrometer is a ruby ball with 3 mm diameter, which measures in the center of the ablation area. The measurement area considered to be point-like. During this study every PMMA plate was measured once. Sixty seconds waiting time has been kept after the ablation and before the measurement to stabilize the surface of the PMMA.

The percent differences between each two ablation depths of the same air-flow velocity were calculated. A collapsed variable from the three measurements were calculated. Linear regression was conducted to predict the ablation depth from the air flow velocity. Statistical analysis was performed using OriginPro 9 (OriginLab Corp., Northampton, MA, USA). A p-value of < 0.05 was considered statistically significant.

Results

As no significant difference was observed between the percent difference of every two measurements (percent differences: 0.00–2.29, M = 1.02, SD = 0.57) a collapsed variable was calculated from the three measurements, which is a mean value (Table 1). A simple linear regression was calculated to predict the central ablation depth based on the air velocity. A significant equation was found (F(1,8) = 552.85, $p < 0.001$). The results of the regression indicated the velocity explained 98.7% of the variance ($R^2 = 0.987$, $R^2_{adj} = 0.986$) (Fig. 2.)

Discussion

One of the most important calibration measures is the preventive, regular maintenance and calibration of the excimer laser devices used by refractive surgery. The other important one is the analysis of optical results of artificial treatments on specific polymer plates. PMMA plates are widely used to test the ablation depth and to guarantee the refractive results of the excimer laser equipment from the first step of the design to the user-side daily calibration procedure [8–11].

Authors in a preliminary study verified that beside the optical outcomes the test treatments on PMMA are able to evaluate the corneal temperature changes during and short by after refractive treatment as well [1].

Other studies show, that shielding effect due to the insufficient air aspiration might be an important cause of

Table 1 Percent difference and descriptive statistical indicators. M refers to the mean of the measured central ablation depths at given air flow velocity

Air flow velocity	Percent difference			Collapsed indicators [μm]		
[m/s]	AB	AC	BC	M	SD	SE
4.6	0.63	0.63	0.00	63.87	0.23	0.13
4.9	0.63	1.56	0.93	64.27	0.50	0.29
5.3	0.31	1.55	1.23	64.60	0.53	0.31
5.5	0.93	2.16	1.23	64.67	0.70	0.41
5.7	0.46	1.84	1.38	65.10	0.62	0.36
6.1	0.77	2.29	1.52	65.37	0.76	0.44
6.4	0.46	1.37	0.91	65.50	0.46	0.26
6.7	0.46	1.36	0.91	65.90	0.46	0.26
7.4	0.15	0.90	1.06	66.27	0.38	0.22

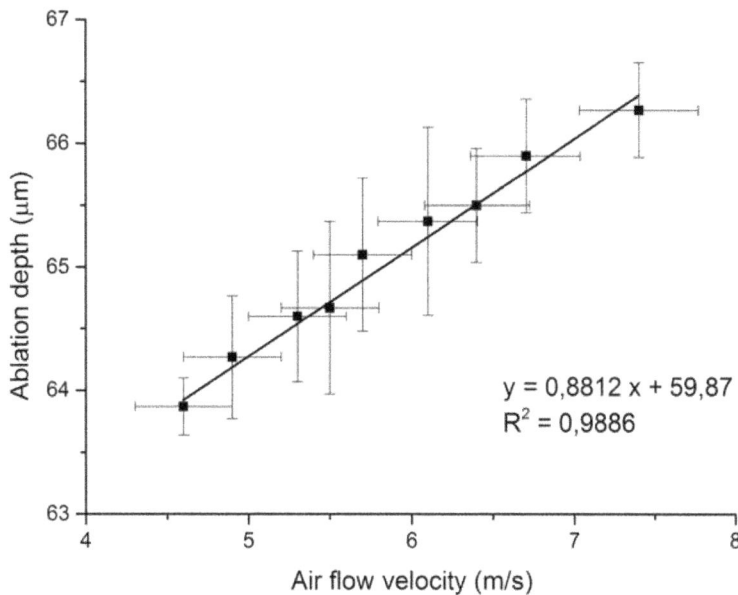

Fig. 2 Correlation between the velocity of air flow and the ablation depth

asymmetrical surface after treatment with undesired refractive outcomes [16].

Others suggest that the circumstances of the treatment could have an influence on the long-term refractive results and biomechanical condition of the cornea [3, 4, 9, 17, 18].

Authors of the current study hypothesized a relationship between the shielding effect and the strength of the air aspiration. A deeper understanding of the effect of the evacuation will help to increase the predictability of the short and long-term refractive outcomes and the quality of vision.

During the study authors observed the ejection of the particles from the surface and the development of the smoke plume column without evacuation. Increasing the evacuation power this smoke plume column begins to be removed by the evacuation system. A stronger evacuation power results more evacuated part of the column and reduces the shielding effect. A linear correlation was found between the air velocity and the shielding effect.

The conclusions found are limited to PMMA and should not be directly applied to the corneal conditions. The corneal smoke plume generation and shielding differs from the PMMA [7], which is one of the limitations of this study. The examination of the repeatability with more measurements and corneal application could be the subject of future studies.

Conclusions

Decreasing ablation effect was found due to the shielding effect of the ejected particles from the surface of PMMA plates which are widely used to calibration of excimer lasers. This effect can be caused by insufficient power of the smoke plume evacuation system. Linear correlation was found between the air flow speed and the ablation depth. It suggests an optimal ratio, and requires the regular check-ups and maintenance of the factory settings of the in-build debris removal equipment of excimer laser devices.

The debris generation, and the scattering and shielding effect depend on the ablated material. The cornea has lower particle ejection, and the dynamics of the corneal smoke plume is faster. Therefore, the obtained conclusions related to the examined PMMA material only and should not be directly extrapolated to the clinical circumstances. However the findings of our study suggest that the effect of the airflow speed to the ablation depth exist by corneal ablation as well.

The results of the study indicate the importance of the maintenance of the proper smoke plume evacuation system, which may have an influence on the short and long-term outcome of the refractive procedures performed on the cornea.

Based on the findings of this study, it is recommended to use air flow setting of the debris suction determined by the manufacturer, which should be measured and tested by every technical security check of the laser equipment.

Abbreviations
HEPA: High-efficiency particulate arrestance; PMMA: Polymethyl methacrylate; PTK: Phototherapeutic keratectomy

Acknowledgements
Many thanks to Dr. Erika Tátrai, Johanna Takács and István E. Ferincz for the valuable advices.

Funding
The authors declare that they have no funding.

Authors' contributions
CS: design of the measurement. CS, TF, HK, NZZ: analysis of the measurement data. All authors read and approved the final manuscript.

Competing interests
The authors declare that they have no competing interests.

Author details
[1]Faculty of Health Sciences, Semmelweis University, Vas u. 17, Budapest 1088, Hungary. [2]Department of Ophthalmology, Semmelweis University, Budapest, Hungary.

References
1. Szekrényesi C, Sándor GL, Gyenes A, Kiss H, Filkorn T, Nagy Z. Relationship between corneal surface temperature and air flow conditions during refractive laser eye surgery using three different excimer lasers. Orv Hetil. 2016;157(43):1717–21.
2. Dantas PE, Martins CL, de Souza LB, Dantas MC. Do environmental factors influence excimer laser pulse fluence and efficacy? J Refract Surg. 2007; 23(3):307–9.
3. Maldonado-Codina C, Morgan PB, Efron N. Thermal consequences of photorefractive keratoectomy. Cornea. 2001;20:509–15.
4. Müller B, Boeck T, Hartmann C. Effect of excimer laser beam delivery and beam shaping on corneal sphericity in photorefractive keratectomy. J Cataract Refract Surg. 2004 Feb;30(2):464–70.
5. Bor Z, Hopp B, Rácz B, Szabó G, Ratkay I, Süveges I, Füst A, Mohay J. Plume emission, shock wave and surface wave formation during excimer laser ablation of the cornea. Refract Corneal Surg. 1993 Mar-Apr;9(2 Suppl):S111–5.
6. Hahn DW, Ediger MN, Pettit GH. Dynamics of ablation plume particles generated during excimer laser corneal ablation. Lasers Surg Med. 1995; 16(4):384–9.
7. Noack J, Tönnies R, Hohla K, Birngruber R, Vogel A. Influence of ablation plume dynamics on the formation of central islands in excimer laser photorefractive keratectomy. Ophthalmology. 1997 May;104(5):823–30.
8. Dorronsoro C, Siegel J, Remon L, Marcos S. Suitability of Filofocon A and PMMA for experimental models in excimer laser ablation refractive surgery. Opt Express. 2008;16(25):20955–67.
9. Szekrényesi C, Réz K, Nagy ZZ. Surface temperature change of PMMA plates in refractive surgery performed with two types of modern excimer lasers. New Med. 2016;20(4):126–9. https://doi.org/10.5604/14270994.1228144.
10. Gottsch JD, Rencs EV, Cambier JL. Excimer laser calibration system. J Refract Surg. 1996;12(3):401–11.
11. Doga AV, Shpak AA, Sugrobov VA. Smoothness of ablation on polymethylmethacrylate plates with four scanning excimer lasers. J Refract Surg. 2004;20(5 suppl):730–3.
12. Naroo SA, Charman WN. Surface roughness after excimer laser ablation using a PMMA model: profilometry and effects on vision. J Refract Surg. 2005;21(3):260–8.
13. Wernli J, Schumacher S, Wuellner C, et al. Initial surface temperature of PMMA plates used for daily laser calibration to control the predictability of corneal refractive surgery. J Refract Surg. 2012;28(9):639–44.
14. Arba-Mosquera S, Shraiki M. Analysis of the PMMA and cornea temperature rise during excimer laser ablation. J Mod Opt. 2010;57(5):400–7.
15. Zhao MH, Wu Q, Jia LL, Hu P. Changes in central corneal thickness and refractive error after thin-flap laser in situ keratomileusis in Chinese eyes. BMC Ophthalmol. 2015;15:86. https://doi.org/10.1186/s12886-015-0083-2.
16. Dorronsoro C, Schumacher S, Pérez-Merino P, Siegel J, Mrochen M, Marcos S. Effect of air-flow on the evaluation of refractive surgery ablation patterns. Opt Express. 2011;19(5):4653–66. https://doi.org/10.1364/OE.19.004653.
17. Kim JM, Kim JC, Park WC, Seo JS, Chang HR. Effect of thermal preconditioning before excimer laser photoablation. J Korean Med Sci. 2004 Jun;19(3):437–46.
18. Kymionis GD, Diakonis VF, Kounis G, Bouzoukis DI, Gkenos E, Ginis H, Yoo SH, Pallikaris IG. Effect of excimer laser repetition rate on outcomes after photorefractive keratectomy. J Cataract Refract Surg. 2008;34(6):916–9. https://doi.org/10.1016/j.jcrs.2008.02.022.

24

Analysis of differences in intraocular pressure evaluation performed with contact and non-contact devices

Michele Lanza[1][*] [iD], Michele Rinaldi[1], Ugo Antonello Gironi Carnevale[1], Silvio di Staso[2], Mario Bifani Sconocchia[1] and Ciro Costagliola[3]

Abstract

Background: To evaluate differences of intraocular pressure (IOP) measurements performed with Goldmann applanation tonometer (GAT), dynamic contour tonometer (DCT), rebound tonometry (RT), Ocular Response Analyzer (ORA) and Corvis ST (CST) in eyes screened for refractive surgery.

Methods: One eye, only the right one, of 146 patients was included in this study. Each participant was submitted to a corneal analysis with Scheimpflug camera and IOP evaluation with GAT, DCT, RT, ORA and CST. Differences in IOP values obtained thanks to each instruments were compared and then correlations between these discrepancies and morphological features such as mean keratometry (MK) and central corneal thickness (CCT) provided by Pentacam were studied. Software used to run statistical evaluations was SPSS, version 18.0.

Results: Study participants had a mean age of 33.1 ± 9.2 years old. IOP values observed in this study were 15.97 ± 2.47 mmHg (GAT), 17.55 ± 2.42 mmHg (DCT), 17.49 ± 2.08 mmHg (RT), 18.51 ± 2.59 mmHg (ORA) and 18.33 ± 2.31 mmHg (CST). The mean CCT was 560.23 ± 31.00 μm, and the mean MK was 43.33 ± 1.35 D. GAT provided significant lower values in comparison to all other devices. DCT and RT gave significantly lower intermediate IOP values than those measured with ORA and CST. All the IOP measures and the differences between devices were significantly correlated with CCT.

Conclusions: According to our data, although our findings should be confirmed in further studies, GAT tonometer cannot be used interchangeably with DCT, RT, ORA and CST.

Keywords: Innovative technology, Scheimpflug camera, Goldmann applanation tonometry, Corvis, naïve eyes, Healthy eyes, Rebound tonometry, ORA, No contact tonometry

Background

Intraocular pressure (IOP) evaluation is a crucial phase of a routine eye examination, particularly for glaucoma patients. Indeed, in these cases, elevated IOP is the only risk factor that physicians are able to modify [1]. This is the reason for the importance of the patient's IOP value: it is a crucial element of glaucoma diagnosis and management [2].

Goldmann applanation tonometry (GAT) represents the "gold standard" method for IOP evaluation [3]. However, many factors may affect its precision. Among these, there are those related to the morphology of the eye, such as central corneal thickness (CCT) or corneal curvature, and those related to corneal biomechanical properties. CCT has been demonstrated to bias IOP measurements by GAT, inducing IOP underestimation in thin corneas and overestimation in thick ones [4]. Different formulas have been used to improve GAT precision, in an attempt to adjust IOP on the basis of CCT, but there is still not one capable of providing reliable and precise results [3, 5]. In order to overcome the problem, new tonometers have been developed. These have been designed to avoid the bias related not only to the corneal morphological

---
* Correspondence: mic.lanza@gmail.com
[1]Multidisciplinary Department of Medical, Surgical and Dental Sciences, Università della Campania, Luigi Vanvitelli, Via de Crecchio 16, 80100 Naples, Italy
Full list of author information is available at the end of the article

properties and ocular surface, but also to corneal biomechanical properties, even though the real influence of the latter has not yet been completely established [6–12]. The most important goal of new devices to measure IOP is to provide accurate evaluations, free from the well-known limitations of GAT [13, 14]. Dynamic contour tonometry [6] (DCT Swiss Microtechnology AG, Port, Switzerland), rebound tonometry [9] (RT, Icare, Tiolat Oy, Helsinki, Finland), Ocular Response Analyzer [7] (ORA, Reichert, Buffalo, NY, USA) and Corvis ST [10] (CST, Oculus, Wetzlar, Germany) are devices capable of measuring IOP in different ways and they have been evaluated and compared to GAT in healthy subjects in this study.

Although studies on repeatability, reproducibility and comparisons among tonometers have already been published [12, 15–24], for the first time we provide a comparison among these 5 devices in naïve eyes and an analysis of differences related to corneal morphological parameters in a large population.

Methods

In this prospective study 146 consecutive healthy subjects (62 females and 84 males), screened for refractive surgery, were included and evaluated. Every participant with any kind of illness (systemic or ocular) which could potentially affect the measurements of the parameters analyzed in the study were excluded, in order to have an unbiased statistical evaluation. Contact lens-wearing participants were asked to stop using them at least one week prior to examination. As protocol of the study, a routine eye examination was performed together with a Pentacam (Oculus, Wezlar, Germany) scan and IOP evaluations with GAT, DCT, RT, ORA and CST.

The Oculus Pentacam is a device which provides information in the form of maps and data regarding anterior and posterior corneal surface, depth of anterior chamber, corneal thickness and details about the lens [25]. Among the parameters it provides to measure anterior corneal power, Sim'K (MK) and CCT at pupil center were selected to be analyzed in this study.

DCT (Swiss MicrotechnologyAG, Port, Switzerland) is a contact tonometry that relies on the law of Blaise Pascal hydrostatic pressure [6].

RT is a contact tonometer that allows the measurement of the IOP thanks to a very small magnetized probe [9].

ORA is a non-contact device able to evaluate IOP by taking into account corneal biomechanical properties [7].

CST (Oculus, Wetzlar, Germany) is a recently introduced non-contact device that analyzes corneal deformation due to a constant air puff impulse. By measuring corneal deformation, this device provides some corneal biomechanical characteristics and IOP evaluations [10].

After Pentacam evaluation, ORA, CST, RT, DCT and GAT measurements were taken in this sequence in order to obtain the most accurate IOP evaluations possible, reducing errors due to potential corneal deformation. Thus, the more "invasive" devices were used at the end. Each measurement was performed 10 min after the previous one, and three consecutive IOP measurements for each instrument were collected and averaged; the mean value was utilized for statistical evaluations.

All IOP evaluations were completed between 2:00 pm and 4:00 pm. Eyes with corneal anomalies, such as corneal thickness increase, corneal disepithelization or corneal curvature alterations, documented at the end of IOP measurements, were also excluded from the study. Each device was associated with an operator who performed the evaluation, unaware of the results obtained by the other physicians with the other equipments.

Study participants signed an informed consent form before starting examinations; this study followed the ethical standards of the 1964 Declaration of Helsinki and approved by the local clinical research ethics committee.

Statistical analysis

Even though both eyes of the participants were evaluated, only the right eye was selected to be used in the statistical analysis in order to avoid any potential intra-subject effect. Normality of distribution of the study population was analyzed with the Kolmogorov-Smirnov test. In this study analysis of differences and correlations of data not reaching the normality standards was performed using non-parametric tests. Particularly, a Friedman test, as a non-parametric alternative to ANOVA, was performed, followed by a post-hoc Wilcoxon signed rank test to evaluate comparisons among values obtained from different instruments. Moreover, considering that we did 10 pairwise comparisons, p-value of each comparison was adjusted using the Bonferroni method (pa = px10). Furthermore, the correlations among CCT and MK vs IOP values obtained with tested devices were evaluated using non-parametric (Spearman) tests. After analysis of the study population and evaluation of the error of the tested devices, the level of significance was set at $p < 0.05$ for all statistical tests. Statistical evaluations were performed using SPSS software (IBM Corp. Armonk, New York) version 18.0.

Table 1 Clinical characteristics of patients included in the study

Characteristic	Mean ± SD	Range
Age (year)	33.10 ± 9.22	from 19 to 55
Spherical equivalent (D)	−4.65 ± 2.03	from − 10.25 to 0
Corneal curvature (D)	43.33 ± 1.35	from 40.1 to 46.6
Corneal pachymetry at pupil center (μm)	560.23 ± 31.00	from 500 to 665

SD standard deviation

Table 2 IOP differences between tested tonometers (mmHg, Wilcoxon test)

	Mean (mmHg)	p_a value
DCT - GAT	+ 1.580	0.0001
ORA - DCT	+ 0.958	0.0001
DCT - RT	+ 0.064	0.62
CST - DCT	+ 0.775	0.0001
ORA - GAT	+ 2.538	0.0001
RT - GAT	+ 1.516	0.0001
CST - GAT	+ 2.355	0.0001
ORA - RT	+ 1.022	0.0001
ORA - CST	+ 0.183	0.194
CST - RT	+ 0.839	0.0001

Legend: Legend: Mean IOP difference between tested devices (pa: Bonferroni adjusted p-value); Corvis ST (CST), Ocular Response Analyzer (ORA), rebound tonometry (RT), dynamic contour tonometer (DCT) and Goldmann applanation tonometer (GAT)

Results

The participants in the study were aged between 19 and 55 years old (mean: 33.1 ± 9.22 years) with a mean refraction, calculated as spherical equivalent (SE), of -4.65 ± 2.03 D (ranging from -10.25 D to 0 D). In particular, there were 47 eyes with myopia, 98 ones with myopic astigmatism and only one with mixed astigmatism. Details of demographical and morphological parameters of the subjects included in this study are shown in Table 1. Table 2 and Fig. 1 show the IOP values obtained with the tested instruments. A preliminary analysis confirmed significant differences among the values of different instruments (F_R: 288.71, d.f. 4, $p < 0.001$; Friedman test). Overall, GAT values showed significantly lower values in comparison with those obtained from other devices. IOP measurements obtained by the tested tonometers were plotted by the means of Bland et Altman plots (Fig. 2). ORA showed the largest IOP overestimation compared to GAT ($+ 2.54$ mmHg; $p_a < 0.001$, Fig. 2b). Differences between CST and GAT ($+ 2.35$ mmHg; $p_a < 0.001$, Fig. 2d), between DCT and GAT ($+ 1.58$ mmHg; $p_a < 0.001$, Fig. 2a) and between RT and GAT ($+ 1.52$ mmHg; $p_a < 0.001$ Fig. 2c) were also significant.

Table 3 shows the correlations and their significances between IOP values provided by the tested devices and other parameters such as age, spherical equivalent, MK and CCT.

Discussion

Lowering IOP is the most important aid that physicians can offer to block or reduce glaucoma progression [1], thus a precise and reliable estimation of this is extremely important. Because glaucoma is a chronic degenerative disease and IOP values must be recorded for a patient's whole life, it is extremely important that a device able to measure IOP without any bias should be available for eye doctors. It is well known that the current gold standard, GAT, does not always provide very precise measurements but new IOP measuring devices haven't shown uniform accuracy, according to previously published papers [12, 21–29].

Each tonometer tested in this study evaluates IOP with different working principles; three are contact tonometers (GAT, DCT and RT) whereas two do not require any contact (ORA and CST). Even though each one

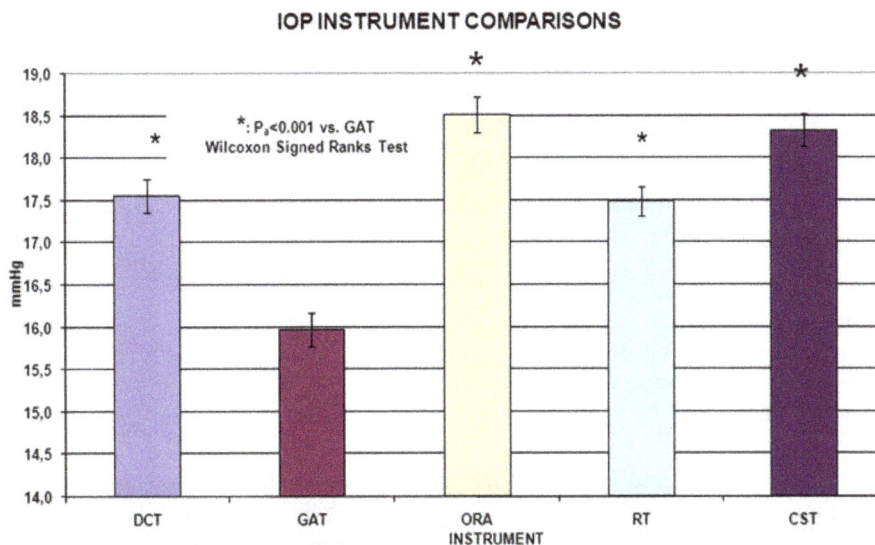

Fig. 1 Range (expressed as mean ± standard deviation) of intraocular pressure measurements in healthy participants observed using Ocular Response Analyzer, Goldmann tonometer, Dynamic Contour Tonometry, Rebound tonometer and Corvis tonometer; statistical differences expressed as * when $p_a < 0.001$

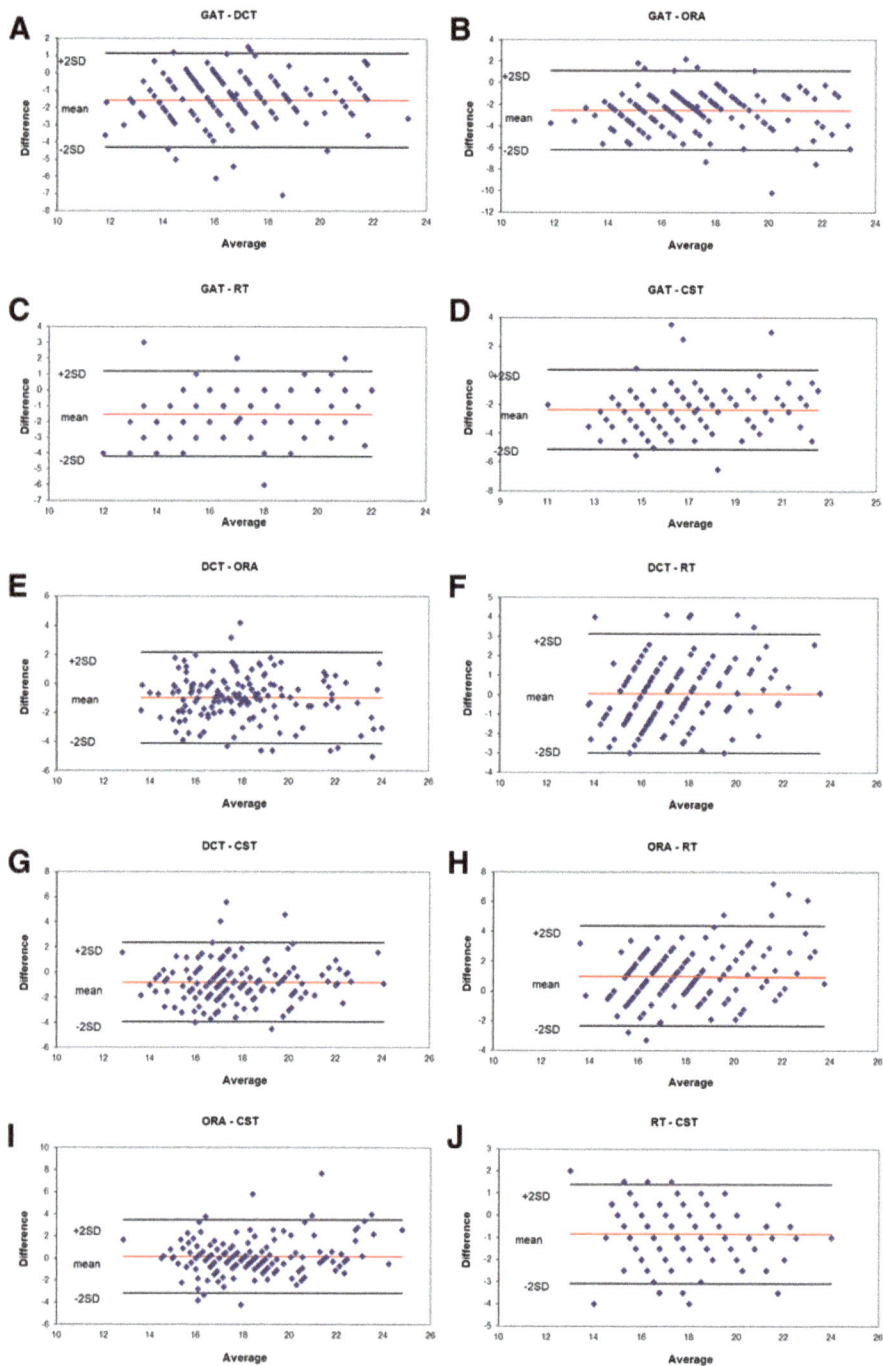

Fig. 2 Bland & Altman plots. **a** Goldman vs Dynamic Contour Tonometry; **b** Goldman vs Ocular Response Analyser; **c** Goldman vs Rebound tonometry; **d** Goldman vs Corvis tonometry; **e** Dynamic Contour Tonometry vs Ocular Response Analyser; **f** Dynamic Contour Tonometry vs rebound tonometry; **g** Dynamic Contour Tonometry vs Corvis; **h** Ocular Response Analyser vs rebound tonometry; **i** Ocular Response Analyser vs Corvis tonometry; **j** Rebound tonometry vs Corvis

resulted in some way as being dependent on CCT, CST seems to be influenced by MK too (Table 3).

DCT, as already reported by Schneider et al. [26], is more suitable for measuring IOP in cooperative patients with sufficient bilateral ocular fixation, however, some patients are not sufficiently compliant. ORA and CST,

being non-contact tonometers, are less invasive for patients and thus they can also be used particularly in clinical situations where it is better to avoid direct corneal contact (corneal infections, recent corneal surgery). RT operates through very soft and well-tolerated contact between the probe and the cornea; however, its results

Table 3 Correlations between IOP, as obtained from tested tonometers, and age, spherical equivalent (SE), corneal curvature (MK) and central corneal thickness (CCT)

Correlations

		AGE	SE	MK	CCT
DCT	Spearman's rho	−0.117	0.025	−0.067	0.470
	Sig. (2-tailed)	0.159	0.762	0.422	**0.0001**
	N	146	146	146	146
GAT	Spearman's rho	−0.143	0.102	−0.043	0.625
	Sig. (2-tailed)	0.085	0.221	0.608	**0.0001**
	N	146	146	146	146
ORA	Spearman's rho	−0.089	−0.029	−0.096	0.413
	Sig. (2-tailed)	0.283	0.732	0.251	**0.0001**
	N	146	146	146	146
RT	Spearman's rho	−0.114	0.072	−0.098	0.519
	Sig. (2-tailed)	0.172	0.389	0.240	**0.0001**
	N	146	146	146	146
CST	Spearman's rho	−0.104	0.040	−0.201	0.522
	Sig. (2-tailed)	0.210	0.633	**0.015**	**0.0001**
	N	146	146	146	146

Legend: Corvis ST (CST), Ocular Response Analyzer (ORA), rebound tonometry (RT), dynamic contour tonometer (DCT) and Goldmann applanation tonometer (GAT). Highlighted values are the correlations resulted to be significant

could be affected by tear film more than the other tested devices [24].

Each tonometer alternative to GAT tested in this study provided significantly higher IOP values, probably because of their working principles. It is not possible to establish which one is the most reliable, since they should be compared with real IOP measurements obtained only by intraocular probe.

The results observed herein agree with most of the previously published papers analyzing the differences among tested devices on healthy subjects [11, 12, 17, 19–22, 24, 26–29]. In this study, a strict measurement order going from the less supposedly "invasive" device for cornea to the one considered to be the most "invasive", was followed, whereas in other papers a random order was often adopted [10, 29]. The order of IOP measurements chosen in this study may introduce some other kind of bias, due to the fixed sequence and to the number of devices tested. In this paper differences between ORA and CST are not statistically significant whereas a statistical difference of 1.25 mmHg was observed in a previous paper by the same group of authors [11]. The explanations for this data could be related to different reasons: the group of healthy subjects analyzed in this paper is larger (146 vs 76) compared to the previous one, no participants of the other study contributed to this one, CST software has changed over time and this could be one of the reasons for these different observed results. It is important to

underline that the refractive defect of the participants in the study is mostly myopic; this need to be considered in comparison with other papers.

Another limit of this study could be related to the long time (about 40 min) which was needed to perform all the IOP measurements on the participants, because an IOP fluctuation occurs during this time. It is important to underline that, in order to minimize this kind of bias, every IOP evaluation was performed between 2:00 pm and 4:00 pm and during this time IOP fluctuation has been demonstrated to be about 0.5 mmHg whereas it is much higher in the early hours of the morning, about 2 mmHg from 7:00 a.m. to 9:00 a.m. [30, 31].

Comparing devices capable of measuring IOP is always a complex procedure, also because physicians are currently using instruments that perform indirect evaluations. There are few studies comparing the IOP obtained with these devices with IOP recorded with invasive intra-cameral manometry of the anterior chamber [32]. Even though both healthy subjects and glaucoma patients are evaluated in this study, the authors found an overestimation of DCT compared to GAT and that manometric IOP values are lower than GAT ones [32]. This could be useful to take in account the differences of the tonometers evaluated in this study.

Conclusions

Results observed in the current study suggest that each device evaluated provides an overestimation of IOP compared to GAT. This is not claiming that one of them is more accurate than the others but, according to this data, it is still not possible to obtain IOP values which are not influenced by corneal morphological parameters and if one of these new tonometers is adopted as the gold standard in the future, new IOP limits need to be set when evaluating the risk of the development of glaucoma.

Funding

This research has not received any specific grants from funding agencies in the public, commercial, or non-profit sectors.

Authors' contributions

ML and CC contributed to the design of this study, and the acquisition and analysis of data. ML drafted and revised the manuscript. MBS and CC critically revised the manuscript. MR, UAGC, SDS and MBS acquired and analysed data. All authors read and approved the final manuscript.

Competing interests

The authors declare that there are no competing interests.

Author details
[1]Multidisciplinary Department of Medical, Surgical and Dental Sciences, Università della Campania, Luigi Vanvitelli, Via de Crecchio 16, 80100 Naples, Italy. [2]Ophthalmology Unit, Department of Life, Health and Environmental Sciences, University of L'Aquila, L'Aquila, Italy. [3]Department of Medicine and Healthy Sciences, Università del Molise, Campobasso, Italy.

References
1. Coleman AL, Miglior S. Risk factors for glaucoma onset and progression. Surv Ophthalmol. 2008;53(Suppl1):S3–10.
2. Arora R, Bellamy H, Austin M. Applanation tonometry: a comparison of the Perkins handheld and Goldmann slit lamp-mounted methods. Clin Ophthalmol. 2014;26(8):605–10.
3. Standardization IOf. Ophthalmic Instruments—Tonometers: ISO8612:2001. Geneva, Switzerland: International Organization for Standardization. 2001.
4. Wang J, Cayer MM, Descovich D, Kamdeu-Fansi A, Harasymowycz PJ, Li G, Lesk MR. Assessment of factors affecting the difference in intraocular pressure measurements between dynamic contour tonometry and goldmann applanation tonometry. J Glaucoma. 2011;20(8):482–7.
5. Brandt JD, Gordon MO, Gao F, Beiser JA, Miller JP, Kass MA. Adjusting intraocular pressure for central corneal thickness does not improve prediction models for primary open-angle glaucoma. Ophthalmology. 2012;119:437–42.
6. Kanngiesser HE, Kniestedt C, Robert YC. Dynamic contour tonometry: presentation of a new tonometer. J Glaucoma. 2005;14:344–50.
7. Luce DA. Determining in vivo biomechanical properties of the cornea with an ocular response analyzer. J Cataract Refract Surg. 2005;31:156–62.
8. Medeiros FA, Weinreb RN. Evaluation of the influence of corneal biomechanical properties on intraocular pressure measurements using the ocular response analyzer. J Glaucoma. 2006;15:364–70.
9. Kontiola AI. A new induction-based impact method for measuring intraocular pressure. Acta Ophthalmol Scand. 2000;78:142–5.
10. Hong J, Xu J, Wei A, Deng SX, Cui X, Yu X, Sun X. A new tonometer--the Corvis ST tonometer: clinical comparison with noncontact and Goldmann applanation tonometers. Invest Ophthalmol Vis Sci. 2013;54(1):659–65.
11. Lanza M, Iaccarino S, Mele L, Carnevale UA, Irregolare C, Lanza A, Femiano F, Bifani M. Intraocular pressure evaluation in healthy eyes and diseased ones using contact and non contact devices. Cont Lens Anterior Eye. 2016;39(2):154–9.
12. Lanza M, Iaccarino S, Cennamo M, Irregolare C, Romano V, Carnevale UA. Comparison between Corvis and other tonometers in healthy eyes. Cont Lens Anterior Eye. 2015;38(2):94–8.
13. Brandt JD, Beiser JA, Kass MA, Gordon MO. Central corneal thickness in the ocular hypertension treatment study (OHTS). Ophthalmology. 2001;108:1779–88.
14. Whitacre MM, Stein R. Sources of error with use of Goldmann-type tonometers. Surv Ophthalmol. 1993;38:1–30.
15. Hon Y, Lam AK. Corneal deformation measurement using Scheimpflug noncontact tonometry. Optom Vis Sci. 2013;90:e1–8.
16. Reznicek L, Muth D, Kampik A, Neubauer AS, Hirneiss C. Evaluation of a novel Scheimpflug-based non-contact tonometer in healthy subjects and patients with ocular hypertension and glaucoma. Br J Ophthalmol. 2013;97:1410–4.
17. Lanza M, Borrelli M, De Bernardo M, Filosa ML, Rosa N. Corneal parameters and difference between goldmann applanation tonometry and dynamic contour tonometry in normal eyes. J Glaucoma. 2008;17:460–4.
18. Fogagnolo P, Figus M, Frezzotti P, Iester M, Oddone F, Zeppieri M, et al. Test-retest variability of intraocular pressure and ocular pulse amplitude for dynamic contour tonometry: a multicentre study. Br J Ophthalmol. 2010;94:419–23.
19. Ceruti P, Morbio R, Marraffa M, Marchini G. Comparison of Goldmann applanation tonometry and dynamic contour tonometry in healthy and glaucomatous eyes. Eye (Lond). 2009;23:262–9.
20. Heinrich MA, Eppig T, Langenbucher A, Walter S, Behrens-Baumann W, Viestenz A. Comparison of Goldmann applanation and dynamic contour tonometry before and after cataract surgery. J Cataract Refract Surg. 2012;38:683–9.
21. Hsu SY, Sheu MM, Hsu AH, Wu KY, Yeh JI, Tien JN, Tsai RK. Comparisons of intraocular pressure measurements: Goldmann applanation tonometry, noncontact tonometry, Tono-pen tonometry, and dynamic contour tonometry. Eye (Lond). 2009;23(7):1582–8.
22. Mollan SP, Wolffsohn JS, Nessim M, Laiquzzaman M, Sivakumar S, Hartley S, Shah S. Accuracy of Goldmann, ocular response analyser, Pascal and TonoPen XL tonometry in keratoconic and normal eyes. Br J Ophthalmol. 2008;92(12):1661–5.
23. Kotecha A, White E, Schlottmann PG, Garway-Heath DF. Intraocular pressure measurement precision with the Goldmann applanation, dynamic contour, and ocular response analyzer tonometers. Ophthalmology. 2010;117:730–7.
24. Avitabile T, Longo A, Rocca D, Amato R, Gagliano C, Castaing M. The influence of refractive errors on IOP measurement by rebound tonometry (ICare) and Goldmann applanation tonometry. Graefes Arch Clin Exp Ophthalmol. 2010;248(4):585–91.
25. Rosa N, De Bernardo M, Borrelli M, Filosa ML, Lanza M. Effect of oxybuprocaine eye drops on corneal volume and thickness measurements. Optom Vis Sci. 2011;88(5):640–4.
26. Schneider E, Grehn F. Intraocular pressure measurement-comparison of dynamic contour tonometry and goldmann applanation tonometry. J Glaucoma. 2006;15:2–6.
27. Ito K, Tawara A, Kubota T, Harada Y. IOP measured by dynamic contour tonometry correlates with IOP measured by Goldmann applanation tonometry and non-contact tonometry in Japanese individuals. J Glaucoma. 2012;21:35–40.
28. Realini T, Weinreb RN, Hobbs G. Correlation of intraocular pressure measured with goldmann and dynamic contour tonometry in normal and glaucomatous eyes. J Glaucoma. 2009;18:119–23.
29. Martinez-de-la-Casa JM, Garcia-Feijoo J, Fernandez-Vidal A, Mendez-Hernandez C, Garcia-Sanchez J. Ocular response analyzer versus Goldmann applanation tonometry for intraocular pressure measurements. Invest Ophthalmol Vis Sci. 2006;47:4410–4.
30. Lau W, Pye DC. Associations between diurnal changes in Goldmann tonometry, corneal geometry, and ocular response analyzer parameters. Cornea. 2012;31:639–44.
31. Hamilton KE, Pye DC, Aggarwala S, Evian S, Khosla J, Perera R. Diurnal variation of central corneal thickness and Goldmann applanation tonometry estimates of intraocular pressure. J Glaucoma. 2007;16:29–35.
32. Riva I, Quaranta L, Russo A, Katsanos A, Rulli E, Floriani I. Dynamic contour tonometry and goldman applanation tonometry: correlation with intracameral assessment of intraocular pressure. Eur J Ophthalmol. 2012;22:55–62.

25

Universal ocular screening of 481 infants using wide-field digital imaging system

Yan Ma, Guangda Deng, Jing Ma, Jinghua Liu, Songfeng Li and Hai Lu*

Abstract

Background: Universal ocular screening of infants is not a standard procedure in children's health care system in China. This pilot study investigated prevalence of ocular abnormalities of 6 weeks-age infants using wide-field digital imaging system.

Methods: Infants aged 6 weeks around were consecutively enrolled in a public hospital between April 2015 and August 2016. All the infants who were enrolled in the study underwent vision assessment, eye position examination, external eye check, pupillary light reflex, red reflex examination, anterior and posterior ocular segments were examined using flashlight, ophthalmoscope, and wide-field digital imaging system.

Results: A total of 481 infants at 45.1 ± 6.1 days after birth were enrolled in the study. 198 infants had abnormal findings (41.2%). Retinal white spots and retinal white areas were the most common findings (42.9% of abnormalities and 17.7% of all infants screened). The second major finding was retinal hemorrhage (16.2% of abnormalities and 6.7% of all infants screened). Other abnormal findings include retinal pigmentation, concomitant exotropia, neonatal dacryocystitis, retinopathy of prematurity, 'albinism-like fundus', congenital nasolacrimal duct obstruction, familial exudative vitreoretinopathy, immature retina, corneal dermoid tumor, large physiologic cupping of optic disc, congenital persistent pupillary membrane, entropion trichiasis, subconjunctival hemorrhage, congenital cataract, vitreous hemorrhage, ptosis and choroidal nevus. Intervention of any form was required in 22 infants, which accounted for 11.1% of abnormalities detected and 4.6% of all infants screened.

Conclusion: Universal ocular screening is not only necessary for preterm infants but also for full-term infants. Addition of red reflex examination with wide-field digital imaging system can enhance the sensitivity of screening for ocular fundus abnormities. Further study with a long-term follow-up is needed in the future.

Keywords: Infant, Ocular screening, Wide-field imaging, RetCam

Background

Ocular problems in infants, especially visual impairment has to be detected passively since infants cannot convey their discomfort verbally. The American Academy of Pediatrics recommends red reflex examination as a component of ophthalmic evaluation of children. Ideally it should be started in the neonatal period and continued during the routine periodic well health visits by the children's primary care provider. [1]. During the routine well health visits if any abnormality is detected the primary care provider should refer the child to an ophthalmologist. Currently in

China and other developing counties, ocular screening for infants is not a strict requirement during the well health check-ups.

In China, infants go through their first well child check-up at about six weeks of age in some big cities and tertiary hospitals. But even in these places, sometimes the pediatricians are not comfortable using the ophthalmoscope to perform red reflex examination in infants and thus in most cases only an external examination of the eye is performed during the well child check-up. Therefore, some full-term infants with eye diseases are not detected in a timely manner. The condition can worsen and result in impaired vision. In some instances, by the time parents become aware of the visual impairment in their children,

* Correspondence: hailu2017@163.com
Department of Ophthalmology, Beijing Tongren Eye Center, Beijing Tongren Hospital, Capital Medical University, Beijing Ophthalmology and Visual Sciences Key Lab, 1 Dongjiaominxiang, Dongcheng District, Beijing 100730, China

the ideal time for treatment would have been missed and it could result in life-threatening consequences.

In recent years, as children's healthcare system in China has improved, policies about eye screening and vision care in childhood has been issued. Children in some metropolitan cities have received neonatal eye screening using wide-field digital imaging [2]. Most of these screenings were done in the first 72 h after birth. Previous studies showed that majority of abnormal findings in such screenings were retinal hemorrhages [3]. As most retinal hemorrhages can absorb spontaneously, screening too early may increase patient's economic burden due to multiple revisits. Further, it is very difficult to check for visual functions and eye movements like following light in neonates.

The purpose of this pilot study was to detect the prevalence of ocular abnormalities in infants around 6 weeks of age using red reflex examination and wide-field digital imaging system in a single public hospital and to explore the feasibility and efficacy of using wide-field digital imaging system as an universal tool for ocular screening in infants.

Objectives and methods

Four hundred eighty-one infants who underwent the infant ocular screening program at Beijing Tongren Hospital affiliated to Capital Medical University between April 2015 and August 2016 were enrolled in the study. Infants who were unable to tolerate the eye screening examination conducted by the pediatrician or whose guardians refused to consent were excluded from the study. Clinical Research Ethics Committee of Beijing Tongren Hospital approved this study. All participants were screened according to the Declaration of Helsinki document on human research ethics, and underwent both verbal and written informed consent by their guardians for participation and data publication. The first screening time was around 6 weeks of age. The cost of one-time screening examination is about fifty US dollars. Two ophthalmologists who have been trained in pediatric retinal examinations performed the screening test and reviewed the images. A senior reviewer was consulted if the diagnoses were not consistent. Information about the infants' gestational age at birth, birth weight, Apgar score and hypoxia during birth were collected. Details about the course of mother's pregnancy and delivery were also obtained.

Vision assessment was performed initially by evaluating the ability to fix and follow light and objects binocularly and then monocularly. Following that an external eye examination, test for eye position, regular anterior segment examination and pupillary light reflex were performed. Red reflex examination was performed using a direct ophthalmolscope (mini3000, Heine, Germany). Pupils were then dilated by compound tropicamide eye drops (0.5% Tropicamide and 0.5% phenylephrine), which was administered every 10 min for 3 to 6 times until pupils dilated at least 5 mm. A

wide-angle digital camera (RetCam 3, Clarity Medical System, CA, USA) and 130-degree lens were used to acquire anterior and posterior images from one eye to the other eye. Photographs of the fundus were taken in the following order: posterior pole, temporal, superior, nasal, and inferior retinal fields. Proparacaine hydrochloride eye drops were given for topical anesthesia before using the camera. Corneal lubricating gel and sterile pediatric eyelid speculum were used. Breast milk, formula, and clear liquids were withheld for 1 h before using the eyelid speculum. There were no ocular or systemic complications during or after any of the examination sessions.

Severity of retinal hemorrhage was graded by the number of hemorrhages per eye [4]. Presence of one or two hemorrhage spots was defined as grade 1, three to ten hemorrhage spots was defined as grade 2, and more than ten hemorrhage spots was defined as grade 3. Statistical analysis of the data was performed using a commercially available statistical software package (SPSS for Windows, version 17.0, SPSS Inc., Chicago, Illinois, USA). Data are presented as frequencies or as the mean $\pm$ SD. Logistic regression analysis was performed to identify the risk factors of abnormal findings. Probabilities of less than 0.05 were considered to indicate statistical significance.

Results

Four hundred eighty-one infants were screened during the study period, including 253 (52.6%) males and 228 (47.4%) females. There were 408 (84.8%) full-term infants and 73 (15.2%) premature infants. Of all the infants screened, low birth weigh infants (birth weight less than 2500 g) were 50 (10.4%) and infants with macrosomia (birth weight equal or more than 4000 g) were 41 (8.5%). 276 (57.4%) were delivered vaginally and 205 (42.6%) were delivered by Caesarian section. 11 (2.3%) had hypoxia at birth (Apgar score less than 8) [5]. The birth weight of 73 preterm babies was 2400.0 $\pm$ 459.5 g, the gestational age was 35.2 $\pm$ 1.4 weeks, and the postmenstrual age was 41.5 $\pm$ 1.6 weeks. During the eighteen-month study period, 1785 newborns that met inclusion criteria for study participation were approached. Four hundred and eight-one subjects (962 eyes) participated in the universal ocular screening study, for a participation rate of 26.9%. The most common reasons why babies' guardians chose not to participate in the study were they believed it was not necessary for the babies and they concerned about adverse effects.

Of the 481 infants who underwent eye examination, 198 (41.2%) were found to be abnormal. Retinal whites was the most common finding and was found in at least one eye in 85 infants, accounting for 42.9% of abnormalities and 17.7% of all screened infants (Fig. 1). Retinal hemorrhages were the second majority finding and were found in at least one eye in 32 infants, accounting for 16.2% of abnormalities and 6.7% of all screened infants.

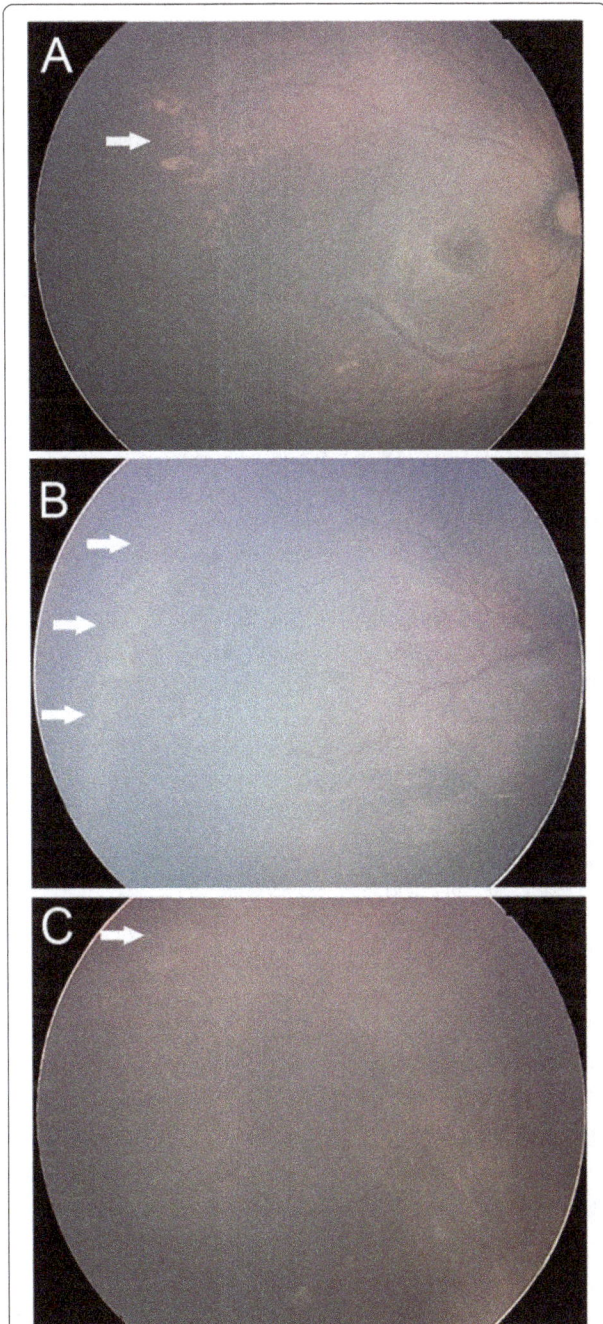

Fig. 1 Retinal white changes were detected in at least one eye in 85 infants, accounting for 42.9% of abnormalities and 17.7% of all screened infants. **a**. Retinal white changes with spot shaped (pointing by white arrow). **b**. Retinal white changes with strip shaped (pointing by white arrows). **c**. Retinal white changes with patch shaped (pointing by white arrow)

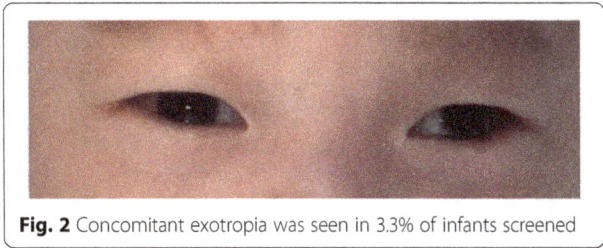

Fig. 2 Concomitant exotropia was seen in 3.3% of infants screened

corneal dermoid tumor, large physiologic cupping of optic disc, congenital persistent pupillary membrane, entropion trichiasis, subconjunctival hemorrhage, congenital cataract, vitreous hemorrhage, ptosis (Fig. 6) and choroidal nevus. These findings are summarized in Table 1. Intervention of any form was required in 22 infants, which accounted for 11.1% (22/198) of abnormalities detected and 4.6% (22/481) of all infants screened (Table 2). Once the ophthalmic diagnosis was made, 8 infants had to be referred to a dermatologist for specific examination towards any systemic condition that the infants could have possibly had.

Of all retinal white changes, 56 cases (69 eyes) were spot shaped, 17 cases (30 eyes) were strip shaped and 12 cases (21 eyes) were patch shaped changes. 22 cases (25 eyes) had changes on the posterior retina and 63 cases (95 eyes) on peripheral retina. No eminence, vascular branching, tortuous vessel, avascular peripheral retina or retinal ridge changes were found in these eyes. Retinal white changes did not relate to sex, family history of high myopia, preterm delivery, low birth weight, macrosomia, fetal distress, history of hypoxia, method of delivery, abnormal stage during labor, pregnancy-induced hypertension, or gestational diabetes ($P > 0.05$). These infants were examined during revisit at 3 months, 6 months and 12 months of age. Excluding 10 individuals who refused for follow up examination, retinal white changes disappeared spontaneously in 58 infants (68.2%) at 3 months of age, in 14

Other abnormalities were concomitant extropia (Fig. 2), retinal pigmentation (Fig. 3), neonatal dacryocystitis, 'albinism-like fundus' (Fig. 4), retinopathy of prematurity (ROP) (Fig. 5), congenital nasolacrimal duct obstruction, familial exudative vitreoretinopathy (FEVR), immature retina,

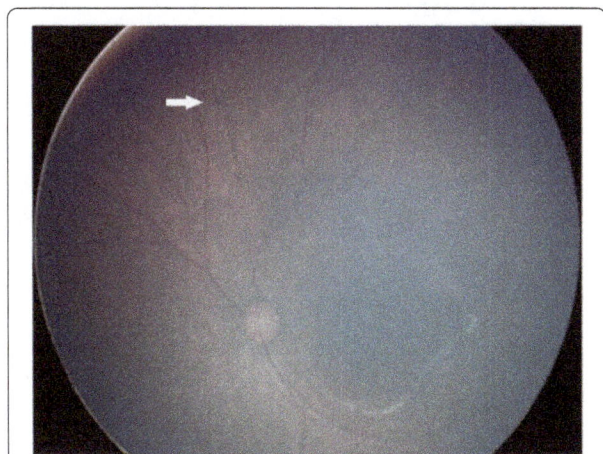

Fig. 3 Retinal pigmentation was found in 3.3% of all screened infants (pointing by white arrow)

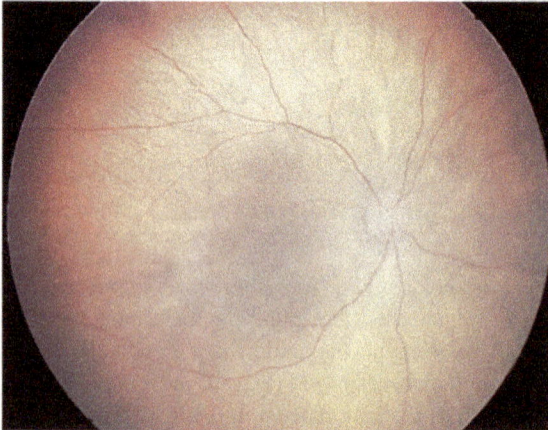

Fig. 4 'Albinism-like fundus' was seen in 1.7% of all infants screened, who was excluded from albinism by Dermatologist consulting

infants (16.5%) at 6 months of age, and in 2 infants (2.4%) at 12 months of age. Only 1 case (1.2%) had the retinal white spot without any change at 12 months of age.

Of 32 cases and 39 eyes with retinal hemorrhages, 29 eyes (74.4%) had grade 1, 9 eyes (23.1%) had grade 2, and one eye (2.6%) had grade 3 hemorrhage. Only one eye had a hemorrhage spot on the macula. All retinal hemorrhages were absorbed spontaneously at 3 months follow-up. Vitreous hemorrhage of one infant had been absorbed spontaneously at 3 months follow-up without any intervention. Two infants had been diagnosed as FEVR after checking their parents' eyes. Both of them were grade 1 [6]. Retinal lesions were stable and without any neovascularization or intervention when followed up to 12 months. All concomitant exotropia were intermittent, and relieved spontaneously at 3 months follow-up. 'Albinism-like fundus' was noted in 8 infants without family history

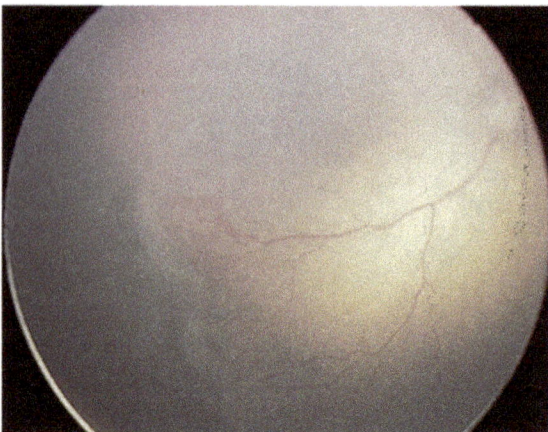

Fig. 5 Threshold retinopathy of prematurity was detected and received laser treatment immediately

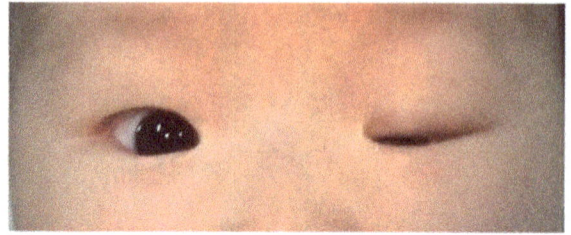

Fig. 6 Ptosis was seen in one eye (0.2% of all screened infants)

of albinism or absence of pigment in the skin, hair, lashes and iris. Albinism was excluded after consultation with a dermatologist. Of 73 preterm infants, ROP was detected in 9 infants (18 eyes), and immature retina was detected in 2 infants (4 eyes). All of them did not have ROP screening before we screened. The stage and zone of ROP in these infants and their gestational age, birth weight are demonstrated in Table 3. One patient with both eyes had threshold ROP and received photocoagulation treatment. Red reflex examination was normal except for one case of unilateral vitreous hemorrhage and one case with congenital cataract.

The patient with vitreous hemorrhage of his right eye could not fix or follow a light or object at the first time screening. At his 3 months follow-up, his right eye with

Table 1 Ocular abnormalities detected in 198 cases out of 481 infants by eye screening

Abnormality	Abnormality cases (%)	Abnormality eyes (%)
Retinal white change	85(17.7%)	120 (12.5%)
Retinal hemorrhage	32 (6.7%)	39 (4.1%)
Concomitant exotropia	16 (3.3%)	32 (3.3%)
Retinal pigmentation	16 (3.3%)	19 (2.0%)
Neonatal dacryocystitis	13 (2.7%)	16 (1.7%)
Retinopathy of prematurity	9 (1.9%)	18 (1.9%)
Albinism-like fundus	8 (1.7%)	16 (1.7%)
Lacrimal duct obstruction	4 (0.8%)	6 (0.6%)
Familial exudative vitreoretinopathy	2 (0.4%)	4 (0.4%)
Immature retina	2 (0.4%)	4 (0.4%)
Corneal dermoid tumor	2 (0.4%)	2 (0.2%)
Large physiologic cupping of optic disc	2 (0.4%)	4 (0.4%)
Congenital persistent pupillary membrane	1 (0.2%)	2 (0.2%)
Entropion trichiasis	1 (0.2%)	2 (0.2%)
Subconjunctival hemorrhage	1 (0.2%)	1 (0.1%)
Congenital cataract	1 (0.2%)	1 (0.1%)
Vitreous hemorrhage	1 (0.2%)	1 (0.1%)
Ptosis	1 (0.2%)	1 (0.1%)
Choroidal nevus	1 (0.2%)	1 (0.1%)
Subtotal	198 (41.2%)	289 (30.0%)

Table 2 Characteristics of infants with diseases who were suggested interventions

Screening Number/ Sex/Laterality	Diagnosis	Intervention Method
025/M/OS	Corneal dermoid tumor	Surgery
030/F/OS	Ptosis	Surgery
077/F/OD	CNLDO	Lacrimal sac massage
093/M/OD	Dacryocystitis	Lacrimal sac massage and topical antibiotics
146/F/OD	Dacryocystitis	Lacrimal sac massage and topical antibiotics
148/F/OS	Dacryocystitis	Lacrimal sac massage and topical antibiotics
176/F/OU	CNLDO	Lacrimal sac massage
252/M/OU	Dacryocystitis	Lacrimal sac massage and topical antibiotics
268/F/OD	Congenital Cataract	Surgery
275/F/OS	Dacryocystitis	Lacrimal sac massage and topical antibiotics
287/M/OS	Dacryocystitis	Lacrimal sac massage and topical antibiotics
294/F/OD	Dacryocystitis	Lacrimal sac massage and topical antibiotics
304/F/OU	ROP	Photocoagulation
342/F/OU	Dacryocystitis	Lacrimal sac massage and topical antibiotics
345/F/OS	Dacryocystitis	Lacrimal sac massage and topical antibiotics
392/F/OD	Dacryocystitis	Lacrimal sac massage and topical antibiotics
394/M/OU	Dacryocystitis	Lacrimal sac massage and topical antibiotics
403/F/OD	Dacryocystitis	Lacrimal sac massage and topical antibiotics
424/F/OU	CNLDO	Lacrimal sac massage
440/F/OS	Dacryocystitis	Lacrimal sac massage and topical antibiotics
445/F/OD	Corneal dermoid tumor	Surgery
474/F/OS	CNLDO	Lacrimal sac massage

Abbreviations: *M* male, *F* female, *OD* right eye, *OS* left eye, *OU* both eyes, *CNLDO* congenital nasolacrimal duct obstruction, *ROP* retinopathy of prematurity

Table 3 Demographic data of patients with retinopathy of prematurity

Screen Number	Gender	Laterality	Stage/Zone	Gestational age (weeks)	Birth Weight (grams)
053	Female	Both Eyes	2/III	32^{+6}	1780
149	Male	Both Eyes	2/II	32^{+5}	1640
161	Male	Both Eyes	1/III	34^{+2}	1720
304	Female	Both Eyes	3+/I	31^{+6}	1320
305	Female	Both Eyes	2/II	31^{+6}	1420
311	Female	Both Eyes	1/III	35	2460
312	Female	Both Eyes	1/II	33^{+5}	2130
342	Female	Both Eyes	1/III	36^{+1}	2020
465	Male	Both Eyes	2/III	33^{+4}	2280

Discussion

Universal ocular screening of infants is not a common practice in most developing countries and even in some developed countries. Recently, national health and family planning commission of China has issued some guidelines about eye screening at an early age. But only a few children can be screened in some big cities. Those who lived in less developed areas cannot be covered by the healthcare system. Red reflex examination is recommended in neonates, infants and children in several developed countries [7, 8]. But red reflex examination still has some limitations in detecting sensitivity of fundus abnormality [9]. In this study, we also found 157 abnormal cases by RetCam but normal by red reflex examination.

The ocular abnormalities can be divided into three types as following: The first type is with no particular clinical significance, such as subconjunctival hemorrhage, retinal pigmentation and self-resolved retinal hemorrhage. The second type is with some clinical significance that should be monitored periodically through revisit check-ups, which include immature retina, FEVR grade 1 and grade 2 and retinal white change. The third part is with important clinical significance and requires some form of intervention, like threshold ROP, dacryocystitis, severe cataract and ptosis. In this pilot study, we found 198/481 (41.2%) had abnormal ocular signs, and 22/481 (4.6%) required at least one form of intervention. Those who required intervention were healthy and normal at the time of universal eye screening.

Congenital nasolacrimal duct obstruction is the most common disorder of the nasolacrimal duct system in infants. Although the diagnosis of a congenital nasolacrimal duct obstruction is usually not difficult, there are still some debatable issues about the timing and methods of intervention among pediatric ophthalmologists. In this study, we prescribed lacrimal sac massage or topical antibiotics for infants with congenital nasolacrimal duct obstruction and dacryocystitis as nonsurgical interventions,

vitreous hemorrhage was absorbed spontaneously. At that time, he can fix and follow a light and object with left eye. But when we tried to assess the visual function of his right eye, he refused to cover his left eye and cannot corporate with fixing or following test. We believed that his right eye had visual impairment because of visual deprivation and suggested him to cover his left eye for two hours every day and asked him to re-check his visual function one month later, but the patient never came back and lost to follow-up.

which are the same as Pediatric Eye Disease Investigator Group did [10]. Although most nasolacrimal duct obstruction can be self-resolved during the first year of life, and there is no proof that massage can elevate the recovery rate, it still seems logical to perform massage as a noninvasive intervention. A survey of common management policies for nasolacrimal duct obstruction among pediatric ophthalmologists showed that 82% respondents preferred to instruct parents to massage nasolacrimal duct during the first year of life [11]. In addition, more than 90% of pediatric ophthalmologists in that survey wait until approximately 1 year old before recommending a surgical intervention for congenital nasolacrimal duct obstruction.

The previous studies of universal eye screening were based on neonates within 72 h after birth [2, 12, 13]. The most common ocular abnormality in their studies was retinal hemorrhage with 21.52%, 2.4%, and 20.3% prevalence respectively. In this pilot study, the prevalence of retinal hemorrhage is 6.7%, and all cases spontaneously resolved by the 3rd month revisit check-ups. The prevalence of subconjunctival hemorrhage is 0.2% compared to 1.4% in previous study [2]. The lower prevalence of retinal hemorrhage and subconjunctival hemorrhage in our study is due to an older age at the time of examination compared to the other study. We believe that ocular examination at an older age can reduce revisit times of the self-resolving hemorrhages. Furthermore, fixation and following light and object can be assessed in infants who are 6 weeks old. In this study, we found only one eye with vitreous hemorrhage that could not fix or follow a light or object.

Congenital cataract is an important treatable disease leading to childhood visual disability. Universal ocular screening is an effective to screening congenital cataracts at an early age. To avoid amblyopia and nystagmus caused by visual deprivation, early intervention is recommended [14]. In infants suffering from congenital cataracts, especially posterior, perinuclear, nucleus, and total cataracts, the crucial time for surgery in order to preventing amblyopia is probably within the first three months of life [15]. FEVR, characterized by congenital anomalous retinal vascularization, is an inherited vitreoretinopathy. The presentation and severity of this disease could be very different even in the same family. The mild and most common lesions often manifest as avascular zone in peripheral retina, supernumerous vascular branching, venous-venous anastomoses and vitreoretinal adhesions, which could be asymptomatic during the entire life. The severe and progressive forms of the diseases are including neovascularization, retinal exudates, retinal hemorrhage, preretinal membranes, retinal folds and retinal detachment [6, 16]. In this study, we found two infants with bilateral avascular peripheral retinas and finally were diagnosed as FEVR. Fluorescein angiogram

(FA) is the most helpful method to confirm and diagnose FEVR, but during routine eye screening we cannot perform FA on the 6 week-old infants under topical anesthesia, so we made the diagnosis based on demographic features, clinical presentations, fundus findings and family history through the following steps. First, we differentiated them from ROP by their full term birth and normal birth weight without supplemental oxygenation. Second, incontinentia pigmenti and Norrie disease can be excluded by their skin manifestations, hearing screening results, genders and family histories. Third, the fundus showed classic vascular anomalies such as avascular zone, supernumerous vascular branching and peripheral exudation, which can be differentiated from avascular retina. Forth, when these two patients were suspicious for FEVR, we checked their parents' fundus by ophthalmoscopy and FA. Two mothers were diagnosed as FEVR, and one of them had bilateral retinal holes and received photocoagulation treatment. Clinical examination alone can be insufficient to identify the subtle and atypical vascular changes of FEVR, which requiring the assistance of FA. Fortunately, the two FEVR patients had classic vascular changes, in addition to the demographic features and positive familial presentations that provided further evidence for the diagnosis. FEVR can be found through universal ocular screening and treated timely to avoid visual impairment consequences. Considering that FEVR is a lifelong disease, FEVR patients should be followed up regularly.

Retinal white spots or area was the most common finding, which was not mentioned in previous studies. All retinal white changes in the posterior area were dot shaped. Peripheral retinal white changes can be spots, strips or patches, and some of them were adjacent to ora serrata. We hypothesize that several reasons could cause this kind of retinal change. The first is because the peripheral retina has poor blood flow as retinal vessels are developing, which causes uneven cellular metabolism and displays retinal malnutrition-like changes. The second speculation is that the development of retinal vessel epithelial cells at the periphery is delayed than the posterior areas, which cause retinal exudations due to the immature development of blood-retina barrier. In addition, subretinal lipid or calcium deposition partially absorbed retinal hemorrhage and local undeveloped retinal pigment epithelium may also attribute to these findings. Undoubtedly, FA is the only way to ascertain the nature of these white changes. But we cannot perform FA on the 6 week-old infants under topical anesthesia during routine eye screening. Therefore, we use rule-out and observation strategy for these findings. Firstly, we ruled-out the potential diseased which could cause visual impairment like ROP, FEVR and retinoblastoma by checking if the white changes were in the vascular area, if the peripheral vascular branching and position are normal, if the white change was protruded into vitreous cavity. Secondly, for the retinal white changes without potential risks, we can wait and observe to find out what they would be. Most retinal white changes were relieved spontaneously as the children grew, and were not related to mother or newborn conditions, so it can be considered as a physiological change. In this study, only one case of a retinal white spot at posterior area remained unchanged at 12 months revisit. This spot was with a clear boundary and without eminence. We considered it as retinal pigment maldistribution. Above were our hypotheses because only retinal FA can ascertain the nature of these changes, which need further researches.

Choroidal vessels can be seen in 'albinism-like fundus'. But none of them had family history of albinism or absence of pigment in the skin, hair, eyelashes and iris. We considered immature retinal pigment epithelial cells to be the etiological factor for 'albinism-like fundus'. All concomitant exotropia were relieved spontaneously by the revisit at 3 months of age, which reflects immaturity of the ocular motor system as the possible etiology [17].

There are certain limitations in this study. Firstly, it is a single center study in a public hospital and it is a pilot study as the sample size is not large. As there is no control group in this study, it is more important to discuss 'how to explain what we find' than report 'what we find'. Secondly, further in-depth study involving multiple centers with large sample size and long time follow-up needs to be done in order to discuss the prevalence and etiology of ocular abnormalities.

Conclusion

To sum up, universal ocular screening is not only necessary for preterm infants but also for full-term infants. In addition to red reflex examination, wide-field digital imaging can enhance the sensitivity of screening ocular fundus abnormities. First screening at around six weeks of age could reduce re-examinations for self-resolved cases. Visual function and eye position can also be checked at this age. The outcomes of our work would help in revising guidelines for children's health screening system.

Acknowledgements
The authors thank Dr. Yonghong Jiao and Dr. Ming Cui for supporting this study. Mr. Jelliffe Jeganathan provided professional writing service.

Funding
This research is supported by Beijing Municipal Science & Technology Commission (No.Z141107002514029) and Beijing Tongren Hospital, Capital Medical University (No. TRZDYXZY201703). The funders were not involved in the design of the study and collection, analysis, and interpretation of data and in writing the manuscript.

Authors' contributions
All authors conceived of and designed the research protocol. YM, GDD, JM and JHL were responsible for data collection. YM, GDD and SFL were involved in the analysis and interpretation of the data. YM and HL was responsible for conception of the manuscript, as well as write the manuscript. All authors read and approved the final manuscript.

Competing interests
The authors declare that they have no competing interests.

References
1. American Academy of Pediatrics, Committee on practice and ambulatory medicine, section on ophthalmology; American Association of Certified Orthopedists; American Association for Pediatric Ophthalmology and Strabismus; American Academy of ophthalmology. Eye examination in infants, children, and young adults by pediatricians. Pediatrics. 2003;111: 902–7.
2. Li LH, Li N, Zhao JY, Fei P, Zhang GM, Mao JB, et al. Findings of perinatal ocular examination performed on 3573, healthy full-term newborns. Br J Ophthalmol. 2013;97:588–91.
3. Zhao Q, Zhang Y, Yang Y, Li Z, Lin Y, Liu R, et al. Birth-related retinal hemorrhages in healthy full-term newborns and their relationship to maternal, obstetric, and neonatal risk factors. Graefes Arch Clin Exp Ophthalmol. 2015;253:1021–5.
4. Emerson MV, Pieramici DJ, Stoessel KM, Berreen JP, Gariano RF. Incidence and rate of disappearance of retinal hemorrhage in newborns. Ophthalmology. 2001;108:36–9.
5. American academy of pediatrics committee on fetus and newborn; American college of obstetricians and gynecologists committee on obstetric practice. The Apgar Score. Pediatrics. 2015;136:819–22.
6. Pendergast SD, Trese MT. Familial exudative vitreoretinopathy. Results of surgical management. Ophthalmology. 1998;105:1015–23.
7. American Academy of Pediatrics; Section on ophthalmology; American Association for Pediatric Ophthalmology and Strabismus; American Academy of ophthalmology; American Association of Certified Orthoptists. Red reflex examination in neonates, infants, and children. Pediatrics. 2008; 122:1401–4.
8. Magnusson G, Bizjajeva S, Haargaard B, Lundström M, Nyström A, Tornqvist K. Congenital cataract screening in maternity wards is effective: evaluation of the Paediatric cataract register of Sweden. Acta Paediatr. 2013;102:263–7.
9. Khan AO, Al-Mesfer S. Lack of efficacy of dilated screening for retinoblastoma. J Pediatr Ophthalmol Strabismus. 2005;42:205–10.
10. Pediatric Eye Disease Investigator Group. Resolution of congenital nasolacrimal duct obstruction with nonsurgical management. Arch Ophthalmol. 2012;130:730–4.
11. Dotan G, Nelson LB. Congenital nasolacrimal duct obstruction: common management policies among pediatric ophthalmologists. J Pediatr Ophthalmol Strabismus. 2015;52:14–9.
12. Vinekar A, Govindaraj I, Jayadev C, Kumar AK, Sharma P, Mangalesh S, et al. Universal ocular screening of 1021 term infants using wide-field digital imaging in a single public hospital in India - a pilot study. Acta Ophthalmol. 2015;93:e372–6.
13. Callaway NF, Ludwig CA, Blumenkranz MS, Jones JM, Fredrick DR, Retinal MDM. Optic nerve hemorrhages in the newborn infant: one-year results of the newborn eye screen test study. Ophthalmology. 2016;123:1043–52.
14. Vaegan, Taylor D. Critical period for deprivation amblyopia in children. Trans Ophthalmol Soc U K. 1979;99:432–9.
15. Elston JS, Timms C. Clinical evidence for the onset of the sensitive period in infancy. Brit J Ophthalmol. 1992;76:327–8.
16. Miyakubo H, Hashimoto K, Miyakubo S. Retinal vascular pattern in familial exudative vitreoretinopathy. Ophthalmology. 1984;91:1524–30.
17. Pediatric Eye Disease Investigator Group. Spontaneous resolution of early-onset esotropia: experience of the congenital esotropia observational study. Am J Ophthalmol. 2002;133:109–18.

26

Prognostic value of ocular trauma score for open globe injuries associated with metallic intraocular foreign bodies

Dilek Yaşa[*] ⓘ, Zeynep Gizem Erdem, Ali Demircan, Gökhan Demir and Zeynep Alkın

Abstract

Background: The prognostic value of the ocular trauma score (OTS) in patients who underwent 23-gauge pars plana vitrectomy (23-G PPV) for surgical removal of posterior segment metallic intaocular foreign bodies (IOFB) was evaluated.

Methods: Patients who underwent 23-G PPV for surgical removal of retained metallic IOFBs were retrospectively analyzed. OTS score for each patient was calculated and raw scores were converted to their corresponding OTS categories. The final VAs in study patients were compared with their respective OTS categories.

Results: Twenty-five eyes from 25 patients were examined. Twenty-four (96%) of the patients were male, and the mean age was 34 ± 12 years. The time from injury to 23-G PPV was 9 ± 4 days. Fourteen (56%) patients had zone 1 trauma, eight (32%) patients had zone 2 trauma, and three (12%) patients had zone 3 trauma. Postoperative visual acuity was $\geq 20/200$ in 14 (56%) of the patients and $\geq 20/40$ in seven (28%) eyes. At the final visit, anatomical success was achieved in 86% of patients with retinal detachment at presentation. No statistically significant differences were found between our final VAs and OTS scores.

Conclusion: OTS, which provides prognostic information after general ocular trauma, may also provide valuable prognostic information for patients who undergo 23-G PPV for the surgical removal of metallic posterior segment IOFBs.

Keywords: OTS, IOFB, Trauma, Pars plana vitrectomy, PPV

Background

Eyes represent only 0.27% of the body's surface area, but they are among the most common trauma-exposed areas and can present with severe morbidity [1]. Ocular trauma is a leading cause of monocular blindness and is an important public health problem [2].

The variablity in clinical characteristics is an inherent property of trauma patients. This variability in clinical characteristics in ocular trauma patients has led several investigators to study the factors that influence both anatomical success and final post-surgical visual acuity. The ocular trauma score (OTS) is a prognostic model developed by Kuhn et al. [3]. More than 2000 cases from the United States and Hungarian Eye Injury Registries were analyzed and > 100 variables were evaluated to identify the best predictors of outcome at 6 months after injury [3]. OTS has been widely used for this purpose in open and closed globe trauma [4, 5], however, only a few studies have evaluated the prognostic value of OTS in patients with retained intraocular foreign bodies (IOFBs) [6–8].

The purpose of this study was to evaluate prognostic OTS values in patients who underwent 23-gauge pars plana vitrectomy (23-G PPV) for removal of metallic IOFBs from the posterior segment of the eyes.

Methods

This study followed the tenets of the Declaration of Helsinki, and approval was obtained from institutional review board of Prof. Dr. N. Resat Belger Beyoglu Eye Training and Education Hospital. Medical records of patients who underwent 23-G PPV for surgical removal of retained IOFBs in the Beyoglu Eye Training and Education Hospital (BEH) during a 1-year period (January

---

[*] Correspondence: dilekyasa2@gmail.com
Beyoğlu Eye Research and Training Hospital, Bereketzade Mah, Bereketzade Sok. No:2, Beyoğlu, İstanbul, Turkey

2016–January 2017) were retrospectively analyzed. Patients who had at least 6 months of follow-up were included in the study. Demographic data of the patients, zones of injury, types of IOFBs, associated ocular pathologies, time from trauma to PPV, follow-up time, and presenting and final visual acuities (VA) were obtained from the patients' records. Zones of injury were classified according to the Birmingham Eye Trauma Terminology System [9]. A zone I wound involves the cornea, a zone II wound extends into the anterior 5 mm of the sclera and a zone III wound involves the sclera extending more than 5 mm from limbus.

All VA examinations were performed with a back-illuminated Early Treatment Diabetic Retinopathy Study (ETDRS) chart. VAs were divided into five groups based on the OTS categories: 1.) no light perception; 2.) light perception/hand motions; 3.) 1/200 to–19/200; 4.) 20/200 to < 20/50; or 5.) ≥ 20/40. The sum of each patient's raw points was calculated, and the numerical value was converted into the corresponding OTS score (shown in Tables 1 and 2) as described by Kuhn et al. [3]. Then, the similarity of final visual acuities by category was compared with those in the OTS study (Table 2).

Surgical technique

All eyes underwent standard 23-G PPV using the Constellation Surgical Vitrectomy System (Alcon Laboratories Inc., Fort Worth, TX, USA). Pars plana lensectomy or phacoemulsification was performed in eyes with lens opacity. In eyes with retinal detachment (RD), perfluorocarbon liquids were used to attach the retina, and retinal breaks were treated with endophotocoagulation. To remove the IOFBs, one of the sclerotomies were enlarged, and IOFBs were removed using intraocular forceps. Air, sulfur hexafluoride (SF6), perfluoropropane (C3F8), or 1000 cSt silicone oil was used at the end of the surgery as an internal tamponade. Sclerotomies were sutured at

Table 1 Ocular Trauma Score (OTS)

Variables	Raw Points
A. Initial Vision	
NLP	60
LP/HM	70
1/200–19/200	80
20/200–20/50	90
≥ 20/40	100
B. Rupture	−23
C. Endophthalmitis	−17
D. Perforating injury	−14
E. Retinal detachment	−11
F: Afferent pupillary defect	−10

NLP No light perception, *LP* Light perception, *HM* Hand motion

the end of the surgery. In eyes with RD, anatomical success was defined as total retinal attachment at the final visit.

Statistical analysis
Continuous data are presented as means and standard deviation while categorical data are presented as percentages. Chi square test was used for comparison of categorical distributions of final visual acuities and OTS scores between OTS study and our series. Mann-Whitney U test was performed for the comparison of final visual acuities between the patients with and without RD. Additionally, Fisher's exact test was used to compare the categorical distribution of VAs in patients with and without RD. A two-tailed p-value < 0.05 was considered statistically significant.

Results
Twenty-five eyes from 25 patients were included in the study. Twenty-four (96%) of the patients were male, and the mean age was 34 ± 12 years (min:12, max: 64, median 37). The mean follow-up time was 10 ± 5 months (min: 6, max: 21, median 6). Presenting and final VAs of each patient are shown in Table 3. Cumulative VAs are presented in Fig. 1. At the final visit VA was 20/200, or better in 56% and 20/40, or better in 28% of the eyes. Cumulative VAs in patients with or without a RD are shown in Table 4. Our hospital is a tertiary referral eye hospital and most of our patients are referred from rural areas of Turkey or from other hospitals. Accordingly, 7 (28%) eyes had RD at presentation, and although anatomical success was achieved in 6 (85.7%) of these, only 14.3% of the eyes had a final VA of 20/40. Cumulative VAs were better in eyes without RD. However, the difference was not statistically significant (Table 4). Work-related trauma (96% of eyes) was the most common cause of the injury, which was followed by car accidents (4% of eyes). None of the patients was wearing protective safety glasses during trauma. Mechanism of injury are presented in Table 5.

There were 14 (56%), eight (32%), and three (12%) cases of zones 1, 2, and 3, respectively. The mean time from injury to 23-G PPV was 9 ± 4 days. Associated ocular pathologies are shown in Table 6 and injured intraocular structures are shown in Table 7. A metallic IOFB was found in all eyes. Posterior segment IOFBs were observed in 10 (40%) eyes. In the remaining 4 (16%) eyes, IOFB located in the vitreous cavity, 9 (36%) in the peripheral retina, and 2 (8%) nasal relative to the optic disc in the posterior pole of the eye. A total of 13 (52%) eyes had cataract at the presentation. Of the 6 eyes with visually significant cataracts, 3 underwent pars plana lensectomy without intraocular implantation and 3 underwent phacoemulsification and intraocular lens implantation.

Table 2 Comparison of final visual acuities and OTS categorical distributions between OTS study and our series

Sum of raw points	OTS	NLP A/B	LP/HM A/B	1/200–19/200 A/B	20/200–20/50 A/B	≥20/40 A/B	P^a
0-44	1	74/0	15/0	7/100	3/0	1/0	0.116
45–65	2	27/7	26/50	18/14	15/22	15/7	0.195
66–80	3	2/0	11/0	15/0	31/50	41/50	0.856
81–91	4	1/0	2/0	3/0	22/33	73/67	0.733
92–100	5	0/0	1/0	1/0	57/0	94/0	N/A

OTS Ocular Trauma Score, *NLP* No light perception, *LP* light perception, *HM* Hand motion, *A* OTS Study results (%), *B* Our study results (%)
[a]Chi-square test

One eye with pars plana vitrectomy underwent intraocular lens placement with scleral fixation 6 months after the first surgery. In the remaining 2 eyes, lens placement was not considered because of the poor visual prognosis. All IOFBs were successfully removed, and anatomical success was achieved at the final visit in 96% of 25 eyes with or without RD at presentation.

Table 3 Presenting and final visual acuities and OTS of individual patients

No	Age	Gender	OTS	OTS Category	VA (admission)	VA (final)
1	40–50	Male	28	1	LP	20/1500
2	40–50	Male	56	2	HM	20/100
3	40–50	Male	56	2	HM	HM
4	20–30	Male	56	2	HM	20/1500
5	60–70	Male	56	2	LP	HM
6	20–30	Male	56	2	LP	20/400
7	10–20	Male	56	2	LP	HM
8	30–40	Male	56	2	LP	HM
9	30–40	Male	56	2	LP	HM
10	30–40	Male	65	2	20/50	20/32
11	30–40	Male	45	2	HM	HM
12	10–20	Female	45	2	HM	HM
13	40–50	Male	45	2	LP	20/200
14	30–40	Male	55	2	5/200	20/100
15	10–20	Male	45	2	LP	NLP
16	40–50	Male	76	3	20/63	20/200
17	10–20	Male	76	3	0.16	20/20
18	30–40	Male	76	3	20/50	20/200
19	40–50	Male	76	3	20/50	20/32
20	20–30	Male	86	4	20/32	20/63
21	30–40	Male	86	4	20/40	20/32
22	40–50	Male	86	4	20/25	20/25
23	20–30	Male	86	4	20/20	20/20
24	30–40	Male	86	4	20/20	20/20
25	20–30	Male	86	4	20/32	20/63

OTS Ocular trauma score, *VA* Visual acuity (Snellen), *LP* Light perception, *NLP* No light perception, *HM* Hand motion

The most common postoperative complication was an increase in intraocular pressure (12%), but it was controlled with medical treatment in all patients. One eye with RD at baseline had macula-off RD and no light perception at the final visit. In one patient, who had a culture that was negative for endophthalmitis at presentation, recurrent RD occurred, but anatomical success was achieved after the second 23-G PPV. Air was used as an internal tamponade in 8 (32%) eyes, SF6 in 2 (8%) eyes, C3F8 in 3 (12%) eyes, and silicone oil in 12 (48%) eyes. One eye with RD at the presentation treated with PPV and silicone oil injection and 1 eye without RD treated with PPV and C3F8 injection showed RD during follow-up. They underwent second PPV to achieve retinal reattachment. At the final visit, retina was still attached in those 2 patients. Silicone oil was removed in 12 eyes in the mean time of 5.7 months after PPV. In the remained one eye with cyclodialysis at the presentation, silicone oil was not removed because of the chronic hypotonia. Final VAs based on OTS categories and the OTS scores are presented in Table 2.

All patients were administered systemic antibiotics (moxifloxacin) until IOFB removal with PPV. Only 3 patients were given intravitreal antibiotics (vancomycin and ceftazidime), solely based on surgeon preference, not signs of endophthalmitis. Topical antibiotics were applied as an appropriate adjuvant to intravitreal and systemic antibiotic use once the wound was closed following PPV.

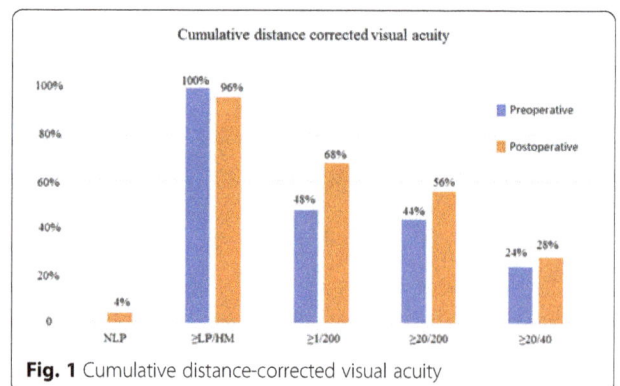

Fig. 1 Cumulative distance-corrected visual acuity

Table 4 Visual acuities in eyes with and without retinal detachment

	Eyes with RD n = 7	Eyes without RD n = 18	p
VA (Mean ± SD, logMAR)	1.64 ± 1.24	1.26 ± 1.27	0.398*
VA ≥ LP/HM (%)	85.7	100	0.280**
VA ≥ 1/200 (%)	57.1	72.7	0.640**
VA ≥ 20/200 (%)	42.9	61.1	0.656**
VA ≥ 20/40 (%)	14.3	33.3	0.626**

HM Hand motions, *LP* Light perception, *n* Number of eyes, *SD* Standard deviation, *RD* Retinal detachment, *VA* Visual acuity
*: Mann Whitney U test, two-tailed *p* value
**: Fisher's Exact Test, two tailed *p* value

Discussion

IOFBs may be associated with up to 40% of open globe injuries especially with respect to work related injuries [10, 11]. Male dominance and the peak patient age in the young to middle-aged group in our study was in agreement with reports in the literature in which young to middle-aged working males are at the highest risk for ocular trauma.

Greven et al. reported final VAs of 20/40 of more were obtained in 71% of IOFB-associated open globe injuries [12]. Although their results are superior to those associated with the general functional outcomes in other types of open globe trauma, other investigators have reported that functional success is not more common in eyes with IOFB [4]. Ahmadieh et al. [13] found that IOFB was a poor predictor of visual outcome. These conflicting findings probably result from the fact that the patients with IOFB are a heterogeneous group with different clinical characteristics that are dependent on the nature of the injury and the foreign body.

Anatomical and visual outcomes, as well as postoperative complications in this study were comparable to those reported in the literature [4–6]. The final visual acuity of eyes with RD was lower when compared to eyes without a RD. However, it did not reach the level of statistical significance. The reason for the lack of statistically significant difference between the groups (eyes with RD and eyes without RD) may be the low number of patients (only seven patients had RD), the complex nature of trauma, heterogeneity of this patient group, and other factors limiting functional success in patients who do not have RD at presentation.

Table 5 Mechanism of injury

	n (%)
Hammering	11 (44)
Chisseling	3 (12)
Drilling	4 (16)
Cutting metal	6 (24)
Car crash	1 (4)

n Number of eyes

Table 6 Associated ocular pathologies

Ocular Pathology	n (%)
Cyclodialysis	3 (12)
Iridodialysis	1 (4)
Traumatic Cataract	13 (52)
Intravitreal hemorrhage	8 (32)
Choroidal detachment	1 (4)
Retinal detachment	7 (28)
Endophtalmitis	1 (4)

n Number of eyes

OTS has been widely in open and closed globe trauma [4, 5, 13–15]. However, it had been validated in only a few subgroups of patients with IOFBs. Unal et al. [6] reported the prognostic value of OTS in cases of deadly weapon-related open-globe injuries with IOFB, Purtskhvanidze et al. [7] in rotating wire brush injuries with IOFB, and Zhu et al. [8] in siderosis bulbi with retained IOFB. Although all of them were associated with IOFBs, the mechanism of injury, presenting clinical characteristics, and distribution of OTS scores were very different among these studies. On one hand, 40% of the patients in the Purtskhvanidze et al. [7] study were OTS 5, whereas none of the patients in the Unal et al. [6] study were OTS 5. Results from Unal et al. [6] were similar to those in this OTS study, except for OTS category 2; results from Purtskhvanidze et al. [7] were similar to those in this OTS study, except for OTS category 1. Results from the study by Zhu et al. [8] were similar to those in this OTS study in all categories.

Our study group was different from the others in the literature in that we only included cases of metallic posterior segment IOFBs that required PPV. However, we obtained similar results and showed that OTS can successfully predict the functional outcome after successful removal of the IOFB with 23-G PPV. We had no patient in OTS category 5, but the final VAs were similar to the OTS categories.

One limitation of our study was the low number of patients and retrospective study design. Also, we evaluated

Table 7 Injured intraocular structures

	n (%)
Zone 1	14 (56)
Zone 2	8 (32)
Zone 3	3 (12)
Iris/ciliary body	4 (16)
Crystalline lens	13 (52)
Macula	2 (8)
Peripheric retina	9 (36)
Sclera	11 (44)

n Number of eyes

pediatric and adult patients together due to the low number of patients. In addition, there may be a geographical bias that is inherent to trauma studies. This fact underlies the need for a National Eye Registry and multicenter studies for trauma patients in Turkey. However, the relatively homogeneous patient group in this study showed that OTS was useful for this special subgroup of IOFB.

Conclusions

In conclusion, we found that OTS, which provides prognostic information after general ocular trauma, may also provide reliable prognostic information on patients who undergo 23-G PPV for the surgical removal of metallic posterior segment IOFBs. OTS may offer the possibility of approximation of the functional result in these patients before the surgery.

Abbreviations
23 G PPV: 23-gauge pars plana vitrectomy; C3F8: Perfluoropropane; HM: Hand motion; IOFB: Intraocular foreign body; IOP: Intraocular pressure; LP: Light perception; OTS: Ocular trauma score; PPL: Pars plana lensectomy; RD: Retinal detachment; SF6: Sulfur hexafluoride; VA: Visual acuity

Funding
The authors declare that no funding was received.

Authors' contributions
Involved in conceptualization of the manuscript and design of the study (DY, ZTA, AD,); acquisition, analysis and interpretation of data of data (ZGE, GD); drafting the manuscript (ZGE, GD); critical review and revision of the manuscript for important intellectual content (DY, ZTA, AD). All authors read and approved the final manuscript.

Competing interests
The authors declare that they have no competing interests.

References
1. Nordber E. Injuries as a public health problem in sub-Saharan Africa: epidemiology and prospects for control. East Afr Med J. 2000;77:1–43.
2. Negrel AD, Thylefors B. The global impact of eye injuries. Ophthalmic Epidemiol. 1998;5:143–69.
3. Kuhn F, Maisiak R, Mann L, Mester V, Morris R, Witherspoon CD. The ocular trauma score (OTS). Ophthalmol Clin N Am. 2002;15:163–5. vi
4. Ünver YB, Kapran Z, Acar N, Altan T. Ocular trauma score in open-globe injuries. J Trauma. 2009;66:1030–2.
5. Serdarevic R. The ocular trauma score as a method for the prognostic assessment of visual acuity in patients with close eye injuries. Acta Inform Med. 2015;23:81–5.
6. Unal MH, Aydin A, Sonmez M, Ayata A, Ersanli D. Validation of the ocular trauma score for intraocular foreign bodies in deadly weapon-related open-globe injuries. Ophthalmic Surg Lasers Imaging. 2008;39:121–4.
7. Purtskhvanidze K, Rüfer F, Klettner A, Borzikowsky C, Roider J. Ocular trauma score as prognostic value in traumatic ocular injuries due to rotating wire brushes. Graefes Arch Clin Exp Ophthalmol. 2017;255:1037–42.
8. Zhu L, Shen P, Lu H, Du C, Shen J, Gu Y. Ocular trauma score in Siderosis bulbi with retained intraocular foreign body. Medicine (Baltimore). 2015;94(39):e1533.
9. Kuhn F, Morris R, Witherspoon CD, Heimann K, Jeffers JB, Treister G. A standardized classification of ocular trauma. Ophthalmology. 1996;103:240–3.
10. Palioura S, Eliott D. Traumatic endophthalmitis, retinal detachment, and metallosis after intraocular foreign body injuries. Int Ophthalmol Clin. 2013;53:93–104.
11. Kıvanç SA, Akova Budak B, Skrijelj E, Tok ÇM. Demographic characteristics and clinical outcome of work-related open globe injuries in the most industrialised region of Turkey. Turk J Ophthalmol. 2017;47:18–23.
12. Greven CM, Engelbrecht NE, Slusher MM, Nagy SS. Intraocular foreign bodies: management, prognostic factors, and visual outcomes. Ophthalmology. 2000;107:608–12.
13. Ahmadieh H, Soheilian M, Sajjadi H, Azarmina M, Abrishami M. Vitrectomy in ocular trauma. Factors influencing final visual outcome. Retina. 1993;13:107–13.
14. Shah MA, Agrawal R, Teoh R, Shah SM, Patel K, Gupta S, Gosai S. Pediatric ocular trauma score as a prognostic tool in the management of pediatric traumatic cataracts. Graefes Arch Clin Exp Ophthalmol. 2017;255:1027–36.
15. Kutlutürk Karagöz I, Söğütlü Sarı E, Kubaloğlu A, Elbay A, Çallı Ü, Pinero DP, Özertürk Y, Yazıcıoğlu T. Characteristics of pediatric and adult cases with open globe injury and factors affecting visual outcomes: a retrospective analysis of 294 cases from Turkey. Ulus Travma Acil Cerrahi Derg. 2018;24:31–8.

27

Changes in anterior chamber volume after implantation of posterior chamber phakic intraocular lens in high myopia

Yi Zhu[1,2], Haobin Zhu[1,2], Yan Jia[1,3]* and Jibo Zhou[1,2]*

Abstract

Background: The present study aimed to assess changes in, and the factors that influence, anterior chamber volume (ACV) after implantable contact lens (ICL) implantation in high myopia eyes using a Pentacam.

Methods: The study sampled 26 high myopia patients (45 eyes) who were treated with ICL implantation. These patients were followed for an average of 4.28 months postoperatively. ACV was measured with a Pentacam preoperatively and at 3 months postoperatively. The data were analyzed by paired samples Wilcoxon signed-rank test. Generalized estimating equation (GEE) model adjusting within-patient intereye correlations in addition to Pearson's and Spearman's correlation tests were performed to determine associations.

Results: The mean ACV was 198.33 ± 33.08 mm^3 before surgery and 118.65 ± 17.70 mm^3 after surgery. A significant decrease of 79.68 mm^3 (40.18%) ($Z = 5.841$, $P < 0.001$) was detected. Positive correlations were found between ACV changes and ICL central vault ($r = 0.528$, $P < 0.001$) and preoperative anterior chamber depth (ACD) ($r = 0.665$, $P < 0.001$). There were positive correlations between postoperative ACV and postoperative anterior chamber angle (ACA) at 3:00 o'clock ($r = 0.448$, $P = 0.002$) and at 9:00 o'clock ($r = 0.405$, $P = 0.006$). GEE regression model showed that postoperative ACV significantly positively correlated with preoperative ACV ($P = 0.002$), ACD ($P = 0.002$) and horizontal ACA ($P = 0.005$) and negatively correlated with ICL central vault ($P < 0.001$).

Conclusion: Complementary to vault and ACD, ACV is a sensitive parameter with certain value of preoperative assessment and postoperative monitoring in ICL implantation.

Keywords: Anterior chamber volume, Implantable collamer lens, High myopia

Background

The implantable collamer lens (ICL V4; STAAR Surgical, Nidau, Switzerland) is a sulcus-placed posterior chamber phakic intraocular lens that can correct high myopia. Compared with keratorefractive surgeries, ICL V4 implantation has several advantages, including faster visual recovery, more stable refraction, better visual quality, reversibility of the surgical procedure and exchangeability of the ICL. However, ICL V4 implantation creates an artificial situation of a shallow anterior chamber and pupillary block. Therefore, laser peripheral iridectomy (LPI) is routinely performed before ICL V4 implantation to prevent intraocular

hypertension and glaucoma. It is important to monitor changes in intraocular pressure (IOP) and the anterior chamber angle (ACA) after surgery.

Although gonioscopy and ultrasonic biomicroscopy can provide direct observation of the ACA, they share the drawback of being contact procedures. As a widely applied non-contact procedure used in the clinic, the Pentacam system (Oculus Inc., Wetzlar, Germany) allows measurement of the ACA, anterior chamber volume (ACV), axial anterior chamber depth (ACD) and ICL vault. ACV and ACD measurements obtained from the Pentacam are more useful in screening for angle closure, because they are less dependent on the configuration of the peripheral part of the ACA [1]. Moreover, the ACV has been described as a sensitive parameter for monitoring ACA width and LPI efficacy [2, 3].

* Correspondence: jiayan_ylyh@sina.com; zhoujibo1000@aliyun.com
[1]Department of Ophthalmology, Shanghai Ninth People's Hospital, Shanghai Jiao Tong University School of Medicine, 639 Zhizaoju Road, Shanghai 200011, China
Full list of author information is available at the end of the article

The exact changes in the ACV after ICL implantation with an LPI cannot be determined from previous studies. A majority of studies involving ICL implantation have focused on changes in postoperative central vault. Since postoperative ACA was determined not only by central vault but also by iris root thickness and iris curvature, ACV is a useful parameter for a more comprehensive assessment of anterior chamber after ICL implantation. In the current study, we investigated the ACV, ACA, ACD and central vault after ICL implantation for the management of high myopia. In addition, we characterized ACV changes and the correlating factors after ICL implantation.

Methods
Patients
In this study, 45 eyes of 26 Chinese patients (8 males and 18 females) with a mean age of 32.47 ± 8.67 years (range 20–47 years) were assessed. The average preoperative spherical equivalent (SE) of all patients was -15.27 ± 4.61 diopters (D). All patients were relatively healthy with no systemic diseases such as kidney diseases, hematologic diseases, immune diseases or a history of drug use. The Institutional Review Board at the Shanghai Ninth People's Hospital, Shanghai JiaoTong University School of Medicine approved the study, and the study was performed in accordance with the Declaration of Helsinki. All patients signed an informed consent form.

Indications for ICL implantation included myopia of at least -5.0 D, stable refraction for at least 1 year before surgery, 20 years of age or older, no pre-existing ocular pathologic features, no previous ocular surgery, IOP between 10 and 21 mmHg, corneal endothelial cell density (ECD) of more than 2000 cells/mm^2, an ACA greater than grade III by gonioscopy and a clear crystalline lens.

Preoperative examination
Before refractive surgery, all patients underwent a complete ophthalmic examination, including the logarithm of the minimal angle of resolution (logMAR) of the uncorrected visual acuity (UCVA), the logMAR of the best spectacle-corrected visual acuity (BSCVA), SE, ACV (Pentacam; Oculus, Wetzlar, Germany), ECD (Topcon-SP; Tokyo, Japan), corneal topography, slit-lamp microscope evaluation, biometry (IOL Master; Carl Zeiss Meditec, Jena, Germany) measurements and a dilated fundus evaluation. White-to-white diameter (WTW) using a surgical compass was also measured in ICL patients. Corneal horizontal diameter and axial length were measured by the IOL-Master.

Surgical implantation of the collamer lens
To avoid postoperative pupillary block, which may result from ICL insertion, a single peripheral laser iridotomy at 12:00 o'clock (1×1 mm^2) was performed 2 to 3 days before surgery. In all patients, 0.5% levofloxacin was topically applied for 3 days preoperatively. One hour before surgery, all pupils were dilated with cycloplegic agents (tropicamide and phenylephrine, Mydrin P; Santen, Osaka, Japan). Topical anesthesia was applied three times, 30 min before surgery, using 4% oxybuprocaine eye drops. ICLs were placed in the lens insertion cartridge under direct visualization using an operating microscope. A lid speculum was placed, a 3.2 mm temporal and vertical clear corneal incision was performed, and sodium hyaluronate (CP, Shandong, China) was injected into the anterior chamber. The injector tip was then placed on the incision, and the lens was slowly injected anterior to the iris plane to ensure proper orientation. Pupillary constriction was induced by acetylcholine injection into the anterior chamber. The remaining viscoelastic material was removed with gentle irrigation and washing with the injector. After surgery, topical tobramycin-dexamethasone eye ointment was applied.

Postoperative follow-up
The mean follow-up time was 4.28 months (3–6 months). The assessed outcome parameters included the logMAR of the UCVA and BSCVA at the last visit, refraction, ECD, lens vault and silt-lamp examination for lens transparency and inflammation. In addition, a Pentacam was used to observe ACD, ACV and the position of the ICL. As shown in Fig. 1, the ACV and ACA were automatically measured and calculated by the Pentacam. ACV was defined by Pentacam software as the volume of the anterior chamber from endothelium down to iris and lens evaluated in a zone of 12 mm around the anterior corneal apex. The ACD and vault were manually identified from images scanned by the Pentacam. The same clinician operated Pentacam and recorded the average value of 3-time measurements for each examination. Postoperative outcome data at 3 months after surgery was collected and analyzed.

Statistical analysis
The data were analyzed using SPSS, version 22.0 for Windows (SPSS, Chicago, IL, USA). The normality of the samples was determined using the Kolmogorov–Smirnov test and homoscedasticity was determined using Levene's test. The Kruskal–Wallis test was used for the comparison of several independent samples. The paired samples Wilcoxon signed-rank test was used for the comparison of two related samples. Pearson's correlation test was used when samples fit the normal distribution; otherwise Spearman's

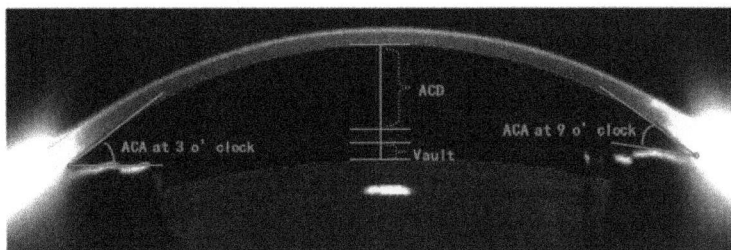

Fig. 1 Postoperative image of the anterior segment taken by the Pentacam at the horizontal meridian. The anterior chamber angle (ACA) of the temporal and nasal quadrants (at 9:00 o'clock and 3:00 o'clock) and the anterior chamber volume (ACV) were automatically measured by the device's software. The postoperative anterior chamber depth (ACD) was defined as the distance between the central posterior corneal endothelium and the anterior implantable contact lens (ICL) surface. The vault was measured as the central distance between the posterior ICL surface and the anterior crystalline lens capsule

correlation test was performed. Generalized estimating equation (GEE) model adjusting within-patient intereye correlations was used to determine the correlative parameters of postoperative ACV. A two-tailed value of $P < 0.05$ was considered to be statistically significant.

Results

Successful implantation was achieved in all patients. No complications occurred during the surgical procedures or follow-up period. None of the surgical cases required a second surgical procedure or prolonged topical medication. Visual acuity, SE, ACV, ACA, ACD and ICL central vault were demonstrated in Table 1.

After surgery, ACV significantly decreased by 79.68 mm^3 (40.18%); ACD decreased by 0.92 mm (28.40%); ACA at 3 and 9 o'clock respectively decreased by 15.80°(34.70%) and 15.58°(36.75%).

Scatterplots showed positive correlations between ACV change value and central vault ($r = 0.528$, $P < 0.001$) and between ACV change value and preoperative ACD ($r = 0.665$, $P < 0.001$) (Fig. 2). Positive correlations between postoperative ACV and postoperative ACA at 3:00 o'clock ($r = 0.448$, $P = 0.002$) and 9:00 o'clock ($r = 0.405$, $P = 0.006$) were showed in Fig. 3.

Generalized estimating equation (GEE) model of postoperative ACV adjusting for within-patient intereye correlations was performed using preoperative ACV, preoperative ACD, preoperative ACA and central vault as independent variables.

The following GEE model was obtained:

$$y = 0.218\chi_1 + 0.030\chi_2 + 0.669\chi_3 - 0.038\chi_4 - 30.217$$

where y, $\times 1$, $\times 2$, $\times 3$ and $\times 4$ are the postoperative ACV (mm^3), preoperative ACV (mm^3), preoperative ACD (μm), preoperative ACA(°) (automatically measured by Pentacam defined as the smaller value of horizontal anterior chamber angles) and ICL central

Table 1 Demographics of the study population undergoing implantable contact lens (ICL) implantation (x ± SD)

Variant	Preoperative	Postoperative	Z	P
logMAR UCVA	1.56 ± 0.45	0.20 ± 0.17	5.848	< 0.001
Spherical equivalent (D)	−15.27 ± 4.61	−0.66 ± 1.14	5.842	< 0.001
ACV (mm^3)	198.33 ± 33.08	118.65 ± 17.70	5.841	< 0.001
	range, 145–270	range, 81–150		
ACA at 3:00 o' clock (°)	43.23 ± 5.72	27.44 ± 5.24	5.841	< 0.001
	range, 32.1–55.4	range, 15.5–41.3		
ACA at 9:00 o' clock (°)	42.40 ± 5.81	26.82 ± 4.73	5.841	< 0.001
	range, 34.7–56.6	range, 16.1–39.0		
ACD (mm)	3.24 ± 0.25	2.32 ± 0.27	5.842	< 0.001
	range, 2.82–3.81	range, 1.54–2.78		
Vault (μm)		460 ± 250		
		range, 130–1110		

Data are expressed as means ± standard deviation

UCVA Uncorrected visual acuity, *D* Diopters, *ACV* Anterior chamber volume, *ACA* Anterior chamber angle, *ACD* Anterior chamber depth, *Z* Z value for Wilcoxon signed-rank test between preoperative and postoperative parameters, *P* P value for Wilcoxon signed-rank test between preoperative and postoperative parameters

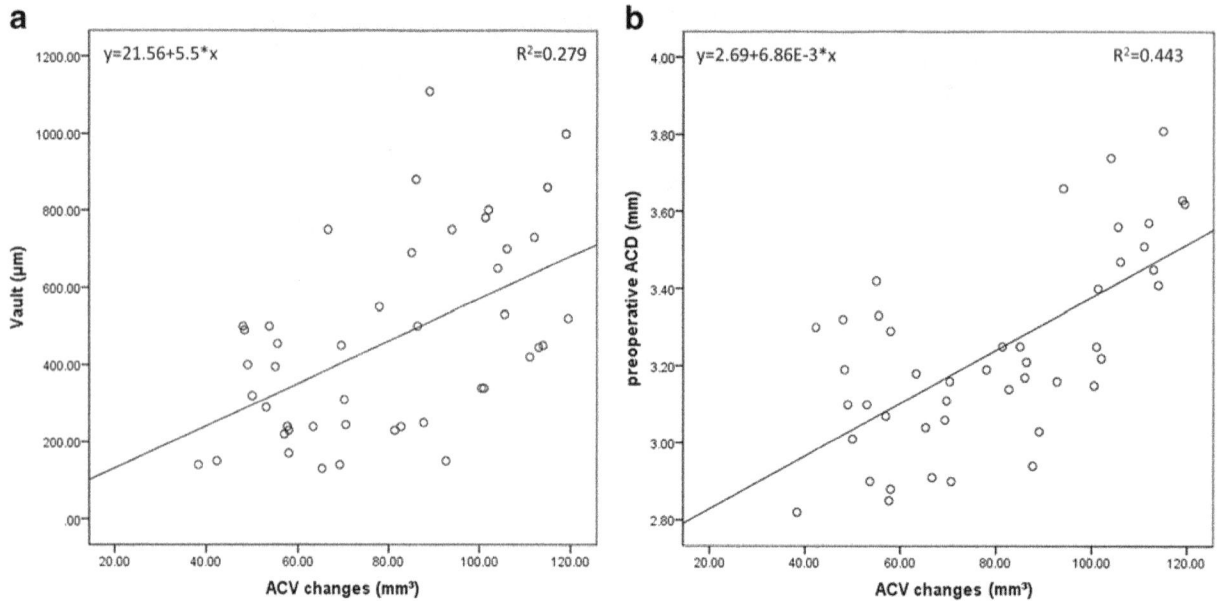

Fig. 2 a A scatterplot revealed a statistically significant correlation between ACV change value (mm^3) and ICL central vault (µm) (Pearson's correlation coefficient $r = 0.528$, $P < 0.001$). Linear regression equation: $y = 21.56 + 5.5 \cdot x$. **b** Spearman's correlation analysis revealed a positive and significant correlation between ACV change value (mm^3) and preoperative ACD (mm) ($r = 0.665$, $P < 0.001$). Linear regression equation: $y = 2.69 + 0.00686 \cdot x$

vault (µm) respectively. Detailed information were demonstrated in Table 2. The predicted postoperative ACV values calculated from the deduced model were in agreement with the measured values (Pearson's correlation coefficient $r = 0.886$, $P < 0.001$).

Discussion

The results of current study showed a decrease of ACV after ICL implantation. The change value of ACV was positively correlated with vault and preoperative ACD. It can be seen from the regression model that postoperative

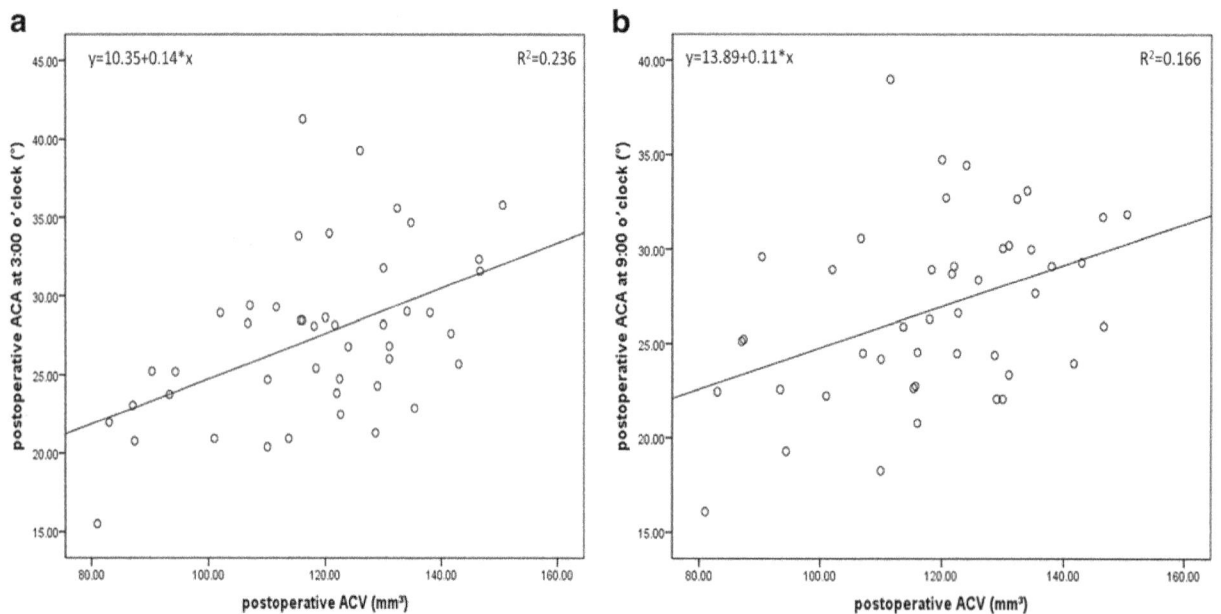

Fig. 3 Scatterplots revealed statistically significant correlations between postoperative ACV and postoperative ACA at 3:00 o'clock (Spearman's correlation $r = 0.448$, $P = 0.002$) (**a**) and at 9:00 o'clock (Spearman's correlation $r = 0.405$, $P = 0.006$) (**b**). Linear regression equations were: $y = 10.35 + 0.14 \cdot x$ (**a**) and $y = 13.89 + 0.11 \cdot x$ (**b**)

Table 2 Factors predicting postoperative ACV determined by generalized estimating equation model adjusting for within-patient intereye correlations

Independent variable	Coefficient	SE	OR	P
Preoperative ACV (mm^3)	0.218	0.0694	1.244	0.002
Preoperative ACD (μm)	0.030	0.0096	1.030	0.002
Preoperative ACA (°)	0.669	0.2387	1.952	0.005
Vault (μm)	−0.038	0.0076	0.962	< 0.001

SE Standard error, *OR* Odds ratio, *P* Significance probability, *ACV* Anterior chamber volume, *ACD* Anterior chamber depth, *ACA* The smaller value of horizontal anterior chamber angles automatically determined by Pentacam

ACV significantly positively correlated with preoperative ACV, ACD and horizontal ACA and negatively correlated with ICL central vault. Complementary to vault and ACD, ACV is a sensitive parameter for postoperative monitoring and complications predicting after ICL implantation.

The change in postoperative ACV was the result of two contrary effects on anterior segment structure changes: one was an increase in ACV caused by iris flattening after LPI, and the other was a decrease in ACV caused by forward movement of the iris under the push from the ICL. Unterlauft and colleagues showed that the mean ACV increased from 48.2 ± 3.6 to 60.6 ± 2.4 mm^3 in acute angle closure eyes and from 60.4 ± 4.6 to 74.1 ± 3.7 mm^3 in fellow eyes after LPI [4]. LPI can lead to iris flattening, angle widening and an increase in ACV in eyes with and without angle closure [4–7]. However, our study showed a 40.2% decrease in ACV, even after LPI, indicating that the decrease in the ACD after ICL insertion plays a more dominant role in the change in ACV than does LPI. A study conducted on healthy Chinese adults reported that the ACV was correlated with most of the anterior segment parameters, especially ACD, which accounted for approximately 85% of the variation in the ACV [8], consistent with the findings in the current study.

Previous studies suggested that the ACV is the strongest determinant and the most sensitive parameter among all of the established and newly identified factors associated with angle width [1–3, 9, 10]. A smaller ACV was reported to be independently associated with narrow angles, even after controlling for other known ocular risk factors, and it performs better than the ACD as a screening parameter for narrow angles [10]. Another Chinese Singaporean population-based study showed that the strongest determinants for angle width among anterior segment optical coherence tomography (ASOCT) and A-scan independent variables were the ACV, followed by anterior chamber area (the cross-sectional area of the ACV) [2]. Compared with Caucasians, ethnic Chinese individuals have a smaller ACV (independent of ACD, anterior chamber width, iris curvature, iris area, pupil diameter, corneal radius of curvature and axial length) [9], which may explain the higher rate of angle closure in the Chinese

population. The ACV was the most prominent contributor to angle width variation in both Chinese and Caucasians in that previous study [9]. Lam et al. reported that middle-aged female Chinese subjects are more likely to have angle closure than are their male counterparts. Female subjects had a smaller ACV but a similar ACD compared with those observed in male subjects. Thus, they concluded that the ACV is a more sensitive parameter to screen for a crowded anterior chamber than is a linear measurement of the ACD [3]. One explanation for this phenomenon may be that eyes with similar ACDs differ in their corneal radius of curvature, peripheral iris thickness and/or iris curvature, which contributes to angle width. Information provided by ACD evaluation is quite limited, because the ACD is a measure along just one axis. The eye is not perfectly spherical; therefore, the measured parameters may be influenced by the measurement plane, whereas the ACV is a more comprehensive parameter of anterior chamber evaluation involving corneal and iris morphologies and allowing for a three-dimensional assessment.

Moreover, the ACV is the only parameter that changed significantly after LPI, and it has the potential to be used as a numerical proxy for iris position when evaluating and monitoring patients after LPI [11–13]. Previous studies have revealed that LPI can lead to iris flattening, angle widening and an increase in the ACV in eyes with and without angle closure [4–7]. However, LPI was not effective in all eyes throughout the follow-up period [14]. He et al. reported that approximately 60% of Chinese eyes with primary angle closure suspects (PACS) exhibited persistent appositional closure in at least one quadrant after LPI [15], and Ang et al. reported that approximately 11% of Caucasian eyes with PACS were closed in at least one quadrant after LPI [16]. Ethnic and individual differences in iris thickness and flexibility likely account for the varying responses to LPI [17]. Therefore, ACV is a useful and necessary parameter that can help identify eyes that respond poorly to LPI and monitor the efficacy of LPI throughout the postoperative follow-up period after ICL implantation.

Despite a 40.18% decrease in ACV after ICL implantation, no angle closure or narrow angle condition required intervention in our study. Several previous studies have reported threshold values for discriminating between healthy eyes and eyes with narrow angles using the Pentacam system. The threshold values reported from a German study were 90.5 mm^3 for ACV, 2.1 mm for ACD and 27.25° for ACA [18]. In another study from Italy, the threshold values were 84 mm^3 for ACV, 1.93 mm for ACD and 22.4° for ACA [19]. The threshold values from an Iran study were 100 mm^3 for ACV, 2.1 mm for ACD and 26° for ACA [20]. In our study, the postoperative values were 118.65 mm^3 for ACV and 2.32 mm for ACD, which are higher than those previously reported threshold values. For eyes with postoperative parameter values under the threshold detected by Pentacam, additional examinations, such as gonioscopy and ultrasonic biomicroscopy, should be appointed.

Our results showed a positive correlation between postoperative ACV and horizontal ACA, it provided clinical evidence of postoperative monitoring value of ACV after ICL implantation. As preoperative ACD positively correlates with postoperative ACV, ICL lens of larger diameter could be considered in condition of large preoperative ACD. A negative correlation was detected between postoperative ACV and central vault as expected. Since postoperative ACV reflected iris root thickness, iris curvature and peripheral vault in addition to central vault, a more comprehensive anterior chamber assessment can be achieved by including ACV as a complementary parameter besides central vault and ACD.

There are some limitations to this study. Firstly, ACV, ACD and AVA can also be determined by pupil diameter and accommodation status. Measurements were taken in the non-mydriatic state, and the room lighting conditions were kept constant. Moreover, the internal fixation target of Pentacam may not provide good accommodation control, especially for young subjects with relatively more active accommodation. In addition, based on an accurate measurement of the IOP, the relationship between ACV changes and IOP after ICL surgery requires further investigation. Thus, in future studies, a large-scale sample study with a long-term follow-up period is needed.

Conclusions

In conclusion, this study found that, in addition to vault and ACD, ACV is a sensitive parameter with certain value of preoperative assessment and postoperative monitoring in ICL implantation. Further studies are needed to confirm its predictive application in the diagnosis and treatment of glaucoma.

Abbreviations
ACA: Anterior chamber angle; ACD: Anterior chamber depth; ACV: Anterior chamber volume; ASOCT: Anterior segment optical coherence tomography; BSCVA: Best spectacle-corrected visual acuity; D: Diopters; ECD: Endothelial cell density; ICL: Implantable contact lens; IOP: Intraocular pressure; LPI: Laser peripheral iridectomy; PACS: Primary angle closure suspects; SE: Spherical equivalent; UCVA: Uncorrected visual acuity; VIF: Variance inflation factor; WTW: White-to-white diameter

Acknowledgements
The English in this document has been checked by at least two professional editors, both native speakers of English. For a certificate, please see: http://www.textcheck.com/certificate/ahwC42.

Funding
This work was partially supported by The Science and Technology Commission of Shanghai (17DZ2260100). The funding agency had no role in the design or conduct of the study; data collection; management, analysis, or interpretation of the data; preparation; review; approval of the manuscript; or in the decision to submit the manuscript for publication.

Authors' contributions
YZ analyzed the patient data and wrote the manuscript. HZ performed the ophthalmologic examinations and collected patient data. YJ made critical revisions of the manuscript. JZ performed ICL implantation surgeries and supervised the study. All authors read and approved the final manuscript.

Competing interests
The authors declare that they have no competing interests.

Author details
[1]Department of Ophthalmology, Shanghai Ninth People's Hospital, Shanghai Jiao Tong University School of Medicine, 639 Zhizaoju Road, Shanghai 200011, China. [2]Shanghai Key Laboratory of Orbital Diseases and Ocular Oncology, Shanghai, China. [3]Department of Ophthalmology, Children's Hospital of Fudan University, Shanghai, China.

References
1. Kurita N, Mayama C, Tomidokoro A, et al. Potential of the pentacam in screening for primary angle closure and primary angle closure suspect. J Glaucoma. 2009;18(7):506–12.
2. Foo LL, Nongpiur ME, Allen JC, et al. Determinants of angle width in Chinese Singaporeans. Ophthalmology. 2012;119(2):278–82.
3. Lam AK, Tse JS. Pentacam anterior chamber parameters in young and middle-aged Chinese. Clin Exp Optom. 2013;96(1):85–91.
4. Unterlauft JD, Yafai Y, Wiedemann P. Changes of anterior chamber architecture induced by laser peripheral iridotomy in acute angle closure crisis. Int Ophthalmol. 2015;35(4):549–56.
5. Razeghinejad MR, Lashkarizadeh H, Nowroozzadeh MH, et al. Changes in ocular biometry and anterior chamber parameters after pharmacologic mydriasis and peripheral iridotomy in primary angle closure suspects. J Optom. 2016;9(3):189–95.
6. Ang BC, Nongpiur ME, Aung T, et al. Changes in Japanese eyes after laser peripheral iridotomy: an anterior segment optical coherence tomography study. Clin Exp Ophthalmol. 2016;44(3):159–65.
7. Jain R, Grewal D, Grewal S P. Quantitative analysis of anterior chamber following peripheral laser iridotomy using Pentacam in eyes with primary angle closure. Eur J Ophthalmol. 2013;23(1):55–60.
8. Zong Y, Xu Q, Jiang C, et al. Measurement of and factors associated with the anterior chamber volume in healthy Chinese adults. J Ophthalmol. 2017; 2017:6762047.
9. Wang D, Qi M, He M, et al. Ethnic difference of the anterior chamber area and volume and its association with angle width. Invest Ophthalmol Vis Sci. 2012;53(6):3139–44.
10. Wu RY, Nongpiur ME, He MG, et al. Association of narrow angles with anterior chamber area and volume measured with anterior-segment optical coherence tomography. Arch Ophthalmol. 2011;129(5):569–74.
11. Acet Y, Yigit FU, Onur IU, et al. The course of the changes in anterior chamber parameters after laser peripheral iridotomy: follow-up for 6 months with a Scheimpflug-Placido disc topographer. J Glaucoma. 2016; 25(1):14–21.
12. Vryonis N, Nikita E, Vergados I, et al. Anterior chamber morphology before and after laser peripheral iridotomy determined by Scheimpflug technology in white patients with narrow angles. J Glaucoma. 2013;22(9):679–83.
13. Talajic JC, Lesk MR, Nantel-Battista M, et al. Anterior segment changes after pilocarpine and laser iridotomy for primary angle-closure suspects with Scheimpflug photography. J Glaucoma. 2013;22(9):776–9.
14. He M, Friedman DS, Ge J, et al. Laser peripheral iridotomy in primary angle-closure suspects: biometric and gonioscopic outcomes: the Liwan Eye Study. Ophthalmology. 2007;114(3):494–500.
15. He M, Friedman DS, Ge J, et al. Laser peripheral iridotomy in eyes with narrow drainage angles: ultrasound biomicroscopy outcomes. The Liwan Eye Study. Ophthalmology. 2007;114(8):1513–9.
16. Ang GS, Wells AP. Changes in Caucasian eyes after laser peripheral iridotomy: an anterior segment optical coherence tomography study. Clin Exp Ophthalmol. 2010;38(8):778–85.
17. Lee RY, Kasuga T, Cui QN, et al. Comparison of anterior segment morphology following prophylactic laser peripheral iridotomy in Caucasian and Chinese eyes. Clin Exp Ophthalmol. 2014;42(5):417–26.

28

Involvement of HDAC6 in ischaemia and reperfusion-induced rat retinal injury

Haihong Yuan[1], Hui Li[2,3], Ping Yu[2], Qichen Fan[2], Xuan Zhang[2], Wei Huang[2], Junyi Shen[2], Yongyao Cui[2*] and Wei Zhou[4,5*]

Abstract

Background: The role of histone deacetylases 6 (HDAC6) has been elucidated in various neurodegenerative diseases. However, the effect of HDAC6 on retinal degenerative processes remains unknown. The aim of this study was to elucidate the potential role of HDAC6 in the retinal ischaemia and reperfusion (I/R) injury model.

Methods: The retinal pathological lesion was evaluated by haematoxylin and eosin (H&E) staining. HDAC expression or activity was detected by immunohistochemistry, Western blotting assays or colorimetric assays. The expression of apoptotic- and autophagic- related proteins were quantified by Western blotting and RT-PCR. The expression of peroxiredoxin 2 (Prx2) was determined by RT-PCR and ELISA. The levels of acetylated α-tubulin and acetylated histone 3 in the retina were assayed by Western blotting.

Results: We found that I/R-induced reduction of the retinal thickness was ameliorated, and the survival of RGCs was increased by the histone deacetylase (HDAC) inhibitor Trichostatin A (TSA) as well as by tubacin (an HDAC6 selective inhibitor). The decreased expression of THY (thymus cell antigen) in the I/R-induced retinas was also reversed by TSA and tubacin. Elevated HDAC6 expression and activity in the retina from I/R injury were significantly inhibited by tubacin, which also attenuated I/R-mediated apoptosis by decreasing TUNEL-positive RGCs and Bax expression and increasing Bcl-2 expression. Additionally, tubacin increased the expression of autophagy-related gene Beclin 1 and microtubule-associated protein 1 light chain 3B (LC3B) and the levels of Prx2. Furthermore, the protective effect of tubacin was associated with acetylated α-tubulin and was independent of acetylated histone 3.

Conclusions: Our findings suggest that tubacin exhibits neuroprotective effects after I/R retinal injury, and HDAC6 may be a potential therapeutic target for the retinal neurodegenerative disease of glaucoma.

Keywords: Glaucoma, Ischaemia and reperfusion, Neuroprotection, HDAC6, Tubacin

Background

Glaucoma is recognized as a collection of neurodegenerative diseases that result in retinal ganglion cell (RGC) degeneration and death [1]. Intraocular pressure (IOP) is regarded as the major risk factor. This is a multifactorial disease, and although intraocular hypertension remains an important risk factor, glaucomatous damage results from a combination of intraocular hypertension and IOP-independent risk factors [2]. Despite efforts to understand the pathological processes in the retina, few prophylaxis treatments are available to prevent glaucoma.

Retinal ischaemia/reperfusion (I/R) injury is a common clinical condition that represents the main cause of visual impairment and blindness [3]. In addition to glaucoma, retinal ischaemia likely contributes to the aetiology of many retinal diseases, such as retinal artery occlusion, optic neuropathy and diabetic retinopathy [4]. In these situations, retinal I/R results in the dysfunction or death of retina cells and retinal degeneration [5, 6]. An animal model of retinal I/R injury, which mimics acute glaucoma, is continually used to study RGC dysfunction or loss following ischaemic injury [7].

* Correspondence: yongyaocui@hotmail.com; sweetzw@hotmail.com
Haihong Yuan and Hui Li are co-first authors.
[2]Department of Pharmacology, Shanghai Jiao Tong University School of Medicine, 280 South Chongqing Road, Shanghai 200025, China
[4]Laboratory of Oral Microbiota and Systemic Diseases, Shanghai Research Institute of Stomatology, Ninth People's Hospital, Shanghai Jiao Tong University School of Medicine, 115 Jin Zun Road, Shanghai 200125, China
Full list of author information is available at the end of the article

Much evidence has indicated that I/R injury is improved via the modulation of anti-inflammatory factors and pro- and anti-apoptotic and upregulation of heat-shock proteins [8, 9]. Recent researches on retinopathy-induced epigenetic changes have advised new therapeutic methods [6, 10–12]. Epigenetic modifications have suggested a promising new approach to modulate cell function as observed in neurodegenerative diseases [13]. Histone deacetylases (HDACs) have been regarded as a therapeutic target in different diseases from neurodegeneration to cancer [14]. HDACs are enzymes that deacetylate lysine residues on histones as well as on several other cytoplasmic mitochondrial and nuclear non-histone proteins [15]. HDACs assure the reversible acetylation of histones and play an essential role in histone metabolism and transcriptional regulation. Considering the importance of HDACs to biological and pathophysiological processes in neurodegeneration and cancer, various medicinal chemistry studies have developed HDAC inhibitors to treat cancer and other malignant tumours [16, 17].

Recently, scientists studying neurodegeneration have devoted attention to HDACs, especially to HDAC6, because it could be a crucial player in various neurodegenerative diseases. HDAC6, a unique class IIb HDAC, plays an essential role in protein quality control because of its unique characteristics [16]. First, HDAC6 involves two functional N-terminal catalytic sites that are combined with a ubiquitin-binding domain at the C-terminus. Second, HDAC6 is located in the cytoplasm, indicating that its activity neither depends on histone nor influences transcriptional processes [16]. After injury to neurons, the expression of HDAC6 is elevated. Genetic and pharmacological methods have demonstrated that HDAC6 inhibition can promote the survival and regeneration of injured neurons, suggesting that HDAC6 acts as a target for the protection and regeneration in neurodegenerative disorders [18]. However, the effect of HDAC6 on the retina remains largely unknown.

Few reports exist on the effect of HDAC inhibition on RGCs. Crosson et al. [19] and Fan et al. [20] demonstrated that the inhibition of HDAC protected the retina from ischaemic injury. HDAC is involved in the neuroprotection of valproic acid (VPA) on RGCs [6, 21–23]. However, they could not verify changes in the histone acetylation levels. The interpretation of this discrepancy is that VPA-induced neuroprotection may be independent of histone acetylation [24]. Considering a histone acetylation-independent mechanism, HDAC6 could play a crucial role in the neuroprotection provided by HDAC inhibitors in the retina. Therefore, it greatly interested us whether the HDAC6 inhibitor has neuroprotective properties and its mechanism of action in a glaucoma model.

In the present study we used an in vivo retinal I/R injury model to explore the potential role of HDAC6 in glaucoma. Our results showed that HDAC activity and HDAC6 expression were significantly elevated over baseline in the retina from I/R injury in association with pathological retinal events. The HDAC6 inhibitor tubacin exerted retinal neuroprotective effects that were associated with enhanced autophagy, the inhibition of apoptosis, anti-oxidative stress. The protective effects of tubacin may be independent of acetylated histone 3 and rely on acetylated tubulin. Tubacin is a selective HDAC6 inhibitor, and Trichostatin A (TSA) is a pan-HDAC inhibitor.

Materials and methods
Animals
Adult male SD rats, whose weight ranged from 200 to 300 g in the study, were provided by the Department of Laboratory Animal Science of Shanghai Jiao Tong University School of Medicine. The rats were kept under ambient temperature (24 ± 2 °C) with a day-night rhythm of twelve hours and were given free water and food intake. All the experimental protocols were approved by the ethical committee of the Animal Care and Experimental Committee of Shanghai Jiao Tong University School of Medicine. All protocols of the animals were in accordance with the ARVO Statement for the Use of Animals in Ophthalmic and Vision Research. For neuroprotection studies, tubacin (1.33 mg/kg), vehicle or TSA (2.5 mg/kg) was administered to rats by intraperitoneal injection once per day for 6 days (3 days before and after ischaemia) [19, 20].

Animal model of retinal ischaemia and reperfusion
The animal model of retinal ischaemia/reperfusion was established based on a previously described protocol [5]. Briefly, 3% sodium pentobarbital was intraperitoneally injected into rats for anaesthesia, while 0.5% phenylephrine hydrochloride and 0.5% tropicamide were used for full dilation of pupils. A 30-gauge needle in connection with a vessel filled with saline was applied to the cannulating anterior chamber. The vessel was raised to form a hydrostatic pressure ranged from 110 to 120 mmHg for fifty minutes to increase IOP and induce retinal ischaemia. Each pressure was then returned to normal, and the eye was examined to ensure that retinal blood flow was re-established. The experimental rats were divided into four groups—sham group, I/R plus vehicle group, I/R plus tubacin group, and I/R plus TSA group—with five to eight rats in each group.

Histopathologic study
The rats were anaesthetized with chloral hydrate and were perfused with physiological saline before sacrifice.

The experimental globes were enucleated three days after the ischaemia-reperfusion operation. The eyes were fixed with PBS containing 4% paraformaldehyde and were subsequently washed with PBS. After dissecting foreparts and lens, the eye cups were dewatered and embedded using paraffin and were cut into slices horizontally through optic discs at 3-μm thickness. Haematoxylin and eosin (H&E) were used to stain the slices. In each slice, the layers of the retina apart from the centre of the optic nerve head (ONH) for approximately 1.5 mm were collected as picture data and were written into a disk using an optical microscope in connection with a digital camera. The retinal injuries were evaluated by measuring the quantity of cells in the ganglion cell layer (GCL) and thickness of each layer. The nuclear cells in GCL were quantified every 200 μm, and the average value was applied to determine a typical cell quantity in GCL.

TUNEL staining

Four-percent paraformaldehyde was utilized to fix freshly isolated retinas, and paraffin was used for embedding. The retina sections were mounted on glass slides and then were de-paraffinized/hydrated for TUNEL staining. The TUNEL assay was performed using the In Situ Cell Death Detection Kit (Roche, Penzberg, Germany) according to the manufacturer's instructions. The retina slides were permeabilized with 0.1% Triton X-100 and blocked with 3% H_2O_2. After incubation with the TUNEL reaction mixture for 60 min at 37 °C in a humid chamber, the slides were incubated in Converter-peroxidase (POD) for 30 min at 37 °C and were stained with diaminobenzidine (DAB) POD substrate. Images were acquired by microscopy.

Measurement of HDAC6 expression and retinal HDAC activity in the retina

The avidin-biotin-peroxidase complex (ABC) technique and HDAC6 antibody (1:50; Cell Signalling Technology, Beverly, MA, USA) were used to process frozen sections of retinas in the I/R + Vehicle, I/R + tubacin, I/R + TSA and sham groups to conduct immunohistochemical analyses at 4 °C overnight. Subsequently, the slices were incubated with ABC complex and biotinylated rabbit anti-goat IgG purified by affinity at ambient temperature for 1 h. In the experiment, 0.1 M PBS containing 0.5% Triton X-100 was used to dilute all antisera. After DAB staining, images were acquired by microscopy.

To assess the fluctuations in HDAC activity affected by tubacin, the retinae dissected free after euthanization was stored at − 80 °C for subsequent experiments. The retinal lysates were sonicated and centrifuged. The supernatant was used to determine the HDAC activity using a HDAC Activity Colorimetric Assay Kit (BioVision,

Mountain View, CA, USA) according to the manufacturer's instruction. The HDAC activity in the samples was calculated based on a standard curve and was normalized to total proteins in the retinae measured using the BCA protein assay kit (Pierce, Rockford, IL, USA).

Total RNA extraction and quantitative real-time PCR (RT-PCR)

Total RNA was extracted from the retinae using the DNA/RNA/Protein Isolation kit (Omega Bio-Tek, Norcross, USA), and RT-PCR was conducted using M-MLV Reverse Transcriptase (Invitrogen, Carlsbad, USA). The cDNA sequences obtained from the reverse transcription of three parallel samples were utilized to determine the level of target mRNA quantitatively through qRT-PCR with SYBR® Premix Ex TaqTM using a LightCycler® 480IIsequence detector (Roche, Forrenstrasse CH-6343, Rotkreuz, Switzerland). The RT-PCR primer sequences are listed in Table 1. β-Actin was used as a control. The 20-μl sample contained 10 μl of PCR using the SYBR® Premix Ex TaqTM (TaKaRa Biotechnology, Dalian, China), 8 pmol of primer and 1.2 μl of RT reaction. The experiments were triplicated in the LightCycler® 480 Multiwell Plate 96 (Roche, Mannheim, Germany). The cycling parameters consisted of 95 °C for 30 s, followed by 40 cycles of 95 °C for 10 s, 60 °C for 20 s, and 72 °C for 15 s. The relative levels of target mRNA expression were calculated using the $2^{-\Delta\Delta Ct}$ method.

Western blotting analysis

Retinae were washed twice in PBS and were lysed in ice-cold RIPA buffer (Beyotime Institute of Biotechnology, Shanghai, China, followed by dispersion ultrasonically. The BCA assay kit (Pierce, Rockford, USA) was utilized to determine the concentration of proteins. The samples were mixed with 0.0125% bromophenol blue and 2.5% β-mercaptoethanol and were boiled for five minutes before being subjected to SDS-PAGE. After transferring the protein blots onto PVDF membranes (Merck Millipore, Billerica, USA), the membranes were incubated at 4 °C overnight with the following primary antibodies: HDAC6 (1:500; SANTA CRUZ Biotechnology, Dallas, USA), Beclin1, LC3, Bax, Bcl2 (1:1000; Cell Signal Technology, Danvers, USA), peroxiredoxin 2 (Prx2, 1:500; Sigma, St. Louis, USA), Acetylated-α-tubulin, α-tubulin (1:500; Beyotime Institute of Biotechnology, Shanghai, China), THY (1:500; Merck Millipore, Billerica, USA) and β-actin (1:1000; Zhongshan Biotechnology, Beijing, China). After incubating the membranes with the appropriate secondary antibody conjugated to horseradish peroxidase (1:8000, Zhongshan Biotechnology, Beijing, China), an enhanced chemiluminescence detection kit (Pierce Chemical,

Table 1 The RT-PCR primer sequences are listed

Gene name	Primer sequence	
	Forward	Reverse
actin	5'-AATCCTGTGGCATCCATGAA-3'	5'-GGACAGTGAGGCCAGGATAGA-3'
beclin-1	5'-AGGAGTTGGCCTTGGAGGA-3'	5'-CCGCTGTGCCAGATATGGA-3'
lc3	5'-CGTCCTGGACAAGACCAAGTT-3'	5'-GGTGCCTACGTTCTGATCTGTG-3'
bax	5'-GAGCGGCTGCTTGTCTGGAT-3'	5'-CAAGGCAGCAGGAAGCCTCA-3'
bcl-2	5'- GCAGATGCCGGTTCAGGTA-3'	5'-ACGGTGGTGGAGGAACTCTT-3'
Prx2	5'-AGGACTTCCGAAAGCTAGGC-3'	5'- TTGACTGTGATCTGGCGAAG-3'
HDAC6	5'-GCACGCTGTCTCATCCTACCT-3'	5'-CCCGAGTTTTCATCTTTTCTGTG-3'

Rockford, IL, USA) was utilized to visualize the protein blots.

Enzyme-linked immunosorbent assay (ELISA) of Prx2

Rats injected with vehicle, TSA or tubacin 1 h before ischaemia of a single retina, aiming to determine whether Prx2 activity was affected by HDAC inhibition. After I/R, the retina was cut open and immersed into lysing buffer containing proteinase inhibitors and then were stored at – 80 °C. Subsequently, ELISA (Xi'tang Biotechnology, Shanghai, China) was conducted to analyse Prx2 activity using the supernatant from the centrifuged extract of retinae. The total protein of retinae was measured using the BCA protein assay (Pierce Chemical, Rockford, IL, USA) and was applied to normalizing the concentration of prx2 in samples which was calculated based on the standard curve. Prx2 activity can be expressed as the concentration per mg protein sample.

Statistically analysis of the data

All data were represented as mean ± SEM. One-way analysis of variance (ANOVA) and Dunnett's post hoc tests were successively applied to result analyses. P value less than 0.05 was accepted as the threshold of statistical significance. An image-analysis programme (IPP, Olympus, Japan) was used to perform all measurements.

Results

Effect of tubacin on retinal morphological injury after I/R injury

The morphological changes induced by 50-min ischaemia in each group were assessed on days 3 after I/R injury (Fig. 1a; Table 2). Table 2 showed the overall retinal thickness in the I/R-plus-vehicle group had significantly decreased at 3 days after I/R injury compared with that in the sham-operated group. The inner nuclear layer (INL) thickness and inner plexiform layer (IPL) thickness in the I/R-plus-vehicle group were both reduced. A significantly decreased cell count in the I/R-plus-vehicle group was observed in the ganglion cell layer (GCL) that was reduced by 26.2% compared with

that in the sham-operated group. By contrast, the overall retinal thickness in the I/R-plus-tubacin group or in the I/R-plus-TSA group was significantly increased compared with that in the I/R-plus-vehicle group. Tubacin or TSA could significantly restore the IPL thickness. The loss of the GCL cells was restored only by tubacin, while the INL thickness was recovered only by TSA.

Additionally, Western blotting (Fig. 1b, c) results demonstrated that I/R-induced down-regulation of protein expression of THY gene, a ganglion cell-specific marker in rodent retina, could be antagonized by tubacin. These above results demonstrated that HDAC6 is involved in I/R-induced retinal morphological injury.

HDAC6 expression and HDAC activity in normal or I/R injury retinas

Immunohistochemical staining revealed that HDAC6 is primarily localized in the INL and GCL, with little expression in the ONL, OPL and IPL (Fig. 2a). HDAC activity in normal retinas was low but was increased significantly after I/R injury. The increased retinal HDAC activity after retinal I/R injury can be attenuated either by the pan-HDAC inhibitor TSA (26.5%) or HDAC6 inhibitor tubacin (20.7%) compared with that in the I/R group (Fig. 2b). Immunohistochemical staining (Fig. 2a) and Western blot analysis (Fig. 2c) revealed that HDAC6 expression was significantly increased after I/R injury compared with that in the sham-operated retinas. The high expression of HDAC6 after retinal I/R injury could be attenuated either by TSA or tubacin.

Effect of tubacin on retinal cell apoptosis and autophagy after I/R injury

Because cell apoptosis and autophagy are the prominent features of axonal degeneration in the optic nerve, we next evaluated whether HDAC6 is involved in the regulation of cell apoptosis and autophagy after I/R injury. The apoptotic cells were counted by the TUNEL assay (Fig. 3a). The number of TUNEL-positive cells in the I/R-plus-vehicle group was obviously higher than that in the sham group. However, a decrease occurred in the

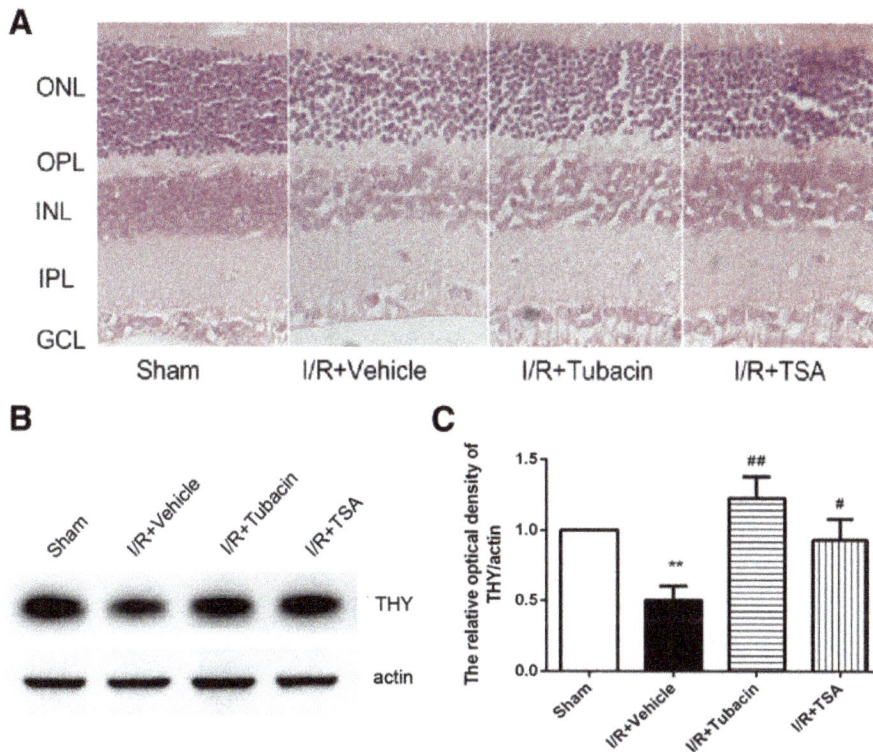

Fig. 1 Effect of tubacin on retinal morphologic changes after I/R injury. (**a**) Photomicrographs of retinal cross-sections. Five well-organized retinal layers: ONL, outer nuclear layer; OPL, outer plexiform layer; INL, inner nuclear layer; IPL, inner plexiform layer; and GCL, ganglion cell layer. Analysis of the overall retinal thickness includes ONL, OPL, INL, IPL, and GCL. Analysis of the cell body counts from the retinal ganglion cell layer (GCL) over 200-μm distances. (**b**, **c**) Expression of THY as detected by Western blotting and quantitative analyses. The data are presented as means ± SEM ($n = 5$–8 rats per group). $*P < 0.05$, $**P < 0.01$ vs. Sham group; $^{\#}P < 0.05$, $^{\#\#}P < 0.01$ vs. I/R-plus-vehicle

density of apoptotic cells in the I/R-plus-tubacin group compared with that in the I/R-plus-vehicle group. This result suggested that I/R-induced apoptotic cell death can be alleviated by the HDAC6 inhibitor tubacin in the rat model.

RT-PCR (Fig. 3b, c) and Western blotting (Fig. 3d, e, f) showed that I/R injury activated Bax and attenuated the expression of Bcl-2. By contrast, tubacin significantly inhibited the activation of Bax and increased the expression of Bcl-2. These data suggested that tubacin suppressed I/R injury-induced retinal cell apoptosis.

The expression of autophagy-related genes and proteins were evaluated by RT-PCR (Fig. 4a, b) and Western blotting (Fig. 4c, d, e). The levels of LC3B and Beclin1 were decreased in the retina of the I/R-plus-vehicle group,

indicating autophagy was diminished after I/R. However, the levels of LC3B and Beclin1 in the retina could be significantly upregulated by pretreatment with tubacin. These results demonstrated that the I/R injury-induced autophagy activity could be reversed by attenuating HDAC6.

Effect of tubacin on increasing Prx2 after I/R injury

Several studies have suggested that Prx2 is related to the development of neurodegenerative disease and confirmed that Prx2 is a specific target of HDAC6; thus, we observed the expression of Prx2 in the retinal I/R injury animal model and role of HDAC6. RT-PCR (Fig. 5a) and ELISA (Fig. 5b) analyses revealed that Prx2 was significantly decreased after I/R, whereas TSA, as well as

Table 2 Effect of tubacin on ischaemia-induced depth of overall retina, inner retina, and number of cells in GCL

	Overall retinal thickness (μm)	Inner nuclear layer (μm)	Inner plexiform layer (μm)	Number of cells in GCL (per mm)
Sham	300.56 ± 61.82	49.01 ± 7.94	69.98 ± 15.25	42.65 ± 1.68
I/R + Vehicle	224.44 ± 25.33**	41.64 ± 8.04*	45.95 ± 11.85**	31.47.± 1.47**
I/R + Tubacin	283.89 ± 54.12$^{\#\#}$	44.76 ± 4.37	62.15 ± 18.20$^{\#\#}$	37.04 ± 1.66$^{\#}$
I/R + TSA	287.22 ± 51.56$^{\#\#}$	49.02 ± 5.89$^{\#\#}$	71.58 ± 8.60$^{\#\#}$	34.39 ± 1.30

At 3 days after I/R, the eyes were enucleated, and cross-sections were prepared. Retinal I/R induced a significant decrease in the overall retinal thickness from GCL to ONL, inner retina thickness including INL and IPL, and cell number of GCL. The alteration in overall retinal thickness, inner retina including INL and IPL, and in cell number of GCL was partially prevented by tubacin. The values are expressed as means ± SEM ($n = 5$–8 rats per group). $**P < 0.01$ vs. Sham; $^{\#}P < 0.05$ vs. I/R + vehicle

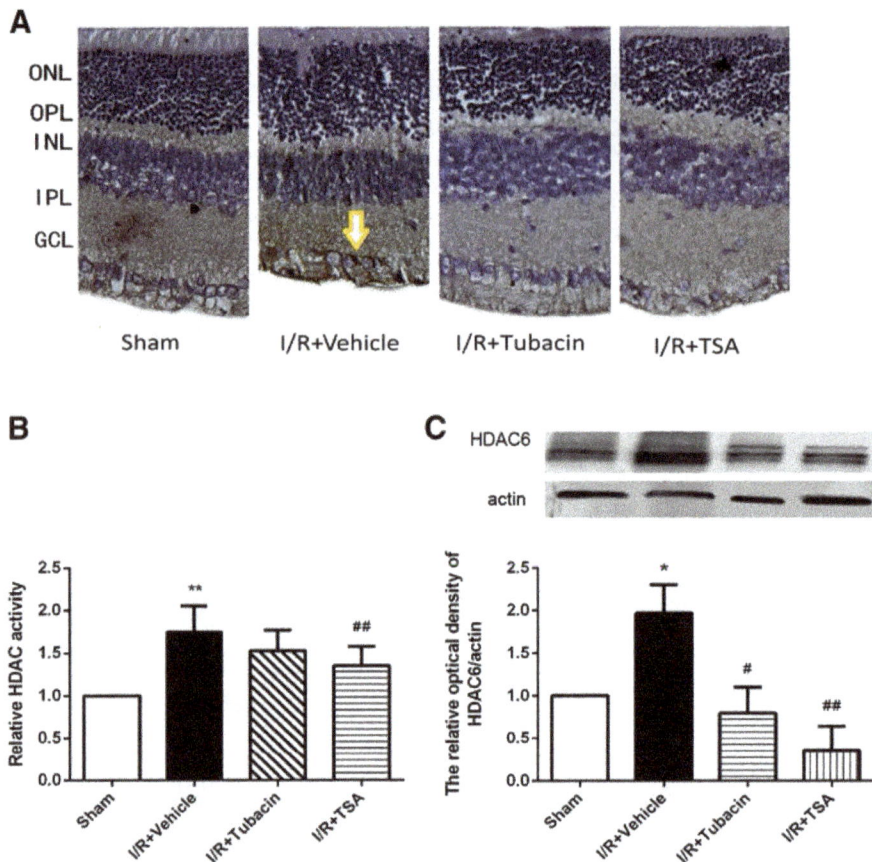

Fig. 2 HDAC6 expression and effect of tubacin in the retina. (**a**) Immunohistochemical staining of HDAC6 in the retina (brown). HDAC6 immunoreactivity in the sham-operated retina, I/R-plus-vehicle retina, I/R-plus-tubacin retina and I/R-plus-TSA retina. (**b**) HDACs activity of retinas in different group. (**c**) Western blotting analysis of HDAC6 expression in retinal lysates. The values are expressed as means ± SEM ($n = 5$–8 rats per group). *$P < 0.05$, **$P < 0.01$ vs. Sham group; #$P < 0.05$, ##$P < 0.01$ vs. I/R-plus-vehicle

tubacin, could reverse I/R-induced events that decrease Prx2. These results indicated that manipulating HDAC6 by tubacin could increase the expression of Prx2 influenced by I/R injury.

Effect of tubacin on restoring the α-tubulin acetylated levels

To evaluate whether treatment with tubacin could result in the hyperacetylation of retinal proteins, the expression of acetylated histone-3 in the retina was determined by Western blot analysis. The result showed that the level of acetylated histone-3 in the retinas of tubacin-treated animals was relatively lower than that of the sham group. However, the level of retina histone-3 acetylation in the TSA-treated group was markedly increased (Fig. 6a, c). The relatively high expression of acetylated α-tubulin was detected in the retinas of both tubacin-treated and TSA-treated animals (Fig. 6a, b). These results indicated that the neuroprotection of tubacin did not involve the histone acetylation but tubulin stabilization.

Discussion

It was confirmed that the HDAC6 inhibitor tubacin could protect the retina from I/R injury, as indicated by the preservation of retinal morphology and neurons in the GCL. Moreover, tubacin pretreatment inhibited the expression of pro-apoptotic proteins and inflammatory mediators and enhanced the expression levels of Bcl-2, which inhibits apoptosis. Tubacin treatment also upregulated the expression of autophagy-related proteins and anti-oxidative proteins. Furthermore, the protective role of tubacin was associated with acetylated α-tubulin rather than acetylated histone. These results demonstrated that HDAC6 plays an important role in I/R-induced neurodegenerative disorders of the retina.

Until now, eighteen human HDACs of four categories were discovered, the functions of are involved in apoptosis, differentiation, the cell cycle and transcription. HDAC1, HDAC2, HDAC3 and HDAC8 in Class I are distributed ubiquitously, while HDAC4, HDAC 5, HDAC6, HDAC7, HDAC9 and HDAC10 in class II are distributed specifically. HDAC6 belongs to class IIb

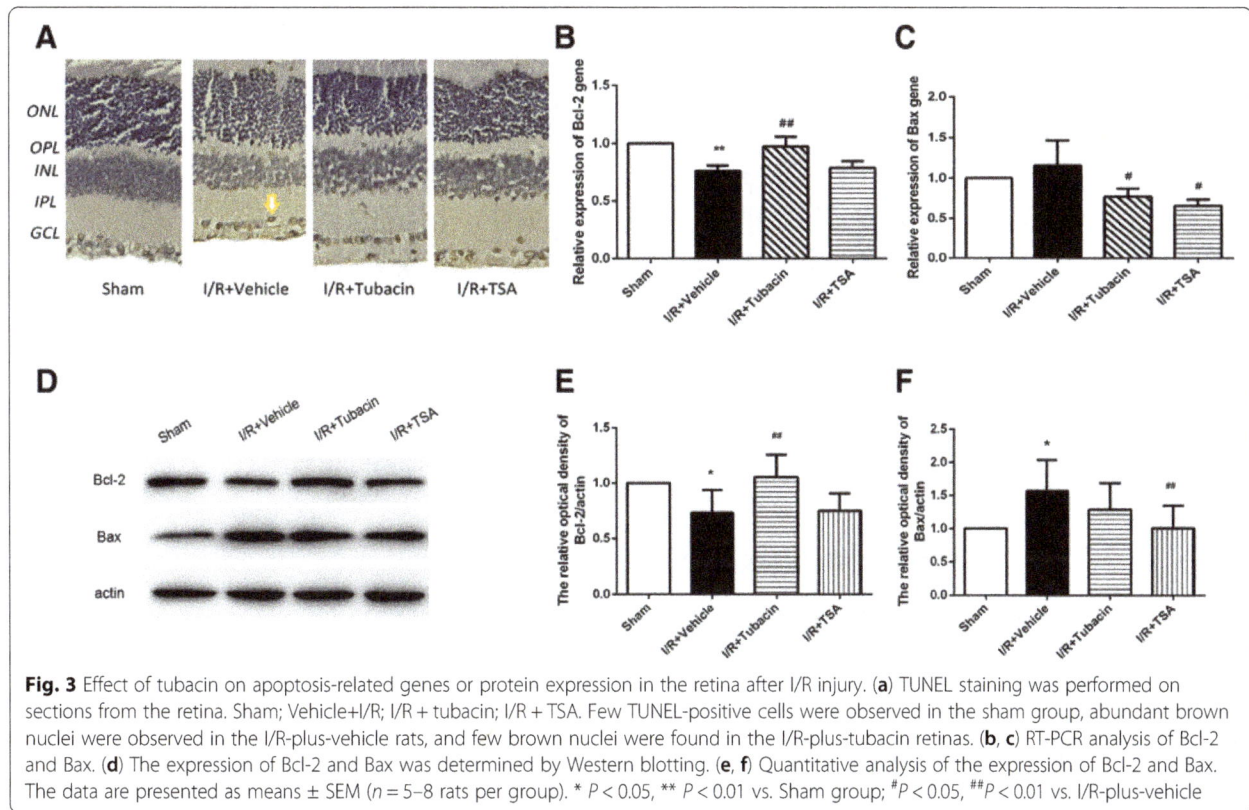

Fig. 3 Effect of tubacin on apoptosis-related genes or protein expression in the retina after I/R injury. (a) TUNEL staining was performed on sections from the retina. Sham; Vehicle+I/R; I/R + tubacin; I/R + TSA. Few TUNEL-positive cells were observed in the sham group, abundant brown nuclei were observed in the I/R-plus-vehicle rats, and few brown nuclei were found in the I/R-plus-tubacin retinas. (b, c) RT-PCR analysis of Bcl-2 and Bax. (d) The expression of Bcl-2 and Bax was determined by Western blotting. (e, f) Quantitative analysis of the expression of Bcl-2 and Bax. The data are presented as means ± SEM ($n = 5$–8 rats per group). * $P < 0.05$, ** $P < 0.01$ vs. Sham group; #$P < 0.05$, ##$P < 0.01$ vs. I/R-plus-vehicle

HDACs and is unique in that it is a cytoplasmic microtubule-associated enzyme. HDAC6 deacetylates tubulin, HSP90, and cortactin, forms complexes with other partner proteins and is involved in numerous biological processes, such as cell migration and cell-to-cell interactions [17, 20, 24, 25]. Preliminary studies on the retina of mice proved the expression of HDAC1 3, 4, 5, 6, 16, and 17. These isoforms play essential roles in the development of Müller cells and neurocytes in the retina that include ganglia and bipolar and rod cells. Our present study agreed with these studies and showed that HDAC6 is expressed in the cytosol of the retina and is mainly localized in the inner retinal layer and GCL. Furthermore, I/R injury significantly increased the expression of HDAC6, which could be inhibited by the selective HDAC6 inhibitor tubacin and pan-HDAC inhibitor TSA. Our study suggests that HDAC6 may be involved in I/R-induced retinal neurodegeneration, and inhibiting HDAC6 may exert a neuroprotective effect.

Glaucoma is a primary cause of global blindness. The disease is characterized by the progressive degeneration of RGCs and their axons, resulting in irreversibly damaged visual function in the end [26, 27]. All the programmed cell death (PCD) types, including apoptosis and autophagy, play important roles in the development of the glaucomatous retina of glaucoma patients and mammalian models. It is crucial to better understand the molecular mechanism of retinal PCD and develop better therapies. The methods aimed at understanding the molecular mechanisms of PCD and its regulation may be helpful for neuronal survival and preservation of visual function. The understanding of the potential principle of the deaths of retinal neurons in glaucoma are probably increased; thus, the relevant therapies are improved by using the model of I/R injury in the retina, mimicking the clinical manifestations of acute angle closure glaucoma. Our study also indicated that the HDAC6 inhibitor tubacin could attenuate I/R-induced RGC loss.

Autophagy is an evolutionarily conserved process that is involved in regulating organelles and proteins [28]. It plays a key role in maintaining intracellular homeostasis [29] and cell survival in a stressful environment. According to different circumstances, autophagy can have beneficial or deleterious effects on neurons [3]. Thus far, little is known about the role of the autophagic pathway in RGC death. Activation of autophagy was investigated in RGCs following optic nerve transection, and a protective role was indicated in RGC-5 cells in starvation [18]. The persistent accumulation of autophagosomes, concurrent with injury-induced axonal degradation and secondary to lesion-induced calcium influx, was reported in the optic nerve following optic nerve crushing.

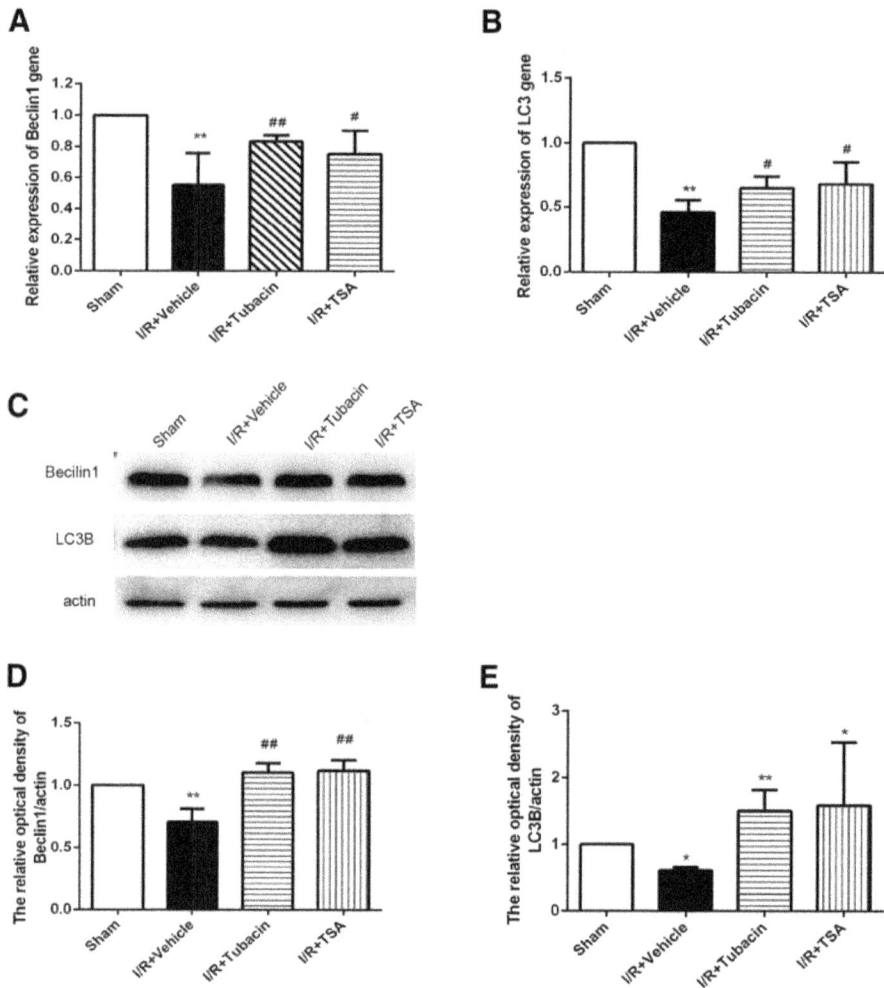

Fig. 4 Effect of tubacin on autophagy-related genes after I/R injury. (**a**, **b**) RT-PCR analysis of LC3B and Beclin1 expression in the retina of different groups. (**c**, **d**, **e**) The expression of LC3B and Beclin1 was determined by Western blotting. The data are presented as means ± SEM ($n = 5$–8 rats per group). $*P < 0.05$, $**P < 0.01$ vs. Sham group; $^{\#}P < 0.05$, $^{\#\#}P < 0.01$ vs. I/R-plus-vehicle

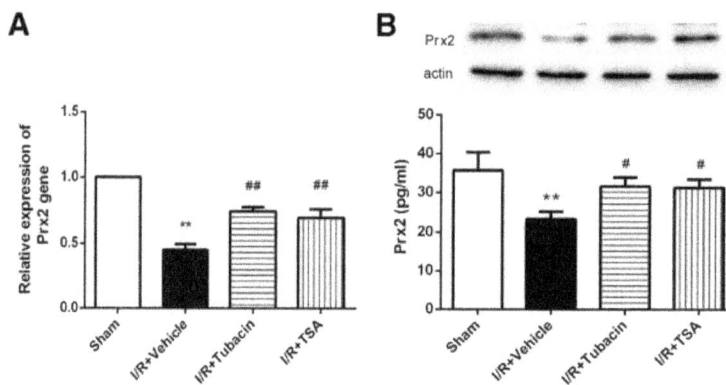

Fig. 5 Effect of tubacin on Prx2 after I/R injury. The animals were treated with vehicle or tubacin, and Prx2 was measured 8 h after ischaemia. (**a**) PCR analysis of Prx2 expression. (**b**) Prx2 level detected by ELISA. The data are expressed as means ± SEM. $**P < 0.01$ vs. Sham group; $^{\#}P < 0.05$, $^{\#\#}P < 0.01$ vs. I/R-plus-vehicle

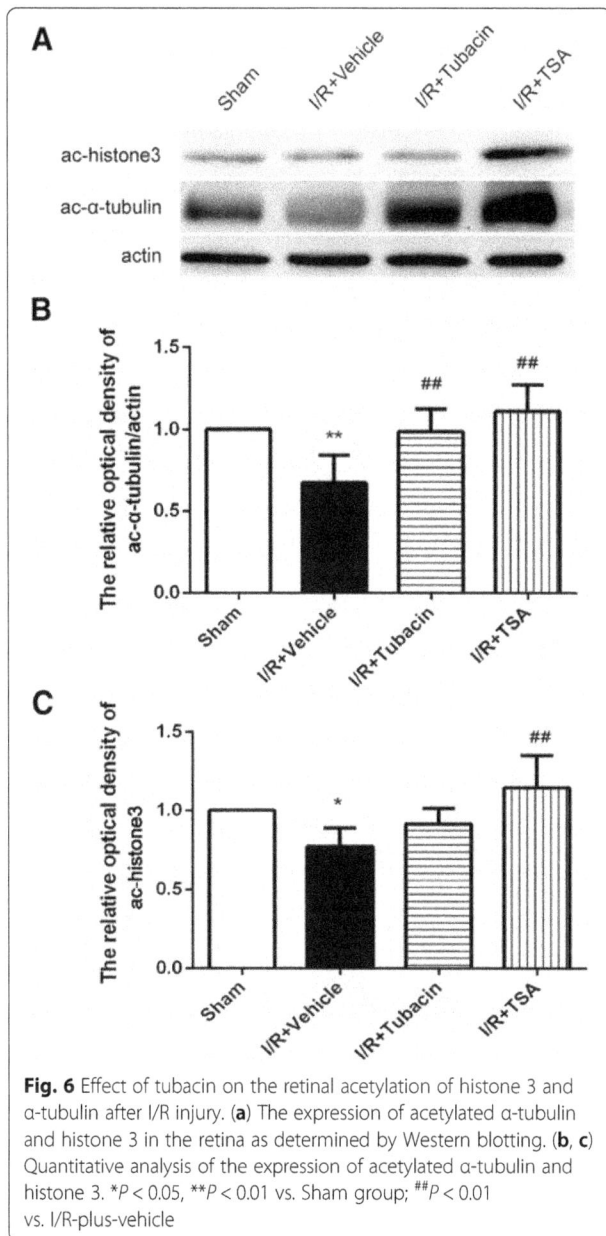

Fig. 6 Effect of tubacin on the retinal acetylation of histone 3 and α-tubulin after I/R injury. (a) The expression of acetylated α-tubulin and histone 3 in the retina as determined by Western blotting. (b, c) Quantitative analysis of the expression of acetylated α-tubulin and histone 3. *$P < 0.05$, **$P < 0.01$ vs. Sham group; ##$P < 0.01$ vs. I/R-plus-vehicle

Presently, the role of autophagy in I/R injury remains controversial. The effect of inhibiting autophagy was considered as protection for neurocytes and potentially as an innovative approach to preventing ischaemia injuries. Nevertheless, activated autophagy was also considered as protective for neurocytes in the ischaemic brain and I/R retina [3]. Our results support the view that autophagy plays a protective role in retinal I/R. Beclin1 plays an important role in the induction of autophagy, and LC3 is involved in the maturation process of autophagosomes. A significant decrease in Beclin1 and LC3 expression was observed in retinas subjected to I/R injury, suggesting impaired autophagic activity that seemingly agreed with the conclusion of a previous study [3].

Additionally, the multifarious effect of HDAC6 on stimulating autophagy was unrevealed yet and disputable to a certain extent. Despite abundant facts indicating the stimulative role of HDAC6 in autophagic activity, the latest results suggested the necessity of hyper-acetylated α-tubulin in generating an assembly platform for autophagosomes [30–32]. HDAC6 is indispensable to fusing autophagosomes and lysosomes instead of causing autophagy [33]. The significance of HDAC6 in selective autophagy was probably superior to that in other types of autophagy—for example, autophagy caused by starvation—because HDAC6 has domains that bind ubiquitin and could modulate the responses to unfolded proteins [33]. Our results also showed that tubacin administration increased the expression levels of retinal Beclin1 and LC3B after I/R injury, indicating that tubacin reversed retinal autophagic activity, which was probably related to the principle of tubacin preventing I/R injury. We noted that the observed increase in autophagy may be traced back to the inhibition of HDAC6-mediated tubulin deacetylation [34]. Further research is needed to clarify the mechanism of the regulation of tubacin in the autophagy activity of the retina and to identify new targets for autophagy pathways to establish new treatment strategies for I/R injury.

RGC deaths induced by I/R were postponed by tubacin treatment, a finding that agreed with the results of former studies that tubacin effectively protected neurons in other neurodegenerative disorders of the central nervous system [35, 36]. However, recent studies on cancer therapy have demonstrated that HDAC6 inhibitors inhibit proliferation and induce apoptosis in multiple myeloma cells. This consistency presumes that tubacin could indirectly exert anti-apoptotic activity via HSP90 or Prxs. This protective effect was accompanied by tubacin-mediated inhibition of a pro-apoptosis molecule (Bax) and induction of anti-apoptotic factors (Bcl-2). Bcl-2 is associated with apoptosis [37] and can be induced via various stimuli, including glucose deprivation, growth factor deprivation and lipid peroxidation [38]. The induction of Bcl-2 has been indicated to protect against apoptosis [39]. Bax, a pro-apoptotic protein of the Bcl-2 family of proteins, could strongly facilitate mitochondrial membrane permeabilization and the activation of nucleases and caspases. This can result in irreversible damage to the mitochondria and acceleration of programmed cell death [40, 41]. The anti-apoptosis effect of tubacin was confirmed by the attenuation of cell death due to I/R in this study.

Prxs belong to a superfamily of thiol peroxidases that act as the catalyst in the reactions of reducing reactive oxygen species (ROS) and consequently play a crucial role in oxidation resistance and redox signalling pathways. Prx2 is especially essential to protect the nerve system, and it has cytoprotective effects in response to transient brain ischaemia and oxidative stress [42–45]. Parmigiant et al. reported that HDAC6 is a specific deacetylase of Prxs and is involved in redox regulation [46]. Previous studies have revealed that, after being intensively exposed to ROS, cysteine in the active sites of Prx2 was hyper-oxidized into derivatives of cysteine sulfonic acid or sulfinyl (Cys-SO2/3) and the activity of peroxidase for protection was lost [47, 48]. Our study agrees with the above studies. HDAC6 and Prxs may be targets to modulate the intracellular redox status in neurodegenerative diseases, and the HDAC6 inhibitor exerted retinal neuroprotection due to I/R injury.

Conclusions

Our studies demonstrate that pretreatment with the HDAC6 inhibitor against I/R injury in the retina may exert potential retinal neuroprotection by enhancing autophagy, inhibiting apoptosis, and modulating anti-oxidative stress. Furthermore, its protective effect may be independent of histone acetylation and mediated by acetylated tubulin. These findings support the view that the regulation of acetylation in the retina is not only histone dependent but also histone-independent regulation, with potential beneficial effects as a neuroprotectant. Our findings may provide a potential neuroprotective strategy for the treatment of glaucoma.

Abbreviations

ABC: Avidin-biotin-perosidase complex; Bax: Bcl-2 Assaciated X protein; Bcl-2: B-cell lymphoma-2; Cys-SO2/3: cysteine sulfonic acid or sulfinyl; DAB: Diaminobenzidine; GCL: Ganglion cell layer; H&E: Hematoxylin and eosin; HDAC: Histone deacetylase; HSP: Heat Shock Proteins; I/R: Ischemia and reperfusion; INL: Inner nuclear layer; IOP: Intraocular pressure1; IPL: Inner plexiform layer; LC3: light chain 3; ONH: Optic nerve head; ONL: Outernuclear layer; OPL: Outer plexiform layer; PCD: Programmed cell death; POD: Peroxidase; Prx2: Peroxiredoxin 2; RGC: Retinal ganglion cell; ROS: Reactive oxygen species; TSA: Trichostatin A; VPA: Valproic acid

Acknowledgments

We thank Lin Zheng for technical support in immunohistochemistry.

Funding

This study was supported by the National Natural Science Foundation of China (No. 81273519, 30700280 and 81370144), National Science and Technology Major Projects for Major New Innovation and Development (No.2014ZX09104002–005) and the Shanghai Education Commission (No.12YZ037, 12YZ200).

Authors' contributions

WZ and YC designed the study, analyzed the data, and wrote the manuscript. HY and HL carried out most of the experimental work and prepared the manuscript. PY, QF and XZ performed the animal study and the partial histological analysis. JYS and WH revised the manuscript. All authors read and approved the final manuscript.

Competing interests

The authors declare that they have no competing interests.

Author details

[1]Department of Pharmacy, Shanghai University of Medicine & Health Science, Shanghai, China. [2]Department of Pharmacology, Shanghai Jiao Tong University School of Medicine, 280 South Chongqing Road, Shanghai 200025, China. [3]Department of Pharmacy, Qingpu Branch of Zhongshan Hospital, Fudan University School of Medicine, Shanghai, China. [4]Laboratory of Oral Microbiota and Systemic Diseases, Shanghai Research Institute of Stomatology, Ninth People's Hospital, Shanghai Jiao Tong University School of Medicine, 115 Jin Zun Road, Shanghai 200125, China. [5]Shanghai Key Laboratory of Stomatology & Shanghai Research Institute of Stomatology, National Clinical Research Center of Stomatology, Shanghai, China.

References

1. Chang EE, Goldberg JL. Glaucoma 2.0: neuroprotection, neuroregeneration, neuroenhancement. Ophthalmology. 2012;119(5):979–86.
2. Mozaffarieh M, Flammer J. New insights in the pathogeesis and treatment of normal tension glaucoma. Curr Opin Pharmacol. 2013;13(1):43–9.
3. Russo R, Berliocchi L, Adornetto A, et al. Calpain-mediated cleavage of Beclin-1 and autophagy deregulation following retinal ischemic injury in vivo. Cell Death Dis. 2011;2:e144.
4. Osborne NN, Schmidt KG. Neuroprotection against glaucoma remains a concept. Ophthalmologe. 2004;101(11):1087–92.
5. Tan PP, Yuan HH, Zhu X, Cui YY, Li H, Feng XM, Qiu Y, Chen HZ, Zhou W. Activation of muscarinic receptors protects against retinal neurons damage and optic nerve degeneration in vitro and in vivo models. CNS Neurosci Ther. 2014;20(3):227–36.
6. Zhang Z, Qin X, Tong N, Zhao X, Gong Y, Shi Y, Wu X. Valproic acid-mediated neuroprotection in retinal ischemia injury via histone deacetylase inhibition and transcriptional activation. Exp Eye Res. 2012;94(1):98–108.
7. Wei T, Kang Q, Ma B, Gao S, Li X, Liu Y. Activation of autophagy and paraptosis in retinal ganglion cells after retinal ischemia and reperfusion injury in rats. Exp Ther Med. 2015;9(2):476–82.
8. Shi Y, Wu X, Gong Y, Qiu Y, Zhang H, Huang Z, Su K. Protective effects of caffeic acid phenethyl ester on retinal ischemia/reperfusion injury in rats. Curr Eye Res. 2010;35(10):930–7.
9. Xie J, Jiang L, Zhang T, Jin Y, Yang D, Chen F. Neuroprotective effects of Epigallocate- chin-3-gallate (EGCG) in optic nerve crush model in rats. Neurosci Lett. 2010;479(1):26–30.
10. Pelzel HR, Schlamp CL, Nickells RW. Histone H4 deacetylation plays a critical role in early gene silencing during neuronal apoptosis. BMC Neurosci. 2010;11:62.
11. Wallace DM, Cotter TG. Histone deacetylase activity in conjunction with E2F-1 and p53 regulates Apaf-1 expression in 661W cells and the retina. J Neurosci Res. 2009;87(4):887–905.
12. Zhong Q, Kowluru RA. Role of histone acetylation in the development of diabetic retinopathy and the metabolic memory phenomenon. J Cell Biochem. 2010;110(6):1306–13.
13. Didonna A, Opal P. The promise and perils of HDAC inhibitors in neurodegeneration. Ann Clin Transl Neurol. 2015;2(1):79–101.
14. Haberland M, Montgomery RL, Olson EN. The many roles of histone deacetylases in development and physiology: implications for disease and therapy. Nat Rev Genet. 2009;10(1):32–42.
15. Simões-Pires C, Zwick V, Nurisso A, Schenker E, Carrupt PA, Cuendet M. HDAC6 as a target for neurodegenerative diseases: what makes it different from the other HDACs ? Mol Neurodegener. 2013;8:7.
16. d'Ydewalle C, Bogaert E, Van Den Bosch L. HDAC6 at the intersection of neuroprotection and neurodegeneration. Traffic. 2012;13(6):771–9.
17. Seidel C, Schnekenburger M, Dicato M, Diederich M. Histone deacetylase 6 in health and disease. Epigenomics. 2015;7(1):103–18.
18. Rivieccio MA, Brochier C, Willis DE, et al. HDAC6 is a target for protection and regeneration following injury in the nervous system. Proc Proc Natl Acad Sci USA. 2009;106(46):19599–604.
19. Crosson CE, Mani SK, Husain S, et al. Inhibition of histone deacetylase protects the retina from ischemic injury. Invest Ophthalmol Vis Sci. 2010;51(7):3639–45.
20. Fan J, Alsarraf O, Dahrouj M, et al. Inhibition of HDAC2 protects the retina from ischemic injury. Invest Ophthalmol Vis Sci. 2013;54(6):4072–80.

21. Biermann J, Grieshaber P, Goebel U, Martin G, Thanos S, Di Giovanni S, Lagrèze WA. Valproic acid-mediated neuroprotection and regeneration in injured retinal ganglion cells. Invest Ophthalmol Vis Sci. 2010;51(1):526–34.

22. Biermann J, Boyle J, Pielen A, Lagrèze WA. Histone deacetylase inhibitors sodium butyrate and valproic acid delay spontaneous cell death in purified rat retinal ganglion cell. Mol Vis. 2011;17:395–403.

23. Zhang ZZ, Gong YY, Shi YH, Zhang W, Qin XH, Wu XW. Valproate promotes survival of retinal ganglion cells in a rat model of optic nerve crush. Neuroscience. 2012;224:282–93.

24. Valenzuela-Fernández A, Cabrero JR, Serrador JM, Sánchez-Madrid F. HDAC6: a key regulator of cytoskeleton, cell migration and cell-cell interactions. Trends Cell Biol. 2008;18(6):291–7.

25. Sancho-Pelluz J, Paquet-Durand F. HDAC inhibition prevents Rd1 mouse photoreceptor de- generation. Adv Exp Med Biol. 2012;723:107–13.

26. Semba K, Namekata K, Kimura A, Harada C, Mitamura Y, Harada T. Brimonidine pre- vents neurodegeneration in a mouse model of normal tension glaucoma. Cell Death Dis. 2014;5:e1341.

27. Glaucoma QHA. Lancet. 2011;377(9774):1367–77.

28. Glick D, Barth S, Macleod KF. Autophagy: cellular and molecular mechanisms. J Pathol. 2010;221(1):3–12.

29. Klionsky DJ, Emr SD. Autophagy as a regulated pathway of cellular degradation. Science. 2000;290(5497):1717–21.

30. Pandey UB, Nie Z, Batlevi Y, et al. HDAC6 rescues neurodegeneration and provides an essential link between autophagy and the UPS. Nature. 2007;447(7146):859–63.

31. Geeraert C, Ratier A, Pfisterer SG, et al. Starvation-induced hyperacetylation of tubulin is required for the stimulation of autophagy by nutrient deprivation. J Biol Chem. 2010;285(31):24184–94.

32. Zhao G, Zhang W, Li L, Wu S, Du G. Pinocembrin protects the brain against ischemia- reperfusion injury and reverses the autophagy dysfunction in the penumbra area. Molecules. 2014;19(10):15786–98.

33. Lee JY, Koga H, Kawaguchi Y, et al. HDAC6 controls autophagosome maturation essential for ubiquitin-selective quality-control autophagy. EMBO J. 2010;29(5):969–80.

34. McLendon PM, Ferguson BS, Osinska H, et al. Tubulin hyperacetylation is adaptive in cardiac proteotoxicity by promoting autophagy. Proc Natl Acad Sci U S A. 2014;111(48):E5178–86.

35. Dompierre JP, Godin JD, Charrin BC, et al. Histone deacetylase 6 inhibition compensates for the transport deficit in Huntington's disease by increasing tubulin acetylation. J Neurosci. 2007;27(13):3571–83.

36. Parmigiani RB, Xu WS, Venta-Perez G, et al. HDAC6 is a specific deacetylase of peroxiredoxins and is involved in redox regelation. Proc Natl Acad Sci U S A. 2008;105(28):9633–8.

37. Thomas S, Quinn BA, Das SK, et al. Targeting the Bcl-2 family for cancer therapy. Expert Opin Ther Targets. 2013;17:61–75.

38. Reed JC. Bcl-2 and the regulation of programmed cell death. J Cell Biol. 1994;124:1–6.

39. Kelly PN, Strasser A. The role of Bcl-2 and its prosurvival relatives in tumourigenesis and cancer therapy. Cell Death Differ. 2011;18:1414–24.

40. Liu Z, Ding Y, Ye N, et al. Direct activation of bax protein for cancer therapy. Med Res Rev. 2016;36:313–41.

41. Gross A, Jockel J, Wei MC, et al. Enforced dimerization of BAX results in its translocation, mitochondrial dysfunction and apoptosis. EMBO J. 1998;17:3878–85.

42. Boulos S, Meloni BP, Arthur PG, et al. Peroxiredoxin 2 overexpression protects cortical neuronal cultures from ischemic and oxidativeinjury but not glutamate excitotoxicity, whereas cu/Zn superoxide dismutase1 overexpression protects only against oxidative injury. J Neurosci Res. 2007;85(14):3089–97.

43. Gan Y, Ji X, Hu X, et al. Transgenic overexpression of peroxiredoxin-2 attenuates ischemicneuronal injury via suppression of a redox-sensitive pro-death signaling pathway. Antioxid Redox Signal. 2012;17(5):719–32.

44. Sung JH, Gim SA, Koh PO. Ferulic acid attenuates the cerebral ischemic injury-induced decrease in peroxiredoxin-2 and thioredoxin expression. Neurosci Lett. 2014;566:88–92.

45. Hu X, Weng Z, Chu CT, et al. Peroxiredoxin-2 protects against 6-hydroxydopamine induced dopaminergic neurodegeneration via attenuation of the apoptosis signal regulating kinase (ASK1) signaling cascade. J Neurosci. 2011;31(1):247–61.

46. Parmigiani RB, Xu WS, Venta-Perez G, et al. HDAC6 is a specific deacetylase of peroxiredoxins and is involved in redox regulation. Proc Natl Acad Sci U S A. 2008;105(28):9633–8.

47. Fang J, Nakamura T, Cho DH, Gu Z, Lipton SA. S-nitrosylation of peroxiredoxin 2 promotes oxidative stress induced neuronal cell death in Parkinson's disease. Proc Natl Acad Sci U S A. 2007;104(47):18742–7.

48. Rezaie T, McKercher SR, Kosaka K, et al. Protective effect of carnosic acid, a pro-electrophilic compound, in models of oxidative stress and light-inducedretinal degeneration. Invest Ophthalmol Vis Sci. 2012;53(12):7847–54.

29

Studying the factors related to refractive error regression after PRK surgery

Mehdi Naderi[1], Siamak Sabour[1*] ⓘ, Soheila Khodakarim[1] and Farid Daneshgar[2]

Abstract

Backgtound: Photorefractive keratectomy (PRK) is used for a wide range of refractive errors such as low to moderate myopia, hyperopia and astigmatism. While many improvements have been made in laser application and accuracy as well as the modes of corneal flap removal, and although the results are somewhat predictable, regression of refractive errors is still a common complaint among the patients undergoing refractive surgery with Excimer Laser. We aimed to determine related factors of regression following photorefractive keratectomy (PRK) in different types of refractive errors.

Methods: This cross-sectional study included patients who had undergone PRK more than 6 months previously and investigated refractive error regression and related factors. The participants were those who had PRK eye surgery for the first time from 2013 to 2016 using Technolas 217z100. A refraction value of spherical equivalent > 0.75 D after cycloplegic refraction was defined as refractive error regression.

Results: A total of 293 eyes on 150 subjects were studied. The preoperative refractive error of the eyes were as follows: 5.5% were myopic, 1% were hyperopic, 4.8% had astigmatism, 76% had myopic astigmatism and 12.6% had hyperopic astigmatism. Regressed and non-regressed eyes were assessed using the generalized estimating equations for the probabilistic variables of demographic characteristics, topography and eye refraction. The variables of simulated keratometry astigmatism (simK) (OR = 2.8; $p = 0.04$), 5 mm irregularity (OR = 3.56; $p = 0.01$) and sphere value (OR = 1.98; $p = 0.01$) were significantly related to refractive error regression. There was no significant relationship between the regressed and non-regressed eyes of the same person ($p \geq 0.05$).

Conclusion: There was a positive relationship between the increase of 5 mm irregularity, simK, sphere value before surgery and refractive error regression. Age, sex and type of refraction error of the patient and the expertise of the PRK surgeon could change the general results; therefore, not all cases should be dealt with identically.

Keywords: Refractive error regression, PRK surgery, Related factors

Background

Current advances in refractive surgery have caused dramatic changes in ophthalmology. Excimer laser photorefractive keratectomy (PRK) is accepted as an effective and desirable method of treating refractive error [1, 2]. PRK is used for a range of refractive errors, including low to moderate myopia, hyperopia and astigmatism [2, 3]. While many improvements have been made in laser applications and accuracy as well as the mode of corneal flap removal,

regression of refractive error is still a common complaint among patients undergoing refractive surgery with excimer laser. Recent estimates showed that 3.8% to 20.8% of patients require retreatment after myopia correction. Generally, the need for retreatment after surgery with an excimer laser is 6.8% [4–9]. This is why some patients are not satisfied with this type of surgery.

The factors associated with the need for retreatment after LASIK surgery include a small optical zone [10–12], flap thickness [13], high correction [14], keratometry readings [15], significant astigmatism [6, 10, 16], age over 40 years [16]. In PRK, they include the use of Mitomycin [17], refractive correction > − 5.00 D, smaller optical zone (< 6.00 mm) and unstable fixation during

* Correspondence: s.sabour@sbmu.ac.ir
[1]Department of Clinical Epidemiology, School of Public Health, Safety Promotion and Injury Prevention Research Center, Shahid Beheshti University of Medical Sciences, Chamran Highway, Velenjak, Daneshjoo Blvd, Tehran, I.R. Iran
Full list of author information is available at the end of the article

laser ablation [18]. It can be said that the stability of PRK is less satisfactory than with LASIK surgery [19, 20]. Determining the factors associated with regression in PRK surgery can help select the best case for this type of surgery and reduce the financial burden of the patient.

The number of studies have comprehensively that have examined the factors relating to regression of refractive error after PRK is insufficient. The current study was carried out to identify the factors associated with refractive error regression in individuals who had undergone PRK because of refractive error. The prevalence of refractive error regression was examined using the variables of sex and age as well as the medical specialty of the surgeon. The relationships between the factors related to refractive error regression in each subgroup were assessed to determine the moderating effects.

Methods

The study protocol was approved by the Department of Epidemiology, School of Public Health, at Shahid Beheshti University of Medical Sciences and was conducted at Kermanshah University of Medical Sciences. The cross-sectional study was designed to examine the results of PRK at the Lasik Clinic of Imam Khomeini Hospital in Kermanshah province. The medical records of each patient who had undergone PRK for correction of myopia, myopic astigmatism, astigmatism, hyperopia and hyperopic astigmatism were investigated. The procedures had been done by surgeons having different specialties from 2013 to 2016.

A code was employed to prevent identification of the patient for each record. About 2400 patients (roughly 4600 eyes) had undergone PRK with Technolas 217z100 (Bausch & Lomb) over the course of 3 years. The participants were patients who had undergone PRK at least 6 months in the past. Their medical records were randomly selected and they were invited to undergo supplementary examinations. If an individual had not undergone a follow-up examination or there were defects in the data in his/her medical record, another person was randomly selected. This study received ethical approval from the Institutional Review Board of Shahid Beheshti University of Medical Sciences.

Photorefractive keratectomy surgery

In PRK, the eye is first anesthetized and the cornea is exposed to alcohol 20% for 15 s. A disk of epithelium with a diameter of 8–9 mm is removed with a sponge. The excimer laser then is applied according to the nomogram that the surgeons have prepared with respect to patient age and amount of refraction. The surgeons applies the nomogram in all cases of myopia, then adds 0.25 D to the myopia value to prevent under-correction. The procedure is performed for astigmatism and hyperopia

according to the nomogram. After excimer ablation, a sponge soaked with MMC 0.02% is placed on the stroma (according to amount and type of refractive error at 10 s per 1.0 D of correction). The eye is rinsed with balanced saline solution (30 cc) to dilute and remove residual MMC and a bandage contact lens is placed over the cornea.

Postoperatively, all patients receive a topical antibiotic, corticosteroids and artificial tears. The patients are prescribed chloramphenicol 0.5% drops (four times daily for 5 days), betamethasone 0.1% drops (four times a day for 1 week, decreasing to 3 times a day for 3 weeks) and artificial tears (Artelac; Bausch & Lomb) four times a day for 9 weeks. The bandage contact lens is removed when epithelial healing is complete (5 to 7 days postoperative).

Regression

Cases of regression refers to eyes recording a spherical equivalent cycloplegic refraction of greater than 0.75 D after 6 months upon examination using an auto kerato-refractometer (Topcon 8900; Japan). The information contained in the patients' preoperative medical records (eye topography variables, eye refraction variables and demographic variables), surgical records (eye movement rate, optical zone size and surgeon specialty) and the post-surgery information, including the cycloplegic refraction value, were included in the data analysis. Eye refraction variables included the type of refractive error, refractive error value and, in case of astigmatism, eye astigmatism axis.

Preoperative refractive error was considered to be myopia, hyperopia, astigmatism, myopic astigmatism and hyperopic astigmatism. The demographic variables chosen were age, sex and level of education (which is indicative of rate of study, computer use and following postoperative medical advice). These were used as quantitative, qualitative-nominal and qualitative-ordinal variables, respectively. An Orbscan IIz device (Bausch & Lomb; USA) was used to draw the thickness, posterior Diff, irregularity (3 and 5 mm) and simK on the topographic map. Orbscan IIz was used to detect corneal irregularities with radii of 3 and 5 mm and the average high and low corneal points as irregularities. To calculate simK, the Orbscan Ilz found the highest and lowest points on two perpendicular axes and converted the difference between them into the unit of power (D). It also calculated the posterior Diff as the distance between the highest point of the cornea and the BFS surface (ideal spherical surface of the cornea). The thickness (of the central part of the cornea) was measured in microns.

The variables in the surgery files were eye movement rate, optical zone size and surgeon specialty. The eye tracker device recorded the changes in eye movement from the steady state during surgery as positive or negative on the coordinate axes. The optical zone is the area on the cornea which is determined based on pupil size and is influenced by the excimer laser. It is classified into groups of 5.5, 6 and 6.5 mm diameters. The surgeon chose one depending on the situation. Surgeon specialty was classified qualitatively-nominally into four groups: ophthalmologists and strabismus, cornea and retina subspecialists. The confounding effect of age and sex was considered, particularly the moderating role of sex, age and surgeon specialty, was dealt with using stratified analysis.

Power and Sample Size Calculation (version 3.1.2) was used to calculate the sample size at a significance level of < 5% and a power of 80% taking into consideration the 60% prevalence of females in the study. To detect an OR value of 2.5 (clinically important) between exposure and refractive error regression after PRK, a total sample size of 195 eyes was required. Given the 25% probability of data loss and non-compliance of the participants to determine the refraction, 50 eyes were added to the sample size in order to preserve the validity of the results. To increase the power of the study, the surgery files of 150 patients were randomly selected and each was invited to undergo another examination. Of the 2400 who underwent PRK surgery, 1535 were women. For this reason, the proportion of males and females was preserved as much as possible.

The variables of irregularity (3 and 5 mm) and posterior Diff were applied quantitatively and continuously (in mm) and simK was applied quantitatively and continuously (in D). The change in eye movement was recorded by the eye tracker device and its absolute value was used in the analysis. Refractive error regression as the main outcome was divided into regressed and non-regressed groups at a cut-off value of 0.75. To determine the effect of an increase in the sphere and astigmatism value before surgery on regression, their refractive errors were considered as absolute values.

The preliminary survey assessed about 2400 people. After removal of persons with incomplete case files (67), pregnant women (16) and those who had not been referred for follow-up examinations (272), 2045 eligible

people entered the study (Fig. 1). Out of these, 150 were randomly selected.

Statistical analysis

The statistical analysis was done using SPSS, version 24. Depending on the distribution of the variables, the quantitative variables were described as mean, standard deviation, median, range of change. Qualitative and ordinal variables were described as numerical values and related percentages. The variables of thickness, 3 and 5 mm irregularity, simK, posterior Diff and age were assessed as regressed or non-regressed with regard to the sample size and variable distribution using Mann-Whitney test and t-test. Generalized estimating equations (GEEs) were used to determine the neighbor effect of refractive error regression between the right and left eyes and assess the relationship between all variables and refractive error regression. The moderating role of sex, type of refractive error, age group and surgeon specialty were assessed using stratified analysis.

Results

The participants totaled 150 patients representing 293 eyes. Seven patients were assessed for one eye each and the remaining 143 had both eyes assessed (286). The participants were 61% female and 39% male. Using the definition of refractive error regression, 56 eyes demonstrated regression. The regression frequency was about 19%. Of the 56 regressed eyes, 16 belonged to 16 patients (one regressed eye per individual) and 40 eyes belonged to 20 patients (both eyes were regressed). The prevalence of regression was 21.1% among females and 15.9% among males. The prevalence of regression for each specialty was 20.7% among general ophthalmologists, 21.6% among strabismus subspecialists, 14.7% among retina subspecialists and 16.4% cornea subspecialists. The prevalence of regression was 17.4% in the under 30 year age group and 21.4% in the over 30 year age group. The prevalence of regression for myopia was 5.9%, hyperopia was 1.3%,

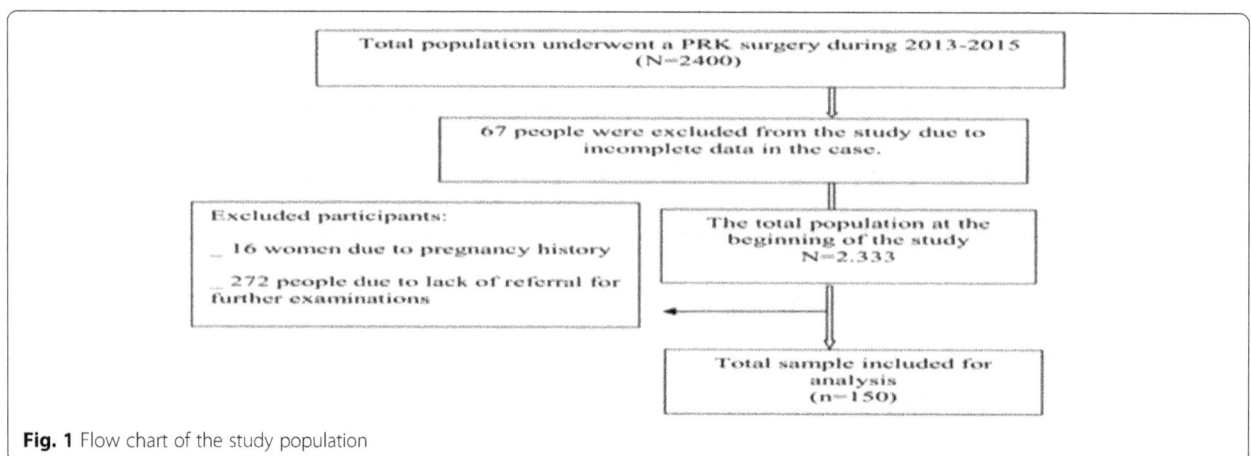

Fig. 1 Flow chart of the study population

astigmatism was 4.2%, myopic astigmatism was 78.1% and hyperopic astigmatism was 10.5%. The preoperative refractive error in the eyes that had undergone PRK were as follows: 5.5% myopia, 1% hyperopia, 4.8% astigmatism, 76% myopic astigmatism and 12.6% hyperopic astigmatism. The characteristics of the patient in terms of other qualitative variables are shown in (Table 1).

The mean age of those who had undergone PRK was 31.4 ± 7.7 years. The characteristics of the subjects in terms of other quantitative variables are shown in Table 2.

Table 1 Preoperative characteristics in 293 eyes that undergo PRK Surgery

Factor	Frequency	Percent
Female	180	61.4
Men	113	38.6
Education degree		
Under diploma	47	16
Diploma	91	31.1
Bachelor	115	39.2
Post graduate	40	13.7
Optical zone		
5.5 (mm)	7	2.1
6.00 (mm)	20	6.8
6.50 (mm)	267	91.1
Refraction type		
Myopia (D)	16	5.5
Hyperopia (D)	3	1
Astigmatism (D)	14	4.8
Myopic astigmatism (D)	223	76.1
Hyperopic astigmatism (D)	37	12.6
Surgeon specialty		
Ophthalmologist	135	46.1
Deviation specialty	51	17.4
Retina specialty	34	11.6
Cornea specialty	73	24.9
Astigmatism category (D)		
Astigmatism category (0–2) D	243	82.9
Astigmatism category (2–4) D	47	16
Astigmatism category (4–6) D	3	1
Sphere category (D)		
Sphere category (0–2) D	93	31.7
Sphere category (2–4) D	110	37.5
Sphere category (4–6) D	50	17.1
Sphere category (6–8) D	22	7.5
Sphere category (8<) D	18	6.1
Total	293	100

PRK photorefractive keratectomy, D Diopter

Table 2 Preoperative characteristics in 293 eye that undergo PRK surgery

Factor	Minimum	Maximum	Mean	Std. deviation
Age (y)	20	60	31.4	7.7
Irregularity 3 (mm)	0.4	2.4	1.02	0.33
Irregularity 5 (mm)	0.80	4.90	1.41	0.44
Diff posterior (mm)	0.01	0.04	0.02	0.01
SimK (D)	0.1	3.8	1.2	0.7
Thickness (µm)	453	610	543.6	32.8
Eye movement (mm)	0	24	3.9	2.9
Sphere value (D)	0	12	3.4	2.3
Astigmatism value (D)	0	4.75	1.3	0.94

PRK Photorefractive keratectomy, Diff posterior: steepest posterior point difference from Best fit sphere, simulated k astigmatism: keratometry astigmatism, D Diopter, y year

The comparison between the variables in both the regressed and non-regressed groups showed a significant difference in the mean 3 mm irregularity ($\bar{x} = 1.16$ vs. $\bar{x} = 0.99$, $p = .001$), 5 mm irregularity ($\bar{x} = 1.61$ vs. $\bar{x} = 1.36$, $p = 0.001$) and simK ($\bar{x} = 1.69$ vs. $\bar{x} = 1.06$, $p = 0.001$) (Table 3). In the eyes with astigmatism, there was no significant relationship between refractive error with type of astigmatism axis (WTR, oblique and ATR; $p > 0.05$).

The astigmatism value, 5 mm irregularity, simK and sphere value in the individuals with both eyes regressed and those with both eyes non-regressed showed no significant difference between medians for the left and right eyes (Table 4). Comparison was made of the variables of astigmatism, thickness, 5 mm irregularity, simK and sphere value in right eyes showing regression after PRK for individuals with non-regressed left eyes and vice versa. The only significant difference was observed between the median 5 mm irregularity in the right eye (2.20 vs. 1.80,

Table 3 Comparison of preoperative characteristics of the eyes with and without regression

Characteristics	Mean		P value
	No regression (n = 237)	Regression (n = 56)	
Age (y)	31.4	31.8	0.72
Thickness(µm)	535.7	529.7	0.21
Irregularity 3 (mm)	0.99	1.16	0.001
Irregularity 5 (mm)	1.36	1.61	0.001
Diff posterior (mm)	0.02	0.02	0.34
SimK (D)	1.06	1.69	0.001
Eye movement (mm)	3.80	4.56	0.07
Sphere value (D)	3.07	5.17	0.001
Astigmatism value (D)	1.09	2.05	0.001

PRK Photorefractive keratectomy, Diff posterior: steepest posterior point difference from Best fit sphere, Sim k astigmatism: *simulated keratometry* astigmatism, P value: Independent T test

Table 4 Relationship between Refractive error regression after PRK Surgery and preoperative variables in people with both eyes regressed and both eyes non-regressed

Variables	People whose both eyes were non regressed after surgery			People whose both eyes were regressed after surgery		
	Right eye N = 107	Left eye N = 107	Test	Right eye N = 20	Left eye N = 20	Test
	Mean ± SD	Mean ± SD	P value[§]	Mead(min-max)	Mead(min-max)	P value[®]
Thickness (μm)	536.7 ± 32.6	537.6 ± 34.7	0.84	537.5 (499–572)	531 (501–575)	0.49
Irregularity5(mm)	1.33 ± 0.31	1.36 ± 0.38	0.55	1.35 (1.00–2.70)	1.25 (0.9–2.6)	0.45
Astigmatism(D)	0.99 ± 0.70	1.07 ± 0.73	0.43	1.62 (0–3.75)	1.87 (0–4.25)	0.43
Sphere (D)	3.17 ± 1.69	3.12 ± 1.70	0.84	6.25 (0.25–12)	7.87 (0–11.50)	0.41
SimK (D)	0.97 ± 0.49	1.04 ± 0.51	0.30	1.25 (0.25–2.90)	1.50 (0.50–2.90)	0.92

PRK Photorefractive keratectomy, Sim k astigmatism: simulated keratometry astigmatism, P value: [§]: Independent sample t. test [®]; Mann –Whitney U independent sample test

$p = 0.03$) and in the left eye (1.60 vs. 1.20, $p = 0.08$) (Table 5).

The GEEs showed that simK (OR = 2.8, $p = 0.04$), 5 mm irregularity (OR = 3.56, $p = 0.01$) and sphere value (OR = 1.98, $p = 0.01$) were significantly related to refractive error regression after considering the potential confounding variables. Refractive error regression was not influenced by the variables of the other eye of the individual and there was no significant relationship between the regressed and non-regressed eyes of one individual (Table 6).

The results of stratified analysis on the moderating role of sex, age group, type of refractive error and surgeon specialty showed that the regression of refractive error in females was related to the 5 mm irregularity (OR = 4.2, $p = 0.02$) and simK (OR = 3.6, $p = 0.04$). There was a significant negative relationship between thickness and refractive error regression in males (OR = 0.97, $p = 0.02$). The 5 mm irregularity and simK showed a much weaker relational power and was not statistically significant. As the sphere value increased in females and males, a significant relationship with refractive error regression was observed (Table 7).

The relationship between the variables and the regression of refractive error was examined for the myopic astigmatism and hyperopic astigmatism groups. It was found that results of the simK and 5 mm irregularity differed between groups (Table 8). The relationship between these variables was also examined by age group. It was found that only the 5 mm irregularity in the under 30 age group (OR = 3.98, $p = 0.03$) had a significant relationship with refractive error regression. In both groups, a significant relationship with refractive error regression was found with an increase in sphere value.

The refractive error regression versus surgeon specialty was also examined. For ophthalmologists, only the 5 mm irregularity (OR = 2.7, $p = 0.04$) and simK (OR = 7.8, $p = 0.03$) had a significant relationship with refractive error regression. No significant relationship was found between these variables and refractive error regression for strabismus, cornea and retina subspecialists. A positive relationship was observed between the increase in sphere and astigmatism values and regression of refractive error for all specialties.

The relationship between variables was examined according to type of refractive error. For myopic astigmatism, only the 5 mm irregularity (OR = 5.11, $p = 0.02$) and simK

Table 5 Relationship between refractive error regression after PRK surgery and preoperative variables in 16 patients who had one regressed and one non-regressed eyes

Variables	People whose right eyes were regressed after surgery but their left eyes were not surgery			People Whose left eyes were regressed after surgery but their right eyes were not		
	Right eye N = 7	Left eye N = 7	Test	Right eye N = 9	Left eye N = 9	Test
	Mead(minmax)	Mead(minmax)	P value[§]	Mead(min-max)	Mead(min-max)	P value[§]
Thickness (μm)	526 (466–573)	520 (474–588)	0.94	505 (470–558)	514 (461–562)	0.72
Irregularity 5 (mm)	2.20 (1.70–4.90)	1.80 (1.20–2.10)	0.03	1.20 (1.00–2.30)	1.60 (1.10–2.40)	0.08
Astigmatism (D)	3.00 (1.50–4.75)	2.25 (1.00–3.75)	0.36	1.5 (1.25–2.75)	2.25 (0.50–4.25)	0.14
Sphere (D)	0.50 (0–5.00)	0.50 (0–4.25)	0.79	2.25 (0.25–7.00)	2.00 (0.50–8.25)	0.82
SimK (D)	2.50 (0.6–3.80)	2.7 (0.9–3.00)	0.94	1.30 (0.80–2.10)	1.75 (0.70–2.90)	0.21

PRK Photorefractive keratectomy, Sim k astigmatism simulated keratometry Astigmatism, D Diopter, P value: [§]: Mann –Whitney Uindependent sample test

Table 6 Generalized Estimating Equations of independent variable of regression after PRK

Factor	OR (%95 C. I)	P value
Age (years)	1.01 (0.95 to 1.06)	0.69
Sex (male vs. female)	1.28 (0.29 to 1.91)	0.79
Thickness (μm)	0.99 (0.98 to 1.03)	0.12
Irregularity 5 (mm)	3.56 (1.32 to 9.22)	0.01
SimK (D)	2.80 (1.01 to 8.20)	0.04
Astigmatism value (D)	2.01 (0.98 to 4.92)	0.06
Sphere value (D)	1.98 (1.59 to 2.54)	0.01
Right or Left	1.07 (0.69 to 1.87)	0.80

Adjusted odds ratio: age, sex, thickness, irregularity 5 mm, simulated keratometry astigmatism, Astigmatism value, Sphere value

(OR = 4.4, p = 0.02) had significant relationships with refractive error regression. For hyperopic astigmatism, no significant relationship was found between these variables and refractive error regression. In both types, a significant relationship was observed between an increase in the probability of refractive error regression and an increase in sphere value.

Discussion

The current study found a relationship between simK and 5 mm irregularity and refractive error regression after PRK. An increase in these variables increased the likelihood of refractive error regression after PRK. These results emphasize that the overall results cannot be generalized to all patients. For example, unlike for females, no males showed a significant relationship between the 5 mm irregularity and simK and refractive error regression. Although the relational power of thickness and regression was stronger in males than in females, there was a significant negative relationship between thickness and refractive error regression. In the assessment of factors related to refractive error regression versus age group, the 5 mm irregularity was the only variable that had a positive and significant relationship with regression. This underlines why the age, sex and type of refractive error of the individual are important during decision-making.

In addition, the specialty of the surgeon performing PRK showed a relationship with the regression of refractive error. Only general ophthalmologists showed an effect for simK and 5 mm irregularity. The other subspecialties showed no effect. As in previous studies, there was a positive relationship between an increase in sphere value and astigmatism. An increase in refractive error increased the likelihood of refractive error regression [6, 13, 18].

No significant relationship was found between refractive error regression and education level, type of refractive error, surgeon specialty, type of astigmatism axis or posterior Diff. Studies also have reported no significant relationship between age, sex and the thickness and regression of refractive error after PRK [6, 18], although some studies have shown age as a risk factor for regression of refractive error after LASIK surgery [13]. In the present study, although the surgeon specialty showed no significant association, it could be said that surgical decisions such as patient selection, surgical technique and nomogram selection for PRK is very important [6, 21].

No relationship was found between the rate of eye movement and regression of refractive error. These results are inconsistent with the findings of Mohammadi et al. [18] The reason for this discrepancy in the results may be that, in Mohammadi et al., the eye movement rate was qualitatively affected by the surgeon observation and view, but the present study used the range of change (the eye movement rate as recorded by the eye tracking device).

As in previous studies, no relationship was found between the optical zone and refractive error regression [21, 22]. This is inconsistent with the results of Mohammadi et al [18] As in Pokroy et al., the present study observed a relationship between the preoperative refractive error high and the regression of the refractive error. The greater the preoperative refractive error, the greater the likelihood of refractive error regression [10].

Although PRK is safe and effective, it is usually recommended for patients with mild to moderate refractive

Table 7 Comparing the results of GEE analysis in women and men to examine the role of gender moderating

Factor	Male (n = 113)		Female (n = 180)	
	P value	OR (%95 C. I)	P value	OR (%95 C. I)
Age (years)	0.25	1.04 (0.81 to 4.05)	0.71	0.98 (0.90 to 1.06)
Left or right eye	0.75	0.88 (0.30 to 2.35)	0.67	1.18 (0.53 to 2.64)
Thickness (μm)	0.02	0.97 (0.94 to 0.99)	0.66	0.99 (0.98 to 1.03)
Irregularity 5 (mm)	0.09	4.00 (0.85 to 19.48)	0.02	4.14 (1.17 to 14.58)
SimK (D)	0.54	1.71 (0.39 to 10.8)	0.04	3.61 (1.05 to 12.43)
Astigmatism value (D)	0.10	4.78 (0.72 to 33.01)	0.23	1.81 (0.86 to 4.84)
Sphere value (D)	0.01	1.90 (1.39 to 2.60)	0.01	2.30 (1.66 to 3.18)

Odds ratio: age, thickness, irregularity 5 mm, simulated keratometry astigmatism, astigmatism value, sphere value, *D* Diopter

Table 8 Comparing the results of GEE analysis in eyes hyperopic astigmatism and myopic astigmatism

Factor	Myopic astigmatism		Hyperopic astigmatism	
	P value	OR (%95 C. I)	P value	OR (%95 C. I)
Sex (male vs. female)	0.80	1.18 (0.31 to 4.39)	0.65	1.61 (0.19 to 13.41)
Age (years)	0.80	0.98 (0.89 to 1.09)	0.75	0.98 (0.89 to 1.08)
Left or right eye	0.50	0.79 (0.40 to 1.56)	0.96	0.95 (0.15 to 6.09)
Thickness (μm)	0.13	0.98 (0.97 to 1.03)	0.51	0.98 (0.93 to 1.03)
Irregularity 5 (mm)	0.02	4.04 (1.24 to 13.13)	0.74	1.43 (0.16 to 12.98)
SimK (D)	0.02	5.11 (1.26 to 20.58)	0.66	0.69 (0.13 to 3.60)
Astigmatism value (D)	0.58	1.33 (0.48 to 3.59)	0.17	4.37 (0.51 to 37.44)
Sphere value (D)	0.01	2.41 (1.72 to 3.36)	0.01	2.16 (1.51 to 3.11)

Odds ratio: age, thickness, irregularity 5 mm, simulated keratometry astigmatism, astigmatism value, sphere value, *D* Diopter

error [23–25]. This study was focused on the factors related to refractive error regression after PRK and had some weaknesses in terms of the use of variables indicating refractive error regression. One weakness was the lack of assessment of the relationship between epithelium tissue repair disorder and hyperplasia of epithelium tissue in refractive error regression after PRK [26–28].

Because of insufficient information about the amount and administration of medication as well as dryness of the eyes after surgery [29, 30], it was not possible investigate the relationship between these variables and refractive error regression after PRK. Technological advances in corneal imaging have made the precise measurement of anterior and posterior corneal curvature and corneal thickness possible [31]. The careful use of this data can help in the planning of refractive surgery such as PRK.

Insufficient information about employment, history of eye infection and visual activities such as computer use and reading time per day prevented investigation of a relationship between these variables and refractive error regression after PRK. The similarities between the study population and the population targeted by PRK in other communities in terms of gender and age groups mean that the results could be generalized to all except pregnant women, who were excluded from the study.

Conclusion

The current study showed that, in general, a relationship exists between the variables of 5 mm irregularity, simK and sphere value before surgery and the regression of refractive error; however, the variables of age, sex and type of refractive error and surgeon specialty could change the general results. Therefore, not all individuals should be treated alike. It is recommended that general ophthalmologists consider these variables before intervention in order to determine the best candidates for PRK. It is recommended that insurance companies takes measures to prevent the waste of financial resources on candidates for PRK with a high risk of post-surgery refractive error

regression. In addition, the health system should propose a protocol for advising candidates of PRK based on age, sex and other characteristics to the type of surgery that will minimize the likelihood of regression.

Abbreviations
CI: Confidence interval; D: Diopters; Diff posterior: steepest posterior point difference from Best fit sphere; OR: Odds ratio; PRK: Photorefractive keratometry; SD: Standard deviation; SE: Spherical equivalent; SimK: Simulated keratometry astigmatism; y: year

Acknowledgements
The authors thank the subjects who participated in the study. The authors thank Hadis Pourchamani and Saeed Fathi for their help to data collection and patient's examinations.

Authors' contributions
MN, SS, SK and FD conceived and designed the study protocol. MN and FD collected the data. SS, MN and SK were involved in the analysis. SS, MN wrote the first draft of the manuscript. FD and SS and MN reviewed and revised the manuscript and produced the final version. All authors have read and approved the final manuscript.

Competing interests
The authors declare that they have no competing interests.

Author details
¹Department of Clinical Epidemiology, School of Public Health, Safety Promotion and Injury Prevention Research Center, Shahid Beheshti University of Medical Sciences, Chamran Highway, Velenjak, Daneshjoo Blvd, Tehran, I.R, Iran. ²Department of Ophthalmology, School of Medicine, Kermanshah University of Medical Sciences, Kermanshah, Iran.

References

1. Lee JB, Choe CM, Seong GJ, Gong HY, Kim EK. Laser subepithelial Keratomileusis for low to moderate myopia: 6-month follow-up. Jpn J Ophthalmol. 2002;46(3):299–304.
2. Liu YL, Tseng CC, Lin CP. Visual performance after excimer laser photorefractive keratectomy for high myopia. Taiwan J Ophthalmol. 2017;7(2):82–8.
3. Sher NA, Barak M, Daya S, DeMarchi J, Tucci A, Hardten DR, Frantz JM, Eiferman RA, Parker P, Telfair WB, et al. Excimer laser photorefractive keratectomy in high myopia. Arch Ophthalmol. 1992;110(7):935–43.
4. Shojaei A, Mohammad-Rabei H, Eslani M, Elahi B, Noorizadeh F. Long-term evaluation of complications and results of photorefractive keratectomy in myopia: an 8-year follow-up. Cornea. 2009;28(3):304–10.
5. Vaddavalli PK, Yoo SH, Diakonis VF, Canto AP, Shah NV, Haddock LJ, Feuer WJ, Culbertson WW. Femtosecond laser-assisted retreatment for residual refractive errors after laser assisted in situ keratomileusis. J Cataract Refract Surg. 2013;39(8):1241–7.
6. Randleman JB, White AJ Jr, Lynn MJ, Hu MH, Stulting RD. Incidence, outcomes, and risk factors for retreatment after wavefront-optimized ablations with PRK and LASIK. J Refract Surg. 2009;25(3):273–6.
7. Yuen LH, Chan WK, Koh J, Mehta JS, Tan DT, SingLasik Research Group. A 10-year prospective audit of LASIK outcomes for myopia in 37,932 eyes at a single institution in Asia. Ophtalmology. 2010;117(6):1236–44.
8. Wagoner MD, Wickard JC, Wandling GR Jr, Milder LC, Rauen MP, Kitzmann AS, Sutphin JE, Goins KM. Initial resident refractive surgical experience: outcomes of PRK and LASIK for myopia. J Refract Surg. 2011;27(3):181–8.
9. D'Arcy FM, Kirwan C, O'keefe M. Ten year follow up of laser in situ keratomileusis for all levels of myopia. Acta ophtalmol. 2012;90(4):335–6.
10. Pokroy R, Mimouni M, Sela T, Munzer G, Kaiserman I. Myopic laser in situ keratomileusis retreatment: incidence and associations. J Cataract Refract Surg. 2016;42(10):1408–14.
11. Chen YI, Chien KL, Wang IJ, Yen AM, Chen LS, Lin PJ, Chen TH. An interval-censored model for predicting myopic regression after laser in situ keratomileusis. Invest Ophthalmol Vis Sci. 2007;48(8):3516–23.
12. Lian J, Zhang Q, Ye W, Zhou D, Wang K. An analysis of regression afterlaser in situ keratomileusis for treatment of myopia. Zhonghua Yan Ke Za Zhi. 2002;38(6):363–6.
13. Flanagan GW, Binder PS. Role of flap thickness in laser in situ keratomileusis enhancement for refractive undercorrection. J Cataract Refract Surg. 2006;32(7):1129–41.
14. Gazieva L, Beer MH, Nielsen K, Hjortdal J. A retrospective comparison of efficacy and safety of 680 consecutive LASIK treatments for high myopia performed with two generations of flying-spot excimer lasers. Acta ophtalmol. 2011;89(8):729–33.
15. Christiansen SM, Neuffer MC, Sikder S, Semnani RT, Moshirfar M. The effect of preoperative keratometry on visual outcomes after moderate myopic LASIK. Clin Ophthalmol. 2012;6:459–64.
16. Kruh JN, Garrett KA, Huntington B, Robinson S, Melki SA. Risk factors for retreatment following myopic LASIK with femtosecond laser and custom ablation for the treatment of myopia. Semin Ophthalmol. 2017;32(3):316–20.
17. Sy ME, Zhang L, Yeroushalmi A, Huang D, Hamilton DR. Effect of mitomycin-C on the variance in refractive outcomes after photorefractive keratectomy. J Cataract Refract Surg. 2014;40(12):1980–4.
18. Mohammadi SF, Nabovati P, Mirzajani A, Ashrafi E, Vakilian B. Risk factors of regression and undercorrection in photorefractive keratectomy. Int J Ophthamol. 2015;8(5):933–7.
19. Dirani M, Couper T, Yau J, Ang EK, Islam FM, Snibson GR, Vajpayee RB, Baird PN. Long-term refractive outcomes and stability after excimer laser surgery for myopia. J Cataract Refract Surg. 2010;36(10):1709–17.
20. Hashemi H, Ghaffari R, Miraftab M, Asgari S. Femtosecond laser-assisted LASIK versus PRK for high myopia: comparison of 18-month visual acuity and quality. int ophtalmol. 2016;37(4):995–1001.
21. Pokroy R, Mimouni M, Sela T, Munzer G, Kaiserman I. Predictors of myopic photorefractive keratectomy retreatment. J Cataract Refract Surg. 2017;43(6):825–32.
22. Frings A, Richard G, Steinberg J, Druchkiv V, Linke SJ, Katz T. LASIK and PRK in hyperopic astigmatic eyes: is early retreatment advisable. Clin Ophthalmol. 2016;10:565–70.
23. Bricola G, Scotto R, Mete M, Cerruti S, Traverso CE. A 14-year follow-up of photorefractive keratectomy. j Refract surg. 2009;25(6):545–52.
24. Goes FJ. Photorefractive keratectomy for myopia of −8.00 to-24.00 diopters. J Refract Surg. 1996;12(1):91–7.
25. Guerin MB, Darcy F, O'Connor J, O'Keeffe M. Excimer laser photorefractive keratectomy for low to moderate myopia using a 5.0 mm treatment zone and no transitional zone: 16-year follow-up. J Cataract Refract Surg. 2012;38(7):1246–50.
26. Gauthier CA, Holden BA, Epstein D, Tengroth B, Fagerholm P, Hamberg-Nyström H. Role of epithelial hyperplasia in regression following photorefractive keratectomy. Br J Ophthalmol. 1996;80:545–8.
27. Ramirez-Florez S, Maurice DM. Inflammatory cells, refractive regression, and haze after excimer laser PRK. J Refract Surg. 1996;12(3):370–81.
28. Kim TI, Tchah H, Lee SA, Sung K, Cho BJ, Kook MS. Apoptosis in Keratocytes caused by Mitomycin C. Invest Ophthalmol Vis Sci. 2003;44(5):1912–7.
29. Bower KS, Sia RK, Ryan DS, Mines MJ, Dartt DA. Chronic dry eye in photorefractive keratectomy and laser in situ keratomileusis: manifestations, incidence, and predictive factors. J Cataract Refract Surg. 2015;41(12):2624–34.
30. Kymionis GD, Tsiklis NS, Ginis H, Diakonis VF, Pallikaris I. Dry eye after photorefractive keratectomy with adjuvant mitomycin C. J Refract Surg. 2006;22(5):511–3.
31. Fan R, Chan TC, Prakash G, Jhanji V. Applications of corneal topography and tomography: a review. Clin Exp Ophthalmol. 2018;46(2):133–46.

30

Effect of incision on visual outcomes after implantation of a trifocal diffractive IOL

Shasha Xue, Guiqiu Zhao*, Xiaoni Yin, Jing Lin, Cui Li, Liting Hu, Lin Leng and Xuejiao Yang

Abstract

Background: To evaluate visual acuity, corneal astigmatism and corneal higher-order aberrations (HOAs) after implantation of trifocal diffractive IOLs operated with either a corneal steep-axis incision or 135° incision.

Method: This prospective study enrolled patients randomly assigned to different groups. According to preoperative corneal astigmatism, 101 eyes of 77 patients were assigned into group A_1 (0 ~ 0.50 D) or A_2 (0.51 ~ 1.00 D) with a corneal steep-axis incision or group B_1 (0 ~ 0.50 D) or B_2 (0.51 ~ 1.00 D) with a 135° incision. Visual acuity, corneal astigmatism and corneal higher-order aberrations (HOAs) were followed-up for 3 months.

Results: Corneal astigmatism in group A_2 significantly decreased 3 months after surgery ($P < 0.01$) and was significantly lower than that in group B_2 1 day, 2 weeks, 1 month, and 3 months postoperatively (all values of $P < 0.01$). The following parameters were better in group A_2 than in group B_2: uncorrected intermediate visual acuity (UIVA) at 1 day, 2 weeks, 1 month, and 3 months ($P = 0.00, 0.00, 0.01, 0.01$, respectively);uncorrected distance visual acuity (UDVA) at 1 day and 2 weeks ($P = 0.00, 0.01$); and uncorrected near visual acuity (UNVA) at 1 day, 2 weeks, and 1 month postoperatively ($P = 0.00, 0.01, 0.02$, respectively).

Conclusions: After a corneal steep-axis incision, patients with preoperative corneal astigmatism of 0.51 D to 1.00 D exhibited reduced corneal astigmatism and achieved better UIVA and early postoperative UDVA/UNVA.

Keywords: Cataract, Incision, Trifocal IOL, Corneal astigmatism

Background

Patients' expectations regarding refractive outcomes and spectacle independence have increased substantially, and both cataract patients and refractive patients have the same demands [1]. Multifocal IOLs were developed with the target of reducing spectacle dependence, which can provide patients with near and distance visual restoration after cataract surgery [2]. However, intermediate vision is limited because no specific focus is provided for this distance. Trifocal diffractive IOL designs have shown their capability to provide effective uncorrected intermediate visual acuity (UIVA) restoration without degradation of uncorrected distance visual acuity (UDVA) or uncorrected near visual acuity (UNVA). This new concept of IOL has confirmed good performance for visual outcomes, patient satisfaction and spectacle independence [3–10].

Patients' preoperative corneal astigmatism is critical to the choice of trifocal diffractive IOL, which is a key factor influencing the visual acuity and refractive outcomes postoperatively. Many studies have shown that the location of the corneal incision has an impact on postoperative corneal astigmatism and higher-order aberrations (HOAs), such as degradation of vision at night, halos and glare [11]. However, there is no research on the effect of incisions on visual outcomes after implantation of trifocal diffractive IOLs. This study aimed to evaluate visual acuity, corneal astigmatism and corneal HOAs after implantation of a trifocal diffractive IOL operated with either a corneal steep-axis incision or a 135° incision.

Methods
Patients

In this prospective comparative study, 101 eyes of 77 patients undergoing cataract surgery with implantation

* Correspondence: zhaoguiqiu_good@126.com
The Affiliated Hospital of Qingdao University, No.16, Jiangsu Road, Qingdao, China

of a trifocal diffractive IOL (AT LISA tri 839MP, Carl Zeiss Meditec, Germany) at the Affiliated Hospital of Qingdao University between January 2016 and December 2017 were enrolled. All eyes were divided into two groups: group A including 49 eyes of 37 patients with a 2.8 mm clear corneal incision at the steep-axis and group B including 52 eyes of 40 patients with a 2.8 mm clear corneal incision at 135°. According to the preoperative corneal astigmatism, groups A and B were separated into two subgroups: A_1 (0 ~ 0.50 D with 22 eyes), A_2 (0.51 ~ 1.00 D with 27 eyes), B_1 (0 ~ 0.50 D with 23 eyes), and B_2 (0.51 ~ 1.00 D with 29 eyes).The inclusion criteria were cataract or presbyopia patients who had preexisting corneal astigmatism of less than 1.00 D and seeking spectacle independence suitable for refractive lens exchange. The exclusion criteria were patients with a history of previous ocular surgery or ocular diseases, such as ocular inflammation, keratopathy, glaucoma, retinopathy or optic neuropathy.

The research adhered to the tenets of the Declaration of Helsinki and was approved by the ethics committee of the Affiliated Hospital of Qingdao University. A consent form were signed by all patients who were adequately informed and voluntary participated in the study.

Examination protocol

Complete preoperative and 1-day, 2-week, 1-month, and 3-month postoperative ophthalmological examinations were performed in all cases, including monocular visual acuity (logMAR), Goldmann applanation tonometry, slit-lamp examination, funduscopy, manifest refraction, optical biometry (IOL Master 500; Carl Zeiss Meditec), and measurement of total corneal astigmatism and corneal aberration (both with a Galilei G2, Ziemer ophthalmic systems AG, Port, Switzerland). Visual acuities including preoperative corrected distance visual acuity (CDVA), postoperative UDVA, UIVA and UNVA were measured. The classifications of astigmatic axial length with the rule (WTR) (90° ± 30°), against the rule (ATR) (0° to 30° or 150° to 180°), and oblique (30° to 60° or 120° to 150°) were used. The calculation of surgically induced astigmatism (SIA) adopted the Jaffe/Clayman vector analysis [12]. The corneal aberrations considered a pupil aperture of 3.5 mm and were calculated and recorded with the Zernike coefficient.

Surgical procedure

All surgeries were performed by the same experienced surgeon who was masked to the patients' data before the surgery. Sutureless 2.8-mm main corneal incisions either on the corneal steep-axis or at 135° were set up in the navigation system by the same experimenter prior to the surgical procedure. After manual capsulorhexis and phacoemulsification, the trifocal diffractive IOL was inserted

into the capsular bag through the main corneal incision using a specific injector. A postoperative topical therapy based on a combination of levofloxacin, nebcin and dexamethasone eye drops were prescribed to be applied four times daily for 1 week.

Intraocular lens

The AT Lisa tri 839MP is a diffractive trifocal preloaded IOL with a 6.0 mm biconvex optic, an overall length of 11.0 mm, and a posterior surface with a sphericity of − 0.18 μm. The near add is + 3.33D, and the intermediate add is + 1.66D. Its design allocates 50% of light to far, 20% to intermediate, and 30% to near vision. The central 4.34 mm follows the described trifocal design, and the peripheral part is only bifocal.

Statistical analysis

SPSS statistics software package version 22.0 was used for statistical analysis. Kolmogorov–Smirnov test was used to check the normality of the data distribution. When parametric analysis was possible, Student's t-tests for paired data were performed for all parameter comparisons. Otherwise, the Wilcoxon signed rank test was applied to assess the significance of differences between examinations. A power analysis was performed with G*Power software, and figures were made by GraphPad Prism. In all cases, the same level of significance ($P < 0.05$) was used.

Results

The study enrolled 101 eyes of 77 patients with a mean age of 59.33 years ranging from 43.00 to 77.00 years. There was no significant difference in age between the groups. The mean preoperative anterior chamber depth (ACD) and axial length (AL) were 3.21 mm (standard deviation [SD]: 0.40; median: 3.33; range: 2.54 to 3.94 mm) and 23.99 mm (SD: 1.42; median: 23.54; range: 21.91 to 27.51 mm), respectively. There were no statistically significant differences in preoperative ACD or AL between groups (Table 1).

Corneal astigmatism

There were no statistically significant differences between 3-month postoperative and preoperative corneal astigmatism in groups A_1, B_1, or B_2 ($P = 0.17$, 0.15, 0.22, respectively). However, corneal astigmatism in group A_2 3 months postoperatively was significantly lower than preoperatively ($P < 0.01$). There were no statistically significant differences between group A_1 and group B_1 1 day, 2 weeks, 1 month, or 3 months postoperatively ($P = 0.32$, 0.73, 0.42, 0.29, respectively), but corneal astigmatism in group A_2 was significantly lower than group B_2 1 day, 2 weeks, 1 month, and 3 months postoperatively (all $P < 0.01$) (Table 2).

The proportion of WTR in group A_1 declined from 59.1% preoperatively to 40.9% 3 months postoperatively,

Table 1 Preoperative and Postoperative Clinical Date

Parameters mean ± SD median (range)	Group A₁	Group B₁	A₁/B₁ (P)	Group A₂	Group B₂	A₂/B₂ (P)
Age (y)	59.23 ± 7.12 57.00 (51.00 to 74.00)	61.52 ± 7.86 62.00 (43.00 to 77.00)	0.31	57.22 ± 10.86 55.00(51.00 to 76.00)	59.62 ± 7.54 59.00 (43.00 to 75.00)	0.28
ACD (mm)	3.15 ± 0.36 3.26 (2.60 to 3.78)	3.24 ± 0.41 3.34 (2.54 to 3.81)	0.45	3.29 ± 0.41 3.36 (2.54 to 3.94)	3.17 ± 0.43 3.33 (2.54 to 3.78)	0.89
AL (mm)	23.68 ± 1.16 23.49 (21.96 to 26.45)	24.29 ± 1.53 24.37 (22.00 to 26.84)	0.14	24.21 ± 1.56 24.44 (21.91 to 27.51)	23.78 ± 1.36 23.53 (21.96 to 26.74)	0.30
Preoperative UDVA	0.52 ± 0.18 0.52 (0.22 to 1.00)	0.58 ± 0.16 0.60 (0.30 to 0.82)	0.23	0.56 ± 0.16 0.60 (0.22 to 0.82)	0.56 ± 0.17 0.52 (0.22 to 0.92)	0.85
Preoperative CDVA	0.40 ± 0.14 0.40 (0.10 to 0.70)	0.47 ± 0.12 0.40 (0.20 to 0.70)	0.24	0.49 ± 0.15 0.52 (0.22 to 0.82)	0.50 ± 0.18 0.52 (0.10 to 0.82)	0.34
Spherical Refraction[a] (D)	−0.11 ± 0.21 0.00 (−0.50 to 0.25)	−0.13 ± 0.24 0.00 (−0.50 to 0.25)	0.67	−0.07 ± 0.25 0.00 (−0.50 to 0.25)	−0.07 ± 0.23 0.00 (−0.50 to 0.25)	0.94
Cylindrical Refraction[a] (D)	−0.34 ± 0.21 −0.38 (−0.75 to 0.00)	−0.37 ± 0.24 −0.50 (−0.75 to 0.00)	0.81	−0.34 ± 0.16 −0.25 (−0.50 to 0.00)	−0.54 ± 0.25 −0.50 (−1.00 to 0.00)	0.00
SE[a] (D)	−0.28 ± 0.22 −0.25 (−0.63 to 0.25)	−0.32 ± 0.23 −0.38 (−0.75 to 0.13)	0.59	−0.25 ± 0.24 −0.25 (−0.63 to 0.25)	−0.34 ± 0.26 −0.38 (−1.00 to 0.13)	0.18

[a]3 months postoperation

while ATR increased from 27.3 to 45.5%.The WTR of group B₁ decreased from 52.2 to 39.1%, while ATR increased from 34.8 to 43.5%. The WTR of group A₂ decreased from 48.1 to 37.0%, while ATR increased from 29.6 to 37.1%.The WTR of group B₂ decreased from 48.3 to 27.6%, while ATR increased from 27.6 to 34.5%. However, the oblique of group B₂ increased from 24.1% preoperatively to 37.9% 3 months postoperatively, but no obvious changes were found in groups A₁, B₁, or A₂ (13.6 to 13.6%, 13.0 to 17.4%, 22.2 to 25.9%, respectively). (Fig. 1).

No significant differences in surgically induced astigmatism (SIA) were detected between group A₁ and group B₁ nor between group A₂ and group B₂ 3 months postoperatively (P = 0.61, 0.82, respectively). (Fig. 2).

Visual acuity

There were no significant differences in preoperative UDVA and CDVA between the subgroups (Table 1). Postoperative visual acuity in each group was definitely better than preoperatively. No statistically significant differences in UDVA, UIVA, or UNVA between group A₁ and B₁ were found 1 day, 2 weeks, 1 month, or 3 months postoperatively (all values of P > 0.05). However, the UIVA of group A₂ was significantly better than that of group B₂ 1 day, 2 weeks, 1 month, and 3 months postoperatively (P = 0.00, 0.00, 0.01, 0.01, respectively), while UDVA 1 day and 2 weeks (P = 0.00, 0.01) and UNVA 1 day, 2 weeks, and 1 month postoperatively (P = 0.00, 0.01, 0.02, respectively)in group A₂ were better than those in group B₂.However, there were no significant differences in UDVA

Table 2 Preoperative and Postoperative Corneal Astigmatism Data (D)

Groups mean ± SD median (range)	Preoperation	1 Day Postoperation	2 Weeks Postoperation	1 Month Postoperation	3 Months Postoperation	P[a]
A₁	0.37 ± 0.07 0.39 (0.23 to 0.49)	0.68 ± 0.32 0.82 (0.20 to 1.26)	0.64 ± 0.22 0.60 (0.26 to 1.05)	0.55 ± 0.17 0.55 (0.25 to 0.86)	0.42 ± 0.12 0.44 (0.22 to 0.61)	0.17 (power = 50.64%)
A₂	0.73 ± 0.11 0.70 (0.58 to 0.99)	0.63 ± 0.26 0.66 (0.26 to 1.27)	0.48 ± 0.12 0.45 (0.29 to 0.86)	0.49 ± 0.09 0.54 (0.36 to 0.60)	0.44 ± 0.09 0.45 (0.25 to 0.56)	0.00 (power = 100%)
B₁	0.40 ± 0.07 0.41 (0.27 to 0.49)	0.80 ± 0.46 0.88 (0.20 to 1.87)	0.66 ± 0.23 0.62 (0.26 to 1.00)	0.60 ± 0.22 0.57 (0.25 to 1.00)	0.47 ± 0.18 0.53 (0.12 to 0.88)	0.15 (power = 52.65%)
B₂	0.73 ± 0.12 0.68 (0.58 to 0.99)	1.01 ± 0.38 0.91 (0.66 to 2.16)	0.79 ± 0.30 0.69 (0.48 to 1.54)	0.79 ± 0.28 0.83 (0.45 to 1.83)	0.69 ± 0.21 0.70 (0.43 to 1.35)	0.22 (power = 31.10%)
A₁/B₁ (P)	0.21 (power = 40.89%)	0.32 (power = 25.94%)	0.73 (power = 8.83%)	0.42 (power = 21.03%)	0.29 (power = 28.57%)	–
A₂/B₂ (P)	0.98 (power = 5.00%)	0.00 (power = 99.61%)	0.00 (power = 99.96%)	0.00 (power = 99.99%)	0.00 (power = 100%)	–

[a]Comparison between preoperation and 3 months postoperation

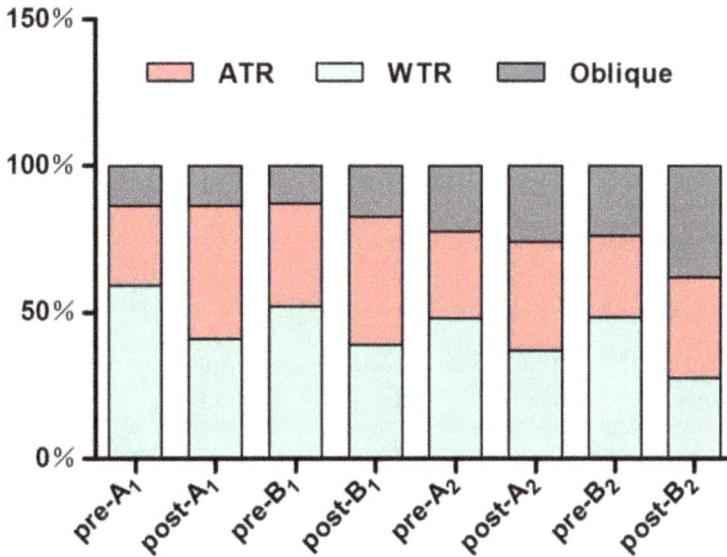

Fig. 1 Preoperative and postoperative proportion of WTR, ATR, Oblique in each subgroup

1 month or 3 months postoperatively ($P = 0.26, 0.44$) or in UNVA 3 months postoperatively ($P = 0.45$) (Table 3).

Corneal aberration

There were no significant differences in preoperative total corneal wave-front aberration, root mean square value of corneal higher-order aberrations (RMS HOAs), spherical aberration (SA), coma, or trefoil between group A and group B. Total corneal wave-front aberrations were much higher 1 day, 2 weeks, and 1 month postoperatively in group B than in group A (all $P < 0.01$). There were no statistically significant differences in total corneal wave-front aberrations 3 months postoperatively or in RMA HOAs, SA, coma, or trefoil 1 day, 2 weeks,

1 month, and 3 months postoperatively between group A and group B (all $P > 0.05$). (Fig. 3).

In group A, RMS HOAs and trefoil 1 day and 2 weeks postoperatively increased apparently (all $P < 0.05$), while there were no differences in RMS HOAs or trefoil 1 month or 3 months postoperatively. There were no obvious changes in total corneal wave-front aberrations, SA or coma after surgery (all $P > 0.05$). (Fig. 3).

In group B, the level of total corneal wave-front aberrations, RMS HOAs, and trefoil 1 day and 2 weeks postoperatively (all values of $P < 0.01$) significantly increased, but there were no differences 1 month or 3 months postoperatively. There were no obvious changes in SA or coma after surgery (all $P > 0.05$). (Fig. 3).

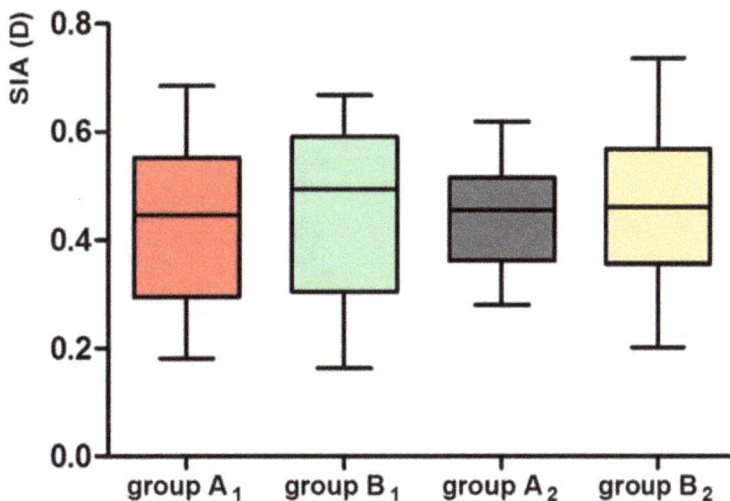

Fig. 2 SIA at 3 months postoperation in group A_1, B_1, A_2, B_2

Table 3 Postoperative Visual Acuity Data (logMAR)

Visions *mean ± SD median (range)*	Group A$_1$	Group B$_1$	A$_1$/B$_1$ (*P*)	Group A$_2$	Group B$_2$	A$_2$/B$_2$ (*P*)
UDVA (1 day)	0.06 ± 0.05 0.10 (0.00 to 0.15)	0.03 ± 0.06 0.00 (− 0.08 to 0.20)	0.11 (power = 55.88%)	−0.01 ± 0.04 0.00 (− 0.08 to 0.10)	0.06 ± 0.08 0.00 (0.00 to 0.22)	0.00 (power = 99.27%)
UDVA (2 weeks)	0.01 ± 0.06 0.00 (− 0.08 to 0.10)	0.00 ± 0.05 0.00 (− 0.08 to 0.10)	0.72 (power = 14.75%)	−0.01 ± 0.03 0.00 (− 0.08 to 0.05)	0.02 ± 0.05 0.00 (− 0.08 to 0.10)	0.01 (power = 85.12%)
UDVA (1 month)	−0.01 ± 0.04 0.00 (− 0.08 to 0.05)	0.00 ± 0.05 0.00 (− 0.08 to 0.10)	0.65 (power = 17.99%)	−0.01 ± 0.03 0.00 (− 0.08 to 0.05)	0.00 ± 0.05 0.00 (− 0.08 to 0.10)	0.26 (power = 22.68%)
UDVA (3 months)	−0.02 ± 0.04 0.00 (− 0.08 to 0.05)	−0.01 ± 0.04 0.00 (− 0.08 to 0.05)	0.40 (power = 20.62%)	−0.01 ± 0.03 0.00 (− 0.08 to 0.00)	0.00 ± 0.05 0.00 (− 0.08 to 0.10)	0.44 (power = 22.68%)
UIVA (1 day)	0.10 ± 0.06 0.10 (0.00 to 0.22)	0.09 ± 0.06 0.10 (0.00 to 0.20)	0.59 (power = 13.68%)	0.03 ± 0.05 0.00 (0.00 to 0.15)	0.12 ± 0.11 0.10 (0.00 to 0.30)	0.00 (power = 98.76%)
UIVA (2 weeks)	0.06 ± 0.05 0.10 (− 0.08 to 0.10)	0.03 ± 0.06 0.00 (− 0.08 to 0.20)	0.14 (power = 55.88%)	0.02 ± 0.04 0.00 (0.00 to 0.10)	0.07 ± 0.05 0.10 (0.00 to 0.15)	0.00 (power = 99.25%)
UIVA (1 month)	0.03 ± 0.05 0.00 (− 0.08 to 0.15)	0.02 ± 0.05 0.00 (− 0.08 to 0.15)	0.55 (power = 16.24%)	0.02 ± 0.03 0.00 (0.00 to 0.10)	0.07 ± 0.08 0.10 (− 0.08 to 0.20)	0.01 (power = 92.08%)
UIVA (3 months)	0.01 ± 0.03 0.00 (− 0.08 to 0.05)	0.01 ± 0.04 0.00 (− 0.08 to 0.10)	0.57 (power = 5.00%)	0.00 ± 0.04 0.00 (− 0.08 to 0.10)	0.04 ± 0.06 0.05 (− 0.08 to 0.10)	0.01 (power = 89.46%)
UNVA (1 day)	0.11 ± 0.07 0.10 (0.00 to 0.20)	0.12 ± 0.05 0.10 (0.00 to 0.20)	0.50 (power = 13.52%)	0.10 ± 0.05 0.10 (0.00 to 0.20)	0.19 ± 0.09 0.20 (0.10 to 0.30)	0.00 (power = 99.82%)
UNVA (2 weeks)	0.08 ± 0.04 0.10 (0.00 to 0.15)	0.09 ± 0.03 0.10 (0.00 to 0.15)	0.22 (power = 23.84%)	0.10 ± 0.05 0.10 (0.00 to 0.20)	0.14 ± 0.05 0.10 (0.00 to 0.20)	0.01 (power = 90.47%)
UNVA (1 month)	0.06 ± 0.06 0.05 (0.00 to 0.15)	0.08 ± 0.03 0.10 (0.00 to 0.10)	0.19 (power = 40.00%)	0.09 ± 0.04 0.10 (0.00 to 0.15)	0.12 ± 0.05 0.10 (0.00 to 0.20)	0.02 (power = 78.86%)
UNVA (3 months)	0.05 ± 0.06 0.05 (− 0.08 to 0.15)	0.04 ± 0.05 0.00 (− 0.08 to 0.10)	0.59 (power = 14.75%)	0.09 ± 0.05 0.10 (0.00 to 0.20)	0.10 ± 0.05 0.10 (0.00 to 0.20)	0.45 (power = 18.24%)

Discussion

The trifocal diffractive IOLs have shown perfect visual restoration of intermediate vision without degradation of distance or near vision. It's worth noting that its efficacy is affected by many factors, among which incision location, SIA and preoperative corneal astigmatism are of great importance. Owing to personal surgical practice, some surgeons tend to choose a habitual incision location.

Mojzis et al. [13] adopted temporal clear corneal incision, Florian et al. [14] chose incision at the corneal steep-axis, and Matthias Müller et al. [1] used incisions at twelve o'clock on the cornea. Effective restoration of postoperative distance vision, intermediate vision, and near vision was obtained in their studies. However, the influence of the location of corneal incision on postoperative residual corneal astigmatism and visual acuities after implantation

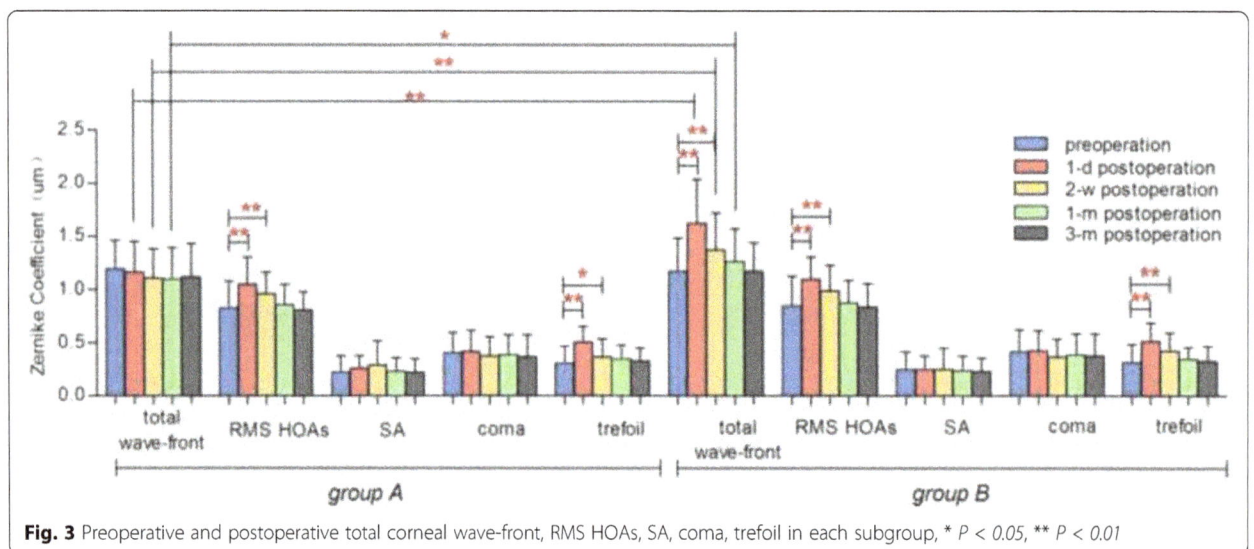

Fig. 3 Preoperative and postoperative total corneal wave-front, RMS HOAs, SA, coma, trefoil in each subgroup, * *P < 0.05*, ** *P < 0.01*

of the trifocal diffractive IOLs was unclear. Therefore, we comprehensively assessed the performance of a steep-axis incision and 135° incision. We found that after a corneal steep-axis incision, patients with preoperative corneal astigmatism of 0.51 D to 1.00 D achieved reduced corneal astigmatism and better UIVA and early postoperative UDVA/UNVA.

In our study, we found that when patients' preoperative corneal astigmatism was under 0.50 D, there were no significant differences in postoperative vision or corneal astigmatism between a steep-axis incision and 135° incision. Because currently used incision sizes are small, even on the micro scale, their interference with the cornea is not significant. Therefore, surgeons can select an appropriate incision based upon their own operational preferences. As for patients with preoperative corneal astigmatism of 0.51 D to 1.00 D, making a corneal incision at the steep-axis can reduce postoperative corneal astigmatism and provide patients with better UIVA and better early postoperative UDVA/UNVA. This kind of trifocal IOL design allocates 50% of light to far, 20% to intermediate and 30% to near vision. Owing to the proportion of light allocation, the influence of corneal astigmatism on visual acuity after implantation with the trifocal diffractive IOLs is UDVA > UNVA > UIVA, but the sensitivity of corneal astigmatism is UIVA > UNVA > UDVA.

Corneal astigmatism was much higher in the early period after the surgery due to corneal edema, but the steep-axis incision shaped the cornea more regularly than the 135° incision after cataract operation. This difference produced early postoperative UDVA, UIVA, and UNVA that were much better in patients with corneal steep-axis incision. With the healing of the corneal incision and fading of corneal edema, corneal astigmatism reduced and gradually became steady, and intermediate vision was more susceptible to corneal astigmatism, which maybe small but is indeed important for UIVA. This study is the first clinical study comparing the visual outcomes obtained with either corneal steep-axis incision or 135° incision and showing the realistic benefits of corneal steep-axis incision in patients implanted with trifocal diffractive IOLs.

There were no significant differences in the SIA between a steep-axis incision and 135° incision in our study. Postoperative astigmatism depends on preoperative corneal astigmatism and SIA. Since incisions currently are small or even on a micro scale in cataract surgery, the value of SIA is not large enough to markedly affect visual acuity [11]. There is an inseparable relationship between corneal astigmatism and vision quality after implantation with a trifocal diffractive IOL. The recommended corneal astigmatism from cataract surgery with trifocal diffractive IOL is no more than 0.75 D. However, Elizabeth et al. [5] chose

patients with preoperative corneal astigmatism under 1.00 D, and Peter Mojzis [15] and Florian Tobias selected 1.25 D [16] at most, but Thomas et al. [17] expanded the range to 1.50 D. Our study opted for preoperative corneal astigmatism equal to or less than 1.00 D. Excellent visual outcomes were obtained, and a significant improvement in UDVA, UIVA, and UNVA was found in all these studies with appropriate incision locations. Whether there is an acceptable range of preoperative corneal astigmatism with implantation of trifocal diffractive IOLs needs further study.

We found a drift phenomenon from WTR to ATR postoperatively with a corneal steep-axis incision and135° incision. This finding was consistent with Cui Y's [18, 19] studies, which showed the same phenomenon after cataract surgery. However, the impact of the astigmatic axial on visual acuity was oblique> ATR > WTR astigmatism [20]. In our study, a higher percentage of oblique astigmatism but a much lower percentage of WTR astigmatism was found postoperatively in group B_2 compared with those in group A_2. This finding maybe another factor that contributed to better outcomes in group A_2 than in group B_2.

We detected that there was no difference in corneal HOAs between steep-axis incision and 135° incision, but both corneal HOAs from the different incisions were much higher in the early period after the surgery. Some patients achieved vision of 0.00 logMAR or better but still suffered from degradation vision at night, halos and glare. This phenomenon may be due to the increase in postoperative HOAs. Mojzis et al. [3] reported that after surgery for trifocal diffractive IOLs, there was a significant decrease in ocular aberrations and internal aberrations, while there was no statistically significant difference between preoperative and postoperative corneal aberrations. In our study, corneal HOAs increased with steep-axis and 135° incisions due to the existence of a surgical incision and early postoperative corneal edema. However, it reduced gradually and was not different compared to preoperative HOAs 3 months postoperatively. This finding was consistent with Florian T.A Kretz's discovery [14] that negative effects were not disturbing and were a temporary phenomenon that reduced over time. However, total corneal wave-front aberration was much higher with the 135° incision because of its larger, early postoperative corneal astigmatism than that with the steep-axis incision that shaped the cornea more regularly.

Conclusions

In summary, steep-axis incision may be an ideal incision choice for patients with preoperative corneal astigmatism of 0.51 D to 1.00 D for trifocal diffractive IOL implantation. However, for patients with preoperative corneal astigmatism under 0.50 D, surgeons can select the appropriate incision based on their own preferences.

Abbreviations
ACD: Anterior chamber depth; AL: Axial length; ATR: Against the rule; CDVA: Corrected distance visual acuity; HOAs: Higher-order aberrations; RMS HOAs: Root mean square value of corneal higher-order aberrations; SA: Spherical aberration; SE: Spherical equivalent; SIA: Surgically induced astigmatism; UDVA: Uncorrected distance visual acuity; UIVA: Uncorrected intermediate visual acuity; UNVA: Uncorrected near visual acuity; WTR: With the rule

Acknowledgments
We acknowledge the professional help of American Journal Experts for correcting all linguistic errors in the manuscript, including the section of the abstract.

Funding
It was funded by the National Natural Science Foundation of China (81470609, 81300730) and the National Natural Science Foundation of Shandong (ZR2017BH025). The funders played an important role in study design, data collection and analysis, decision to publish, or preparation of the manuscript.

Authors' contributions
SSX was responsible for its design, collection of data, analysis and interpretation of results and wrote the first draft of the manuscript. GQZ participated in its design and revise of manuscript. XNY was involved in data collection. JL, CL, XJY and LL helped revise of manuscript; LTH conceived the study design. All authors have read and approved the final manuscript.

Competing interests
The authors declare that they have no competing interests.

References

1. Kretz FT, Müller M, Gerl M, et al. Binocular function to increase visual outcome in patients implanted with a diffractive trifocal intraocular lens. BMC Ophthalmol. 2015;15:110.
2. Calladine D, Evans JR, Shah S, Leyland M. Multifocal versus monofocal intraocular lenses after cataract extraction. Sao Paulo Med J. 2015 Feb;133(1):68.
3. Mojzis P, Peña-García P, Liehneova I, Ziak P, Alió JL. Outcomes of a new diffractive trifocal intraocular lens. J Cataract Refract Surg. 2014;40:60–9.
4. Alió JL, Montalbán R, Peña-García P, Soria FA, Vega-Estrada A. Visual outcomes of a trifocal aspheric diffractive intraocular lens with micro incision cataract surgery. J Refract Surg. 2013;29:756–61.
5. Law EM, Aggarwal RK, Kasaby H. Clinical outcomes with a new trifocal intraocular lens. Eur J Ophthalmol. 2014;24:501–8.
6. Cochener B, Vryghem J, Rozot P, et al. Visual and refractive outcomes after implantation of a fully diffractive trifocal lens. Clin Ophthalmol. 2012;6:1421–7.
7. Sheppard AL, Shah S, Bhatt U, Bhogal G, Wolffsohn JS. Visual outcomes and subjective experience after bilateral implantation of a new diffractive trifocal intraocular lens. J Cataract Refract Surg. 2013;39:343–9.
8. Lesieur G. Outcomes after implantation of a trifocal diffractive IOL [article in French]. J Fr Ophthalmol. 2012;35:338–42.
9. Voskresenskaya A, Pozdeyeva N, Pashtaev N, Batkov Y, Treushnicov V, Cherednik V. Initial results of trifocal diffractive IOL implantation. Graefes Arch Clin Exp Ophthalmol. 2010;248:1299–306.
10. Mendicute J, Kapp A, Lévy P, Krommes G, Arias-Puente A, Tomalla M, Bouchut P. Evaluation of visual outcomes and patient satisfaction after implantation of a diffractive trifocal intraocular lens. J Cataract Refract Surg. 2016;42(2):203–10.
11. He W, Zhu X, Du Y, Yang J, Lu Y. Clinical efficacy of implantation of toric intraocular lenses with different incision positions: a comparative study of steep-axis incision and non-steep-axis incision. BMC Ophthalmol. 2017;17(1):132.
12. Jaffe NS, Clayman HM. The pathophysiology of corneal astigmatism after cataract extraction. Trans Am Acad Ophthalmol Otolaryngol. 1975;79:615–30.
13. Mojzis P, Kukuckova L, Majerova K, Liehneova K, Piñero DP. Comparative analysis of the visual performance after cataract surgery with implantation of a bifocal or trifocal diffractive IOL. J Refract Surg. 2014 Oct;30(10):666–72.
14. Kretz FT, Breyer D, Diakonis VF, et al. Clinical Outcomes after Binocular Implantation of a New Trifocal Diffractive Intraocular Lens. J Ophthalmol. 2015;2015:962891.
15. Mojzis P, Majerova K, Hrckova L, Piñero DP. Implantation of a diffractive trifocal intraocular lens: one-year follow-up. J Cataract Refract Surg. 2015;41:1623–30.
16. Kretz FT, Choi CY, Müller M, Gerl M, Gerl RH, Auffarth GU. Visual outcomes, patient satisfaction and spectacle independence with a trifocal diffractive intraocular Lens. Korean J Ophthalmol. 2016;30(3):180–91.
17. Kohnen T, Titke C, Bohm M. Trifocal intraocular Lens implantation to treat visual demands in various distances following Lens removal. Am J Ophthalmol. 2016;161:P71–7.
18. Cui Y, Meng Q, Guo H, Zeng J, Zhang H, Zhang G, Huang Y, Lan J. Biometry and corneal astigmatism in cataract surgery candidates from southern China. J Cataract Refract Surg. 2014;40(10):1661–9.
19. Özyol E, Özyol P. Analyses of surgically induced astigmatism and axis deviation in microcoaxial phacoemulsification. Int Ophthalmol. 2014;34(3):591–6.
20. Remón L, Monsoriu JA, Furlan WD. Influence of different types of astigmatism on visual acuity. J Optom. 2017;10(3):141–8.

31

Comparison of a new swept-source optical biometer with a partial coherence interferometry

Hyo Kyung Lee[1,2] and Mee Kum Kim[1,2]* (ORCID)

Abstract

Background: The purpose of this study is to compare the biometric parameters and intraocular lens (IOL) power calculation by a new swept-source optical coherence tomography (SS-OCT) biometer with those by a partial coherence interferometry (PCI) biometer.

Methods: Medical records of 175 eyes from 175 patients were retrospectively reviewed. One of two monofocal IOLs (Tecnis ZCB00 or Acrysof SA60AT) were implanted in the eyes. Axial length (AL), mean keratometry (Km), J0, J45 and anterior chamber depth (ACD) were compared between PCI and SS-OCT biometers. The refractive mean error (ME) and refractive mean absolute error (MAE) were also compared. Examination failure rates were calculated in each device.

Results: Out of 175 eyes, 150 eyes were successfully examined by both devices. AL was measured slightly shorter when using SS-OCT than PCI biometer, while Km was measured higher ($P < .0001$, $P = .03$, respectively, paired t-test). J0, J45 and ACD were not significantly different between two devices. ME and MAE calculated using SRK-T, Hoffer Q, and Haigis formula were not significantly different except MAE calculated with Haigis formula for Tecnis ZCB00 IOLs ($P = .03$, paired t-test). The examination failure rates were 14.29 and 1.14% when using the PCI and SS-OCT biometers, respectively.

Conclusions: AL and Km don't seem to be comparable between two devices, while J0, J45, and ACD do. IOL power calculation using SRK-T and Hoffer Q was correlated between the devices. The penetration ability of a SS-OCT biometer is superior.

Keywords: Swept-source optical coherence tomography, IOLMaster 700, Optical biometer, Intraocular lens power calculation

Background

As technology has been developed to produce better refractory outcomes, cataract surgery has become a part of refractory surgery [1]. For an accurate intraocular lens (IOL) power calculation, accurate ocular biometry, use of an appropriate calculation formula, and careful optimization of the individual component parts should be considered. Of those, the most important factor is the accuracy of ocular biometric measurements [2]. In the current market, various types of biometric devices based on different technologies are available to provide more accurate ocular biometric measurements.

To our knowledge, a partial coherence interferometry (PCI)-based optical biometer is considered as gold standard for axial length (AL) measurement [3]. In a PCI biometer, optical length is measured from the anterior surface of the cornea to the retinal pigment epithelium with a 780 nm laser diode infrared light. Keratometry (K) is calculated from measurements taken at 6 reference points on the corneal surface in an optical zone with a diameter of 2.4 mm. Anterior chamber depth (ACD) is measured with the lateral slit illumination technique. However, in some cases such as subcapsular lens opacity, dense cataracts, and poor fixation, measuring AL is

* Correspondence: kmk9@snu.ac.kr
[1]Department of Ophthalmology, Seoul National University College of Medicine, 103 Daehak-Ro, Jongno-Gu, Seoul 110-799, Republic of Korea
[2]Laboratory of Ocular Regenerative Medicine and Immunology, Seoul Artificial Eye Center, Seoul National University Hospital Clinical Research Institute, Seoul, Republic of Korea

impossible. For these reasons, the examination failure rate when using a PCI biometer has been reported to be as high as 35.47% [4].

Recently, a swept-source optical coherence tomography (SS-OCT)-based optical biometer was introduced to the market. The SS-OCT technology enables a 44 mm scan depth with 22 μm resolution in corneal tissue using a rapid-cycle, tunable wavelength laser source. Compared with a PCI biometer, an SS-OCT biometer can scan a deeper area and produce a better quality image [5]. Also, it allows for cross-sectional visualization along the visual axis and shows good cataract penetration [6].

The present study was performed to compare biometric parameters and IOL power calculations by a new SS-OCT biometer, the IOLMaster 700® (Carl Zeiss Meditec AG), with those by a PCI biometer, the IOLMaster 500® (Carl Zeiss Meditec AG). Penetration ability was also compared between the two devices.

Methods

Patients and methods

The protocol of this study adhered to the tenets of the Declaration of Helsinki. This study protocol was approved and the need for informed consent was waived by our Institutional Review and Ethics Board (No. 1684–174-790). The medical records of the patients who underwent uneventful cataract surgery at Seoul National University Hospital, Seoul, Korea from June 2016 to January 2017 were retrospectively reviewed. Subjects who had been followed for more than 1 month after the surgery were included. The following cases were excluded: those with eventful surgeries, postoperative complications, and other accompanying ocular pathologies such as zonular weakness or macular lesions.

Before the surgery, all individuals were examined in detail using both optical biometers in a random order. The optical parameters of AL, mean K (Km), J0, J45 and ACD were recorded and compared between the devices. Km was calculated as the average of flat K and steep K. Astigmatism was evaluated using Jackson cross-cylinder such as J0 and J45, calculated by power vector analysis [7]. The formula to calculate Jackson cross-cylinder was as follows;

$$J0 = -c/2 \times \cos2\theta.$$

$$J_{45} = -c/2 \times \sin2\theta$$

(c: negative astigmatism = flat K − steep K; θ = flat meridian)

To determine the appropriate IOL power, four formulas, SRK-T, Hoffer Q, Holladay, and Haigis, were employed, and the results were compared. Among the formulas, the embedded Holladay formulas were different between the devices used in the present study. Whereas the Holladay 1

formula was embedded in the PCI biometer, the Holladay 2 formula was embedded in the SS-OCT biometer.

A single experienced surgeon (MKK) performed cataract surgeries on all participants enrolled in the present study with a 2.7 mm long, steep-on axis incision technique. For all eyes, one of the two types of monofocal IOLs (Tecnis ZCB00, Acrysof SA60AT) was inserted into the bag without any complications. Target refractive error was from emmetropia to − 2.0 Dsph. We determined the power of the implanted IOL whose predicted refractive error is the targeted one or the negative refraction which is the closest to the emmetropia. The differences between the predicted errors were compared as the refractive mean error (ME) and refractive mean absolute error (MAE), respectively, at 1 week and 1 month after the surgery. ME was defined as the difference between postoperative and predicted spherical equivalents.

Statistical analysis

The paired t-test was used to compare preoperative biometric parameters between the two devices. Agreement of the parameters was evaluated with a Bland-Altman plot. To assess the accuracy of IOL power calculation, ME and MAE were compared between the devices with paired t-test 1 week and 1 month postoperatively. The examination failure rate was calculated for each device to compare penetration capability. All statistical tests were performed using SPSS version 18.0 (SPSS Inc., Chicago, Illinois, USA). Statistical significance was defined as $P < .05$.

Results

A total of 175 eyes from 175 patients were enrolled in this study. Twenty-five eyes were excluded from the main analysis because examination by at least one device had failed. Finally, 150 eyes from 150 patients were eligible for the main analysis. The study subjects consisted of 54 men and 96 women. Their mean age was 69.49 ± 9.55 years. Tecnis ZCB00 and Acrysof SA60AT IOLs were implanted in 102 and 48 eyes, respectively.

Table 1 shows the ocular parameters obtained by the two devices. The AL were measured as 23.99 ± 1.61 mm and 23.98 ± 1.60 mm when using a PCI and SS-OCT biometers, respectively. The AL measured by a SS-OCT was significantly shorter than a PCI biometer, with a mean difference of 0.0098 ± 0.03 mm ($P < .0001$, paired t-test). Km was measured significantly higher by SS-OCT with a mean difference of − 0.0365 ± 0.20 D ($P = .03$, paired t-test). The two devices provided comparable values for J0, J45 and ACD without significant differences ($P = .96$, .41, and .06, respectively, paired t-test). Figure 1 shows Bland-Altman plots illustrating good agreement for all parameters.

To assess the accuracy of IOL power calculation, ME and MAE at 1 week (data not shown) and 1 month

Table 1 Comparison of biometric measurements between two devices (*n* = 150)

Parameter	PCI biometer		SS-OCT biometer			
	Mean ± SD	Range	Mean ± SD	Range	Difference	P value*
AL (mm)	23.99 ± 1.61	21.23 30.47	23.98 ± 1.60	21.19 30.43	0.0098 ± 0.03	< .0001
Km (D)	44.20 ± 1.53	40.99 48.36	44.24 ± 1.55	40.99 48.10	−0.0365 ± 0.20	.03
J0 (D)	−0.007 ± 0.33	−0.995 0.772	−0.005 ± 0.32	−0.794 0.811	−0.0019 ± 0.44	.96
J45 (D)	0.008 ± 0.35	−1.117 0.908	−0.022 ± 0.33	−0.789 1.041	0.0309 ± 0.46	.41
ACD (mm)	3.11 ± 0.41	2.14 4.35	3.08 ± 0.41	2.03 4.15	0.0232 ± 0.15	.06

PCI partial coherence interferometry, *SS-OCT* swept-source optical coherence tomography, *SD* standard deviation, *AL* axial length, *Km* mean keratometry, *ACD* anterior chamber depth
*Paired *t*-test

postoperatively were compared between the two devices (Tables 2 and 3). For Tecnis ZCB00 IOLs, ME was not significantly different between the devices in the SRK-T, Hoffer Q, and Haigis formulas. However, ME in Holladay formula showed a significant difference at 1 week and 1 month postoperatively (all *P* < .0001, paired *t*-test). MAE for Tecnis ZCB00 IOLs was not significantly different between two devices in all the formula except Haigis which was significantly lower in SS-OCT (*P* = .03, paired *t*-test). Meanwhile, for Acrysof SA60AT IOLs, ME and MAE in all the formula at postoperative 1 week and 1 month were not significantly different between the devices except MAE in Holladay formula (*P* = .02, paired *t*-test).

Table 4 shows the examination failure rate for both devices. The examination failure rate was higher in the PCI biometer than the SS-OCT biometer. The types of

cataracts in eyes that could not be examined by at least one device are summarized in Table 5.

Discussion

This study showed significant differences in AL and Km measurements between SS-OCT and PCI biometers. Meanwhile, J0, J45 and ACD were not significantly different between the devices. The IOL power calculation in both devices was comparable when using SRK-T and Hoffer Q formula. The examination failure rate was lower when the SS-OCT rather than the PCI biometer was used.

A few studies have recently been published that evaluated a SS-OCT biometer compared with another one. Srivannaboon et al. [5] and Kathleen et al. [6] reported good agreement and excellent correlation between optical

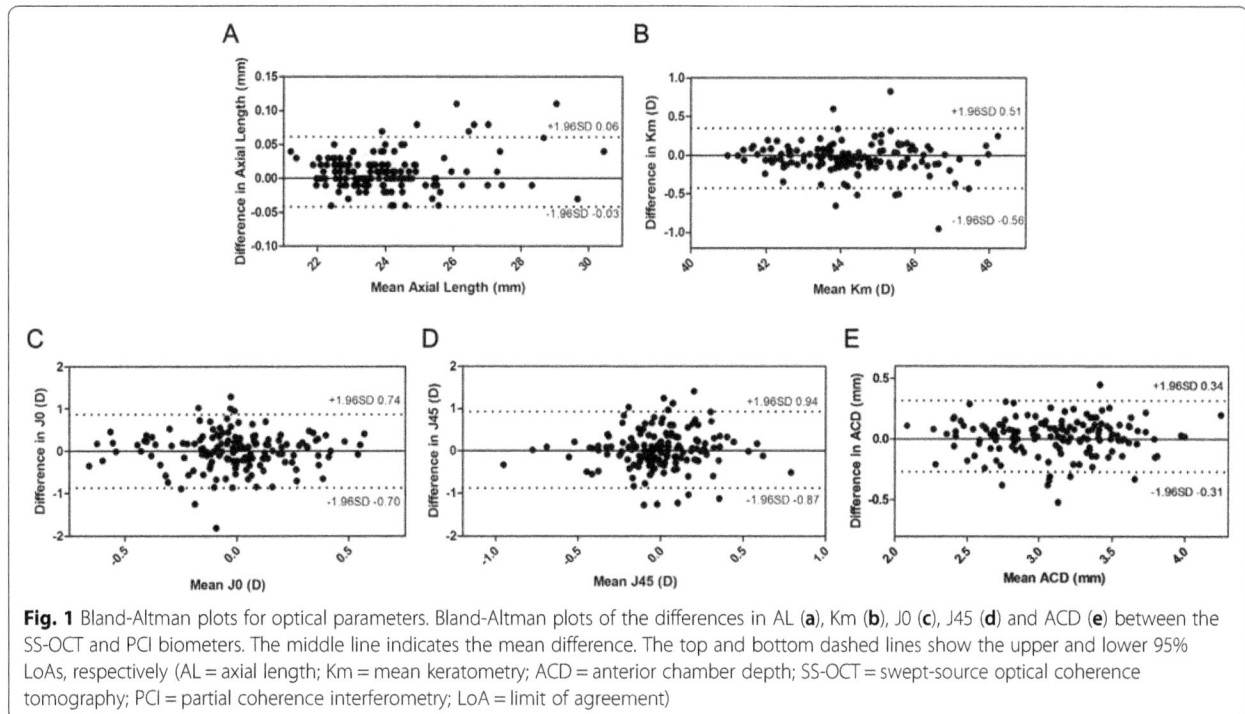

Fig. 1 Bland-Altman plots for optical parameters. Bland-Altman plots of the differences in AL (**a**), Km (**b**), J0 (**c**), J45 (**d**) and ACD (**e**) between the SS-OCT and PCI biometers. The middle line indicates the mean difference. The top and bottom dashed lines show the upper and lower 95% LoAs, respectively (AL = axial length; Km = mean keratometry; ACD = anterior chamber depth; SS-OCT = swept-source optical coherence tomography; PCI = partial coherence interferometry; LoA = limit of agreement)

Table 2 Comparison of refractive mean error[a] at 1 month after the surgery

Formula	PCI biometer	SS-OCT biometer	P value[*]
Tecnis ZCB00 (n = 102)			
SRK-T	− 0.128 ± 0.42	−0.136 ± 0.40	.59
Hoffer Q	−0.036 ± 0.46	−0.028 ± 0.44	.65
Holladay[b]	− 0.070 ± 0.44	−0.157 ± 0.34	.0003
Haigis	−0.046 ± 0.46	−0.038 ± 0.41	.69
AcrySof SA60AT (n = 48)			
SRK-T	0.008 ± 0.53	− 0.019 ± 0.52	.31
Hoffer Q	0.162 ± 0.51	0.126 ± 0.52	.28
Holladay[b]	0.127 ± 0.51	0.069 ± 0.46	.14
Haigis	0.128 ± 0.53	0.115 ± 0.47	.71

PCI partial coherence interferometry, SS-OCT swept-source optical coherence tomography
*Paired t-test
[a]Refractive mean error = postoperative spherical equivalent (SE) – predicted SE
[b]Holladay 1 and 2 formulas were embedded in PCI and SS-OCT biometers, respectively

parameters measured by SS-OCT and PCI biometers. However, Akman et al. [7] and Yoo et al. [8] showed statistically significant differences in AL, K and ACD measurements between the SS-OCT and PCI biometers, although these differences were quite small for clinical significance. Our study supports these reports to some extent.

In this study, AL and ACD measured with the SS-OCT biometer were slightly shorter than those with the PCI biometer, with differences of 0.013 ± 0.03 mm and 0.023 ± 0.15 mm, respectively ($P < .0001$, $P = .06$, respectively, paired t-test). The SS-OCT biometer measures the length of the optical pathway, such as AL,

Table 3 Comparison of refractive mean absolute error[a] at 1 month after the surgery

	PCI biometer	SS-OCT biometer	P value[*]
Tecnis ZCB00 (n = 102)			
SRK-T	0.339 ± 0.28	0.334 ± 0.26	.69
Hoffer Q	0.364 ± 0.28	0.352 ± 0.26	.49
Holladay[b]	0.353 ± 0.27	0.334 ± 0.27	.40
Haigis	0.378 ± 0.26	0.335 ± 0.24	.03
AcrySof SA60AT (n = 48)			
SRK-T	0.399 ± 0.35	0.405 ± 0.31	.79
Hoffer Q	0.409 ± 0.33	0.401 ± 0.35	.77
Holladay[b]	0.410 ± 0.33	0.355 ± 0.30	.02
Haigis	0.417 ± .034	0.372 ± 0.31	.09

PCI partial coherence interferometry, SS-OCT swept-source optical coherence tomography
*Paired t-test
[a]Refractive mean absolute error = I postoperative spherical equivalent (SE) – predicted SE I
[b]Holladay 1 and 2 formulas were embedded in PCI and SS-OCT biometers, respectively

Table 4 Comparison of examination failure rate between the two devices

	Number of eyes			Failure rate (%)
	Failure	Success	Total	
PCI biometer	25	150	175	14.29
SS-OCT biometer	2	173	175	1.14

PCI partial coherence interferometry, SS-OCT swept-source optical coherence tomography

ACD, lens thickness and central corneal thickness, with SS-OCT technology [4]. In contrast, the PCI biometer measures AL and ACD using time-domain OCT technology and slit-imaging technology, respectively [4]. Light scattering by the retinal pigment epithelium and other ocular structures along with the visual axis is less than measured by conventional OCT, as SS-OCT uses a long wavelength of light. Therefore, the difference in AL measurements was likely caused by the difference in laser wavelength used in the two devices. Previous studies reported that 0.1 mm of AL difference would lead to a 0.28 D difference in the IOL power calculation and the minimum detectable change in refraction is 0.25 D with an AL of 0.075 mm [9, 10]. In that regard, even if there was a difference in AL measurements taken with the SS-OCT and PCI biometers in the present study, it was too small to cause a clinically significant error in IOL power calculation.

Measuring the K readings in both devices were based on the distance-independent telecentric keratometry system. SS-OCT measure K readings at 6 points each for 1.3, 2.4 and 3.2 mm diameter optical zones, while PCI-biometer uses only 6 points in a 2.4 mm zone [11, 12]. This would cause the differences in K readings between the devices in this study but those were quite small to make a clinical significance in IOL power calculation. However out data suggests that, in clinical practice, the differences in AL, K readings and ACD should be considered and those parameters could not be interchangeable between two devices.

Table 5 Types of Cataract in eyes that failed to be examined by the devices

Type of cataract	Number of eyes	
	PCI biometer	SS-OCT biometer
Cortical opacity	1	0
ASC	2	0
PSC	18	0
ASC with PSC	2	0
Total white cataract	2	2
Total	25	2

PCI partial coherence interferometry, SS-OCT swept-source optical coherence tomography, ASC anterior subcapsular cataract, PSC posterior subcapsular cataract

Meanwhile, the agreements of all the parameters (AL, Km, J0, J45, and ACD) were generally good.

To assess the accuracy of the IOL power calculation, we compared ME and MAE at postoperative 1 week and 1 month when two different types of monofocal IOLs were used. The SRK-T, Hoffer Q, Holladay, and Haigis formulas are widely used for IOL power calculation. To predict the post-operative refractive error more accurately, the different formulas should be applied depending on the AL. For example, Hoffer Q is more accurate for shorter AL, while SRK-T is more suitable for long AL. However, out of total 47 eyes, only 2 eyes had short AL (< 22 mm) and 6 eyes had long AL (> 26 mm). Because the proportion of the eyes with extreme AL was too small, we didn't divide the eyes depending on the AL. When using Holladay formula, the ME calculated with the SS-OCT biometer for Tecnis ZCB00 IOLs showed a tendency toward more myopia than those with the PCI biometer. This disparity in the tendency in ME between the two devices stemmed from the differences in the embedded Holladay formula in each device used for the present study. The other three formulas, for SRK-T, Hoffer Q, and Haigis, showed no statistically significant difference in either ME for Tecnis ZCB00 IOLs. In contrast, MAE showed a significant difference in Haigis formula for Tecnis ZCB00 IOLs ($p = 0.0271$, paired t-test). Unlike the 3rd generation formula, Haigis formula uses real ACD parameters to predict effective lens position. The tendency of ACD measurements to be shorter in SS-OCT biometer might cause the difference in MAE when using Haigis formula. In the other formulas, the MAE was not significantly different for Tecnis ZCB00 IOLs. In Acrysof SA60AT IOLs, ME and MAE were not significantly different in all formula between the two devices, except MAE calculated using Holladay formula. This disparity was also considered to be originated from the difference of embedded Holladay formula in each device.

In a few published studies, researchers described efforts to evaluate the accuracy of the IOL power calculation made with SS-OCT optical biometry [5, 13]. However, those studies did not use ME or MAE for the analysis. Srivannaboon et al. [5] compared predicted IOL power by the SRK-T and Haigis formulas and showed no significant differences between SS-OCT and PCI biometers. Arriola-Villalobos et al. [13] compared ocular parameters and calculated IOL power with the Holladay 2 and SRK-T formulas in SS-OCT and low-coherence reflectometry biometers. AL, ACD and Km were slightly different between the devices (mean differences = 0.0046 ± 0.022 mm, -0.015 ± 0.038 mm, -0.0546 ± 0.17 D, respectively; P = .09, .001, and .006, respectively). The calculated IOL power was also different when using the SRK-T formula, with a difference of 0.0517 ± 0.186 D (P = .02).

A PCI biometer has been considered as a gold standard for IOL power calculation and widely used across the globe [14]. However, there are concerns over the limitations. One of the major concerns is the penetration ability that affected by the severity and type of cataracts. A PCI biometer uses dual-beam PCI with a 780 nm laser diode infrared light, whereas an SS-OCT biometer uses a 1055 nm tunable laser source [15]. The longer the wavelength a device uses, the less laser scatter it makes with better penetration ability. In this study, two eyes (1.14%) which showed total white cataract could not be examined with the SS-OCT biometer, whereas 25 eyes (14.29%) failed with the PCI biometer. Out of those 25 eyes, 20 had posterior subcapsular lens opacity and 4 had anterior subcapsular opacity. In short, SS-OCT exhibits much better penetration ability, especially in cases of ASC- or PSC-type cataracts. However, in white cataracts, both devices failed to measure AL.

To get a more accurate IOL power calculation, the A constant should be carefully considered. Basically, A constants used in optical biometers were adapted from the ULIB website [5]. However, to adjust the IOL power prediction, personalization by the surgeon based on large-scale clinical data analysis is important [16, 17]. In the present study, the A constant for the PCI biometer was previously optimized for MKK. However, the A constant used in the SD-OCT biometer was not personally optimized in the present analysis. After accumulating a large amount of clinical data on SD-OCT biometers, we can optimize the constant to improve the accuracy of IOL power calculation in clinical practice.

Conclusions

In conclusion, the SS-OCT biometer seems to be comparable to the PCI biometer in measuring J0, J45 and ACD, whereas, AL and K readings were not comparable between two devices. Making IOL power calculation using SRK-T and Hoffer Q was comparable. Penetration ability is better with the SS-OCT biometer than the PCI biometer.

Abbreviations
ACD: Anterior chamber depth; AL: Axial length; ASC: Anterior subcapsular cataract; IOL: Intraocular lens; K: Keratometry; Km: Mean keratometry; MAE: Mean absolute error; ME: Mean error; PCI: Partial coherence interferometry; PSC: Posterior subcapsular cataract; SS-OCT: Swept-source optical coherence tomography

Acknowledgments
There are none to acknowledge.

Authors' contributions
HKL collected and analyzed the data, wrote the manuscript, and gave final approval of the manuscript to publish. MKK designed and made a concept of the study, acquired and analyzed the data, wrote the manuscript, and gave final approval of the manuscript to publish. Both authors read and approved the final manuscript.

Competing interests

The authors declare that they have no competing interests.

References

1. Fontes BM, Fontes BM, Castro E. Intraocular lens power calculation by measuring axial length with partial optical coherence and ultrasonic biometry. Arq Bras Oftalmol. 2011;74(3):166–70.
2. Whang WJ, Jung BJ, Oh TH, Byun YS, Joo CK. Comparison of postoperative refractive outcomes: IOLMaster(R) versus immersion ultrasound. Ophthalmic Surg Lasers Imaging. 2012;43(6):496–9.
3. Bhatt AB, Schefler AC, Feuer WJ, Yoo SH, Murray TG. Comparison of predictions made by the intraocular lens master and ultrasound biometry. Arch Ophthalmol. 2008;126(7):929–33.
4. McAlinden C, Wang Q, Pesudovs K, Yang X, Bao F, Yu A, Lin S, Feng Y, Huang J. Axial length measurement failure rates with the IOLMaster and Lenstar LS 900 in eyes with cataract. PLoS One. 2015;10(6):e0128929.
5. Srivannaboon S, Chirapapaisan C, Chonpimai P, Loket S. Clinical comparison of a new swept-source optical coherence tomography-based optical biometer and a time-domain optical coherence tomography-based optical biometer. J Cataract Refract Surg. 2015;41(10):2224–32.
6. Kunert KS, Peter M, Blum M, Haigis W, Sekundo W, Schutze J, Buehren T. Repeatability and agreement in optical biometry of a new swept-source optical coherence tomography-based biometer versus partial coherence interferometry and optical low-coherence reflectometry. J Cataract Refract Surg. 2016;42(1):76–83.
7. Akman A, Asena L, Gungor SG. Evaluation and comparison of the new swept source OCT-based IOLMaster 700 with the IOLMaster 500. Br J Ophthalmol. 2016;100(9):1201–5.
8. Yoo TK, Choi MJ, Lee HK, Seo KY, Kim EK, Kim T-i. Comparison of ocular biometry and refractive outcomes using IOL master 700, IOL master 500, and ultrasound. J Korean Ophthalmol Soc. 2017;58(5):523–9.
9. Olsen T. Theoretical approach to intraocular lens calculation using Gaussian optics. J Cataract Refract Surg. 1987;13(2):141–5.
10. Norrby S. Sources of error in intraocular lens power calculation. J Cataract Refract Surg. 2008;34(3):368–76.
11. Hoffer KJ, Hoffmann PC, Savini G. Comparison of a new optical biometer using swept-source optical coherence tomography and a biometer using optical low-coherence reflectometry. J Cataract Refract Surg. 2016;42(8):1165–72.
12. Karunaratne N. Comparison of the Pentacam equivalent keratometry reading and IOL master keratometry measurement in intraocular lens power calculations. Clin Exp Ophthalmol. 2013;41(9):825–34.
13. Arriola-Villalobos P, Almendral-Gomez J, Garzon N, Ruiz-Medrano J, Fernandez-Perez C, Martinez-de-la-Casa JM, Diaz-Valle D. Agreement and clinical comparison between a new swept-source optical coherence tomography-based optical biometer and an optical low-coherence reflectometry biometer. Eye (Lon). 2016.
14. Vogel A, Dick HB, Krummenauer F. Reproducibility of optical biometry using partial coherence interferometry : intraobserver and interobserver reliability. J Cataract Refract Surg. 2001;27(12):1961–8.
15. Matsuo Y, Sakamoto T, Yamashita T, Tomita M, Shirasawa M, Terasaki H. Comparisons of choroidal thickness of normal eyes obtained by two different spectral-domain OCT instruments and one swept-source OCT instrument. Invest Ophthalmol Vis Sci. 2013;54(12):7630–6.
16. Sheard R. Optimising biometry for best outcomes in cataract surgery. Eye (Lond). 2014;28(2):118–25.
17. Holladay JT, Prager TC, Chandler TY, Musgrove KH, Lewis JW, Ruiz RS. A three-part system for refining intraocular lens power calculations. J Cataract Refract Surg. 1988;14(1):17–24.

32

Clinical features and outcome of corneal opacity associated with congenital glaucoma

Yu Jeong Kim[1,2], Jin Wook Jeoung[3], Mee Kum Kim[1,3], Ki Ho Park[3], Young Suk Yu[3] and Joo Youn Oh[1,3*]

Abstract

Background: To investigate the clinical features of corneal opacity and the surgical outcome of penetrating keratoplasty (PK) in eyes with congenital glaucoma.

Methods: A retrospective review was made of the records from 320 eyes of 193 patients who were diagnosed with congenital glaucoma between January 1981 and January 2016. Anterior segment photographs at disease presentation were examined for the presence and severity of corneal opacity. Data on patient demographics, intraocular pressure (IOP), ocular and systemic comorbidities, ocular surgery and its outcome were collected.

Results: Overall, corneal opacification was observed in 248 of 320 eyes (77.5%). Out of 248 eyes with corneal opacification, 53 eyes had Haab striae alone, and 195 eyes presented with either nebulomacular corneal opacity (128 eyes, iris details visible through opacity) or leukomatous corneal opacity (67 eyes, iris details invisible through opacity). In 12 eyes with severe leukomatous corneal opacity, PK was performed at the mean age of 18.6 months (range 4–57 months). The grafts failed in 6 eyes (50%) due to endothelial rejection (4 eyes) or graft infection (2 eyes) during the mean 80.6 months of follow-up (range 15–228 months). The median survival time was 36 months. The graft failure was significantly associated with smaller corneal diameter at the time of surgery, but not with the age, IOP, combined aniridia, simultaneous glaucoma or lens surgery.

Conclusion: Congenital glaucoma was combined with corneal opacity in 77.5%. The corneal transplant survival was 50% in eyes with congenital glaucoma and total corneal opacity.

Keywords: Congenital glaucoma, Corneal opacity, Penetrating keratoplasty

Background

Congenital glaucoma (CG) is a rare disease with the incidence largely varying upon the ethnicity [1–3]. Studies reported that the annual incidence of CG was 2.85 to 5.41 in 100,000 live births in Caucasian populations [3, 4], whereas it was higher in South Asian children [3]. Despite its rarity, CG is often associated with poor visual and functional outcome [5, 6], and it is estimated that glaucoma is responsible for 4–18% of childhood blindness [3, 6–8]. Hence, early detection of the disease and

proper treatment are necessary for the vision in pediatric patients with CG.

The classical triad of symptoms in congenital glaucoma includes epiphora, photophobia, and blepharospasm [1]. However, the most common signs first recognized by parents or doctors are corneal abnormalities such as corneal enlargement (buphthalmos) due to increased intraocular pressure (IOP) or corneal clouding as a result of Descemet's membrane tears (Haab striae) or stromal edema [9–13]. In addition, as it is one form of developmental anomaly of anterior segment, CG is often combined with corneal opacity as a sequel to anterior segment dysgenesis. In these cases, corneal opacity can lead to sensory deprivation amblyopia, and the visual outcome can be poor despite optimal control of IOP. One study reported that corneal opacity along with

* Correspondence: bonzoo1@snu.ac.kr; jooyounoh77@gmail.com
[1]Laboratory of Ocular Regenerative Medicine and Immunology, Seoul Artificial Eye Center, Seoul National University Hospital Biomedical Research Institute, Seoul, Korea
[3]Department of Ophthalmology, Seoul National University Hospital, 101 Daehak-ro, Jongno-gu, Seoul 110-744, Korea
Full list of author information is available at the end of the article

anisometropia was responsible for vision loss in 50% of childhood glaucoma patients [14]. Therefore, evaluation for corneal opacity and its management are critical for early diagnosis of the disease and the favorable outcome in patients with CG.

We performed this study to evaluate the incidence and clinical characteristics of corneal opacity combined with CG and to investigate the surgical outcome of penetrating keratoplasty (PK) and clinical factors affecting the outcome in eyes with CG.

Methods

This retrospective study was approved by the Institutional Review Board (IRB No. 1706–094-860). Medical records were reviewed for 320 eyes of 193 Korean patients who were diagnosed with CG between January 1981 and January 2016.

The diagnosis of CG was taken as recorded in the charts. The diagnosis was usually made on the basis of two or more of the following ocular findings: elevated IOP (> 21 mmHg), buphthalmos (enlarged corneal diameter, Fig. 1a), Haab striae, corneal stromal edema, and glaucomatous optic disc change which had been present at birth or shortly after birth. Glaucoma of childhood or juvenile onset was excluded.

Data collected were the patient demographics, laterality of disease, IOP, corneal diameter, ocular comorbidities (aniridia, Peters anomaly, cataract, posterior segment anomalies), systemic abnormalities (Sturge-Weber syndrome, neurofibromatosis, congenital heart disease, TORCH positivity, cerebral palsy, Wilms tumor, chromosomal anomaly), ocular surgery (PK, glaucoma surgery, lens extraction), and last-recorded visual acuity.

In addition, anterior segment photographs at first presentation of a patient were reviewed for the presence of corneal opacity, and the corneal findings were classified as follows: 1) completely clear cornea, 2) Haab striae

only (Fig. 1b, c), and 3) corneal opacity. The severity of corneal opacity was further graded based on both four-stage system and two-scale system. The four-stage system followed the corneal opacity scoring system suggested by Gupta et al. [15, 16] with modification: stage 1 = minimal opacity (Fig. 1d), stage 2 = moderate stromal opacity (anterior chamber and iris both well visualized, Fig. 1e), stage 3 = significant stromal opacity (pupil visible with haze, Fig. 1f), and stage 4 = intense stromal opacity (pupil invisible, Fig. 1g). The two-scale system was composed of nebulomacular corneal opacity (iris details visible through opacity) and leukomatous corneal opacity (unable to visualize iris details through opacity). Overall, nebulomacular corneal opacity included stage 1 and 2 opacities, and leukomatous corneal opacity comprised stage 3 and 4 opacities.

The data were additionally analyzed in 12 eyes of 10 CG patients with stage 4 corneal opacity who underwent PK. The graft failure was determined when corneal clarity was irreversibly lost under slit-lamp examination, and the graft survival time was defined as the period from PK to the day when the graft failure was first noted. When multiple PKs were performed in a patient, the first surgery was taken for analysis. The association of age, IOP at the time of surgery, corneal diameter, donor/recipient trephine sizes, difference of sizes between donor and recipient trephines, presence of ocular comorbidities, and concurrent lens or glaucoma surgeries with corneal graft outcome was evaluated.

Data were presented as mean ± SD. The GraphPad Software (GraphPad Prism, La Jolla, CA) was used for statistical analysis. Comparison of quantitative variables between two groups was made by using Student t test. The correlation between IOP and the severity of corneal opacity was tested by using Pearson r coefficient and two-tailed P value. Survival analysis was performed using the Kaplan–Meier method to estimate the median time

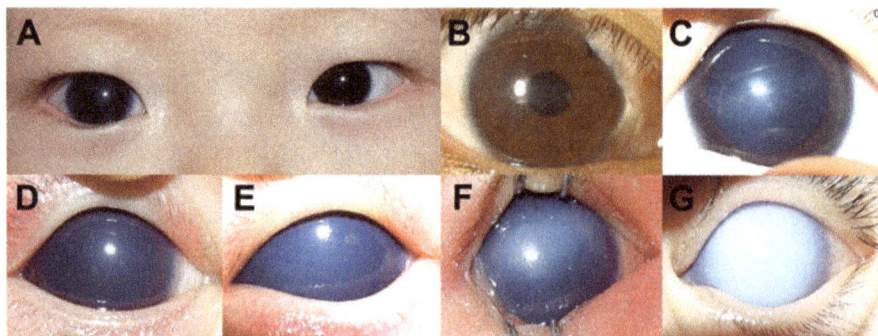

Fig. 1 Representative photographs of corneal abnormalities associated with congenital glaucoma. **a** Enlarged cornea (buphthalmos) in the right eye with congenital glaucoma. **b, c** Horizontal lines of Haab striae are present in the cornea. **d** Grade 1 corneal opacity. Minimal and superficial opacity is observed. **e** Grade 2 corneal stromal opacity. Both anterior chamber and iris are well-visible despite the opacity. **f** Grade 3 corneal stromal opacity. The pupil is still visible but iris details difficult to see through the opacity. **g** Grade 4 corneal stromal opacity. Pupil is invisible due to total stromal opacity of the cornea

to graft failure. The association with the surgical outcome and each clinical factor was analyzed using Fisher's exact test for qualitative variables and two-tailed Student t test for quantitative variables. A P value < 0.05 was considered statistically significant.

Results

Demographical, ocular and systemic features of CG patients

The demographical, ocular and systemic findings of patients are summarized in Table 1. Of a total 320 eyes in 193 Korean patients with CG, 116 patients (60.1%) were male and 77 (39.9%) were female. The disease was bilateral in 127 patients (65.8%) and unilateral in 66 patients (34.2%) (Right: Left = 26: 40).

The IOP at first presentation was 28.3 ± 9.3 mmHg (range 9.0–54.7 mmHg) in eyes with CG and $12.9 \pm$

2.9 mmHg (range 6.0–29.0 mmHg) in eyes without CG ($P < 0.0001$). The horizontal corneal diameter was 12.5 ± 1.2 mm (range 7.0–16.5 mm) at presentation in eyes with CG, which was significantly larger than that of the eye without CG (10.9 ± 0.9 mm, range 9.0–11.5 mm) in the same population ($P < 0.0001$). Thirty-six patients (18.7%) had systemic diseases. Sturge-Weber syndrome was the most common anomaly combined with CG ($n = 25$, 12.9%). Other systemic comorbidities included congenital heart disease ($n = 4$, 2.1%), neurofibromatosis (n = 2, 1.0%), TORCH positivity (n = 2, 1.0%), cerebral palsy ($n = 1$, 0.5%), Wilms tumor (n = 1, 0.5%), and chromosomal anomaly (n = 1, 0.5%).

Congenital ocular comorbidities were observed in 38 patients (19.7%) and included aniridia ($n = 14$, 7.3%), Peters anomaly ($n = 7$, 3.6%), congenital cataract (n = 4, 2.1%), and posterior segment anomaly ($n = 13$, 6.7%).

Table 1 Demographics and clinical feature of patients with congenital glaucoma (193 patients, 320 eyes)

Clinical characteristics		No of patients	%
Gender			
Female		77	39.9
Male		116	60.1
Laterality			
Bilateral		127	65.8
Unilateral	Rt	26	13.5
	Lt	40	20.7
IOP of involved eyes at presentation (mmHg)			
Involved eyes (range)		28.3 ± 9.3 (9.0–54.7)	
Uninvolved eyes (range)		12.9 ± 2.9 (6.0–29.0)	
P value		< 0.0001	
Corneal diameter (Horizontal, mm)			
Involved eyes (range)		12.5 ± 1.2 (7.0–16.5)	
Uninvolved eyes (range))		10.9 ± 0.9 (9.0–11.5)	
P value		< 0.0001	
Systemic comorbidity		36	18.7
Sturge-Weber syndrome		25	12.9
Congenital heart disease		4	2.1
Neurofibromatosis		2	1.0
TORCH		2	1.0
Cerebral palsy		1	0.5
Wilms tumor		1	0.5
Chromosomal abnormality		1	0.5
Ocular comorbidity		38	19.7
Aniridia		14	7.3
Peters anomaly		7	3.6
Cataract		4	2.1
Posterior segment anomaly		13	6.7

Corneal opacification combined with CG

Overall, corneal opacification was observed in 248 of 320 eyes with CG (77.5%), while the cornea was completely clear in 72 eyes (22.5%) (Table 2). Among 248 eyes with corneal opacification, 53 (16.6%) had only Haab striae in the cornea (Fig. 1b, c), and 195 (60.9%) had corneal opacity in the presence or absence of Haab striae (Table 2). The severity of corneal opacity in 195 CG eyes combined with corneal opacity was as follows: grade 1 in 68 eyes (21.2%, Fig. 1d), grade 2 in 60 eyes (18.8%, Fig. 1e), grade 3 in 31 eyes (9.7%, Fig. 1f), and grade 4 in 36 eyes (11.2%, Fig. 1g). When classified based on the two-scale system, nebulomacular corneal opacity was observed in 128 eyes (40%), and leukomatous corneal opacity in 67 eyes (20.9%) (Table 2). There was no significant correlation between the severity of corneal opacity and IOP ($R = 0.012$, $P = 0.887$).

Table 2 Keratopathy combined with congenital glaucoma (320 eyes)

Corneal findings			No of eyes (%)	IOP (mmHg, range)
Completely clear cornea			72 (22.5)	24.0 ± 7.8 (11.0–42.1)
Haab striae only			53 (16.6)	24.3 ± 9.7 (11.0–46.0)
Corneal opacification ± Haab striae			195 (60.9)	28.3 ± 9.9 (9.0–54.7)
Nebulomacular opacity	Grade 1	68 (21.2)		27.1 ± 10.6 (9.0–50.0)
	Grade 2	60 (18.8)		28.5 ± 10.3 (13.0–54.7)
Leukomatous opacity	Grade 3	31 (9.7)		30.5 ± 7.6 (17.0–43.0)
	Grade 4	36 (11.2)		28.6 ± 10.1 (9.0–47.0)

IOP Intraocular pressure

Surgical outcome of corneal transplantation in eyes with CG

We additionally analyzed the data of 12 eyes (10 patients) that underwent PK because of non-resolving grade 4 leukomatous corneal stromal opacity. Eight patients had PK in one eye, and 2 underwent PK in both eyes. The demographical, clinical and surgical data are shown in Table 3. The patients included 4 female and 6 male. CG was bilateral in 2 patients and unilateral in 8 patients (Right: Left = 2: 6). The age at time of PK was 18.6 ± 17.8 months (range 4 to 57 months). Aniridia was combined in 7 eyes (5 with total aniridia and 2 with partial aniridia), Peters anomaly in 5 eyes, cataract in 1 eye, and posterior segment abnormality (retinopathy of prematurity) in 1 eye.

The IOP at time of surgery was 35.5 ± 9.3 mmHg (range 20.0–47.8 mmHg), and all eyes were treated with multiple anti-glaucoma medications. The corneal diameters measured at the time of PK were 11.7 ± 1.8 mm (range 9.5–15.0 mm) horizontally and 10.7 ± 1.7 mm (range 9.0–14.0 mm) vertically. The sizes of trephines used for PK were 6.9 ± 0.8 mm (range 6.0–8.0 mm) for recipient beds and 7.5 ± 0.7 mm (range 6.5–8.5 mm) for donor buttons. In 4 eyes, glaucoma valve implantation surgery was simultaneously performed with PK, and in 3 eyes, lens extraction was done in an open-sky manner during PK.

Over the mean 80.6 ± 77.8 months of follow-up (range 15–228 months), the corneal grafts failed in 6 eyes (50%) whereas they survived in 6 eyes (50%) (Fig. 2). The mean time to graft failure after PK was 7.3 ± 3.5 months (range 1–10 months) in patients with graft failure (Fig. 2), and the mean postoperative follow-up period in those with graft success was 38.2 ± 17.2 months (range 16–62 months). The median survival time of the grafts was 36 months. Out of 6 eyes with graft failure, 4 were caused by endothelial rejection, and 2 were due to graft infection. Among 6 eyes with graft failure, a repeat PK was performed in 4 eyes, 3 of which (66.7%) had the graft failure after regrafting (2 eyes with endothelial rejection and 1 with graft infection), an indication that the outcome of a repeat PK was worse than that of the first surgery. Overall, 4 out of 12 eyes with PK (33.3%) achieved ambulatory vision at the last follow-up as defined by the ability to fixate and follow targets or to count fingers at 3 ft or better [17].

Various clinical and surgical factors were analyzed for their association with corneal graft outcome. Of the factors examined, a smaller diameter of the cornea at the

Table 3 Demographics, clinical and surgical features of patients with penetrating keratoplasty (n = 10, 12 eyes)

Clinical or surgical parameters		
Gender (No of patients, %)		
Female		4 (40%)
Male		6 (60%)
Laterality (No of patients, %)		
Bilateral		2 (20%)
Unilateral	Rt	2 (20%)
	Lt	6 (60%)
Age at time of surgery (months, range)		18.6 ± 17.8 (4–57)
The postoperative follow-up (months, range)		80.6 ± 77.8 (15–228)
Systemic comorbidity (No of patients, %)		
Congenital heart disease		1 (10%)
Ocular comorbidity (No of eyes, %)		
Aniridia	Total	5 (41.7%)
	Partial	2 (16.7%)
Peters anomaly		5 (41.7%)
Cataract		1 (8.3%)
Retinopathy of prematurity		1 (8.3%)
IOP at time of surgery (mmHg, range)		35.5 ± 9.3 (20.0–47.8)
Corneal diameter (mm, range)		
Horizontal		11.7 ± 1.8 (9.5–15.0)
Vertical		10.7 ± 1.7 (9.0–14.0)
Trephine diameter (mm, range)		
Recipient		6.9 ± 0.8 (6.0–8.0)
Donor		7.5 ± 0.7 (6.5–8.5)
Concurrent surgery (No of eyes, %)		
Glaucoma surgery (valve surgery)		4 (33.3%)
Lens extraction		3 (25%)

IOP Intraocular pressure

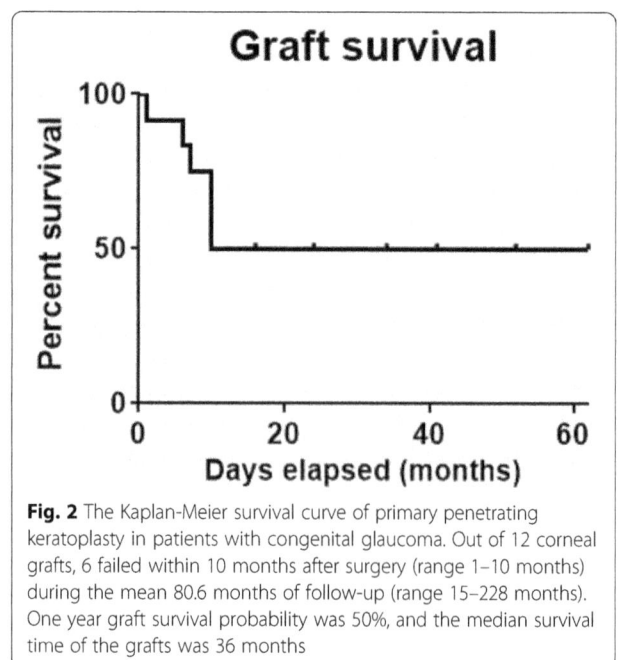

Fig. 2 The Kaplan-Meier survival curve of primary penetrating keratoplasty in patients with congenital glaucoma. Out of 12 corneal grafts, 6 failed within 10 months after surgery (range 1–10 months) during the mean 80.6 months of follow-up (range 15–228 months). One year graft survival probability was 50%, and the median survival time of the grafts was 36 months

time of surgery was significantly associated with the graft failure. The horizontal corneal diameters were 12.8 ± 1.7 mm in the survival group and 10.4 ± 0.9 mm in the failure group (P = 0.0126, Table 4). However, there were no significant associations between the graft survival and other factors such as the age, IOP, the presence of aniridia or Peters anomaly, the difference of sizes between donor and recipient trephines, and simultaneous glaucoma or lens surgery (Table 4).

Discussion

Corneal findings are important for suspicion and diagnosis of CG. Studies reported that cloudy cornea and buphthalmos are the most common presenting signs found in over 40% of patients with CG [11, 12]. In our study, 248 of 320 eyes (77.5%) with CG had corneal opacification at disease presentation, whereas 22.5% had completely clear cornea. However, among 77.5% of CG eyes with corneal opacity, 16.6% presented with Haab striae alone and 21.2% had grade 1 minimal opacity. Therefore, visually significant and recognizable corneal opacity (grade 2, 3 or 4 opacity) was observed in 39.7% of the eyes with CG, which is similar to previous reports [11] [12].

Other notable findings of our study are that male was more prevalent than female in CG patients at a ratio of 60.1 to 39.9, and bilateral involvement was more common compared to unilateral involvement at a ratio of 65.8 to 34.2. Overall, 18.7% of CG patients had

Table 4 Comparison of clinical and surgical factors between the graft survival and failure groups

	Graft survival	Graft failure	P value
Aniridia (No. of eyes)			
O	5	2	0.2424
X	1	4	
Peters anomaly (No. of eyes)			
O	4	1	0.2424
X	2	5	
Concurrrent glaucoma surgery (No. of eyes)			
O	1	3	0.5455
X	5	3	
Concurrrent lens extraction (No. of eyes)			1
O	1	2	
X	5	4	
Corneal diameter (horizontal, mm)	12.8 ± 1.7	10.4 ± 0.9	0.0126
Corneal diameter (vertical, mm)	11.7 ± 1.9	9.6 ± 0.9	0.0354
Age at time of surgery (months)	21.7 ± 15.8	15.5 ± 20.7	0.5739
IOP at time of surgery (mmHg)	36.1 ± 12.5	34.9 ± 5.8	0.8373
Trephine gapping[a] (mm)	0.54 ± 0.3	0.46 ± 0.4	0.8312

aTrephine gapping means the size difference between donor and recipient trephines

combined systemic diseases, and the most common systemic comorbidity was Sturge-Weber syndrome which was found in 12.9% of patients with CG. However, Sturge-Weber syndrome was not associated with severe corneal opacity since no patient with Sturge-Weber syndrome underwent PK because of corneal opacity. Neurofibromatosis was combined in two patients (1.0%) in our study. Quaranta et al. [18] reported that neurofibromatosis patients showed gonioscopic findings characteristic of underdevelopment of the iridocorneal angle, suggesting the vulnerability to glaucoma. Of ocular morbidities combined with CG, aniridia was the most frequent (found in 7.3% of CG patients), followed by Peters anomaly (found in 3.6% of CG patients). Combined aniridia and Peters anomaly predisposed patients with CG to severe non-resolving corneal opacity which required PK. Seven out of 14 patients with CG + aniridia and 5 of 7 patients with CG + Peters anomaly underwent PK.

It is generally accepted that the presence of glaucoma and concurrent glaucoma operation during PK are risk factors for poor graft survival in a pediatric population [19, 20]. However, there have just a few case series evaluating the surgical outcome of PK in CG patients, and the results greatly vary upon studies. In our study, the overall graft survival rate was 50% (6 of 12) in eyes with CG during a mean follow-up of 80.6 months, and 33.3% of patients with PK achieved ambulatory vision at the last follow-up. Of note, in the graft failure group, all grafts failed within 10 months (at the mean 7.3 months) after PK. Ariyasu et al. [21] reported that the graft success occurred in 67% of grafts (6 of 9) in eyes with CG during 24 months of follow-up, and ambulatory vision was achieved in 75% of eyes. In a report by Al-Torbak [22], 43 and 17% of corneal grafts survived at 24 and 48 months, respectively after combined PK and Ahmed valve implantation. In our patients, PK was combined with glaucoma valve implantation in 4 eyes, 3 of which had graft failure. By contrast, 3 of 8 eyes without glaucoma surgery had graft failure. This suggests that concurrent glaucoma valve implant surgery might be associated with poor graft outcome, although it did not reach statistical significance due to the small sample size of the current study. Further study with larger sample size would be necessary to confirm the effect of simultaneous glaucoma surgery on the corneal transplant survival.

The only variable affecting the graft outcome was the corneal diameter in our study. The cornea was significantly smaller in the graft failure group, compared to the graft success group. This result is consistent with our previous findings in patients with Peters anomaly or sclerocornea [23]. The proximity of the donor graft to the recipient limbus and more exposure to the host immune system might be related to the high rate of graft failure in eyes with smaller corneas.

Our study is limited by its retrospective nature. Although we here presented the data on corneal opacity determined from the corneal photography in 320 eyes of 193 patients, it was not possible to evaluate other corneal abnormalities such as topographic changes, endothelial cell counts, or hysteresis. Since it was reported that corneal topographic abnormalities were commonly present in CG [13], further prospective study evaluating the cornea from multiple aspects would be helpful to better understand corneal anomalies associated with CG.

Conclusion

Corneal opacity was a common feature of CG and found in 77.5% of CG patients. The survival rate of corneal allografts in eyes with CG and severe stromal opacity was 50%, and the graft outcome was poorer in eyes with small corneal diameters.

Abbreviations

CG: Congenital glaucoma; IOP: Intraocular pressure; PK: Penetrating keratoplasty

Authors' contributions

YJK analyzed the data and wrote the manuscript. JYO design the study, analyzed the data, and wrote the manuscript. JWJ, KHP, MKK and YSY helped with acquisition of data. All authors read and approved the final manuscript.

Competing interests

The authors declare that they have no competing interests.

Author details

[1]Laboratory of Ocular Regenerative Medicine and Immunology, Seoul Artificial Eye Center, Seoul National University Hospital Biomedical Research Institute, Seoul, Korea. [2]Department of Ophthalmology, Hanyang University Hospital, Hanyang University College of Medicine, Seoul, Korea. [3]Department of Ophthalmology, Seoul National University Hospital, 101 Daehak-ro, Jongno-gu, Seoul 110-744, Korea.

References

1. Ho CL, Walton DS. Primary congenital glaucoma: 2004 update. J Pediatr Ophthalmol Strabismus. 2004;41(5):271–88. quiz 300-1
2. de Luise VP, Anderson DR. Primary infantile glaucoma (congenital glaucoma). Surv Ophthalmol. 1983;28(1):1–19.
3. Papadopoulos M, Cable N, Rahi J, Khaw PT. The British infantile and childhood Glaucoma (BIG) eye study. Invest Ophthalmol Vis Sci. 2007;48(9):4100–6.
4. Bermejo E, Martinez-Frias ML. Congenital eye malformations: clinical-epidemiological analysis of 1,124,654 consecutive births in Spain. Am J Med Genet. 1998;75(5):497–504.
5. Dahlmann-Noor A, Tailor V, Bunce C, Abou-Rayyah Y, Adams G, Brookes J, Khaw PT, Papadopoulos M. Quality of life and functional vision in children with Glaucoma. Ophthalmology. 2017;124(7):1048–55.
6. Taylor RH, Ainsworth JR, Evans AR, Levin AV. The epidemiology of pediatric glaucoma: the Toronto experience. J AAPOS. 1999;3(5):308–15.
7. Franks W, Taylor D. Congenital glaucoma--a preventable cause of blindness. Arch Dis Child. 1989;64(5):649–50.
8. Gilbert CE, Canovas R, Hagan M, Rao S, Foster A. Causes of childhood blindness: results from west Africa, south India and Chile. Eye (Lond). 1993; 7(Pt 1):184–8.
9. Tai TY, Mills MD, Beck AD, Joos KM, Ying GS, Liu C, Piltz-Seymour JR. Central corneal thickness and corneal diameter in patients with childhood glaucoma. J Glaucoma. 2006;15(6):524–8.
10. Thiagalingam S, Jakobiec FA, Chen T, Michaud N, Colby KA, Walton DS. Corneal anomalies in newborn primary congenital glaucoma. J Pediatr Ophthalmol Strabismus. 2009;46(4):241–4.
11. Tamcelik N, Atalay E, Bolukbasi S, Capar O, Ozkok A. Demographic features of subjects with congenital glaucoma. Indian J Ophthalmol. 2014;62(5):565–9.
12. Barsoum-Homsy M, Chevrette L. Incidence and prognosis of childhood glaucoma. A study of 63 cases. Ophthalmology. 1986;93(10):1323–7.
13. Patil B, Tandon R, Sharma N, Verma M, Upadhyay AD, Gupta V, Sihota R. Corneal changes in childhood glaucoma. Ophthalmology. 2015;122(1):87–92.
14. Robin AL, Quigley HA, Pollack IP, Maumenee AE, Maumenee IH. An analysis of visual acuity, visual fields, and disk cupping in childhood glaucoma. Am J Ophthalmol. 1979;88(5):847–58.
15. Gupta N, Kalaivani M, Tandon R. Comparison of prognostic value of roper hall and Dua classification systems in acute ocular burns. Br J Ophthalmol. 2011;95(2):194–8.
16. Choi H, Phillips C, Oh JY, Stock EM, Kim DK, Won JK, Fulcher S. Comprehensive modeling of corneal alkali injury in the rat eye. Curr Eye Res. 2017;42(10):1348–57.
17. Al-Ghamdi A, Al-Rajhi A, Wagoner MD. Primary pediatric keratoplasty: indications, graft survival, and visual outcome. J AAPOS. 2007;11(1):41–7.
18. Quaranta L, Semeraro F, Turano R, Gandolfo E. Gonioscopic findings in patients with type 1 neurofibromatosis (Von Recklinghausen disease). J Glaucoma. 2004r;13(2):90–5.
19. Huang C, O'Hara M, Mannis MJ. Primary pediatric keratoplasty: indications and outcomes. Cornea. 2009;28(9):1003–8.
20. Karadag R, Chan TC, Azari AA, Nagra PK, Hammersmith KM, Rapuano CJ. Survival of primary penetrating Keratoplasty in children. Am J Ophthalmol. 2016;171:95–100.
21. Ariyasu RG, Silverman J, Irvine JA. Penetrating keratoplasty in infants with congenital glaucoma. Cornea. 1994;13(6):521–6.
22. Al-Torbak AA. Outcome of combined Ahmed glaucoma valve implant and penetrating keratoplasty in refractory congenital glaucoma with corneal opacity. Cornea. 2004;23(6):554–9.
23. Kim YW, Choi HJ, Kim MK, Wee WR, Yu YS, Oh JY. Clinical outcome of penetrating keratoplasty in patients 5 years or younger: peters anomaly versus sclerocornea. Cornea. 2013;32(11):1432–6.

33

Fundus images analysis using deep features for detection of exudates, hemorrhages and microaneurysms

Parham Khojasteh, Behzad Aliahmad and Dinesh K. Kumar[*] ⓘ

Abstract

Background: Convolution neural networks have been considered for automatic analysis of fundus images to detect signs of diabetic retinopathy but suffer from low sensitivity.

Methods: This study has proposed an alternate method using probabilistic output from Convolution neural network to automatically and simultaneously detect exudates, hemorrhages and microaneurysms. The method was evaluated using two approaches: patch and image-based analysis of the fundus images on two public databases: DIARETDB1 and e-Ophtha. The novelty of the proposed method is that the images were analyzed using probability maps generated by score values of the softmax layer instead of the use of the binary output.

Results: The sensitivity of the proposed approach was 0.96, 0.84 and 0.85 for detection of exudates, hemorrhages and microaneurysms, respectively when considering patch-based analysis. The results show overall accuracy for DIARETDB1 was 97.3% and 86.6% for e-Ophtha. The error rate for image-based analysis was also significantly reduced when compared with other works.

Conclusion: The proposed method provides the framework for convolution neural network-based analysis of fundus images to identify exudates, hemorrhages, and microaneurysms. It obtained accuracy and sensitivity which were significantly better than the reported studies and makes it suitable for automatic diabetic retinopathy signs detection.

Keywords: Fundus image analysis, Diabetic retinopathy, Deep learning, Convolutional neural networks, Image processing

Background

Diabetic retinopathy (DR) is a leading cause of vision impairment and irreversible blindness in middle-aged and elderly people [1, 2] and is expected to rise to 191 million by 2030 [3–5]. Vision impairment due to DR can be significantly reduced if it is diagnosed in the early stages. It is diagnosed by visual examination of retinal images to detect three most common pathological signs i.e. (i) exudate (ii) hemorrhage and (iii) microaneurysm [6]. However, this is a manual time-consuming procedure and outcomes are subjective and dependent on expertise, thus, there is potential bias of the examiner. The diagnosis can be performed by analysis of color fundus images or fluorescein angiograms (FA) to identify pathological signs. Although FA enables better differentiation

between microaneurisms and micro hemorrhages, due to its invasive nature along with costs and the risk of allergic reactions, fundus images are the preferred modality. For automatic detection of pathological signs, most computer-based studies have developed algorithms for the automatic analysis of the fundus images with the aim to make the diagnosis more objective and easier to access by people in remote communities. However, this is very challenging because of variation in size, color, texture and shape of these signs (Fig. 1).

In computer-based methods, detection of exudate, hemorrhage and microaneurysm can either be done separately for each signs [7–23] or all signs simultaneously [24–31]. For exudate detection, Sánchez et al. [32] used a statistical mixture model-based clustering for dynamic thresholding to separate exudate from background. The algorithm obtained sensitivity of 90.2% and 96.8% for

* Correspondence: Dinesh@rmit.edu.au
Biosignal Lab, School of Engineering, RMIT University, Melbourne, Australia

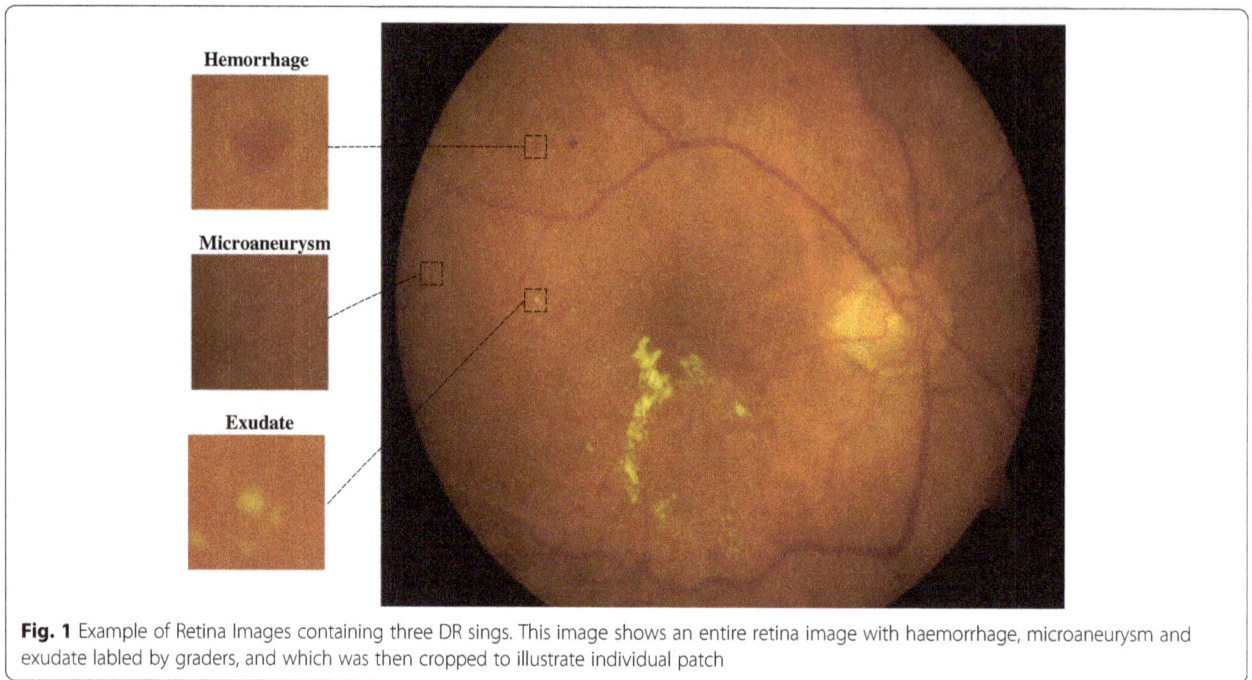

Fig. 1 Example of Retina Images containing three DR sings. This image shows an entire retina image with haemorrhage, microaneurysm and exudate labled by graders, and which was then cropped to illustrate individual patch

lesion and background, respectively. Giancardo et al. [7] proposed a method based on color and wavelet decomposition features from exudate candidates to train classifiers. They achieved the best result using support vector machine (SVM) classifier with areas under the receiver operating characteristics (AUC) between 0.88 and 0.94, depending on different datasets. In 2017, Fraz et al. [8] developed a method to detect exudate based on the multiscale segmentation. They used combination of morphological reconstructions and Gabor filter banks for feature extraction followed by bootstrap decision tree for classification of exudate pixels. In 2018, Kaur and Mittal [3] used a dynamic thresholding method for detection of exudate boundaries. The algorithm obtained sensitivity of 88.85% and 94.62% in lesion-based and image-based, respectively.

Hemorrhage detection was reported by Tang et al. [11] who divided the image into small sub-images (also called splats) for extracting splat features such as texture, splat area, and color. They evaluated their method based on patch and image level analysis and obtained AUC 0.96 and 0.87, respectively. For automatic detection of microaneurysm, Walter et al. [14] used morphological operations and kernel density estimation to extract a feature vector applied to a KNN, Gaussian and Bayesian risk-minimizing classifiers; their method achieved an accuracy of 88.5%.

In the past few years, deep learning approaches have been considered for this application and in 2016, Grinsven et al. [13] presented Convolutional Neural Network (CNN) architecture for detecting hemorrhage with nine layers trained by the selective misclassified negative samples. Their algorithm obtained AUC of 0.89 and 0.97 for two different datasets. In 2016, Shan and Li [15] used a patch-based analysis method to detect microaneurysm and applied a stacked sparse auto-encoder to distinguish between those two groups and they obtained 91.38% accuracy.

The success of diagnosis of DR requires the detection of all the three signs: exudate, hemorrhage and microaneurysm. While some of the studies reported earlier achieved acceptable performance for detection of single pathological sign, they were not suitable for identification of all the three signs simultaneously. Agurto et al. [26] used multiscale amplitude-modulation-frequency-modulation (AM-FM) method for extracting texture features from segmented retinal images to differentiate between groups with and without DR. To distinguish between these two groups, they computed distance metrics between the texture features. While they identified the segments with DR signs, the method did not discriminate between the three DR signs, which is essential for treatment planning. In 2017, Tan et al. [24] proposed a ten layers CNN architecture for DR sign detection. Their proposed network achieved a sensitivity of 0.87 for exudate detection, but this was only 0.62 and 0.46 for detection of hemorrhage and microaneurysm, respectively. Another limitation of this study was that they detected individual patches but did not consider the entire image which may explain the poor sensitivity due to misclassification of the background (with no pathological sign). Table 1 compares performance of the pervious methods for detection of exudate, hemorrhage and microaneurysm.

Table 1 Comparison between performance of the pervious methods for detection of exudate, hemorrhage and microaneurysm

Methodology	Exudate		Hemorrhage		Microaneurysm	
	sensitivity	specificity	sensitivity	specificity	sensitivity	specificity
Tan et al. [24]	0.87	0.98	0.62	0.98	0.46	0.97
Sinthanayothin et al. [29]	0.88	0.99	0.77	0.88	0.77	0.88
Grandet et al. [30]	0.94	–	0.89	–	–	–
Naqvi et al. [43]	0.92	0.81				
Walter et al. [23]	0.92	–	–	–	–	–
Fraz et al. [8]	0.92	0.81	–	–	–	–
Sopharak et al. [18]	0.82	0.99	–	–	–	–
Prentašić et al. [44]	0.78	–	–	–	–	–
Welfer et at. [17]	0.7	0.98	–	–	–	–
Niemeijer et al. [21]	–	–	0.31	–	0.31	–
Fleming et al. [20]	–	–	–	–	0.63	–
Walter et al. [14]	–	–	–	–	0.88	–
Garcia et al. [28]	–	–	0.86	–	0.86	–
Quellec et al. [19]	–	–	–	–	0.89	–
Bae et al. [16]	–	–	0.85	–	–	–
Walter et al. [14]	–	–	–	–	0.88	–

The patch-based analysis has been commonly used for CNN-based retinal image analysis [24, 33]. However, this approach can lead to disparity in the size of the sign due to patch size [24], and the inexact evaluation because of the focus on the pathological signs without considering the neighborhood and the background. While there are studies that have separated the background from the microaneurysm, and there are other studies that have accurately contoured the exudate, these perform analysis for one sign rather than all 3. Such an approach can lead to the detection with overlaps between the three signs. Another shortcoming is that while there are a number of isolated techniques that perform image enhancement, detect the presence of DR signs and perform processing to contour the signs, there is no framework that covers all the aspects.

In this study, the framework for a complete CNN-based system has been described for automatic and simultaneous detection and segmentation of exudate, hemorrhage and microaneurysm from fundus images. A ten-layered CNN architecture was designed and trained using images with annotated patches corresponding to the three signs and the background (No-sign) which was then used to obtain probability maps corresponding to each category (i.e. three sign and background). A post-processing algorithm was developed to differentiate pixels corresponding to a type of pathology from similar-looking cluttered pixels. Receiver Operating Characteristic (ROC) curve analysis was used to find a suitable threshold for differentiating between different types of pathologies This proposed framework was evaluated for both, patch and image-based analysis. Two publicly available databases were used, one was used for training while both were used for evaluation of the proposed method. The performance of the algorithm with and without probabilistic analysis was measured by taking the mean accuracy of ten repetitions.

Materials

In this study, two public databases were used: 1- DIARETDB1, 2- e-Ophtha with total of 284 fundus images. Seventy-five images from DIARETDB1 were used for patch-based analysis, while 209 images were used for image-based analysis.

DIARETDB1

DIARETDB1 database consists of 89 color retinal images with resolution 1500×1152 pixels [34]. Out of this database, 75 images were used for training the CNN while the remaining 14 images were used for testing and validating the performance of this method. In the training data, exudate, hemorrhage and microaneurysm were manually contoured by an experienced grader.

e-Ophtha

e-Ophtha is made up of two subsets: (i) "e-Ophtha EX" which contains 47 color retina images with annotated exudate, (ii) "e-Ophtha MA" which has 148 color retina images with annotated microaneurysm [35]. In this database, there is a variation in the size and resolution of the images, ranging from 1440×960 to 2544×1696 pixels. All images were resized to the size of the DIARETDB1 (1500×1152 pixels).

Methodology

The proposed framework consists of two main phases: 1) patch-based and 2) image-based analysis. The images were enhanced and then segmented in patches which were manually annotated and used to train the CNN. This trained CNN was used to analyze the other images for each pixel and a probability map was created using with which the locations of the pathological signs were identified. These images were processed to remove the isolated signs because these were noise and the spread of the signs which occurs during the earlier stages. The resultant images were compared with the manually annotated images to determine the accuracy of this method. An overview of the proposed method is shown in Fig. 2 and the steps are described below.

Preprocessing

Contrast enhancement (CE) technique was used in this study to enhance the contrast between three DR pathological signs and background. In this study, the first step was to process the images using image enhancement technique [13, 36] described in eq. (1).

$$I_{CE} = \alpha I(x,y) + \beta G(x,y;\sigma) * I(x,y) + \mu \quad (1)$$

where, $I(x,y)$ is the raw image, I_{CE} the enhanced image, $*$ represents the convolution operator, $G(x,y;\sigma)$ is a gaussian filter with the scale σ. The values of the α, β, σ and μ were chosen as 4, −4, 300/30 and 128, respectively based on the works by Van Grinsven [13]. This represents the subtraction of the Gaussian filtered image from the original image and highlights the contrast while μ gives a baseline shift of the gray scale. The result of image enhancement has been shown in Fig. 3 that revealing that some new lesions can be singularized by image enhancement, as specified by the yellow marks.

Convolutional neural network

The enhanced images were segmented into patches of size of S × S which were labeled based on the ground truth images corresponding to the three pathological signs: exudate, hemorrhage, microaneurysm and background (without any pathological sign). These patches were the input to the CNN which was trained against the target labels. The choice of CNN architecture and the parameters have been described in Fig. 4.

In the proposed CNN, four convolutional layers were designed with 16 feature maps in each convolutional layer by the kernel size of 3 × 3 pixels. To avoid saturation, the rectified linear unit (ReLU) was employed in this study. The size of feature maps was reduced using Max-Pooling (MP) layer with a kernel size of 2 × 2 and the values were normalized by the normalization layers (NL) after each MP layer for faster convergence. Sixteen

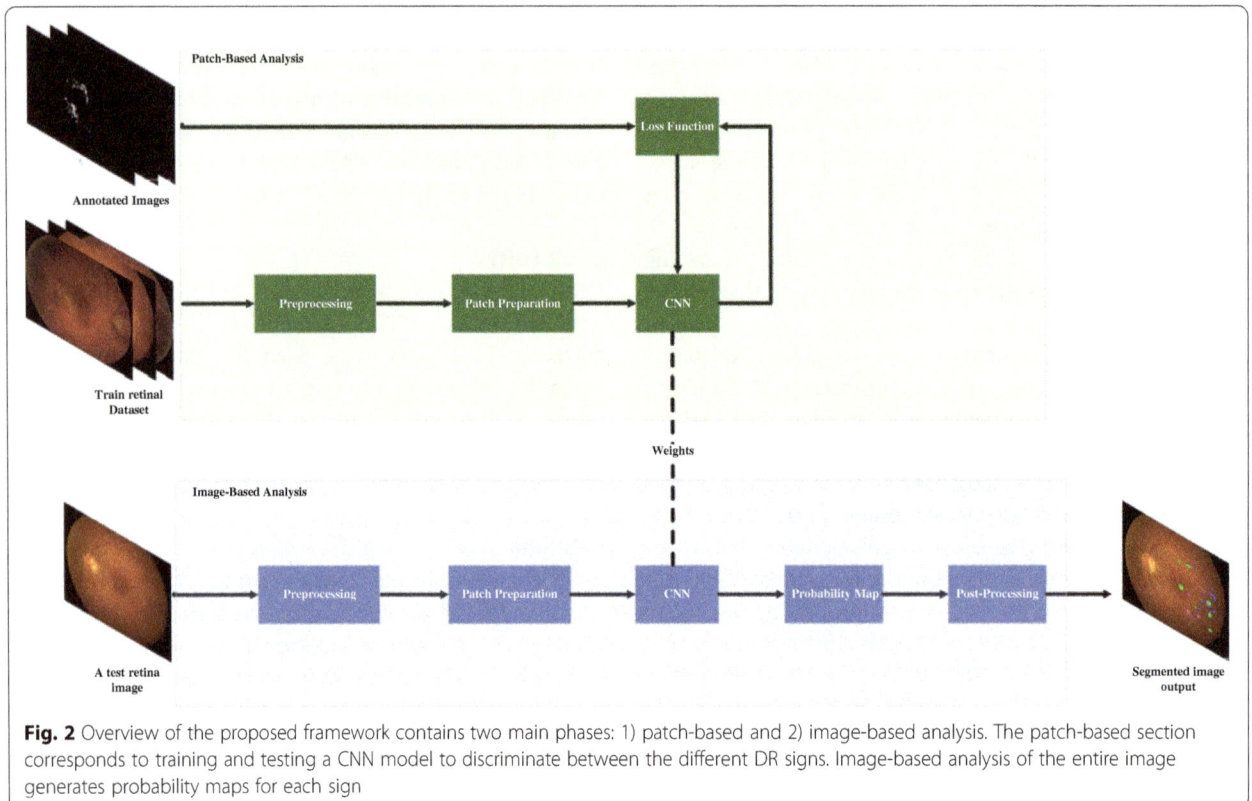

Fig. 2 Overview of the proposed framework contains two main phases: 1) patch-based and 2) image-based analysis. The patch-based section corresponds to training and testing a CNN model to discriminate between the different DR signs. Image-based analysis of the entire image generates probability maps for each sign

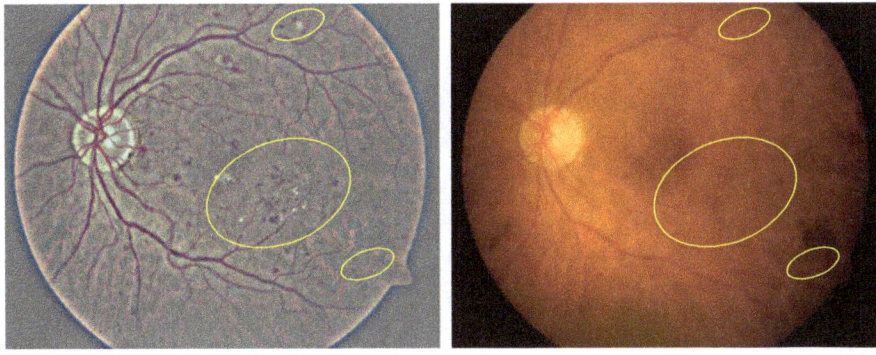

Fig. 3 Applying the image enhancement technique on an example retina image. (**a**) Original retina image; (**b**) After image enhancement. This shows that some new lesions can be singularized by image enhancement shown by yellow annotations)

features were extracted from the last MP layer and fed to a fully-connected (FC) layer with 256 neurons, the output of which was given to the final stage which had four neurons corresponding to the four target classes. To avoid overfitting, drop-out algorithm with a ratio of 0.5 was used in our net design. $\theta = \{W_i, b_i\}$ defined as network parameters, where w and b correspond to weight and bias in the C and FC layers. For the training process, the loss function of L_c was defined as follows:

$$L_c = -\frac{1}{|C|} \sum_{i=1}^{|C|} \ln\left(p\left(D^i | C^i\right)\right) \quad (2)$$

where $|C|$ represents the number of items in the training data, C^i and D^i denote the ith training sample and its label, respectively. To update θ parameters, stochastic gradient descent (SGD) method was used as in:

$$\theta(p+1) = \theta(p) - \gamma\frac{\partial L_c}{\partial \theta} + \vartheta\Delta\theta(p) - a\gamma\theta(p) \quad (3)$$

where γ, ϑ and a denote learning rate, momentum rate and weight delay rate, respectively.

Image analysis

In this study, pixel-based analysis of the image was performed by taking a patch of size S × S centered around pixel (x_i, y_i). This patch is the input to trained CNN which gives membership probabilities (range 0 to 1) at location (x_i, y_i) for the three pathological signs: i.e. exudate, hemorrhage and microaneurysm (shown by $P_{E,xi,yi}$,

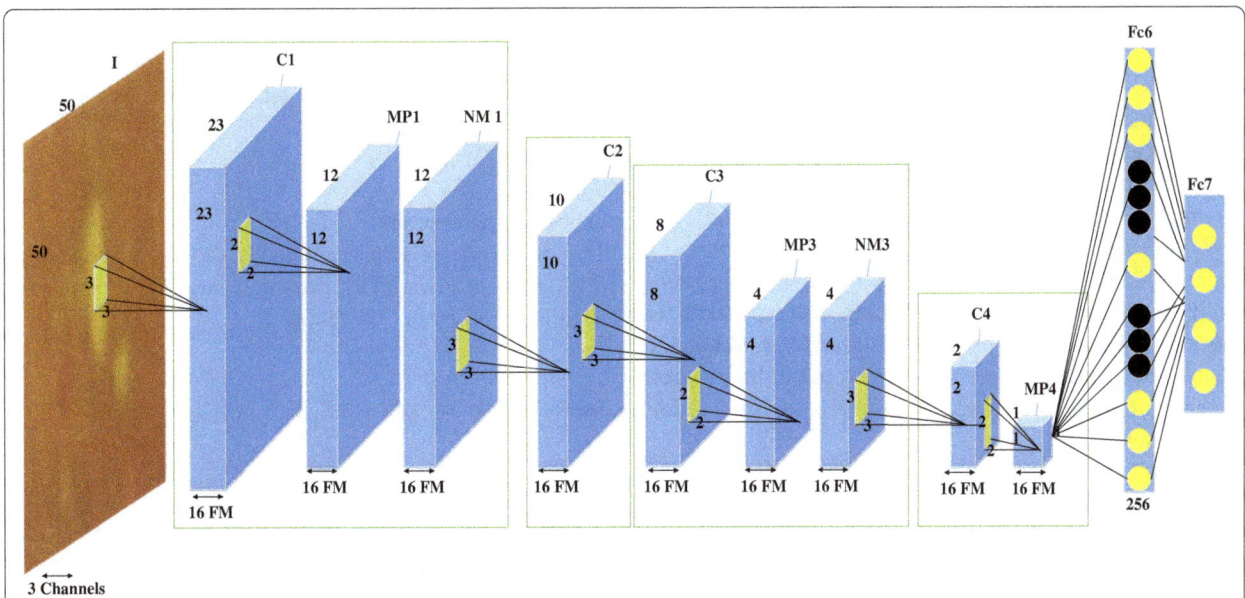

Fig. 4 Hierarchical architecture of the proposed CNN. I: input image, C: convolutional layer, FM: feature map, MP: max pooling, NM: Normalization layer, FC: fully-connected layer

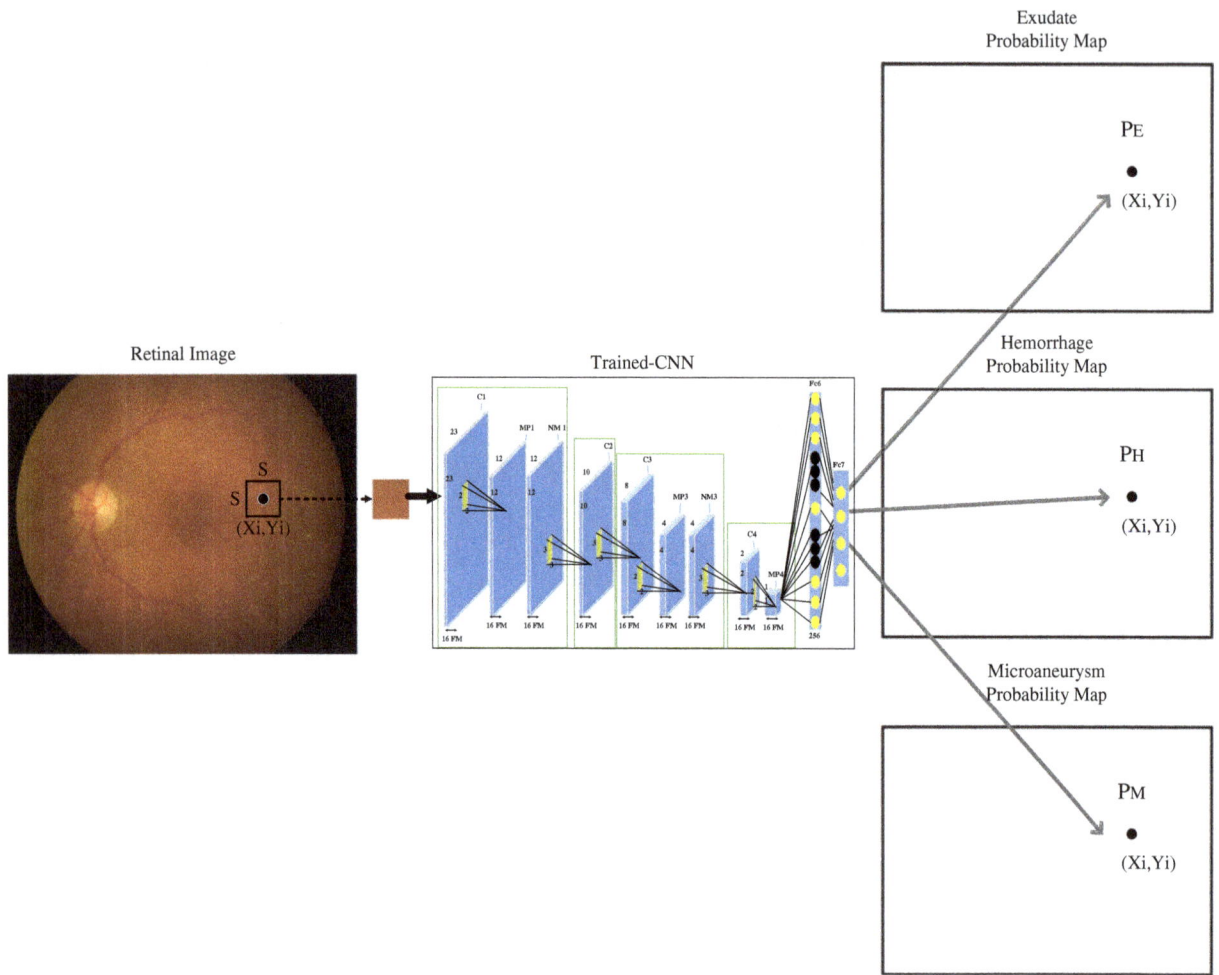

Fig. 5 Process of generating three probability maps corresponding to exudate, hemorrhage and microaneurysm from a retina image. By taking a patch of size S × S centered around pixel (x_i, y_i), each patch is fed to the trained CNN that determines the membership probabilities at location (x_i, y_i) for the three pathological signs: i.e. exudate, hemorrhage and microaneurysm (shown by $P_{E,xi,yi}$, $P_{H,xi,yi}$ and $P_{M,xi,yi}$)

$P_{H,xi,yi}$ and $P_{M,xi,yi}$). Consequently, three probability maps for the image are created and the scheme of this mapping process is shown in Fig. 5.

To identify the signs, a threshold was determined for each of the probability maps. This threshold (Th) was obtained by maximizing the receiver operating characteristics curve and used to binarize each probability map and obtain a binary map corresponding to the three signs. Overlaps were avoided by ranking the points with overlap based on the probability values. Details of this procedure are provided in section "Experiments".

One difficulty that is faced by such methods is the appearance of redundant boundaries and cluttered pixels (False positive pixels) around the segmented signs. To overcome this shortcoming, three morphological operations: closing, opening and erosion were performed with masks of size 5 × 5, 5 × 5 and 4 × 4 pixels, respectively [37, 38]. This was followed by a rule based

post-processing where signs with area of less than $\frac{S^2}{4}$ were removed.

Validation parameters

The performance was evaluated based on false positive (FP), true positive (TP), true negative (TN) and false negative (FN) rates [39] (Table 2).

Table 2 Validation parameters

Parameter	Equation
Accuracy	$\frac{TP+TN}{TP+TN+FP+FN}$
Error rate	$\frac{FP+FN}{TP+TN+FP+FN}$
Positive predict value (PPV)	$\frac{TP}{TP+FP}$
Sensitivity	$\frac{TP}{TP+FN}$
Specificity	$\frac{TN}{TN+FP}$

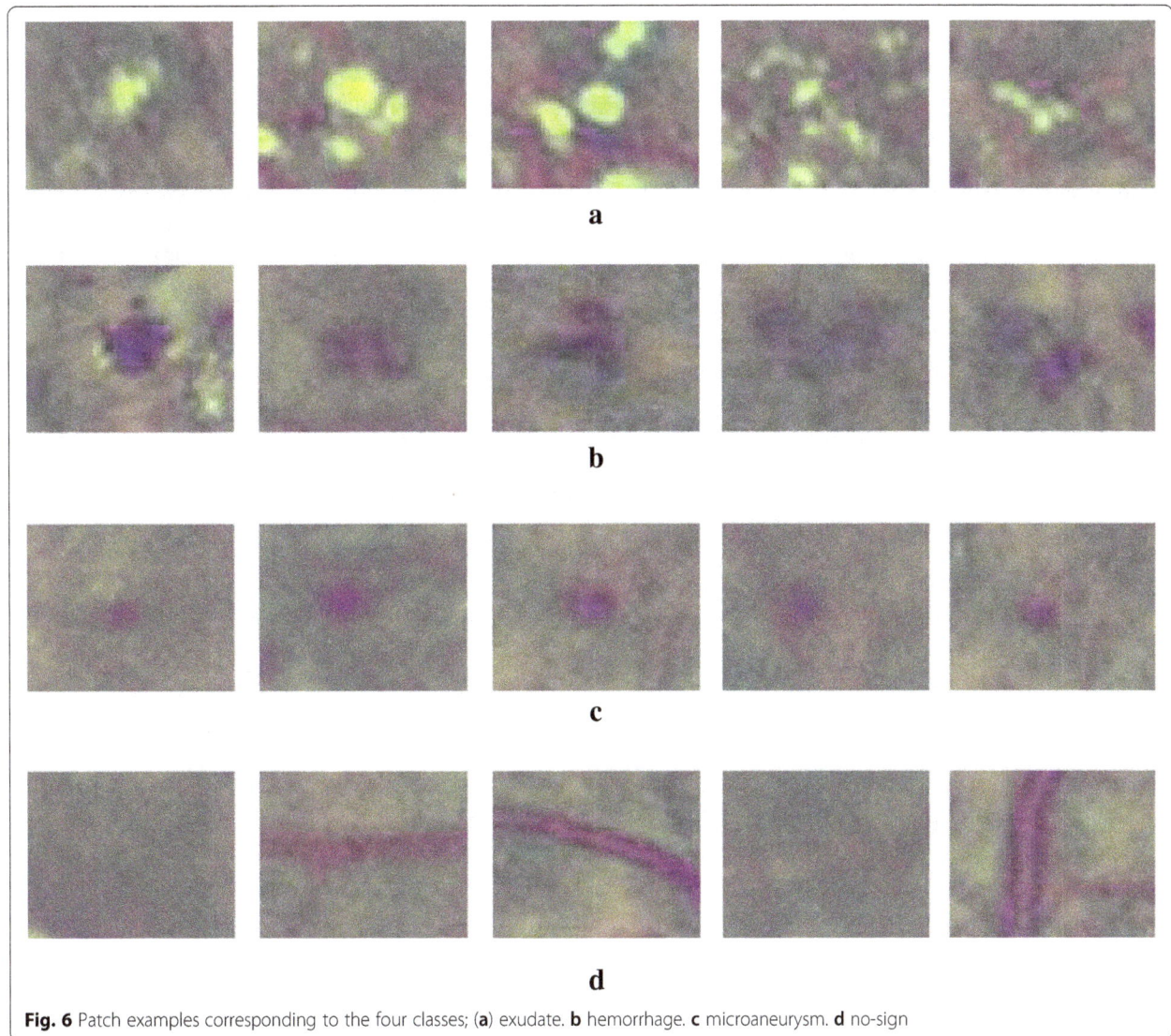

Fig. 6 Patch examples corresponding to the four classes; (**a**) exudate. **b** hemorrhage. **c** microaneurysm. **d** no-sign

Experiments

Data preparation

The image was segmented into patches by the size of $S \times S$, with $S = 50$, which was determined based on the smallest pathological signs in these images. Patches corresponding to the signs were manually extracted from 75 retina images of the DIARETDB1 database and used for the training the network. These resulted in 22,719, 18,882 and 17,824 patches for exudate, hemorrhage and microaneurysm and 50,518 patches with no pathological

Table 3 Statistics information of sign patches

	Exudate	Haemorrhage	Microaneurysm	No-Sign
Training	15,646	13,339	12,477	35,013
Validation	3353	2859	2674	7503
Test	3720	2684	2333	8002
Total Number	22,719	18,882	17,484	50,518

Table 4 CNN setup details

CNN parameters	Optimal value
Learning Rate	0.01
Momentum	0.9
Gaussian Weight Filters	0.01
Training Batch size	128
Validation and Test Batch size	32
Solver Method	SGD
Gamma	0.1
Policy of the SGD	Step-Down
Step size of SGD	33

signs (No-Sign). The No-Sign patches contained vessels, background tissue and optic nerve head. There was no overlap between each to adjacent patch. To increase the robustness of the algorithm, data augmentation was performed using both horizontal and vertical filliping and rotating [40, 41]. Figure 6 shows patch examples corresponding to four classes and Table 3 summarizes the number of patches considered for the training (75%), validation (15%) and testing (15%) CNN.

Network setup

For training the CNN, optimal parameters were heuristically set and shown in Table 4.

The maximum number of epochs was identified by repeating the training from 0 to 100 epochs and recording the accuracy and error using the validation set. It was observed that the accuracy saturated after 43th epoch to 90% and hence was selected as the maximum number of training epochs (Fig. 7). Using a GeForce GTX 1070 and Caffe platform [42] for the CNN implementation, the training process took 8 min and 23 s.

Image analysis

The test image set of DIARETDB1 and all images of e-Ophtha were used to evaluate the performance of the proposed method using image-based analysis. These images were analyzed (section "Materials") and the probability map was created of the all pixels in the image which resulted in three probability maps corresponding to exudate, hemorrhage and microaneurysm. Figure 8 shows an example with the three probability maps. Figure 9 shows the images after applying post-processing (in section "Image analysis"). It can be seen that the algorithm's outcome accurately segmented the actual pixel's signs from the all pixels which were assigned as potential pixels for the signs with different probability.

Results

For the patch-based evaluation, the mean results of ten repetitions for the training are described in Table 5 and Fig. 10 shows the ROC curve for the CNN performance.

Table 5 shows the sensitivity, specificity and accuracy for the proposed method. The best results were for the exudates with sensitivity, specificity and accuracy of 0.96, 0.98 and 0.98, respectively, while that for

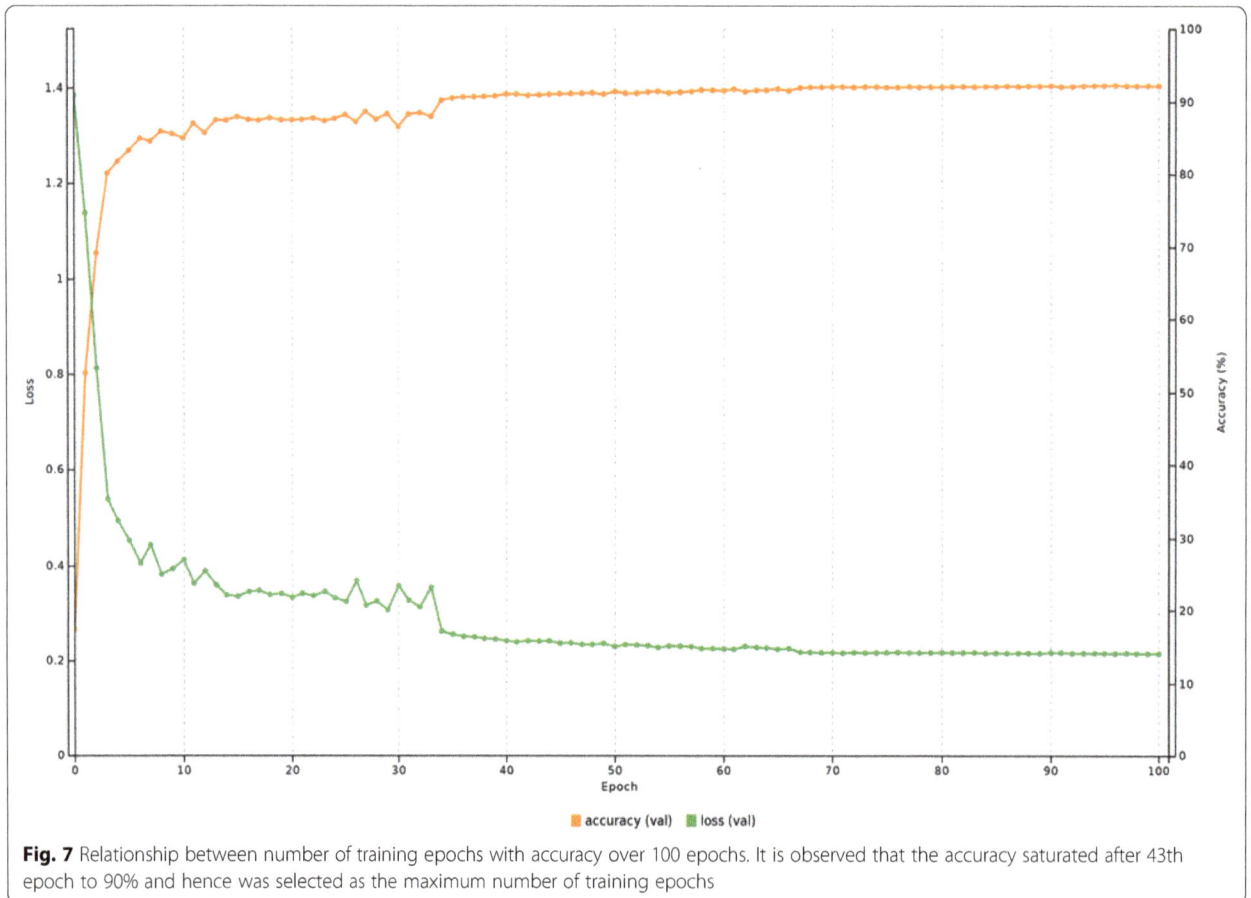

Fig. 7 Relationship between number of training epochs with accuracy over 100 epochs. It is observed that the accuracy saturated after 43th epoch to 90% and hence was selected as the maximum number of training epochs

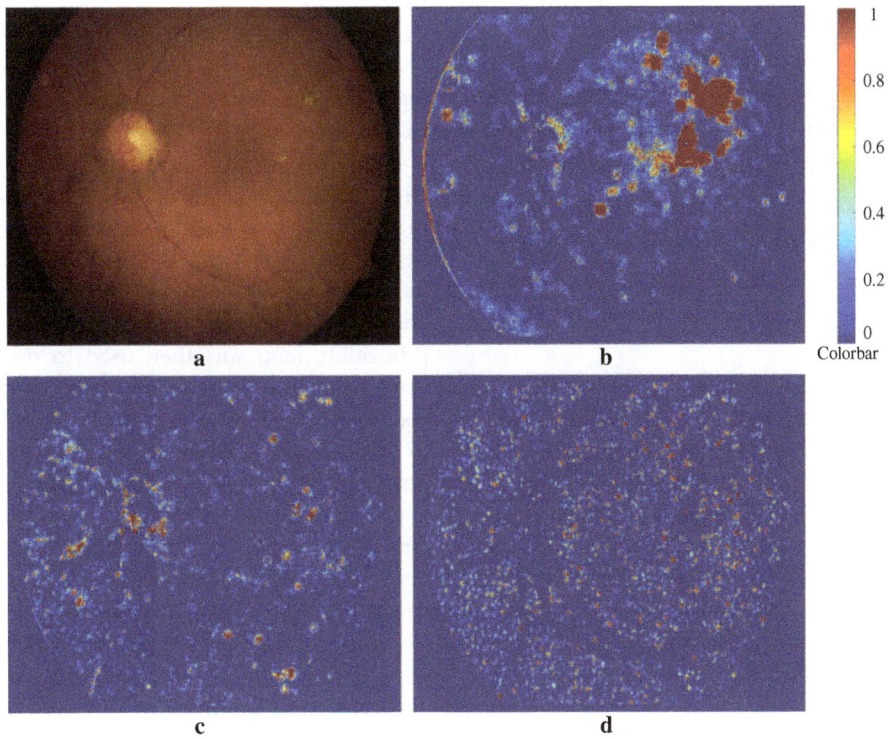

Fig. 8 Three probability maps were generated from an example retina image: (**a**) original retina image; (**b**) Exudate probability map; (**c**) Hemorrhage probability map; (**d**) Microaneurysm probability map. Colorbar shows the severity level of a pixel belong to the sign that is ranging between 0 to 1 corresponding to blue to red color

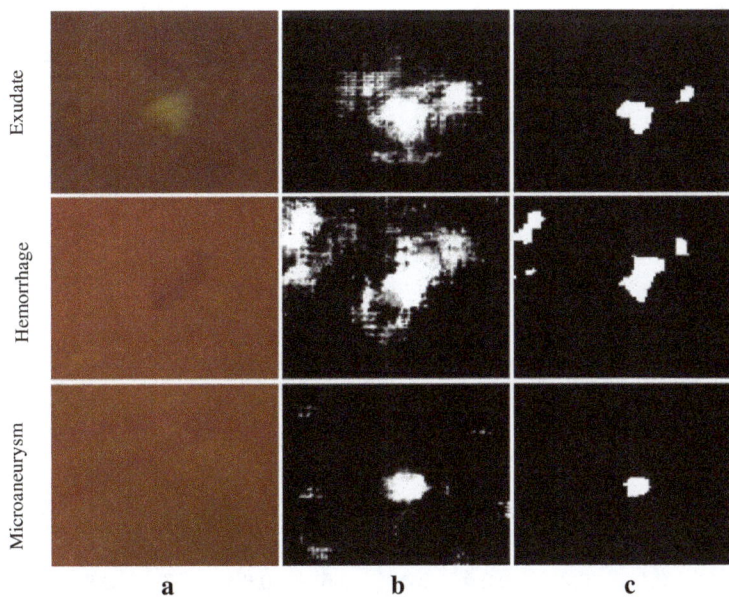

Fig. 9 Three examples of pathological signs before and after post-processing. **a** Original image. **b** Probability map corresponding to the sign. **c** Image output after post-processing

Table 5 Sensitivity, specificity, accuracy and PPV of the proposed method in patch-level evaluation for detection of exudate, hemorrhage and microaneurysm

	Exudate	Hemorrhage	Microaneurysm	No-Sign
Accuracy	0.98	0.90	0.94	0.96
Sensitivity	0.96	0.84	0.85	0.95
Specificity	0.98	0.92	0.96	0.97
PPV	0.94	0.85	0.83	0.96

hemorrhages was 0.84, 0.92 and 0.90, and 0.85, 0.96 and 0.94 for microaneurysm.

For image-level evaluation, performance of the proposed method was compared to the method which used the binary outputs of the network for both datasets and shown in Fig. 11. It is observed that for DIARETDB1, the proposed method achieved the accuracy of 0.96, 0.98 and 0.97 and error rate of 3.9%, 2.1% and 2.04% for segmentation of exudate, hemorrhage and microaneurysm, respectively which shows that this technique outperforms techniques reported in literature. Similarly, there was significant improvement for exudate and microaneurysm detection in the e-Ophtha dataset with accuracy of 0.88, and 3.0 and error rate of 4.2% and 3.1%, respectively. Figure 12 shows example of a retinal image with pathological signs detected by the proposed algorithm.

Discussion

This study has presented a CNN-based framework to analyze the retina fundus images for detection of pathologic signs indicative of DR: exudate, hemorrhage and microaneurysm. The images were first pre-processed to enhance the contrast and then segmented in patches which were then manually annotated and used for training the CNN network. This network was then used to determine the probability for each pixel to belong to the four classes of exudate, haemorrhage, microaneurysm, and background (no pathologic sign). The resultant probability map was then used to determine the locations of all the three types of pathological signs corresponding to DR. The isolated signs and the spread due to convolution were automatically removed in a post-processing step described earlier.

The results show that there was a difference in the accuracy, sensitivity and specificity when using the two databases: DIARETDB1 and e-Ophtha which could be because the CNN was trained using only DIARETDB1. Compared to previous works in which the two databases were used (Table 1), the performance of the proposed approach was higher. It also observed that average sensitivity and specificity for detecting exudates (0.96 and 0.98) is higher than for hemorrhage and microaneurysm. According to Table 1, most of the previous studies suffer from poor sensitivity, particularly for discrimination

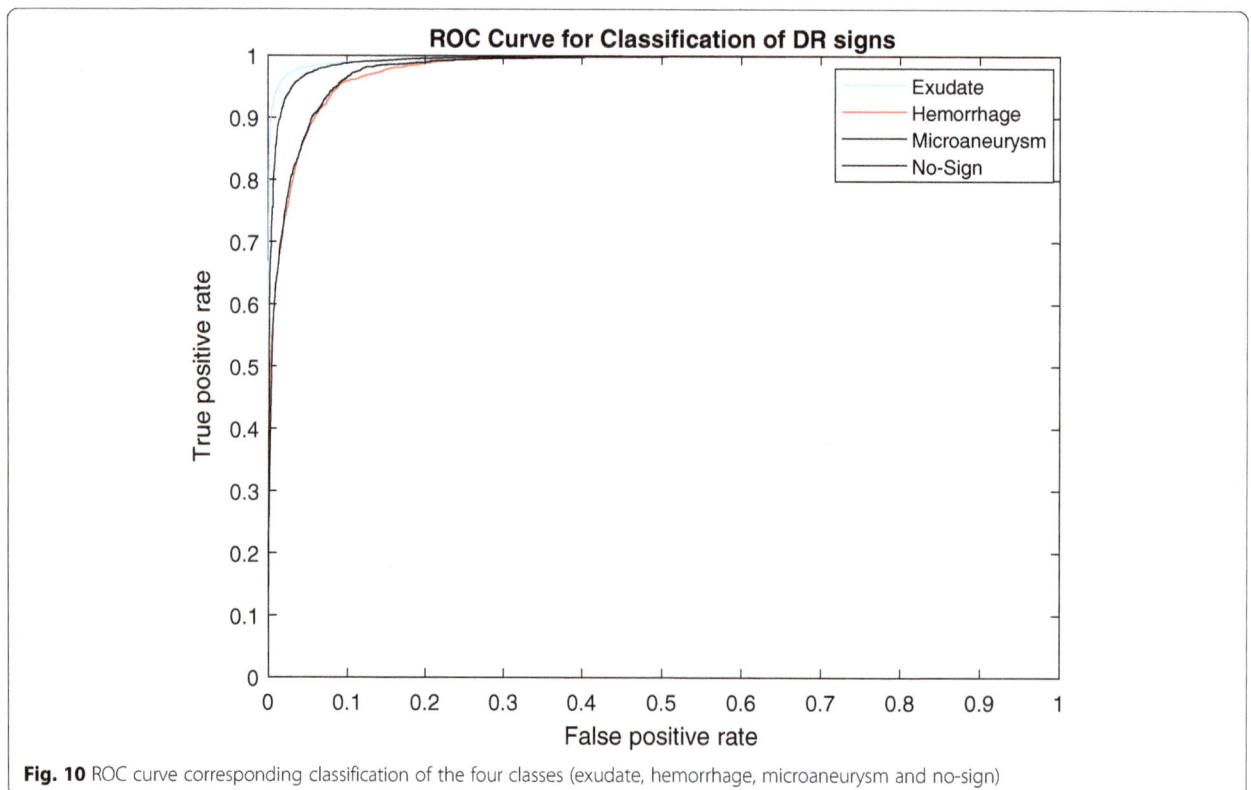

Fig. 10 ROC curve corresponding classification of the four classes (exudate, hemorrhage, microaneurysm and no-sign)

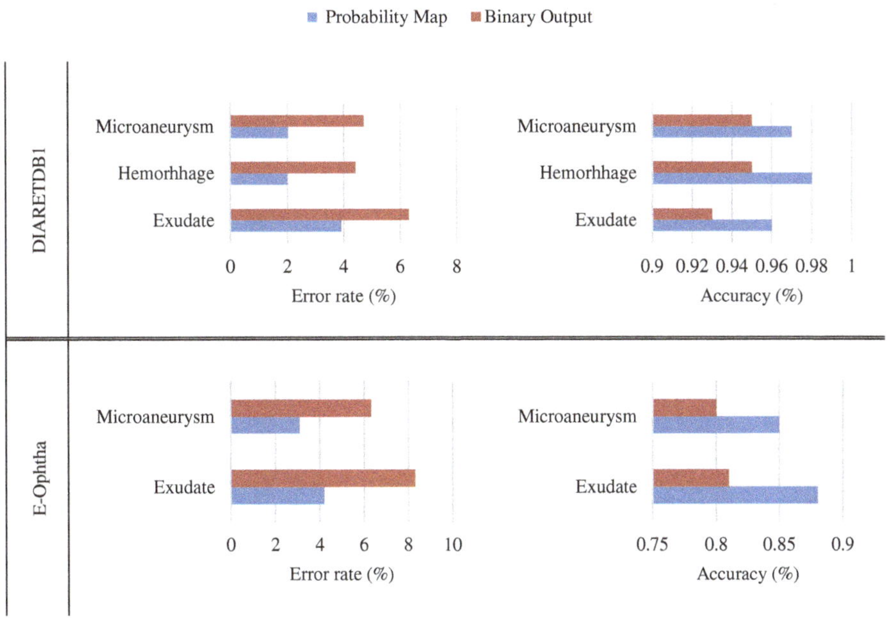

Fig. 11 Performance of proposed framework for the sign detections using two databases (DIARETDB1 and e-Ophtha) compared to the method with binary outputs of the network

between hemorrhages and microaneurysms. Comparing our results with the work by Tan et al. [24] shows that our method achieved significantly better sensitivity for detection of hemorrhage (0.84 vs 0.62) and microaneurysm (0.85 vs 0.46), although the specificity is similar. Our method also obtained better performance for both, sensitivity and specificity, for detection of the three DR signs when compared to the work by Sinthanayothin et al. [29].

Our method simultaneously detects the three pathological signs with improved performance compared to previous studies where only one sign was considered. This makes it suitable for more reliable detection of DR because when the signs are

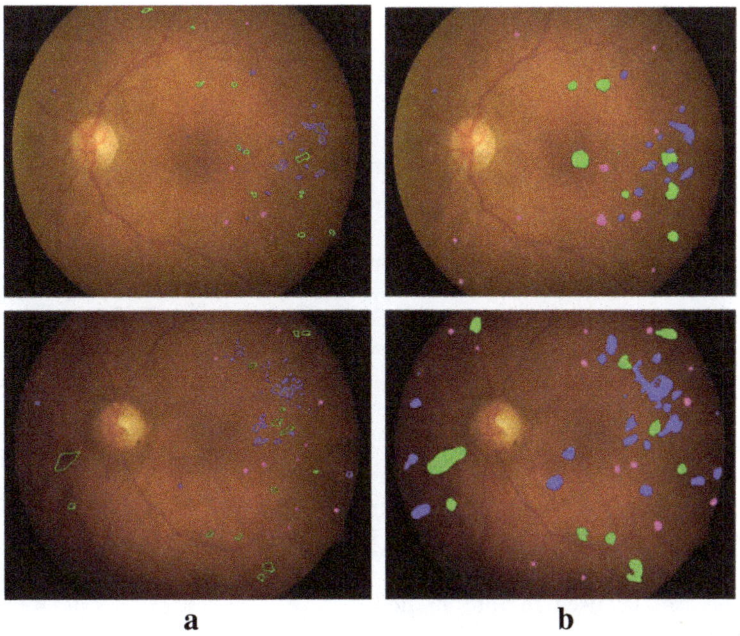

Fig. 12 Segmentation output image of the example retina image. **a** Manually annotated images that exudate, hemorrhage, and microaneurysm signs marked by blue, green and pink color, respectively. **b** Segmented output by the proposed algorithm

identified individually, there is the potential error of identifying the same region for multiple signs. This method performs comprehensive analysis and detects all the three signs simultaneously. The other study that attempted the simultaneous detection of the three signs was by Tan et al. [24] which suffered from poor performance.

One innovation of this method is the use of score values obtained from the softmax layer instead of using the binary output of the network. This results in the generation of the probability map of the locations of the pathological signs on the image, which with suitable post-processing reduces the error rate in the size of the signs.

The first significant strength of this study the significant strength of the study is that we considered two different publicly available databases, with the training done on one and the testing on both with comparable results. The second strength of this study is that fundus images were analyzed using both, patch and image-based analysis, and the results show that this method is significantly better than other studies. The third strength is that this method simultaneously identifies the three different pathological signs on the images which makes it suitable for automatic detection of diabetic retinopathy because when the signs are identified individually, there is potential error when the same region is identified for multiple signs.

A limitation of this study is that it is unable to differentiate between hemorrhages and microaneurysms if there is an overlap between these. This is also a limitation of the dataset because overlaps in the original images have not been labeled. Another limitation is that the database of 284 images was imbalanced with very few images with hemorrhages. There is the need for further testing of this method for databases belonging to different demographics to determine the suitability for different societies.

Conclusion

This paper reports a CNN based framework for the analysis of retinal images to detect the three major signs of diabetic retinopathy: exudates, hemorrhages and microaneurysms. The novelty of this system is that it uses the softmax output of the layers to generate the probability map for the three pathologic signs of DR which is then used to segment the fundus image and identify the signs. The system was trained using one dataset and tested on two datasets which shows the universality of the approach. The results show that such a system can be used for automatic analysis of fundus images for the detection of diabetic retinopathy without requiring a large dataset for training the network.

Abbreviations

AM-FM: Multiscale amplitude-modulation-frequency-modulation; AUC: Receiver operating characteristics; CE: Contrast enhancement; CNN: Convolutional neural network; DR: Diabetic retinopathy; FC: Fully-connected; FN: False negative; FP: False positive; MP: Max-Pooling; NL: Normalization layers; ReLU: Rectified linear unit; ROC: Receiver operating characteristic; SVM: Support vector machine; TN: True negative; TP: True positive

Acknowledgements

We acknowledge RMIT University for funding the PhD scholarship.

Funding

We acknowledge RMIT University for funding the PhD scholarship.

Authors' contributions

PK- conducted the experiment, implemented the methodology and drafted the manuscript. BA- participated in concept, design of the study, analysis, editing and review of the manuscript. DK- participated in concept, editing and review of the manuscript. All authors read and approved the final manuscript.

References

1. Leontidis G. A new unified framework for the early detection of the progression to diabetic retinopathy from fundus images. Comput Biol Med. 2017;90:98–115.
2. Mookiah MRK, Acharya UR, Chua CK, Lim CM, Ng EYK, Laude A. Computer-aided diagnosis of diabetic retinopathy: a review. Comput Biol Med. 2013; 43(12):2136–55.
3. Kaur J, Mittal D. A generalized method for the segmentation of exudates from pathological retinal fundus images. Biocybernetics Biomed Eng. 2018; 38(1):27–53.
4. Shaw JE, Sicree RA, Zimmet PZ. Global estimates of the prevalence of diabetes for 2010 and 2030. Diabetes Res Clin Pract. 2010;87(1):4–14.
5. Mohamed Q, Gillies MC, Wong TY. Management of diabetic retinopathy: a systematic review. JAMA. 2007;298(8):902–16.
6. Hansen MB, Abramoff MD, Folk JC, Mathenge W, Bastawrous A, Peto T. Results of automated retinal image analysis for detection of diabetic retinopathy from the Nakuru study, Kenya. PLoS One. 2015;10(10):e0139148.
7. Giancardo L, Meriaudeau F, Karnowski TP, Li Y, Garg S, Tobin KW Jr, et al. Exudate-based diabetic macular edema detection in fundus images using publicly available datasets. Med Image Anal. 2012;16(1):216–26.
8. Fraz MM, Jahangir W, Zahid S, Hamayun MM, Barman SA. Multiscale segmentation of exudates in retinal images using contextual cues and ensemble classification. Biomed Signal Proc Control. 2017;35:50–62.
9. Akram MU, Tariq A, Khan SA, Javed MY. Automated detection of exudates and macula for grading of diabetic macular edema. Comput Methods Prog Biomed. 2014;114(2):141–52.
10. Lazar I, Hajdu A. Retinal microaneurysm detection through local rotating cross-section profile analysis. IEEE Trans Med Imaging. 2013;32(2):400–7.
11. Tang L, Niemeijer M, Reinhardt JM, Garvin MK, Abramoff MD. Splat feature classification with application to retinal hemorrhage detection in fundus images. IEEE Trans Med Imaging. 2013;32(2):364–75.
12. van Grinsven MJJP, Venhuizen F, van Ginneken B, Hoyng CCB, Theelen T, Sanchez CI. Automatic detection of hemorrhages on color fundus images using deep learning. Invest Ophthalmol Vis Sci 2016;57(12):5966–5966.
13. MJJPv G, Bv G, Hoyng CB, Theelen T, Sánchez CI. Fast convolutional neural network training using selective data sampling: application to hemorrhage detection in color fundus images. IEEE Trans Med Imaging. 2016;35(5):1273–84.
14. Walter T, Massin P, Erginay A, Ordonez R, Jeulin C, Klein J-C. Automatic detection of microaneurysms in color fundus images. Med Image Anal. 2007;11(6):555–66.
15. Shan J, Li L, editors. A Deep Learning Method for Microaneurysm Detection in Fundus Images. 2016 IEEE First International Conference on Connected Health: Applications, Systems and Engineering Technologies (CHASE); 2016 27-29 June 2016.
16. Bae JP, Kim KG, Kang HC, Jeong CB, Park KH, Hwang JM. A study on hemorrhage detection using hybrid method in fundus images. J Digit Imaging. 2011;24(3):394–404.

17. Welfer D, Scharcanski J, Marinho DR. A coarse-to-fine strategy for automatically detecting exudates in color eye fundus images. Comput Med Imaging Graph. 2010;34(3):228–35.

18. Sopharak A, Uyyanonvara B, Barman S, Williamson TH. Automatic detection of diabetic retinopathy exudates from non-dilated retinal images using mathematical morphology methods. Comput Med Imaging Graph. 2008;32(8):720–7.

19. Quellec G, Lamard M, Josselin PM, Cazuguel G, Cochener B, Roux C. Optimal wavelet transform for the detection of microaneurysms in retina photographs. IEEE Trans Med Imaging. 2008;27(9):1230–41.

20. Fleming AD, Philip S, Goatman KA, Olson JA, Sharp PF. Automated microaneurysm detection using local contrast normalization and local vessel detection. IEEE Trans Med Imaging. 2006;25(9):1223–32.

21. Niemeijer M, van Ginneken B, Staal J, Suttorp-Schulten MS, Abramoff MD. Automatic detection of red lesions in digital color fundus photographs. IEEE Trans Med Imaging. 2005;24(5):584–92.

22. Osareh A, Mirmehdi M, Thomas B, Markham R. Automated identification of diabetic retinal exudates in digital colour images. Br J Ophthalmol. 2003;87(10):1220.

23. Walter T, Klein JC, Massin P, Erginay A. A contribution of image processing to the diagnosis of diabetic retinopathy-detection of exudates in color fundus images of the human retina. IEEE Trans Med Imaging. 2002;21(10):1236–43.

24. Tan JH, Fujita H, Sivaprasad S, Bhandary SV, Rao AK, Chua KC, et al. Automated segmentation of exudates, haemorrhages, microaneurysms using single convolutional neural network. Inf Sci. 2017;420:66–76.

25. Imani E, Pourreza H-R, Banaee T. Fully automated diabetic retinopathy screening using morphological component analysis. Comput Med Imaging Graph. 2015;43:78–88.

26. Agurto C, Murray V, Barriga E, Murillo S, Pattichis M, Davis H, et al. Multiscale AM-FM methods for diabetic retinopathy lesion detection. IEEE Trans Med Imaging. 2010;29(2):502–12.

27. Acharya UR, Ng EY, Tan JH, Sree SV, Ng KH. An integrated index for the identification of diabetic retinopathy stages using texture parameters. J Med Syst. 2012;36(3):2011–20.

28. Garcia M, Lopez MI, Alvarez D, Hornero R. Assessment of four neural network based classifiers to automatically detect red lesions in retinal images. Med Eng Phys. 2010;32(10):1085–93.

29. Sinthanayothin C, Boyce JF, Williamson TH, Cook HL, Mensah E, Lal S, et al. Automated detection of diabetic retinopathy on digital fundus images. Diabet Med. 2002;19(2):105–12.

30. Gardner GG, Keating D, Williamson TH, Elliott AT. Automatic detection of diabetic retinopathy using an artificial neural network: a screening tool. Br J Ophthalmol. 1996;80(11):940–4.

31. Roychowdhury S, Koozekanani DD, Parhi KK. DREAM: diabetic retinopathy analysis using machine learning. IEEE J Biomed Health Inform. 2014;18(5):1717–28.

32. Sánchez CI, García M, Mayo A, López MI, Hornero R. Retinal image analysis based on mixture models to detect hard exudates. Med Image Anal. 2009;13(4):650–8.

33. Shuang Yu Y, Di Xiao Y, Kanagasingam Y. Exudate detection for diabetic retinopathy with convolutional neural networks. Conference proceedings : Annual International Conference of the IEEE Engineering in Medicine and Biology Society IEEE Engineering in Medicine and Biology Society Annual Conference. 2017;2017:1744.

34. Kauppi T, Kalesnykiene V, Kamarainen J-K, Lensu L, Sorri I, Raninen A, et al. The DIARETDB1 Diabetic Retinopathy Database and Evaluation Protocol; 2007. p. 1–10.

35. Decencière E, Cazuguel G, Zhang X, Thibault G, Klein JC, Meyer F, et al. TeleOphta: machine learning and image processing methods for teleophthalmology. IRBM. 2013;34(2):196–203.

36. Rasta SH, Partovi ME, Seyedarabi H, Javadzadeh A. A comparative study on preprocessing techniques in diabetic retinopathy retinal images: illumination correction and contrast enhancement. J Med Signals Sens. 2015;5(1):40–8.

37. Soille P. Morphological Image Analysis: Principles and Applications. 2nd ed. Berlin: Springer-Verlag; 2003. https://doi.org/10.1007/978-3-662-05088-0.

38. Zana F, Klein JC, editors. Robust segmentation of vessels from retinal angiography. Proceedings of 13th International Conference on Digital Signal Processing; 1997 2-4 Jul 1997.

39. Dice LR. Measures of the amount of ecologic association between species. Ecology. 1945;26(3):297–302.

40. Roth HR, Lee CT, Shin HC, Seff A, Kim L, Yao J, et al., editors. Anatomy-specific classification of medical images using deep convolutional nets. 2015 IEEE 12th International Symposium on Biomedical Imaging (ISBI); 2015 16-19 April 2015.

41. Pang S, Yu Z, Orgun MA. A novel end-to-end classifier using domain transferred deep convolutional neural networks for biomedical images. Comput Methods Prog Biomed. 2017;140:283–93.

42. Jia Y, Shelhamer E, Donahue J, Karayev S, Long J, Girshick R, et al. Caffe: convolutional architecture for fast feature embedding. Proceedings of the 22nd ACM international conference on multimedia; Orlando, Florida, USA. 2654889: ACM; 2014. p. 675–678.

43. Naqvi SAG, Zafar MF, Haq I. Referral system for hard exudates in eye fundus. Comput Biol Med. 2015;64:217–35.

44. Prentašić P, Lončarić S, editors. Detection of exudates in fundus photographs using convolutional neural networks. 2015 9th International Symposium on Image and Signal Processing and Analysis (ISPA); 2015 7-9 Sept. 2015.

34

Oxidative stress markers in tears of patients with Graves' orbitopathy and their correlation with clinical activity score

Won Choi, Ying Li, Yong Sok Ji and Kyung Chul Yoon[*] 🆔

Abstract

Background: To investigate the concentrations of oxidative stress markers, 8-hydroxy-2′-deoxyquanosine (8-OHdG) and malondialdehyde (MDA), in tears and their correlation with the clinical activity score (CAS) in patients with Graves' orbitopathy (GO) according to disease activity.

Methods: We recruited 27 participants with inactive stage GO, 35 participants with active stage GO, and 25 healthy controls without GO. The tear concentrations of 8-OHdG and MDA were determined by enzyme-linked immunosorbent assay. The correlation between CAS and the concentrations of tear 8-OHdG and MDA were analyzed according to the disease activity in the GO patients.

Results: The levels of 8-OHdG and MDA were 56.30 ± 16.81 ng/mL and 5.39 ± 1.31 pmol/mg, respectively, in the control subjects, and 123.46 ± 22.67 ng/mL and 13.59 ± 3.93 pmol/mg, respectively, in patients with inactive stage GO, and 215.14 ± 35.61 ng/mL and 22.52 ± 4.63 pmol/mg, in patients with active stage GO. The mean concentrations of 8-OHdG and MDA were higher in patients with inactive and active stage GO compared with the control group (all $P < 0.001$). Furthermore, in the active stage group, tear concentrations of 8-OHdG and MDA were higher than those in the inactive stage group (all $P < 0.001$). The level of 8-OHdG ($r = 0.676$, $P < 0.001$) and MDA ($r = 0.506$, $P = 0.002$) correlated with CAS in the active stage GO group.

Conclusions: The concentrations of 8-OHdG and MDA in tears increased in patients with GO, especially in those in the active stage. In patients with active stage GO, CAS correlated significantly with the tear 8-OHdG and MDA levels.

Keywords: Oxidative stress, Graves' orbitopathy, Tear, 8-OHdG, MDA

Background

Thyroid-associated orbitopathy (eye disease), also known as Graves' orbitopathy (GO) and, Graves' ophthalmopathy is partly an autoimmune disease which can affect the periorbital and orbital tissues, and thyroid gland. Clinically detected GO occurs in 25 to 50% of patients with Graves' disease (GD); nevertheless, severe form of GO can be developed only about 5% in patients with GD [1, 2]. GO is characterized by enlargement and inflammatory changes of the extraocular muscles, orbital connective and adipose tissues as a consequence of interactions between different autoantibodies and inflammatory mediators [3].

The pathogenesis of GO in GD considerably rests on the existence of an inflamed cell infiltrate mainly made up of activated T cells that, in turn, trigger secretion of glycosaminoglycans (GAG) by the activated orbital fibroblasts, further inducing orbital fibrosis and edema [4]. However, the detailed pathogenesis of GO is still unclear.

It has been recently reported that oxidative stress is associated with the pathogenesis of GO. Increased levels of extracellular reactive oxygen species (ROS) have been noted in the fibroadipose tissues, blood, orbital fibroblasts, and urine of GO patients [5–12]. Factors known to worsen oxidative stress, including cigarette smoking

---

* Correspondence: kcyoon@jnu.ac.kr
Department of Ophthalmology and Research Institute of Medical Sciences, Chonnam National University Medical School and Hospital, 42 Jebong-ro, Dong-gu, Gwangju 61469, South Korea

and ^{131}I therapy, can also increase the prevalence of GO among GD patients [13, 14]. Cigarette smoking contains radicals and oxidants that cause systemic oxidative weight [15]. Therefore, it has been suggested that elevated ROS production by smoking overcomes oxidation reduction. In addition, Tsai et al. [6] have reveled oxidative deoxyribonucleic acid (DNA) destruction in the urine of GO patients and established a positive interrelation between clinical GO activity and this damage.

Moreover, in vivo and in vitro researches revealed that anti-oxidative parameters of oxidative stress and anti-thyroid drugs both in the whole organism and retro-orbital tissue [16]. In addition, a beneficial property of selenium has been established in patients with mild GO in double blind, placebo-controlled, multicenter clinical trials [17].

Until now, various markers of oxidative damage have been identified. Among these, 8-hydroxy-2′-deoxyquanosine (8-OHdG) and malondialdehyde (MDA) are the most commonly investigated by-products of DNA oxidation and lipid peroxidation [18]. 8-OHdG arises after the assault of the hydroxyl radical (the strongest ROS) at the guanine base in DNA [19]. MDA is generated from the mainly unsaturated fatty acids to their essential chains by oxidative mechanism [20].

To the best of our knowledge, no study has investigated the concentrations of oxidative stress markers in tears from patients with newly diagnosed GO, according to disease activity. The purpose of the current study is to analyze the levels of the oxidative stress markers such as 8-OHdG and MDA in tears according to the disease activity and to evaluate the correlation between these markers and the clinical activity score (CAS) in patients with inactive and active stage GO.

Methods
Subjects
Sixty-two patients with inceptively (< 2 months) diagnosed GD who were mostly consulted from the department of endocrinology and 25 healthy subjects without GD were enrolled in this study between January 2016 and December 2016. This study conducted in accordance with the tenets of the Declaration of Helsinki and performed with approval of the Chonnam National University Hospital institutional review board. Informed consent was acquired from every patients. A diagnosis of GD was made by endocrinologist on the basis of clinical signs and symptoms of thyrotoxicosis, laboratory findings of increased free thyroxine (T4) or triiodothyronine (T3) levels, and decreased thyroid-stimulating hormone levels and/or radiologic feature of diffuse homogeneous increased uptake in both lobes of the thyroid by [99m]Technetium-pertechnetate scan. Every patients received complete ophthalmic examination including

slit-lamp examination, refraction, visual acuity, intraocular pressure, ocular motility, fundus photography, Hertel exophthalmometry, palpebral fissure width, computed tomography, and thyroid hormone status including T3, T4, and free thyroxine (FT4). The diagnosis of GO was based on Bartley and Gorman's criteria [21] that determine the clinical GO diagnosis in patients who have eyelid retraction in conjunction with minimum one of the following signs: proptosis, thyroid dysfunction, optic neuropathy or strabismus, after the elimination of other possible sources. In the cases of no eyelid retraction, the GO diagnosis can be considered even in the absence of other causal factors, if some signs mentioned above are in conjunction with thyroid dysfunction. Patients with a history of previous radioactive iodine therapy, thyroidectomy, any topical medication, ocular surgery or trauma, systemic drugs that may have toxicity of cornea, contact lenses, systemic diseases that can potentially affect the antioxidants levels such as diabetes mellitus, hypertension, coronary artery disease, alcoholism, or liver or kidney disorders, or any systemic disorder that can effect adversely the sub-basal nerve plexus was excluded. Control subjects were enrolled during routine screening visits and had no history of systemic disease, pathologic ocular findings, or ocular disease.

Clinical activity score
The activity of inflammation in GO patients was assessed by the seven-point modification of the CAS, as previously described [22]. This CAS is based on classical signs and symptoms of inflammation (spontaneous pain, pain when moving the globe, redness of eyelids, redness of conjunctiva, swelling of plica/caruncle, swelling of eyelids, and chemosis). For each item present, one point is given. Each item has the same weight. The sum of these points is the CAS (range 0–7). A CAS ≥ 3/7 was indicated as active GO, and CAS < 3/7 was indicated as inactive GO.

Tear collection and detection of 8-OHdG and MDA
As we previously described, basal tear secretions were harvested atraumatically from the both inferior tear meniscus using glass capillary tubes (Corning, Inc., Corning, NY) [23]. Caution was taken not to irritate the surfaces of the conjunctival and corneal. Fifty-microliter of tear materials were harvested and diluted by phosphate-buffered saline. Tear fluids were stored in microtubes and kept at − 70 °C until additional examination.

Total protein levels of the 8-OHdG (Cell Biolabs, San Diego, CA, USA) and MDA (Cell Biolabs) were detected using enzyme-linked immunosorbent assays (ELISA) in accordance with the producer's instructions [24]. Tear specimens were centrifuged at 3000 g during 10 min or filtered through 0.45 mm filter, prior to use in the

ELISA. Both 8-OHdG and MDA protein samples (50 µl) were absorbed onto the 8-OHdG and MDA conjugate coated plate, respectively. The level of 8-OHdG and MDA in an unknown sample was measured by comparing its absorption with the known standard curve. The minimal detectable concentrations of the 8-OHdG and MDA were above 0.078 ng/mL and 6 pmol/mg, respectively.

Statistical analysis

SPSS version 18.0 (SPSS, Chicago, IL) was employed for all statistical analyses. All data are presented as mean ± standard deviation. Groups were compared using the Chi-square, independent t test, and one-way analysis of variance with post hoc test for comparing results between groups; Pearson correlation coefficients were assessed for the correlations between CAS and thyroid hormone status on the one hand and tear 8-OHdG and MDA levels on the other hand. Receiver operator curves (ROCs) were created for analyzing the sensitivity and specificity of active stage GO. A P value of less than 0.05 was considered statistically significant.

Results

Patient clinical features and demographics

Patient clinical features and demographics in the three groups are presented in Table 1. There were 25 patients (9 men and 16 women) in control participants, 27 patients (7 men and 20 women) in the inactive stage group, and 35 patients (13 men and 22 women) in the active stage group. Mean subject age was 38.56 ± 11.78 years (range: 21–59 years), 36.56 ± 13.75 years (range: 20–65 years), and 41.48 ± 14.87 years (range: 20–66 years) in the control and inactive and active stage groups, respectively. There were no statistically significant differences in sex, age, visual acuity, proptosis,

palpebral fissure width, and thyroid hormone state ($P > 0.05$). However, the CAS ($P = 0.001$) and extraocular muscle enlargement in orbital computed tomography ($P = 0.035$) showed significant differences in the active stage group compared to that in the inactive stage group.

Tear 8-OHdG and MDA levels and their correlation with CAS

The mean concentrations of 8-OHdG and MDA were 56.30 ± 16.81 ng/mL and 5.39 ± 1.31 pmol/mL in control subjects, and 123.46 ± 22.67 ng/mL and 13.59 ± 3.93 pmol/mg in inactive stage patients, and 215.14 ± 35.61 ng/mL and 22.52 ± 4.63 pmol/mg, in active stage patients, respectively. The mean levels of 8-OHdG and MDA showed significant differences in the inactive and active stage groups than in the control group (all $P < 0.001$). Moreover, in the active stage GO group, 8-OHdG and MDA levels in tear fluid showed significantly higher results than those in the inactive stage GO group (all $P < 0.001$) (Fig. 1).

In the inactive stage GO patients, the correlations between the CAS and tear 8-OHdG ($r = 0.263$, $P = 0.185$) and MDA ($r = 0.033$, $P = 0.869$) concentrations showed no significant results. On the other hand, in the active stage group, the tear 8-OHdG ($r = 0.676$, $P < 0.001$) and MDA ($r = 0.506$, $P = 0.002$) levels correlated significantly with the CAS (Figs. 2 and 3). In the GO patients, the correlation between tear 8-OHdG and MDA levels in each subject showed significant result ($r = 0.667$, $P < 0.001$).

The cut-off value of the tear 8-OHdG and MDA level were defined as 186 ng/mL and 19.50 pmol/mL. From the ROC curves, these concentrations to predict active stage GO showed 95.2% sensitivity and 85.4% specificity in the 8-OHdG level and 85.7% sensitivity and 87.8% specificity in the MDA level, respectively.

Table 1 Patient demographics and clinical features of the control subjects and patients with inactive and active stages of Graves' orbitopathy

	Control ($n = 25$)	Inactive stage ($n = 27$)	Active stage ($n = 35$)	P value
Sex (M/F)	9/16	7/20	13/22	0.674
Mean age (years)	38.56 ± 11.78	36.56 ± 13.75	41.48 ± 14.87	0.153
Visual acuity (LogMAR)	0.03 ± 0.02	0.04 ± 0.02	0.10 ± 0.14	0.238
Proptosis (mm)	16.12 ± 4.83	18.11 ± 3.38	17.54 ± 5.29	0.513
Palpebral fissure width (mm)	12.28 ± 2.54	11.26 ± 3.38	12.49 ± 3.74	0.911
Clinical activity score		1.33 ± 0.62	4.34 ± 1.30	0.001
EOM enlargement in orbital CT		10 (37.0%)	19 (54.3%)	0.035
Thyroid hormone state				
Hyperthyroid state		16 (59.3%)	20 (57.1%)	0.781
Euthyroid state		10 (37.0%)	13 (40.0%)	0.684
Hypothyroid state		1 (3.7%)	2 (5.7%)	0.305

EOM Extraocular muscle, *CT* Computed tomography

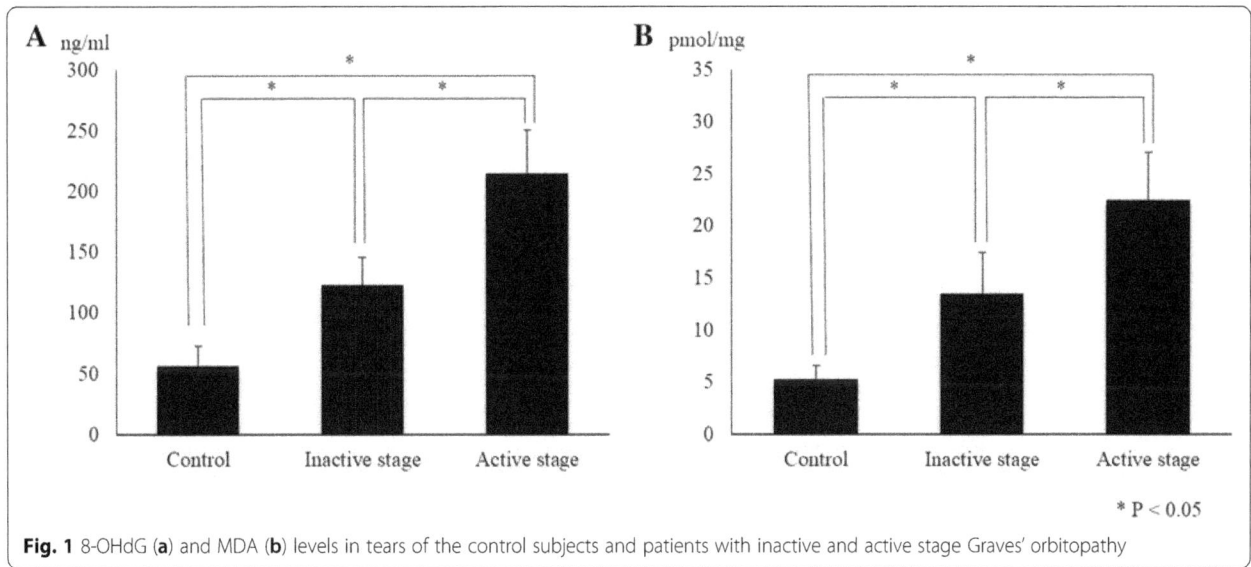

Fig. 1 8-OHdG (**a**) and MDA (**b**) levels in tears of the control subjects and patients with inactive and active stage Graves' orbitopathy

In addition, correlations between tear 8-OHdG levels and serum T3 ($r = 0.104$, $P = 0.381$), T4 ($r = 0.169$, $P = 0.290$), FT4 ($r = 0.255$, $P = 0.213$) status showed no significant results. Similar results were obtained between tear MDA levels and serum T3 ($r = 0.127$, $P = 0.341$), T4 ($r = 0.037$, $P = 0.791$), FT4 ($r = 0.139$, $P = 0.322$) status.

Discussion

The major findings of the present study were as follows. First, compared with the control, increased levels of 8-OHdG and MDA in the tear film were observed in patients with GO, especially with active stage. Second, the levels of the 8-OHdG and MDA were positively correlated with CAS and reflect the disease severity in the active stage GO group. The present study offers interesting and

possibly important findings on the role of 8-OHdG and MDA in the pathogenesis of GO. To the best of our knowledge, this is the first report of increased oxidative stress marker levels in the tear fluid and their correlation with the CAS in GO patients according to disease activity. Our data support the role of oxidative stress in development of GO in accordance with previous findings.

Both 8-OHdG and MDA, in addition to hydrogen peroxide and intracellular superoxide anion, were considerably increased in GO orbital fibroblasts compared with normal controls [5]. The study by Tsai et al. [6] established that the level of 8-OHdG in urine was considerably elevated in GO patients (1.9-fold in comparison with normal subjects). This elevation was remarkable in active GO patients (2.4-fold in comparison with normal

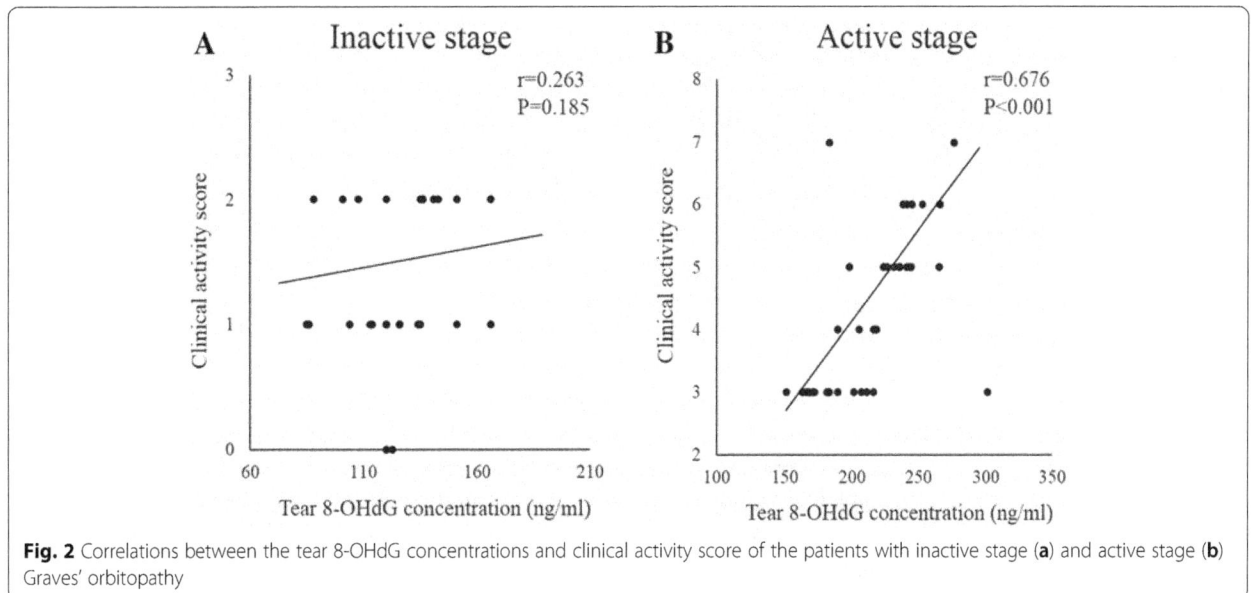

Fig. 2 Correlations between the tear 8-OHdG concentrations and clinical activity score of the patients with inactive stage (**a**) and active stage (**b**) Graves' orbitopathy

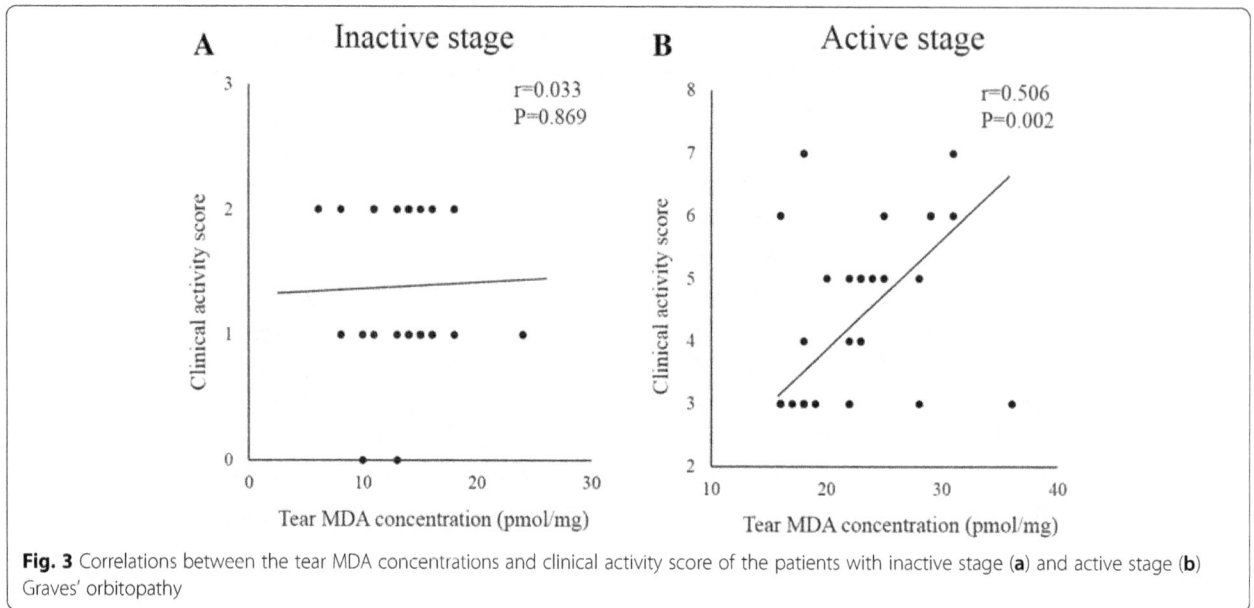

Fig. 3 Correlations between the tear MDA concentrations and clinical activity score of the patients with inactive stage (**a**) and active stage (**b**) Graves' orbitopathy

subjects). Furthermore, 8-OhdG levels in the urine significantly correlated with the TSH receptor antibody levels, CAS, and ophthalmopathy index. They also reported in another study that long term stress-induced ROS overproduction was due to the increase of manganese-dependent superoxide dismutase activity and concomitant decrease of glutathione peroxidase (GPx) activity, resulting in increased accumulation of hydrogen peroxide in GO orbital fibroblasts [25]. Moreover, the prominent decrease of glutathione/oxidized glutathione ratio and the diminished GPx activity in GO orbital fibroblasts indicated a significant redox imbalance in the cells, that in turn led to additional aggregation of endogenous hydrogen peroxide in the orbital fibroblasts with GO patients [25].

ROS (superoxide anions and hydrogen peroxide) trigger the production of pro-inflammatory cytokines that play a pivotal role in the GO development and accelerate proliferation of fibroblast in the orbit by dose-dependent way; the proliferative effect can be decreased with several antioxidants and methimazole [26, 27]. IL-1β induces free radical generation in the fibroblasts of GO and normal control, and enhances superoxide dismutase activity in GO orbital fibroblasts. Moreover, decreasing oxygen-free radicals with superoxide dismutase and catalase partially inhibited GAG production triggered by IL-1β [11].

Based on this mechanism, there have been several articles that antioxidants have a promising role in the prevention of GO progression at mild to moderately active GO. In the first pilot antioxidant supplementation study, allopurinol and nicotinamide therapy decreased total eye score and soft tissue swelling and improved patients' satisfaction in 82% of participants with mild to moderately

severe GO [28]. Selenium is integrated into several selenoproteins and acts as an antioxidant, decreases thyroperoxidase antibodies in patients with autoimmune thyroiditis [29]. A following randomized, double - blind, controlled trial of selenium ingestion for 6 months in GO patients led to an improved appearance, decreased soft tissue inflammation, improved quality of life, and delayed progression of GO compared to the control group [17]. These results indicate increased lipid peroxidation and oxidative DNA damage can play an pivotal role in the pathogenesis of GO.

Several articles report that the tear fluid and lacrimal gland can be directly accompanied in the damage of the ocular surface in GO patients [30–33]. However, the exact mechanisms of increased oxidative stress markers in the tears with GO have not been appropriately explained. We put forward the following hypothesis. Initially, lacrimal glands have been described as the general target organs for the thyroid hormones [34]. This might lead to the binding of autoantibodies to thyrotropin receptor, and antigen-specific response can arouse oxidation and deteriorate the function of lacrimal gland. Finally, the affected lacrimal gland may induce ROS and oxidative markers that are secreted into tears. Therefore, the component of oxidative stress markers in the tears can be altered.

As described above, studies conducted to date about the pathogenesis of GO have focused mostly on orbital tissues obtained by surgery. The disadvantages of this method are that it is invasive, difficult to obtain permission from every patient, and only available from patients through surgery. On the other hand, tear collection is a relatively non-invasive technique used to take samples from the ocular surface to determine oxidative stress markers in GO patients. The advantage of tear sampling method is that it is easy to get permission from most patients, triggers less pain and discomfort, and can be measured repeatedly as time passes.

Conclusions

In summary, we firstly demonstrated the tear 8-OHdG and MDA levels and their correlation with the CAS in patients with GO. The tear 8-OHdG and MDA levels may be used as potential adjuvant biomarkers in the determination of disease activity in patients with active stage GO. In addition, these markers may also be useful for distinguishing between active and inactive stage GO. Modulation of these oxidative stress markers could be considered as a future therapeutic approach for GO.

Abbreviations
8-OHdG: 8-hydroxy-2'-deoxyguanosine; DNA: Deoxyribonucleic acid; GAG: Glycosaminoglycans; GD: Graves' disease; GO: Graves' orbitopathy; GPx: Glutathione peroxidase; MDA: Malondialdehyde; ROCs: Receiver operator curves; ROS: Reactive oxygen species

Funding
The study was supported by the Basic Science Research Program through the National Research Foundation of Korea (NRF) funded by the Ministry of Science, ICT & Future Planning (2017R1A2B4003367) and the Chonnam National University Hospital Biomedical Research Institute (CRI8093-1 and CRI16020-1). The funding organizations had no role in the design or conduct of this research.

Authors' contributions
The work presented here was carried out in collaboration between all authors. WC was the major contributor in writing the manuscript. YL and YSJ were involved in the patient care and edited the manuscript. KCY was the academic advisor. All authors read and approved the final manuscript.

Competing interests
The authors declare that they have no competing interests.

References
1. Abraham-Nordling M, Bystrom K, Torring O, Lantz M, Berg G, Calissendorff J, et al. Incidence of hyperthyroidism in Sweden. Eur J Endocrinol. 2011;165(6): 899–905.
2. Garrity JA, Bahn RS. Pathogenesis of graves ophthalmopathy: implications for prediction, prevention, and treatment. Am J Ophthalmol. 2006;142(1): 147–53.
3. Bahn RS. Current insights into the pathogenesis of Graves' Ophthalmopathy. Horm Metab Res. 2015;47(10):773–8.
4. Weetman AP. Graves' disease. N Engl J Med. 2000;343(17):1236–48.
5. Tsai CC, Wu SB, Cheng CY, Kao SC, Kau HC, Chiou SH, et al. Increased oxidative DNA damage, lipid peroxidation, and reactive oxygen species in cultured orbital fibroblasts from patients with Graves' ophthalmopathy: evidence that oxidative stress has a role in this disorder. Eye (Lond). 2010; 24(9):1520–5.
6. Tsai CC, Cheng CY, Liu CY, Kao SC, Kau HC, Hsu WM, et al. Oxidative stress in patients with Graves' ophthalmopathy: relationship between oxidative DNA damage and clinical evolution. Eye (Lond). 2009;23(8):1725–30.
7. Hondur A, Konuk O, Dincel AS, Bilgihan A, Unal M, Hasanreisoglu B. Oxidative stress and antioxidant activity in orbital fibroadipose tissue in Graves' ophthalmopathy. Curr Eye Res. 2008;33(5):421 7.
8. Bednarek J, Wysocki H, Sowinski J. Oxidative stress peripheral parameters in Graves' disease: the effect of methimazole treatment in patients with and without infiltrative ophthalmopathy. Clin Biochem. 2005;38(1):13–8.
9. Tsai CC, Kao SC, Cheng CY, Kau HC, Hsu WM, Lee CF, et al. Oxidative stress change by systemic corticosteroid treatment among patients having active graves ophthalmopathy. Arch Ophthalmol. 2007;125(12):1652–6.
10. Bednarek J, Wysocki H, Sowinski J. Peripheral parameters of oxidative stress in patients with infiltrative Graves' ophthalmopathy treated with corticosteroids. Immunol Lett. 2004;93(2–3):227–32.
11. Lu R, Wang P, Wartofsky L, Sutton BD, Zweier JL, Bahn RS, et al. Oxygen free radicals in interleukin-1beta-induced glycosaminoglycan production by retro-ocular fibroblasts from normal subjects and Graves' ophthalmopathy patients. Thyroid. 1999;9(3):297–303.
12. Bartalena L, Tanda ML, Piantanida E, Lai A. Oxidative stress and Graves' ophthalmopathy: in vitro studies and therapeutic implications. Biofactors. 2003;19(3–4):155–63.
13. Hegedius L, Brix TH, Vestergaard P. Relationship between cigarette smoking and Graves' ophthalmopathy. J Endocrinol Investig. 2004;27(3):265–71.
14. Bartalena L, Marcocci C, Bogazzi F, Manetti L, Tanda ML, Dell'Unto E, et al. Relation between therapy for hyperthyroidism and the course of Graves' ophthalmopathy. N Engl J Med. 1998;338(2):73–8.
15. Pryor WA, Stone K. Oxidants in cigarette smoke. Radicals, hydrogen peroxide, peroxynitrate, and peroxynitrite. Ann N Y Acad Sci. 1993;686:12–27 discussion 27-18.
16. Zarkovic M. The role of oxidative stress on the pathogenesis of graves' disease. J Thyroid Res. 2012;2012:302537.
17. Marcocci C, Kahaly GJ, Krassas GE, Bartalena L, Prummel M, Stahl M, et al. Selenium and the course of mild Graves' orbitopathy. N Engl J Med. 2011; 364(20):1920–31.
18. Chang YT, Chang WN, Tsai NW, Huang CC, Kung CT, Su YJ, et al. The roles of biomarkers of oxidative stress and antioxidant in Alzheimer's disease: a systematic review. Biomed Res Int. 2014;2014:182303.
19. Karihtala P, Kauppila S, Puistola U, Jukkola-Vuorinen A. Divergent behaviour of oxidative stress markers 8-hydroxydeoxyguanosine (8-OHdG) and 4-hydroxy-2-nonenal (HNE) in breast carcinogenesis. Histopathology. 2011; 58(6):854–62.
20. Ma Y, Zhang L, Rong S, Qu H, Zhang Y, Chang D, et al. Relation between gastric cancer and protein oxidation, DNA damage, and lipid peroxidation. Oxidative Med Cell Longev. 2013;2013:543760.
21. Bartley GB, Gorman CA. Diagnostic criteria for Graves' ophthalmopathy. Am J Ophthalmol. 1995;119(6):792–5.
22. Mourits MP, Prummel MF, Wiersinga WM, Koornneef L. Clinical activity score as a guide in the management of patients with Graves' ophthalmopathy. Clin Endocrinol. 1997;47(1):9–14.
23. Choi W, Li Z, Oh HJ, Im SK, Lee SH, Park SH, et al. Expression of CCR5 and its ligands CCL3, −4, and −5 in the tear film and ocular surface of patients with dry eye disease. Curr Eye Res. 2012;37(1):12–7.
24. Choi W, Lian C, Ying L, Kim GE, You IC, Park SH, et al. Expression of lipid peroxidation markers in the tear film and ocular surface of patients with non-Sjogren syndrome: potential biomarkers for dry eye disease. Curr Eye Res. 2016;41(9):1143–9.
25. Tsai CC, Wu SB, Cheng CY, Kao SC, Kau HC, Lee SM, et al. Increased response to oxidative stress challenge in Graves' ophthalmopathy orbital fibroblasts. Mol Vis. 2011;17:2782–8.
26. Tsai CC, Wu SB, Kao SC, Kau HC, Lee FL, Wei YH. The protective effect of antioxidants on orbital fibroblasts from patients with Graves' ophthalmopathy in response to oxidative stress. Mol Vis. 2013;19:927–34.
27. Burch HB, Lahiri S, Bahn RS, Barnes S. Superoxide radical production stimulates retroocular fibroblast proliferation in Graves' ophthalmopathy. Exp Eye Res. 1997;65(2):311–6.
28. Bouzas EA, Karadimas P, Mastorakos G, Koutras DA. Antioxidant agents in the treatment of Graves' ophthalmopathy. Am J Ophthalmol. 2000;129(5): 618–22.
29. Duntas LH, Mantzou E, Koutras DA. Effects of a six month treatment with selenomethionine in patients with autoimmune thyroiditis. Eur J Endocrinol. 2003;148(4):389–93.
30. Moncayo R, Baldissera I, Decristoforo C, Kendler D, Donnemiller E. Evaluation of immunological mechanisms mediating thyroid-associated ophthalmopathy by radionuclide imaging using the somatostatin analog 111In-octreotide. Thyroid. 1997;7(1):21–9.

Permissions

The contributors of this book come from diverse backgrounds, making this book a truly international effort. This book will bring forth new frontiers with its revolutionizing research information and detailed analysis of the nascent developments around the world.

We would like to thank all the contributing authors for lending their expertise to make the book truly unique. They have played a crucial role in the development of this book. Without their invaluable contributions this book wouldn't have been possible. They have made vital efforts to compile up to date information on the varied aspects of this subject to make this book a valuable addition to the collection of many professionals and students.

This book was conceptualized with the vision of imparting up-to-date information and advanced data in this field. To ensure the same, a matchless editorial board was set up. Every individual on the board went through rigorous rounds of assessment to prove their worth. After which they invested a large part of their time researching and compiling the most relevant data for our readers.

The editorial board has been involved in producing this book since its inception. They have spent rigorous hours researching and exploring the diverse topics which have resulted in the successful publishing of this book. They have passed on their knowledge of decades through this book. To expedite this challenging task, the publisher supported the team at every step. A small team of assistant editors was also appointed to further simplify the editing procedure and attain best results for the readers.

Apart from the editorial board, the designing team has also invested a significant amount of their time in understanding the subject and creating the most relevant covers. They scrutinized every image to scout for the most suitable representation of the subject and create an appropriate cover for the book.

The publishing team has been an ardent support to the editorial, designing and production team. Their endless efforts to recruit the best for this project, has resulted in the accomplishment of this book. They are a veteran in the field of academics and their pool of knowledge is as vast as their experience in printing. Their expertise and guidance has proved useful at every step. Their uncompromising quality standards have made this book an exceptional effort. Their encouragement from time to time has been an inspiration for everyone.

The publisher and the editorial board hope that this book will prove to be a valuable piece of knowledge for researchers, students, practitioners and scholars across the globe.

List of Contributors

André Rosentreter
Department of Ophthalmology, University of Würzburg, Josef-Schneider-Str
11, 97080 Würzburg, Germany

Alexandra Lappas and Thomas Stefan Dietlein
Center of Ophthalmology, University of Cologne, Cologne, Germany

Randolf Alexander Widder
Department of Ophthalmology, St. Martinus-Krankenhaus Düsseldorf, Düsseldorf, Germany

Maged Alnawaiseh
Department Of Ophthalmology, University of Muenster Medical Center, Muenster, Germany

Xin Pan, Zhehui Chen and Yuetian Su
The Second Hospital of Jilin University, No.218, Ziqiang Road, Changchun
130041, China

Daguang Zhang and Zhifang Jia
The First Hospital of Jilin University, No.71, Xinmin Road, Changchun 130021, China

Olivia Xerri, Sawsen Salah, Dominique Monnet and Antoine P. Brézin
Department of Ophthalmology, Hôpital Cochin, Assistance Publique
Hôpitaux de Paris, Université Paris Descartes, Paris, France

Chia-Yu Wang
Department of Ophthalmology, Taipei Tzu Chi Hospital, Buddhist Tzu Chi Medical Foundation, Taipei, Taiwan

Ren-Wen Ho
Department of Ophthalmology, Kaohsiung Chang Gung Memorial Hospital and Chang Gung University College of Medicine, Kaohsiung, Taiwan Graduate Institute of Clinical Medicine, College of Medicine, Kaohsiung Medical University, Kaohsiung, Taiwan

Po-Chiung Fang, Hun-Ju Yu and Ming-Tse Kuo
Department of Ophthalmology, Kaohsiung Chang Gung Memorial Hospital and Chang Gung University College of Medicine, Kaohsiung, Taiwan

Chun-Chih Chien
Department of Laboratory Medicine, Kaohsiung Chang Gung Memorial Hospital and Chang Gung University College of Medicine, Kaohsiung, Taiwan

Chang-Chun Hsiao
Graduate Institute of Clinical Medical Sciences, Chang Gung University, Taoyuan City, Taiwan

Daniel Zapp, Daria Loos, Nikolaus Feucht, Lukas Reznicek and Christian Mayer
Department of Ophthalmology, Klinikum rechts der Isar, Technical University of Munich, Ismaninger Str. 22, 81675 Munich, Germany

Ramin Khoramnia and Tamer Tandogan
Department of Ophthalmology, University of Heidelberg, Heidelberg, Germany

Zhihua Zhang, Minwen Zhou, Kun Liu, Bijun Zhu, Haiyun Liu, Xiaodong Sun and Xun Xu
Shanghai Key Laboratory of Ocular Fundus Diseases, Shanghai, China
Department of Ophthalmology, Shanghai General Hospital, Shanghai Jiao Tong University School of Medicine, 100 Haining Road, Shanghai 200080, China
Shanghai Engineering Center for Visual Science and Photomedicine, Shanghai, China

Aya Takahashi, Kenya Yuki, Sachiko Awano-Tanabe, Takeshi Ono, Daisuke Shiba and Kazuo Tsubota
Department of Ophthalmology, Keio University School of Medicine, Shinanomachi 35, Shinjyuku-ku, Tokyo, Japan

Rui Shi
Department of Ophthalmology, Shaanxi Provincial People's Hospital, No.256 Youyi west Road, Xi'an 710068, Shaanxi Province, China

Lei Zhao
Department of Molecular Physiology and Biophysics, Holden Comprehensive Cancer Center, University of Iowa Carver College of Medicine, Iowa City, IA 52242, USA

Yun Qi
Department of Ophthalmology, the First Affiliated Hospital of Xi'an Jiaotong University, Xi'an 710061, Shaanxi Province, China

Dan Fu, Li Zeng, Jing Zhao and Hua-mao Miao
Department of Ophthalmology, Eye and ENT Hospital, Fudan University,
Shanghai, China

Zhi-qiang Yu and Xing-tao Zhou
Department of Ophthalmology, Eye and ENT Hospital, Fudan University,
Shanghai, China
NHC Key Laboratory of Myopia (Fudan University), No. 83 FenYang Road,
Shanghai 200031, People's Republic of China

Durgul Acan, Duygu Er, Nilufer Kocak and Suleyman Kaynak
Department of Ophthalmology, Dokuz Eylul University School of Medicine, Izmir, Turkey

Mehmet Calan, Tugba Arkan and Firat Bayraktar
Department of Endocrinology and Metabolism, Dokuz Eylul University School of Medicine, Izmir, Turkey

Esther L. Ashworth Briggs and Rajaraman Eri
School of Health Sciences, University of Tasmania, Launceston, Australia

Tze'Yo Toh
Launceston Eye Institute and Launceston Eye Doctors, Launceston, Australia

Alex W. Hewitt
School of Health Sciences, University of Tasmania, Launceston, Australia
Centre for Eye Research Australia, University of Melbourne, Melbourne, Australia

Anthony L. Cook
School of Health Sciences, University of Tasmania, Launceston, Australia
Wicking Dementia Research and Education Centre, University of Tasmania, Hobart 7001, Australia

Zhe Jia, Fei Li, Xiaoyu Zeng, Ying Lv and Shaozhen Zhao
Tianjin Medical University Eye Hospital, Tianjin Medical University Eye Institute and Tianjin Medical University School of Optometry and Ophthalmology, No. 251, Fukang R., Nankai Dist, Tianjin, China

Jing Qiao, Haili Li, Yun Tang, Wenjing Song, Bei Rong, Songlin Yang, Yuan Wu and Xiaoming Yan
Department of Ophthalmology, Peking University First Hospital, Beijing100034, China

Mi Tian, Weijun Jian, Ling Sun, Yang Shen, Xiaoyu Zhang and Xingtao Zhou
Department of Ophthalmology, Eye and ENT Hospital of Fudan University, Myopia Key Laboratory of the Health Ministry, No.19 Baoqing Road, Shanghai 200031, People's Republic of China

Ye He, Xin-jun Ren, Bo-jie Hu and Xiao-rong Li
Department of Retina, Tianjin Medical University Eye Hospital, 251 Fukang Road, Tianjin 300384, China

Wai-Ching Lam
Department of Ophthalmology, The University of Hong Kong, Hong Kong, China

Zequan Xu and Qiang Wu
Department of Ophthalmology, Shanghai Jiao Tong University Affiliated Sixth People's Hospital, No. 600, Yishan Road, Xuhui District, Shanghai 200233, People's Republic of China

Song Wu
School of Integrated Traditional and Western Medicine, Anhui University of Traditional Chinese Medicine, No. 103, Meishan Road, Hefei, Anhui 230038, People's Republic of China

Wenzhe Li
Clinical Medical College, Tianjin Medical University, No. 176 Xueyuan Road, Dagang District, Tianjin 100270, People's Republic of China

Yan Dou
Department of Foreign Languages, Hainan Medical University, No. 3, College Road, Longhua District, Haikou City, Hainan Province 571100, People's Republic of China

Naresh Babu Kannan, Piyush Kohli, Haemoglobin Parida, O. O. Adenuga and Kim Ramasamy
Department of Vitreo-retinal services, Aravind Eye Hospital and Post graduate Institute of Ophthalmology, Madurai, Tamil Nadu, India

Jing-yu Min, Yanan Lv, Lei Mao, Yuan-yuan Gong, Qing Gu and Fang Wei
Department of Ophthalmology, Shanghai General Hospital, Shanghai Jiao Tong University School of Medicine, NO.100, Haining Road, Hongkou District, Shanghai 200080, China. Shanghai Key Laboratory of Ocular Fundus Diseases, NO.100, Haining Road, Hongkou District, Shanghai 200080, China
Shanghai Engineering Center for Visual Science and Photomedicine, NO.100, Haining Road, Hongkou District, Shanghai 200080, China

Giovanni Montesano
ASST Santi Paolo e Carlo, University of Milan, 20142 Milan, Italy
City, University of London, Optometry and Visual Sciences, Northampton

David P. Crabb and Pete R. Jones
City, University of London, Optometry and Visual Sciences, Northampton
Square, EC1V 0HB, London, UK

Paolo Fogagnolo, Maurizio Digiuni and Luca M. Rossetti
ASST Santi Paolo e Carlo, University of Milan, 20142 Milan, Italy

Tessa Hillgrove and Renee Chan
The Fred Hollows Foundation, Level 2, 61 Dunning Avenue, Rosebery, Sydney, NSW 2018, Australia

Camille Neyhouser
The Fred Hollows Foundation, Level 2, 61 Dunning Avenue, Rosebery, Sydney, NSW 2018, Australia
School of Public Health and Community Medicine, Faculty of Medicine, University of New South Wales, Kensington, NSW 2052, Australia

Ingrid Quinn
Siem Reap, Cambodia

Chhorvann Chhea
Phnom Penh, Cambodia

Seang Peou and Pol Sambath
The Fred Hollows Foundation Cambodia, Phnom Penh 12301, Cambodia

Hande Celiker and Haluk Kazokoglu
Department of Ophthalmology, Marmara University School of Medicine,
Fevzi Çakmak Mah. Muhsin Yazıcıoğlu Cad. No:10 Pendik, Istanbul, Turkey

Haner Direskeneli
Division of Rheumatology, Marmara University School of Medicine Fevzi
Çakmak Mah, Muhsin Yazıcıoğlu Cad. No:10 Pendik, Istanbul, Turkey

Danjie Li
Department of Ophthalmology, Gunma University School of Medicine, 3-39-15 Showa-machi, Maebashi, Gunma 371-8511, Japan
Aier eye hospital (Cheng Du), 115 Xiyiduan, Yihuanlu,, Chengdu 610041, China

Hideo Akiyama
Department of Ophthalmology, Gunma University School of Medicine, 3-39-15 Showa-machi, Maebashi, Gunma 371-8511, Japan

Shoji Kishi
Maebashi Central Eye Clinic, Maebashi, Gunma, Japan

Csaba Szekrényesi
Faculty of Health Sciences, Semmelweis University, Vas u. 17, Budapest 1088, Hungary

Huba Kiss and Tamás Filkorn
Department of Ophthalmology, Semmelweis University, Budapest, Hungary

Zoltán Zsolt Nagy
Faculty of Health Sciences, Semmelweis University, Vas u. 17, Budapest 1088, Hungary
Department of Ophthalmology, Semmelweis University, Budapest, Hungary

Michele Lanza, Michele Rinaldi, Ugo Antonello Gironi Carnevale and Mario Bifani Sconocchia
Multidisciplinary Department of Medical, Surgical and Dental Sciences, Università della Campania, Luigi Vanvitelli, Via de Crecchio 16, 80100 Naples, Italy

Silvio di Staso
Ophthalmology Unit, Department of Life, Health and Environmental Sciences, University of L'Aquila, L'Aquila, Italy

Ciro Costagliola
Department of Medicine and Healthy Sciences, Università del Molise, Campobasso, Italy

Yan Ma, Guangda Deng, Jing Ma, Jinghua Liu, Songfeng Li and Hai Lu
Department of Ophthalmology, Beijing Tongren Eye Center, Beijing Tongren Hospital, Capital Medical University, Beijing Ophthalmology and Visual Sciences Key Lab, 1 Dongjiaominxiang, Dongcheng District, Beijing 100730, China

Dilek Yaşa, Zeynep Gizem Erdem, Ali Demircan, Gökhan Demir and Zeynep Alkın
Beyoğlu Eye Research and Training Hospital, Bereketzade Mah, Bereketzade Sok. No:2, Beyoğlu, İstanbul, Turkey

Yi Zhu, Haobin Zhu and Jibo Zhou
Department of Ophthalmology, Shanghai Ninth People's Hospital, Shanghai Jiao Tong University School of Medicine, 639 Zhizaoju Road, Shanghai 200011, China
Shanghai Key Laboratory of Orbital Diseases and Ocular Oncology, Shanghai, China

Yan Jia
Department of Ophthalmology, Shanghai Ninth People's Hospital, Shanghai Jiao Tong University School of Medicine, 639 Zhizaoju Road, Shanghai 200011, China
Department of Ophthalmology, Children's Hospital of Fudan University, Shanghai, China

Haihong Yuan
Department of Pharmacy, Shanghai University of Medicine and Health Science, Shanghai, China

Ping Yu, Qichen Fan, Xuan Zhang, Wei Huang, Junyi Shen and Yongyao Cui
Department of Pharmacology, Shanghai Jiao Tong University School of Medicine, 280 South Chongqing Road, Shanghai 200025, China

Hui Li
Department of Pharmacology, Shanghai Jiao Tong University School of Medicine, 280 South Chongqing Road, Shanghai 200025, China
Department of Pharmacy, Qingpu Branch of Zhongshan Hospital, Fudan University School of Medicine, Shanghai, China

Wei Zhou
Laboratory of OralMicrobiota and Systemic Diseases, Shanghai Research Institute of Stomatology, Ninth People's Hospital, Shanghai Jiao Tong University School of Medicine, 115 Jin Zun Road, Shanghai 200125, China

Shanghai Key Laboratory of Stomatology and Shanghai Research Institute of Stomatology, National Clinical Research Center of Stomatology, Shanghai, China

Mehdi Naderi, Siamak Sabour and Soheila Khodakarim
Department of Clinical Epidemiology, School of Public Health, Safety Promotion and Injury Prevention Research Center, Shahid Beheshti University of Medical Sciences, Chamran Highway, Velenjak, Daneshjoo Blvd, Tehran, I.R, Iran

Farid Daneshgar
Department of Ophthalmology, School of Medicine, Kermanshah
University of Medical Sciences, Kermanshah, Iran

Shasha Xue, Guiqiu Zhao, Xiaoni Yin, Jing Lin, Cui Li, Liting Hu, Lin Leng and Xuejiao Yang
The Affiliated Hospital of Qingdao University, No.16, Jiangsu Road, Qingdao, China

Hyo Kyung Lee and Mee Kum Kim
Department of Ophthalmology, Seoul National University College of Medicine, 103 Daehak-Ro, Jongno-Gu, Seoul 110-799, Republic of Korea
Laboratory of Ocular Regenerative Medicine and Immunology, Seoul Artificial Eye Center, Seoul National University Hospital Clinical Research Institute, Seoul, Republic of Korea

Yu Jeong Kim
Laboratory of Ocular Regenerative Medicine and Immunology, Seoul Artificial Eye Center, Seoul National University Hospital Biomedical Research Institute, Seoul, Korea
Department of Ophthalmology, Hanyang University Hospital, Hanyang University College of Medicine, Seoul, Korea

Jin Wook Jeoung, Ki Ho Park and Young Suk Yu
Department of Ophthalmology, Seoul National University Hospital, 101 Daehak-ro, Jongno-gu, Seoul 110-744, Korea

Mee Kum Kim and Joo Youn Oh
Laboratory of Ocular Regenerative Medicine and Immunology, Seoul Artificial Eye Center, Seoul National University Hospital Biomedical Research Institute, Seoul, Korea
Department of Ophthalmology, Seoul National University Hospital, 101 Daehak-ro, Jongno-gu, Seoul 110-744, Korea

Parham Khojasteh, Behzad Aliahmad and Dinesh K. Kumar
Biosignal Lab, School of Engineering, RMIT University, Melbourne, Australia

Won Choi, Ying Li, Yong Sok Ji and Kyung Chul Yoon
Department of Ophthalmology and Research Institute of Medical Sciences, Chonnam National University Medical School and Hospital, 42 Jebong-ro, Dong-gu, Gwangju 61469, South Korea

Index

www.ingramcontent.com/pod-product-compliance
Lightning Source LLC
Chambersburg PA
CBHW061304190326
41458CB00011B/3764

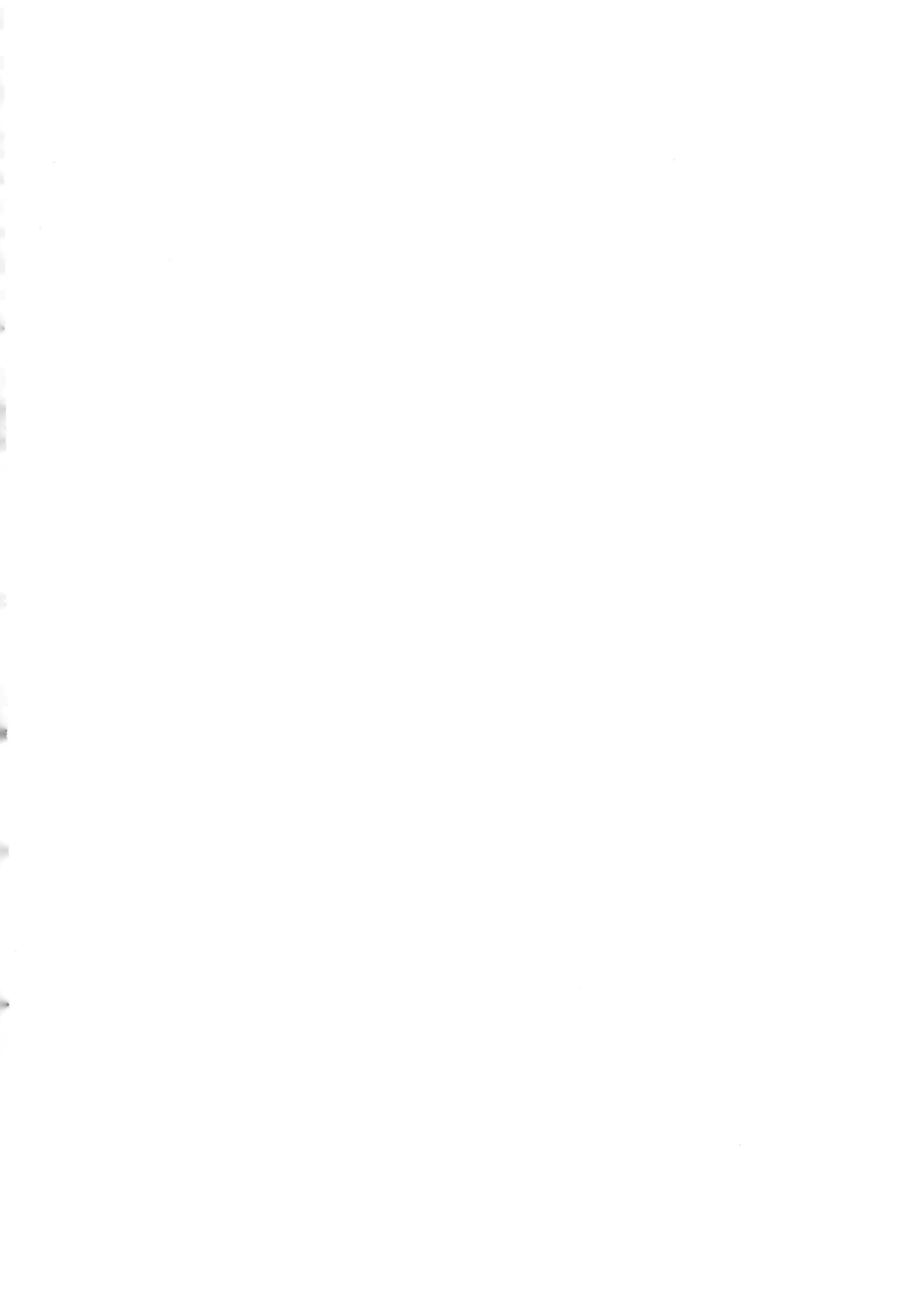